Lateral Ankle Instability

Hélder Pereira • Stéphane Guillo
Mark Glazebrook • Masato Takao
James Calder • Niek Van Dijk
Jón Karlsson
Editors

Lateral Ankle Instability

An International Approach by the Ankle Instability Group

European Society of Sports Traumatology, Knee Surgery & Arthroscopy
ESSKA

Springer

Editors
Hélder Pereira
Póvoa de Varzim-Vila do Conde
Hospital Centre
Minho university
Braga-Guimarães
Portugal

Mark Glazebrook
Queen Elizabeth II Health Sciences
Center & Dalhousie University
Halifax
Nova Scotia
Canada

James Calder
Imperial College London and Fortius
Clinic London
London
UK

Jón Karlsson
Department of Orthopaedics
Sahlgrenska University Hospital
Mölndal
Sweden

Stéphane Guillo
SOS Pied Cheville Bordeaux
Bordeaux-Mérignac
France

Masato Takao
Clinical and Research Institute for Foot
and Ankle Surgery
Jujo Hospital
Kisarazu, Chiba
Japan

Niek Van Dijk
FIFA Medical centre of
excellence Madrid and Porto,
Department of Orthopaedic Surgery
University of Amsterdam, Academic
Medical Centre
Amsterdam
The Netherlands

ISBN 978-3-662-62762-4 ISBN 978-3-662-62763-1 (eBook)
https://doi.org/10.1007/978-3-662-62763-1

This Springer imprint is published by the registered company Springer-Verlag GmbH, DE part of Springer Nature.
The registered company address is: Heidelberger Platz 3, 14197 Berlin, Germany

Preface

Ankle instability is one of the leading causes of disability amongst athletes and general population.

Furthermore, in recent years, there has been a revolution in the research from the pathophysiology, implications, and surgical options which might have no comparison with any other field of orthopedics and sports traumatology.

We are assisting to an arthroscopic revolution in the management of this condition, in a broad and comprehensive perspective.

The European Society for Sports Traumatology, Knee Surgery and Arthroscopy (ESSKA), mainly its section Ankle and Foot Associates (AFAS), founded by Niek Van Dijk, and The Ankle Instability Group (AIG) are proud to present this book.

The AIG study group has been founded by Stéphane Guillo, in 2014, is currently led by Masato Takao and in a short period has been able to produce an incredible amount of quality science on the topic.

Together we were able to gather most of the scientific and clinical leaders in this field.

This was a joint venture with a story to keep, but we must be and we are all very proud of the end result.

This book represents one step, but many more will come from the continuous effort in research and education uprising from ESSKA-AFAS and the very prestigious and productive AIG study Group.

I send a big thank you to all those who have contributed to bring this project to life on behalf of all Editors, Hélder Pereira, Stéphane Guillo, Mark Glazebrook, Masato Takao, James Calder, Niek Van Dijk, and Jón Karlsson.

Hope you will also enjoy.

Braga-Guimarães, Portugal — Hélder Pereira

Preface

Orthopedic and Sports Medicine science has advanced tremendously in the last decades. This is certainly the case with the topic of lateral Ankle Instability.

We who have worked on solutions of ankle problems have all learnt from the classical paper of Lennart Broström, published more than 50 years ago (Broström L. Sprained ankles. VI. Surgical treatment of "chronic" ligament ruptures. Acta Chir Scand 1966;132(5):551–565.). This paper was the cornerstone of the scientific approach towards the unstable ankle. The understanding of basic science, anatomy, and clinical implications as well as treatment options have advanced much since this classic paper was published. Much has changed, but much is in fact still the same. The field has evolved, especially the last 5–10 years with benefits from minimally invasive techniques, arthroscopic evaluation of the entire ankle joint, especially better understanding of cartilage injuries and other concomitant injuries. Lately, advanced arthroscopic techniques are being frequently used for ankle stabilization. Moreover, ankle-specific instruments and implants are commonly used today.

This book combines the efforts of world-leading experts in the field, covering the basics as well as the most updated technical developments and future perspectives, one of the most relevant hot topics in orthopedics today.

This comprehensive book provides a systematic and thorough approach to the topic including classic and updated references, as well as the most recent information about arthroscopic and minimally invasive surgical approaches.

We are confident that this book will serve for the coming years as a "pillar" for all those involved in the treatment of chronic lateral ankle instability. We are equally confident that it will stand out as a reference work for the next decade or more.

It is a must read for all Foot and Ankle surgeons, especially those involved in the treatment of patients with chronic ankle instability.

We hope you all enjoy it as much as we did!

Mölndal, Sweden — Jón Karlsson
Amsterdam, The Netherlands — Niek Van Dijk

Preface

"I disapprove of what you say, but I will defend to the death your right to say it"
Voltaire

We are all, I am sure, inside us driven by the same deep motivation: to improve the care for patients we are responsible in our daily practice. What tool do we have for that?

First of all our individual reflections. We all wonder about our practice and most of the major advances have been based on personal reflections from professionals who "think out of the box" as Niek Van Dijk would say. But these individual reflections are nothing in science if they are not confronted with other opinions. This is why listening to others is a second inseparable component and necessary for our commitments. We are all carriers whatever our "grade," our age, or our geography, possessing our own knowledge 'eminently respectable, which we must cultivate. Exchanging this wealth elevates us. I am convinced that any idea must be shared and confronted by the trials of others. Having had some new ideas on ankle ligamentoplasty, it was therefore natural that I proposed to people who have treated this same subject in recent articles to meet. The Ankle Instability Group was born. This is 2014. This is without a doubt, from a human point of view, one of the most beautiful memories of my professional and scientific life.

The third component on which we must rely to build our own thinking are publications. Scientific journals are responsible for allowing all scientific work to express themselves without judgment other than their scientific quality because they must simply contribute to improving the daily care. Regarding our subject, we all know that it is necessary to publish to increase the evidence of ligamentoplasty, whether it is arthroscopic or not.

Finally, the fourth pillar of our individual reflexion is scientific society. Its role is to federate, organize, and disseminate scientific advances to the whole of society. When a scientific society federates ideas, currents of thought, when it integrates new techniques, when it advances independently of any pressure, it feeds the debate, confronts reflection, disseminates novelty, it is useful for the common interest. As a scientific society, ESSKA trusted us for this work. We cannot thank James Calder and Hélder Pereira enough for their tireless work to bring this book to life.

This book is a collective scientific work which aims to present all the solutions described today to deal with a huge social and economic burden that is chronic ankle instability. The representation of all opinions, even if it is not ours, will always remain in the Voltairean DNA of the Ankle Instability Group.

I join all the members of the AIG in wishing you a good read, hoping that it will help you in your professional life with your patients and that it will be the seed of new collaborations.

Bordeaux-Mérignac, France Stéphane Guillo

Preface

This book has united the work of many global leaders with a common purpose of summarizing and improving our current understanding of ankle instability. It takes the reader from the authoritative anatomy to novel dissection findings and relates them to the various pathological conditions seen in clinical practice. The pathophysiology underlying ankle instability plays an important role in determining which treatments may be appropriate to consider but more importantly may also enable clinicians to discern which individuals may benefit from a particular management pathway. The treatment of elite athletes may differ from that of "normal" individuals or even the "weekend warrior," and this book discusses this controversial area and proffers guidance for treating clinicians.

Ankle injuries are one of the most common to befall recreational and elite athletes and resulting instability is a cause for concern both from the immediate impact on preventing optimal athletic performance and also on the possible long-term adverse sequelae. There has been a rapid evolution of various surgical procedures in recent years aiming to improve speed of recovery and return to sport whilst avoiding postoperative complications or compromising ultimate function for the patients. This book follows the path of these developments, explaining the rationale for their use in individual groups and summarizes their results to date whilst trying to avoid personal preferences and single author series. The surgical treatment of ankle instability (particularly arthroscopic) is very much an evolving sub-specialty. Much may be gained by the Ankle Instability Group (AIG) encouraging scientific advances which can then determine the enhancement of specific surgical procedures in a structured way. It has always been the purpose of AIG through scientific presentations and collaboration with AFAS-ESSKA to promote science, push the boundaries of understanding, and ultimately improve the outcome for our patients following ankle injuries. The book is up to date today, but AIG will continue to grow with experts from across the world helping to "make a difference."

London, UK

James Calder
Daniel Haverkamp

Preface

Activity Report of Ankle Instability Group (AIG)

Surgery for lateral ankle instability has evolved annually from non-anatomical to anatomical, and more recently to arthroscopic anatomic procedure. Arthroscopic surgery for ankle ligaments had been delayed compared to knee and shoulder joints. Ankle instability group (AIG) was established in 2013 for the purpose of development of effective diagnosis and treatment including minimally invasive surgeries for ankle instability. Since 2013, 11 English papers have been published by AIG [1–11]. The first AIG meeting was held at Bordeaux in 2013, second at Chicago in 2014, third at Seoul in 2015, and fourth at Bordeaux again in 2017. The fifth AIG meeting was held in 2018 at Kisarazu, Japan, as a combined meeting of the 43rd annual meeting of the Japanese Society for Surgery of the Foot approved by Ankle & Foot Associates a section of European Society of Sports Traumatology, Knee Surgery and Arthroscopy (ESSKA-AFAS), Arthroscopy Association of North America (AANA), Asian Federation of Foot and Ankle Surgeons (AFFAS), International Society for Cartilage Repair of the Ankle (ISCRA), and French Arthroscopy Society (SFA) with 890 participants from 20 countries. The live demonstration surgeries of minimally invasive surgery for lateral instability of the ankle by ten worldwide experts were also held during the fifth AIG meeting.

In 1966, Broström firstly reported the repair technique for lateral instability of the ankle, and this technique has used as a gold standard still now [12]. In 1987, Hawkins initially described an arthroscopic repair procedure to fix the remnant of anterior talofibular ligament (ATFL) with a staple to the talus [13]. While arthroscopic surgery of other joints has been evolved after the development of suture anchor technique, a procedure for suturing a residual ligament arthroscopically using a suture anchor was introduced to ankle lateral ligament repair by Corte-Real in 2009 [14]. Since then, various procedures have been reported for arthroscopic ligament repair using suture anchors. The arthroscopic repair of the lateral ankle ligament consists of three steps: placement of a suture anchor at ATFL attachment to the lateral malleolus, threading the suture anchor to the remnant, and knotting. Arthroscopic repair procedures can be classified into three types according to the process of threading the suture anchor to the remnant; arthroscopy-assisted mini-open procedure, arthroscopic with percutaneous procedure, and all-inside arthroscopic procedure. Arthroscopy-assisted mini-open procedure reported by Nery in 2011 [15]. Placement of the suture anchor is performed arthroscopically from the portal. But threading the suture anchor to the remnant and knotting are performed via 15 mm extension incision of the portal under direct view. It is easy to operate, but more invasive than following procedures. Nery has improved this procedure to the following arthroscopic with percutaneous procedure [10]. Arthroscopic with percutaneous procedure was firstly reported by Corte-Real in 2009 [14] and has since been developed by several doctors [10, 16–19]. Placement of the suture anchor is performed arthroscopically from the portal. Threading the suture anchor to the remnant are performed by percutaneously inserted needle under arthroscopic view. It is less invasive than arthroscopic assisted mini-open procedure. And it has the advantage of being able to apply sutures to CFL as well as ATFL. On the other hand, it is difficult to apply a thread only to the ligament. Accordingly, it is not an anatomic procedure because the ligament and the inferior extensor ligament are sutured together with the same suture anchor. In addition, the knotting is performed under a small incision or subcutaneously guided to the portal with an additional invasion. In the live demonstration surgery during the fifth AIG meeting, there was a case in which peroneus tertius tendon and a branch of the superficial peroneal nerve were simultaneously knotted with a remnant in dissection after surgery. The risk of above complications cannot be denied. For all-inside arthroscopic procedure, the knotless anchor procedure was firstly reported by Vega in 2013 [20]. It is the most minor invasive procedure because all three steps are performed arthroscopically through one portal. We also reported a suture anchor procedure with lasso-loop stitch technique [4, 21] and developed to modified lasso-loop stitch technique [22]. Since all-inside arthroscopic procedure is possible to suture the ligament in direct arthroscopic view, it can be performed anatomically. On the other hand, since only the ATFL can be observed by arthroscopy, it is impossible to apply a suture directly to CFL. Because CFL is an extra-articular ligament, a wide resection should be required to approach to its attachment to fibula, which is eliminated in minimally invasive surgery. ATFL and CFL are connected with lateral talocalcaneal ligament [8, 23] and detached at these fibular attachment as one unit in most cases of chronic lateral ligament rupture [12]. Although there is a theory that the function of CFL can be restored automatically only with ATFL sutures, the need for suturing CFL and the method how to suture CFL remain as unsolved problems.

For arthroscopic reconstruction of the lateral ligament of the ankle, Lui reported an arthroscopic assisted mini-open ligament reconstruction procedure in 2007 [24]. All-arthroscopic ligament reconstruction technique was firstly reported by Guillo in 2014 [25]. This procedure consisted of seven steps to create bone tunnels at the attachment of ATFL and CFL to fibula, talus, and calcaneus via four portals under ankle arthroscopy, subtalar arthroscopy, and peroneal tendoscopy; and a tendon graft using autologous gracilis tendon was inserted and fixed into each bone tunnels. At the first AIG meeting held in 2013, eight groups were divided to try this procedure using fresh cadaver, but there was only one group to complete surgery because the procedure was complicated and difficult to understand. In addition, there was a discussion about the demerit to release the peroneal tendon sheath under tendoscopically. Accordingly, Guillo developed it simpler as five steps technique via three portals under ankle and subtalar arthroscopy [5.] Wc also developed the AntiRoll (Anatomical Reconstruction of the ankle lateral ligament) method in collaboration with Dr Glazebrook and was published in 2015 [26]. The ankle and subtalar arthroscopic procedure in which the tendon graft is introduced into each bone tunnels by the all inside-out technique and fixed with the interference screw is simple, easy to understand, and reproducible surgery. On the other hand, the process of reconstructing CFL under subtalar arthroscopy is technically demanding. Glazebrook recommends the percutaneous AntiRoll (P-AntiRoLL), which allows the surgery to be easier [27]. On the other hand, since it is not possible to confirm the run of the tendon graft under direct view, the risk remains in particular of reliably passing the tendon graft under the peroneal tendon. In addition, there have been few researches for the suitable placement of each bone tunnels. It is similar to the history of anterior cruciate ligament reconstruction, and biomechanical study should be needed for further development of ankle lateral ligaments' reconstruction.

Kisarazu, Chiba, Japan Masato Takao

References

1. Guillo S, Bauer T, Lee JW, Takao M, Kong SW, Stone JW, Mangone PG, Molloy A, Perera A, Pearce CJ, Michels F, Tourné Y, Ghorbani A, Calder J. Consensus in chronic ankle instability: aetiology, assessment, surgical indications and place for arthroscopy. Orthop Traumatol Surg Res. 2013;99:S411–9.
2. Michels F, Guillo S, Vanrietvelde F, Brugman E, Ankle Instability Group, Stockmans F. How to drill the talar tunnel in ATFL reconstruction? Knee Surg Sports Traumatol Arthrosc. 2016;24:991–7.
3. Michels F, Cordier G, Guillo S, Stockmans F, ESKKA-AFAS Ankle Instability Group. Endoscopic ankle lateral ligament graft anatomic reconstruction. Foot Ankle Clin. 2016;21:665–80.
4. Takao M, Matsui K, Stone JW, Glazebrook MA, Kennedy JG, Guillo S, Calder JD, Karlsson J, Ankle Instability Group. Arthroscopic anterior talofibular ligament repair for lateral instability of the ankle. Knee Surg Sports Traumatol Arthrosc. 2016;24:1003–6.
5. Guillo S, Takao M, Calder J, Karlson J, Michels F, Bauer T, Ankle Instability Group. Arthroscopic anatomical reconstruction of the lateral ankle ligaments. Knee Surg Sports Traumatol Arthrosc. 2016;24:998–1002.
6. Matsui K, Burgesson B, Takao M, Stone J, Guillo S, Glazebrook M, ESSKA AFAS Ankle Instability Group. Minimally invasive surgical treatment for chronic ankle instability: a systematic review. Knee Surg Sports Traumatol Arthrosc. 2016;24:1040–8.
7. Glazebrook M, Stone J, Matsui K, Guillo S, Takao M, ESSKA AFAS Ankle Instability Group. Percutaneous ankle reconstruction of lateral ligaments (Perc-Anti RoLL). Foot Ankle Int. 2016;37:659–64.
8. Matsui K, Oliva XM, Takao M, Pereira BS, Gomes TM, Lozano JM, ESSKA AFAS Ankle Instability Group, Glazebrook M. Bony landmarks available for minimally invasive lateral ankle stabilization surgery: a cadaveric anatomical study. Knee Surg Sports Traumatol Arthrosc. 2017;25:1916–24.
9. Michels F, Pereira H, Calder J, Matricali G, Glazebrook M, Guillo S, Karlsson J, ESSKA-AFAS Ankle Instability Group. Searching for consensus in the approach to patients with chronic lateral ankle instability: ask the expert. Knee Surg Sports Traumatol Arthrosc. 2018;26:2095–102.

10. Nery C, Fonseca L, Raduan F, Moreno M, Baumfeld D, ESSKA AFAS Ankle Instability Group. Prospective study of the "Inside-Out" arthroscopic ankle ligament technique: preliminary result. Foot Ankle Surg. 2018;24:320–5.
11. Takao M, Ozeki S, Oliva XM, Inokuchi R, Yamazaki T, Takeuchi Y, Kubo M, Lowe D, Matsui K, Katakura M, Ankle Instability Group, Glazebrook M. Strain pattern of each ligamentous band of the superficial deltoid ligament: a cadaver study. BMC Musculoskelet Disord. 2020;21:289.
12. Broström L. Sprained ankles. VI. Surgical treatment of "chronic" ligament ruptures. Acta Chir Scand. 1966;132:551–65.
13. Hawkins RB. Arthroscopic stapling repair for chronic lateral instability. Clin Podiatr Med Surg. 1987;4:875–83.
14. Corte-Real NM, Moreira RM. Arthroscopic repair of chronic lateral ankle instability. Foot Ankle Int. 2009;30:213–7.
15. Nery C, Raduan F, Del Buono A, Asaumi ID, Cohen M, Maffulli N. Arthroscopic-assisted Broström-Gould for chronic ankle instability: a long-term follow-up. Am J Sports Med. 2011;39:2381–8.
16. Cottom JM, Rigby RB. The "all inside" arthroscopic Broström procedure: a prospective study of 40 consecutive patients. J Foot Ankle Surg. 2013;52:568–74.
17. Giza E, Shin EC, Wong SE, Acevedo JI, Mangone PG, Olson K, Anderson MJ. Arthroscopic suture anchor repair of the lateral ligament ankle complex: a cadaveric study. Am J Sports Med. 2013;41:2567–72.
18. Acevedo JI, Mangone P. Arthroscopic Brostrom technique. Foot Ankle Int. 2015;36:465–73.
19. Lui TH. Modified arthroscopic Brostrom procedure. Foot Ankle Surg. 2015;21:216–9.
20. Vega J, Golanó P, Pellegrino A, Rabat E, Peña F. All-inside arthroscopic lateral collateral ligament repair for ankle instability with a knotless suture anchor technique. Foot Ankle Int. 2013;34:1701–9.
21. Matsui K, Takao M, Miyamoto W, Innami K, Matsushita T. Arthroscopic Broström repair with Gould augmentation via an accessory anterolateral port for lateral instability of the ankle. Arch Orthop Trauma Surg. 2014;134:1461–7.
22. Takao M, Katakura M, Jujo Y. Arthroscopic ligament repair and reconstruction. Sports injuries of the foot and ankle. New York: Springer; 2019. p. 29–44.
23. DiGiovanni CW, Langer PR, Nickisch F, Spenciner D. Proximity of the lateral talar process to the lateral stabilizing ligaments of the ankle and subtalar joint. Foot Ankle Int. 2007;28:175–80.
24. Lui TH. Arthroscopic-assisted lateral ligament reconstruction in combined ankle and subtalar instability. Arthroscopy. 2007;23:554.e1–5.
25. Guillo S, Archbold P, Perera A, Bauer T, Sonnery-Cottet B. Arthroscopic anatomic reconstruction of the lateral ligaments of the ankle with gracilis autograft. Arthrosc Tech. 2014;22:e593–8.
26. Takao M, Glazebrook M, Stone J, Guillo S. Ankle arthroscopic reconstruction of lateral ligaments (Ankle Anti-ROLL). Arthrosc Tech. 2015;4:e595–600.
27. Glazebrook M, Stone J, Matsui K, Guillo S, Takao M, ESSKA AFAS Ankle Instability Group. Percutaneous ankle reconstruction of lateral ligaments (Perc-Anti RoLL). Foot Ankle Int. 2016;37:659–64.

Acknowledgments

The Editors thank and acknowledge Pontus Andersson from Pontus Art Production for his outstanding contribution, availability, and support in the artwork of this book.

Contents

Part II Non-operative Approach

Part III Surgical Treatment

About the Editors

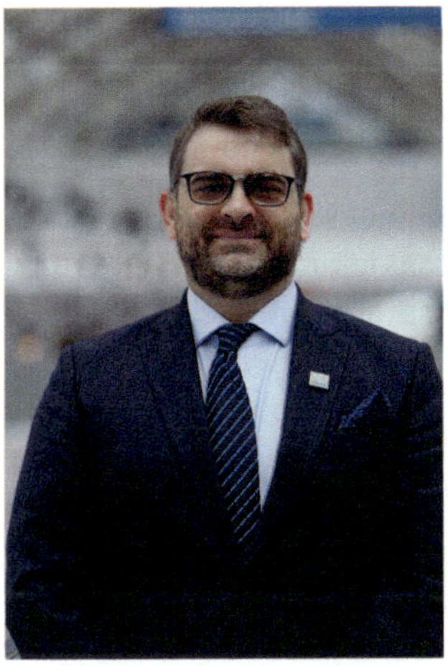

Hélder Pereira, MD, PhD is a Specialist in Orthopaedics and Traumatology at Póvoa de Varzim-Vila do Conde Hospital Centre, Portugal, and he is researcher, PhD candidate, and invited instructor at Minho University, Braga-Guimarães, Portugal.

Moreover, he is member of the Foot and Ankle Unit at Ripoll y De Prado Sports Clinic, FIFA Medical Centre of Excellence, Murcia-Madrid, Spain, where he is Coordinator of Clinical Research. He is past Chairman of ESSKA-AFAS (Ankle and Foot Associates Section) and from 2014 to 2016 chaired the Basic Science Research Committee of ESSKA. He is an editorial board member of *Knee Surgery, Sports Traumatology, Arthroscopy (KSSTA)* and has authored around 100 publications.

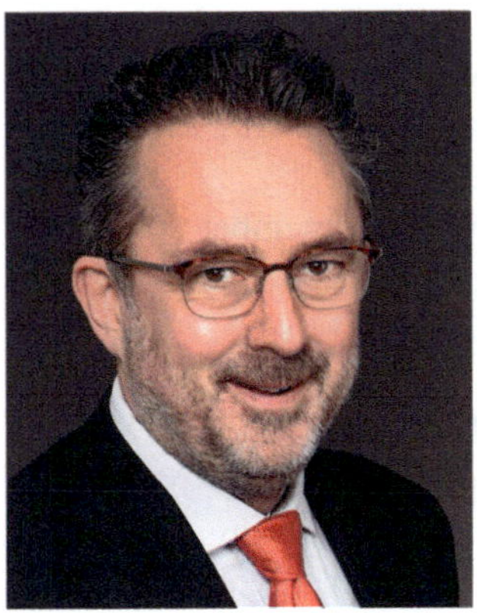

Stéphane Guillo is the Medical Director of SOS Pied Cheville Bordeaux, France, a clinical and research institute for foot and ankle surgery. He is also the founder of the Ankle Instability Group and has held leadership roles in various associations. His research is focused now mainly on ankle ligament treatment.

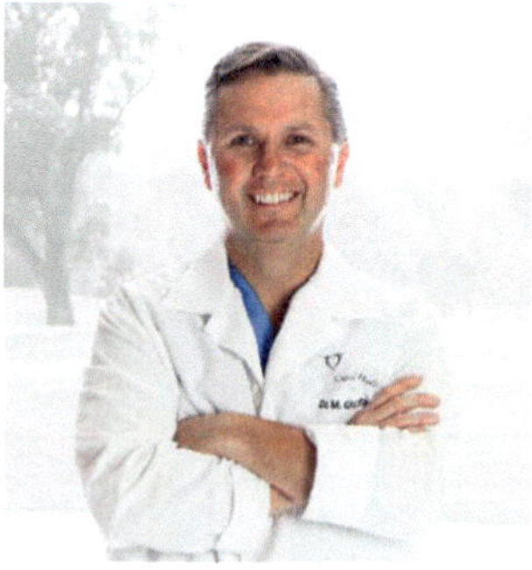

Mark Glazebrook, BSc(H), MSc, PhD, MD, FRCS(C) is a full-time Professor of Orthopaedic Surgery at Dalhousie University. He completed his medical training in 1994 and completed specialty training in Orthopaedic Surgery in 1999 at Dalhousie. He then went on to complete a fellowship in Orthopedic Foot and Ankle and Sports Medicine at the University of Western Ontario. This was followed with a PhD in Achilles Tendon Disease at Dalhousie University. Dr Glazebrook devotes 80% of his working time to clinical practice focusing on Orthopedic Foot and Ankle Reconstruction and Sports Medicine. During research time, focus is on outcome studies on evidence-based medicine, ankle arthritis, MTP arthritis, bone graft substitutes, and Achilles tendon rupture care. He is Past President of the Canadian Orthopaedic Association (COA).

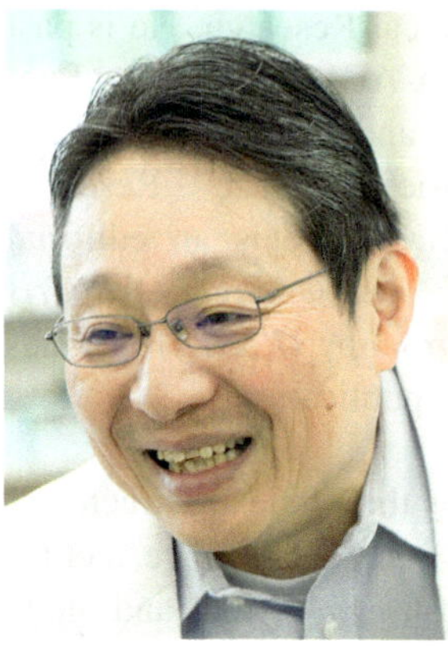

Masato Takao, MD, PhD is Professor and President of Clinical and Research Institute for Foot and Ankle Surgery (CARIFAS), Jujo Hospital, Kisarazu, Chiba, Japan. He has worked at CARIFAS since 2017. His clinical focus is on foot and ankle surgery.

His PhD-thesis in 1999 was devoted to "Anatomy for ankle arthroscopy," and since then he has been the author of more than 250 peer-reviewed publications, more than 50 book chapters and textbooks in orthopedic foot and ankle surgery including English and domestic papers.

He is a founding member of Ankle Instability Group (AIG) and chaired the fifth AIG meeting at 2018.

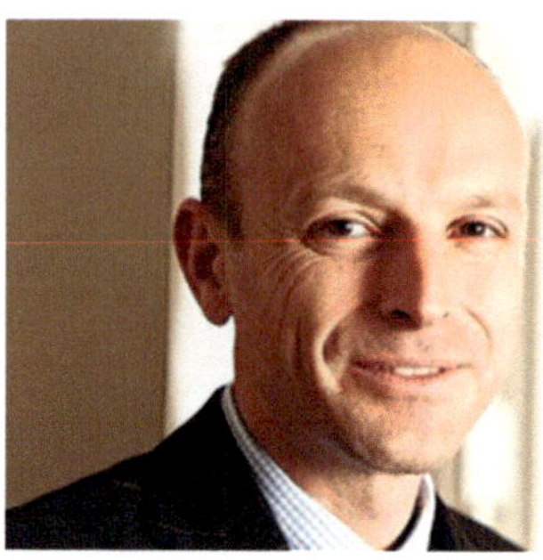

James Calder, TD, MD, PhD, FRCS completed higher surgical training in London before completing a Fellowship in Brisbane, Australia, with Dr Terry Saxby. He was appointed consultant at Hampshire Hospitals and then Chelsea and Westminster Hospital, London. He is Professor in the Department of Bioengineering, Imperial College, London, specializing in sports injury research. He has gained a reputation for his clinical interest in the management of foot and ankle injuries in the elite athlete. He looks after many of the professional football teams across Europe and National Olympic, rugby, and cricket teams as well as the Royal Ballet, Covent Garden, and Birmingham Royal Ballet. He is past chairman of ESSKA-AFAS and the Achilles Tendon Study Group, sub-editor of the *Journal of Bone and Joint* and previously Associate Editor KSSTA. He co-founded the Fortius Clinic, London.

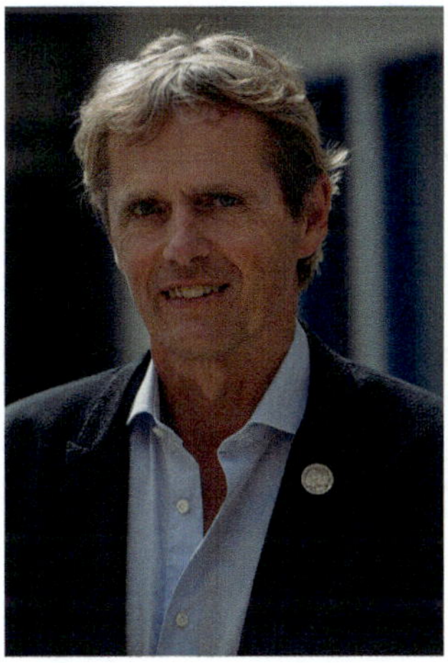

Niek Van Dijk, MD, PhD is a leading authority for surgery of the ankle. He is currently working in the FIFA Medical Centers of Excellence in Madrid, Clinic Ripol&DePrado&VanDijk and in Porto, Clinica de Dragão. Between 2002 and 2016, he was head of the Orthopaedic Department of the AMC Hospital (Amsterdam UMC). He is emeritus professor in Orthopaedic Surgery at the University of Amsterdam.

In 2000, Niek Van Dijk started the first international Amsterdam Foot and Ankle Course. His great interest in teaching and his belief in the techniques of the Amsterdam Foot and Ankle School stimulated him to develop the free access website Amsterdam Foot and Ankle Platform (www.ankleplatform.com). Today, the platform has >4000 members from more than 115 countries. Niek Van Dijk was president of the Dutch Orthopedic Association, president of the Nordic Orthopedic Association, and president of ESSKA and ESSKA-AFAS. He is honorary member of several Societies and Associations. He is the tutor of 50 PhD students who he guided to a successful defense of their PhD-thesis. Niek Van Dijk published over 350 scientific indexed publications, wrote over 100 book chapters, and is editor of several books. He is founding editor of JISAKOS, the *Journal of ISAKOS*.

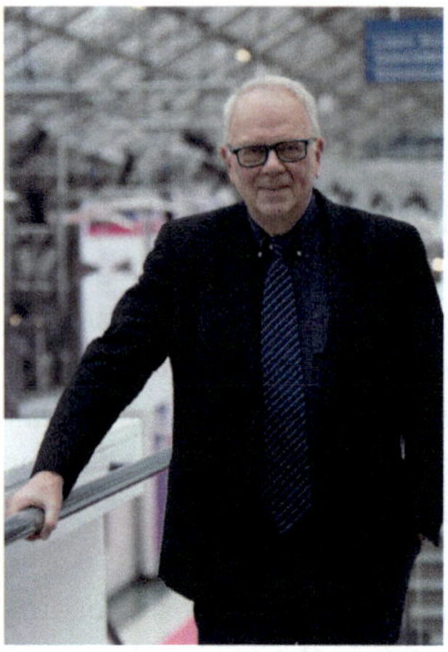

Jón Karlsson, MD, PhD is a Professor of Orthopaedics and Sports Traumatology at the Sahlgrenska Academy, Gothenburg University, Gothenburg, Sweden. Originally from Iceland, he has worked at the Sahlgrenska University Hospital since 1981. His clinical focus is knee surgery, especially complex knee injuries, knee dislocations, and revision surgery. He works as Foot and Ankle surgeon as well.

His PhD-thesis in 1989 was devoted to "Chronic Lateral Ankle Instability," and since then he has been the author of more than 500 peer-reviewed publications, more than 100 book chapters and over 40 textbooks in orthopedics and sports traumatology.

He has mentored 60 PhD students and is currently (since 12 years) the chief Editor of KSSTA (Knee Surgery Sports Traumatology Arthroscopy). He has been the care-taking physician of a professional football club (IFK Göteborg) since 1984.

Part I

Introduction

Anatomy of the Ankle Ligaments

1

Frederick Michels, Miki Dalmau-Pastor,
Jorge Pablo Batista, Xavier Martin Oliva,
Pietro Spennacchio, and Filip Stockmans

1.1 The Lateral Ligament Complex

The lateral joint capsule of the ankle is reinforced by the anterior talofibular ligament (ATFL) and posterior talofibular ligament (PTFL) and the calcaneofibular ligament (CFL) [1]. The increasing popularity of minimally invasive techniques to treat lateral hindfoot instability increases the need for knowledge of the local anatomy [2–6].

1.1.1 Anterior Talofibular Ligament (ATFL)

The ATFL is the first ligament to be injured during an inversion trauma of the ankle. The ATFL is a flat, quadrilateral, and relatively thin ligament (Fact Box 1). Its origin is located on the anterior edge of the lateral malleolus and it inserts on the lateral side of the talus [7, 8]. The ATFL is the main stabilizer during supination and anterior talar translation in all ankle positions [9, 10]. In

F. Michels (✉)
Orthopaedic Department, AZ Groeninge, Kortrijk, Belgium

MIFAS by GRECMIP (Minimally Invasive Foot and Ankle Society), Merignac, France

M. Dalmau-Pastor
MIFAS by GRECMIP (Minimally Invasive Foot and Ankle Society), Merignac, France

Human Anatomy Unit, Department of Pathology and Experimental Therapeutics, School of Medicine, University of Barcelona, Barcelona, Spain

J. P. Batista
Centro Artroscopico Jorge Batista, Buenos Aires, Argentina

Football Department Club Atlético Boca Juniors, Buenos Aires, Argentina

Faculty of Sports Medicine, Universidad Católica, Santiago, Chile

X. M. Oliva
Department of Human Anatomy, Dissection Room, Faculty of Medicine, University of Barcelona, Barcelona, Spain

EFAS educational committee, Barcelona, Spain

Spanisch Foot and Anke Society, Barcelona, Spain

P. Spennacchio
Sports Medicine Department, Centre Hospitalier de Luxembourg, Luxembourg, Luxembourg

F. Stockmans
Orthopaedic Department, AZ Groeninge, Kortrijk, Belgium

Department of Development and Regeneration, Faculty of Medicine, University of Leuven campus Kortrijk, Kortrijk, Belgium

H. Pereira et al. (eds.), *Lateral Ankle Instability*, https://doi.org/10.1007/978-3-662-62763-1_1

Fact Box 1 Dimensions Lateral Ankle Ligaments

Anterior talofibular ligament

Superior band

- Length: 26–31.5 mm
- Fibular insertion area: 6–12 mm
- Talar insertion area: 7–15 mm

Inferior band

- Length: 22–29 mm
- Fibular insertion area: 4–9 mm
- Talar insertion area: 5–10 mm

Calcaneofibular ligament

- Length: 27–52 mm
- Area of fibular insertion into the apex of the lateral malleolus: 3–6 mm
- Area of insertion into the calcaneus: 6–8 mm
- Angle while in neutral position on the floor: 80°

standing position, this ligament runs parallel to the ground. In plantar flexion, its orientation changes and it becomes more tense. In this position, the ATFL is most vulnerable and more prone to injuries [10–15].

According to the literature, ATFL can have 1, 2, or 3 bands [1, 16–21]. Nevertheless, recent publications state it is a 2-bands ligament, and that reported cases where only 1 band is present should be considered pathological (Fig. 1.1) [22]. A small perforating fibular artery separates the superior from the inferior band and anastomoses with the lateral malleolar artery. This small branch is responsible for the bleeding and subsequent hematoma following an ankle sprain, or for postsurgical bleeding, after arthroscopic ATFL repair.

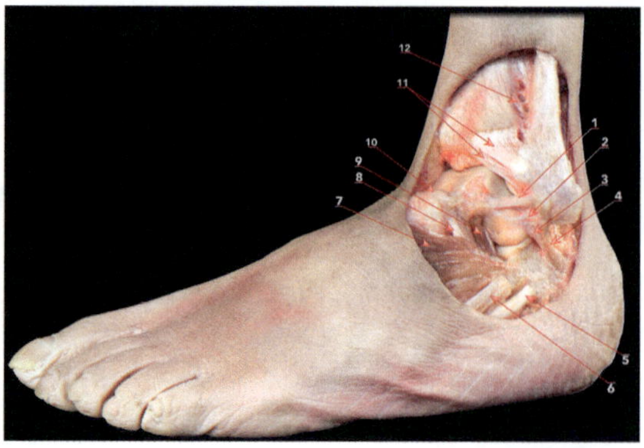

Fig. 1.1 Lateral view of the classical dissecting approach used in this study. (1) ATFL superior fascicle. (2) ATFL inferior fascicle. (3) Arciform fibers of the LFTCL Complex. (4) CFL. (5) Peroneus longus tendon. (6) Peroneus brevis tendon. (7) Extensor digitorum brevis muscle. (8) Cervical ligament. (9) Anterior capsular ligament. (10) Dorsal talonavicular ligament. (11) Anterior tibiofibular ligament and distal fascicle. (12) Interosseous tibiofibular ligament. (Figure reproduced with permission from Vega J, Malagelada F, Manzanares Céspedes MC, Dalmau-Pastor M. The lateral fibulotalocalcaneal ligament complex: an ankle stabilizing isometric structure. Knee Surg Sports Traumatol Arthrosc. 2018 Oct 29. doi: https://doi.org/10.1007/s00167-018-5188-8)

The origin of the superior band is located just below the origin of the anterior tibiofibular ligament (ATiFL). The inferior band is connected with the CFL through arciform fibers in its malleolar origin (Fig. 1.2) [22].

During arthroscopic exploration, the lateral gutter must be recognized and felt, in order to look for injuries in the ATFL. This is possible due to the intra-articular location of ATFL's superior fascicle, which allows for arthroscopic examination and treatment of this ligament (Fig. 1.3) [23]. However, this intra-articular location would possibly impair healing of this band after an ankle inversion sprain, a fact that can explain the very high index of chronic pain after an ankle sprain.

It should not be difficult for the arthroscopist to identify a healthy, whole ligament, or a complete rupture of the ATFL: there are, however, partial injuries associated with the anterolateral soft tissue impingement syndrome, which makes diagnosis difficult (Fig. 1.4).

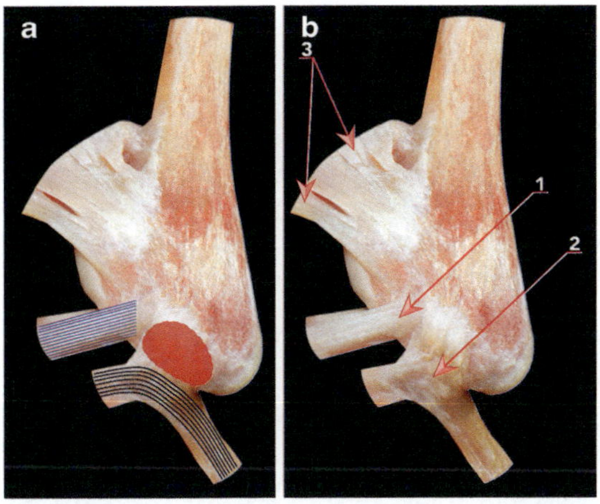

Fig. 1.2 Schematic view of the LFTCL Complex with the lateral malleolus disarticulated from the ankle. (**a**) View with the lateral ankle ligaments highlighted: ATFL superior fascicle (blue lines), LFTCL Complex (black lines), and an area showing the common origin of the LFTCL Complex (red area). (**b**) Classic view of the LFTCL Complex. (1) ATFL superior fascicle. (2) LFTCL Complex. (3) Anterior tibiofibular ligament and distal fascicle. (Figure reproduced with permission from Vega J, Malagelada F, Manzanares Céspedes MC, Dalmau-Pastor M. The lateral fibulotalocalcaneal ligament complex: an ankle stabilizing isometric structure. Knee Surg Sports Traumatol Arthrosc. 2018 Oct 29. doi: https://doi.org/10.1007/s00167-018-5188-8)

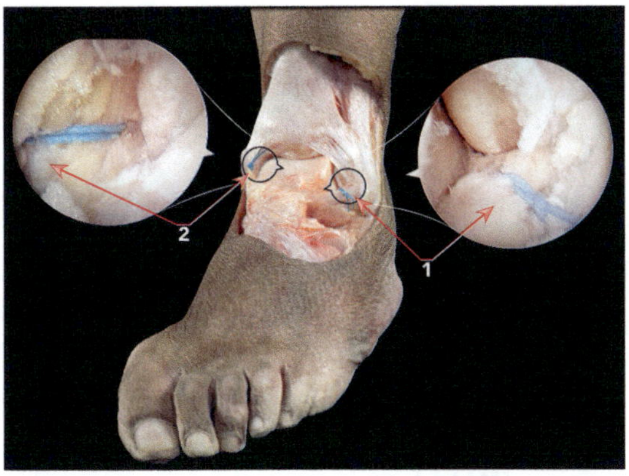

Fig. 1.3 Anterior view of a dissection performed after the arthroscopic procedure. Correlation of the arthroscopically sutured structures was obtained during dissection. (1) ATFL's superior fascicle. (2) Deltoid ligament (Anterior tibiotalar and tibionavicular ligaments). (Figure reproduced with permission from Dalmau-Pastor M, Malagelada F, Kerkhoffs GM, Karlsson J, Guelfi M, Vega J. Redefining anterior ankle arthroscopic anatomy: medial and lateral ankle collateral ligaments are visible through dorsiflexion and non-distraction anterior ankle arthroscopy. Knee Surg Sports Traumatol Arthrosc. 2019 Jul 10. doi: https://doi.org/10.1007/s00167-019-05603-2)

1.1.2 Calcaneofibular Ligament (CFL)

The CFL ligament plays a part in the stability of two joints: the talocrural joint and the subtalar joint. The CFL is a thick and cord-like ligament that is inserted on the anterior side of the lateral malleolus, immediately below, and very close to the insertion of the ATFL, to which it is usually joined by arciform fibers [1, 6, 24]. It is important to recognize that the tip of the lateral malleolus is free of any insertions; this can be clearly seen during ankle arthroscopy. This technical detail is critical when carving a tunnel in the fibula during ligament repair or reconstruction [2, 6, 25, 26].

The direction is oblique, towards posterior and distal, inserting on the lateral side of the calcaneus, almost perpendicularly to the subtalar joint, 13–20 mm dorsally and posterior in relation to the lateral tubercle, involving itself in its medial surface with the talocalcaneal lateral ligament (TCLL) (Fig. 1.5) [16]. Laidlaw studied 750 cadaveric specimens and showed a slight variation in its calcaneal insertion: 64.5% typical location, 25.5% anterior location, 5.5% posterior location, and 4.5% distal location [27]. This variation in its insertion is the result of the obliquity of the ligament in relation to the longitudinal axis of the fibula [27].

Immediately over its anterior edge and separated by a thin fatty tissue which sometimes goes unnoticed, we find the talocalcaneal ligament (TC), which separates it from the subtalar joint. The TC, usually underestimated by most authors, plays an important role in the lateral stability of the ankle [24].

The CFL is an extracapsular ligament that, according to some authors, plays an independent role in the stability of the ankle [28]. During the plantar flexion of the ankle, the CFL is set horizontally; meanwhile, when flexed, it is set vertically, though, in both cases, it is tensed throughout the arc of motion. The only ankle movement during which this ligament is relaxed is in the ankle valgus [1, 17]. In plantar flexion, the CFL limits supination, along with the ATL. In dorsal flexion, the CFL limits supination along with the PTFL. This injury mechanism throughout the

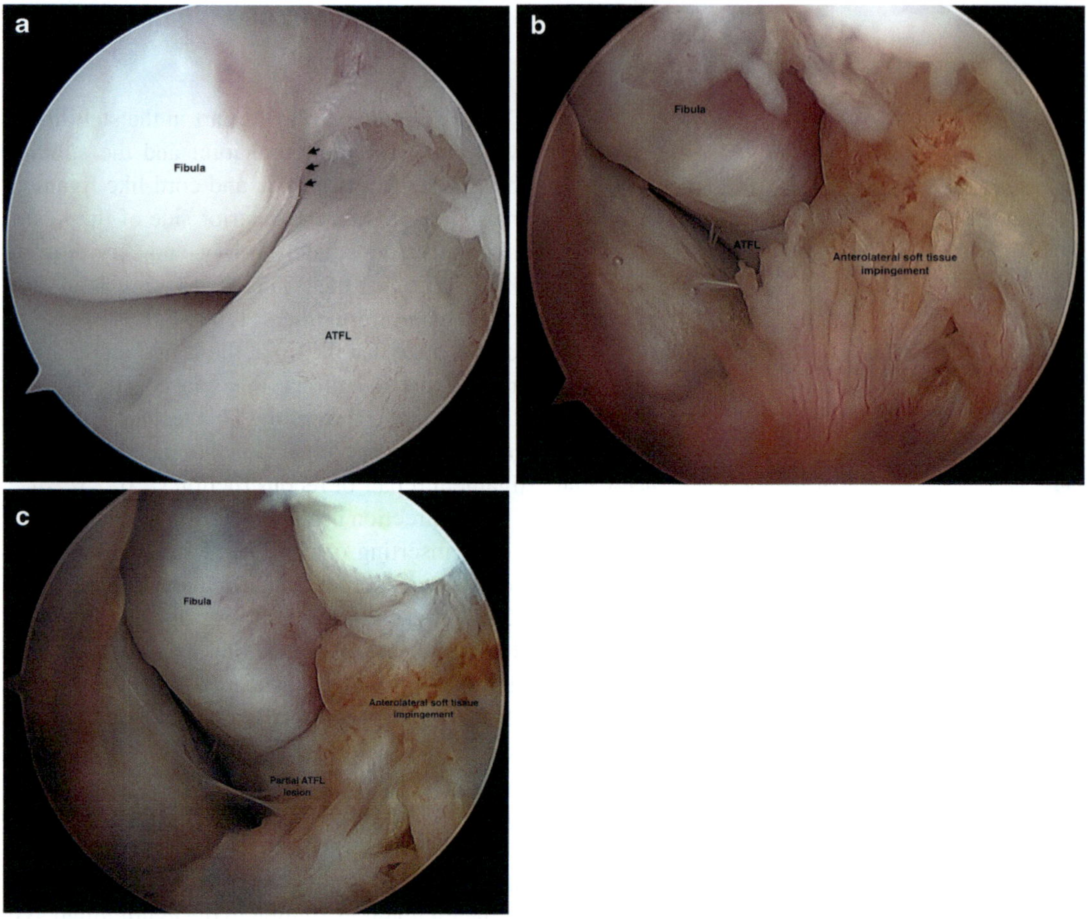

Fig. 1.4 (**a**) Normal ATFL.(**b**) Anterolateral soft tissue impingement. (**c**) Partial lesion ATFL

range of motion of the ankle has been the subject of debate for many years.

This ligament is the second ligament to become injured during an ankle sprain, with an injury incidence of 20% approximately; when it is injured, the ATFL is usually injured as well.

1.1.3 Lateral Talocalcaneal Ligament (LTCL)

This ligament is seldom discussed in publications. It lies in front of the CFL, sometimes parallel to it, and sometimes slightly diverting towards the calcaneus; its orientation varies fundamentally in 35% of the cases in both insertions by the talus and the calcaneus [29]. In 40% of the cases, this ligament is not identified in cadaveric dissections [30]. Usually, its rupture occurs along with the rupture of the CFL, and its pattern of injury is similar to that of the latter [24].

1.1.4 Posterior Talofibular Ligament (PTFL)

The PTFL has a semi cord-like shape, and it is the strongest and most resilient of the ligaments that are part of the lateral structures of the ankle (Fig. 1.6) [7, 17, 24]. Rasmussen states that this structure plays a minor role in the stability of the ankle when the rest of the lateral structures are untouched [28]. The PTFL is rarely injured, except in cases of ankle fracture or dislocation.

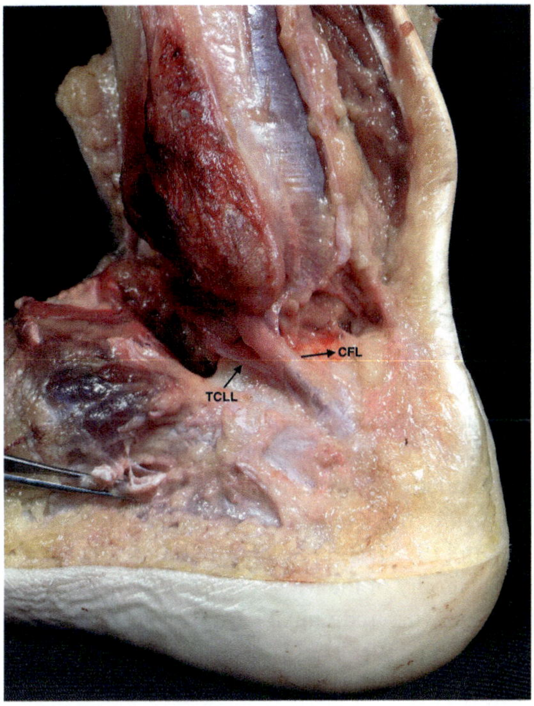

Fig. 1.5 Calcaneofibular ligament (CFL) and talocalcaneal lateral ligament (TCLL)

Golano described the intracapsular but extrasynovial trajectory of the ligament, it explains why it is easily visualized during posterior ankle arthroscopy [1]. This ligament has a conical shape and is 30 mm long, with an average width of 12 mm; its thickness varies depending on the position of the foot. In plantar flexion and neutral position, the ligament is relaxed, while in dorsiflexion, it is tensed. This ligament is much more prominent in sportsmen or dancers [15, 21, 24].

It inserts in the digital fossa, located in the medial, posterior part of the fibular malleolus. It runs medially, almost horizontally towards its insertion in the posterior area of the talus. The footprint on the talus is quite large and must be detached when resecting an os trigonum.

Some fibers of the superior part of the PTFL lie proximally and medially, inserting themselves into the posterior edge of the tibia, and are fused with the fibers of the deep layer of the posterior tibiofibular ligament.

In cadaveric dissections, it has been noted that these fibers reach, in 90% of the cases, the posterior surface of the medial malleolus, creating a labrum on the posterior margin of the tibia. This cluster of fibers is the posterior intermalleolar ligament (or capsular reinforcement bundle, or tibial bundle of PTFL) [1]. Desinsertion of these distal fibers of the PTFL ligament does not generate residual instability.

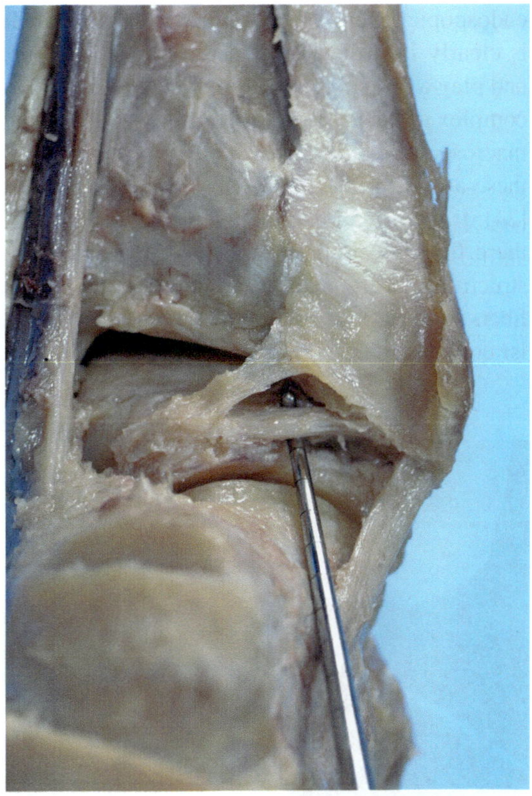

Fig. 1.6 Posterior Talofibular Ligament (PTFL)

1.1.5 Arciform Fibers (AF)

These fibers are an expansion of the regular, collagenous, and elastic dense connecting tissue, in the shape of a triangle or a semicircle, with an anteroinferior base that connects the inferior band of the ATFL, the lateral talocalcaneal ligament, and the CFL, in a constant way (Fig. 1.7). This structure has been clearly described by Sarrafian, and has been confirmed by Pau Golano, but has attracted attention again in recent years due to the critical role it is believed to play in endoscopic repairs of the ATFL [1, 17, 19–21]. It is clearly identified in all cadaveric dissections, and play a critical role within the lateral ligament complex of the ankle. A recent study assessed the macroscopic and microscopic morphology of these arciform fibers, through different colorings [24]. It was found that the histologic structure of these fibers is similar to that of the ligamentous structures, with an abundance of collagenous fibers, low adipose cell content, plus high vascular content (Fig. 1.8) [24].

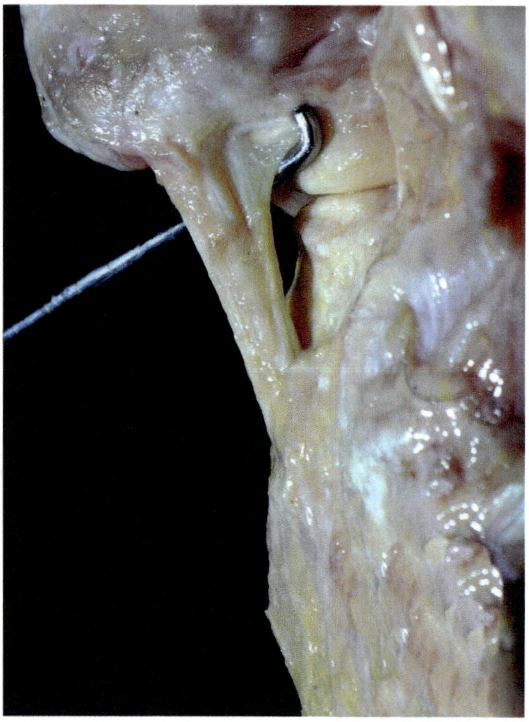

Fig. 1.7 Anterior view of CFL with arciform fibers

1.2 The Medial Ligament Complex

1.2.1 Anatomy

The deltoid ligament, or medial collateral ligament (MCL), is a strong broad multibanded complex, made up of a group of ligaments that span out from the medial malleolus towards the talus, calcaneus, and navicular bones. The characteristic deltoid shape explains the commonly used term.

The different ligaments of the deltoid complex are anatomically difficult to distinguish, due to the tight continuity of the components and the close relation with surrounding structures, as the posterior tibial and flexor digitorum tendon sheath [19, 31, 32]. Golano found that the inherent anatomy of the MCL complex makes the distinction in individual bands artificial and inconstant [19]. These observations explain the variable and sometimes confusing anatomical descriptions of the MCL available in the literature [32–35].

The MCL can roughly be divided into a superficial and deep group of fibers, separated by a fat pad, each one formed by multiple components (Figs. 1.9 and 1.10) [19, 31, 32]. The superficial layer crosses both the ankle and subtalar joint, while the deep layer crosses solely the tibiotalar joint [21, 32, 34, 36]. The variations reported in the literature about the prevalence and size of each component have been summarized by Yammine et al. in a meta-analysis [32]. In order to offer surgical landmarks for deltoid ligament repair or reconstruction, Campbell et al. furnished a thorough description of the anatomical attachment sites of the ligamentous bands of the

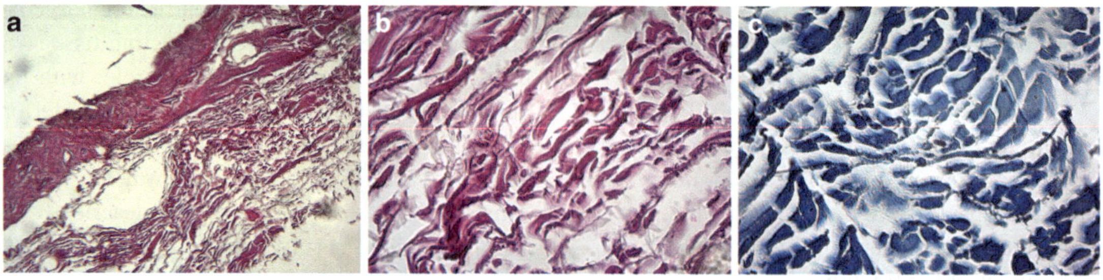

Fig. 1.8 Histological image of arciform fibers with different colorings

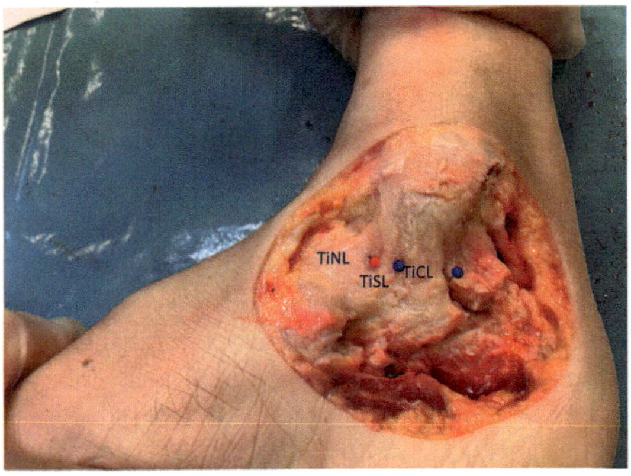

Fig. 1.9 Superficial layer with tibionavicular ligament, tibiospring ligament, and tibiocalcaneal ligament

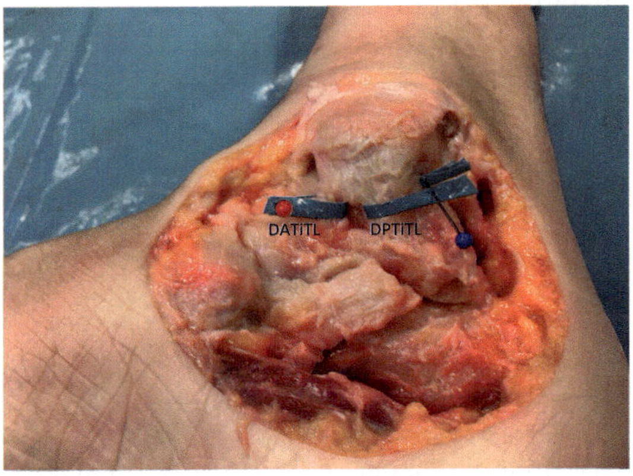

Fig. 1.10 Deep layer with deep anterior tibiotalar ligament (DATiTL) and deep posterior tibiotalar ligament (DPTiTL)

deltoid complex, analyzing 14 non-paired ankle cadaveric specimens (Fact Box 2) [34].

Fact Box 2 Characteristics of the Deltoid Ligament as Described by Yammine and Campbell [32, 34]

Superficial layer
Tibiospring ligament

- Prevalence: 94%
- Origin: tibial attachment slightly proximal and posterior to the tibial attachment of the tibionavicular ligament
- Insertion: onto the spring ligament, usually within its posterior half. The width of its insertion at the spring ligament averaged 5.9 mm.

Tibionavicular ligament

- Prevalence: 90%
- Origin: on the anterior colliculus of the medial malleolus
- Insertion: in an expansive manner onto the dorsomedial surface of the navicular

Superficial posterior tibiotalar ligament

- Prevalence: 80%
- Origin: from the distal center of the intercollicular groove
- Insertion: the posteroinferior medial talar body

Tibiocalacaneal ligament

- Prevalence: 85%
- Origin: near the intercollicular groove of the medial malleolus
- Insertion: at the most posterior aspect of the sustentaculum tali on the calcaneus

Deep layer
Deep posterior tibiotalar ligament

- Constantly (100%) the largest and thickest band of the whole deltoid ligamentous complex
- Origin: near the center of the medial malleolus intercollicular groove
- Insertion: on the posterosuperior aspect of the medial talar body inferior to the articular cartilage of the trochlea

Deep anterior tibiotalar ligament

- Prevalence: 63%

- Origin: from the most inferior and anterior areas of the medial malleolus immediately deep to the tibionavicular and tibiospring ligaments of the superficial deltoid layer
- Insertion: the anterosuperior portions of the medial talus body.

1.2.2 Functional Anatomy and Biomechanics

The deltoid ligament is a primary medial stabilizer of the ankle and serves multiple functions by attaching the medial malleolus to the tarsal bones of the foot.

Through its multiple tibiotalar and tibiocalcaneal attachments, the MCL restrains against pronation and lateral translation of the talus, and contributes, with the lateral ligamentous structures to limit anterior translation of the talus [36–38].

The anatomical separations in different ligamentous bands are guided by its functional importance, as shown in studies investigating the biomechanical behavior of the MCL complex. Both cadaveric studies and finite element analysis suggest that the superficial structures of the deltoid complex mainly resist external rotation of the talus relative to the tibia and the deep deltoid resists valgus angulation and lateral displacement of the talus [31, 39, 40].

Additionally, the broad insertion on the “spring ligament complex” through the tibiospring ligament, the MCL complex is supposed to have a role in medial column stability [36].

Acute lesion of the MCL is much less frequent than lateral ligament injury, representing only 5% of ligamentous ankle injuries [31]. Accepted injury mechanisms involve a pronation/eversion trauma or an excessive inward rotation of the tibia during simultaneous outward rotation of the foot [36, 41, 42].

Other than direct post-traumatic involvement, MCL injuries are also hypothesized as a secondary consequence of the talar instability in the mortise following lateral ankle injuries, which causes a progressive wearing out of the superficial anterior bundle of the deltoid ligament [36, 42].

The existence of this latter mechanism is supported by the clinical observation of combined medial and lateral ligament injuries in patients suffering from chronic functional ankle instability after primary lateral ligament injury [36, 42, 43]. The clinical relevance of MCL lesions remains unclear [40]. However, some authors agree that untreated medial ligamentous injuries could explain why some patients with ankle instability remain symptomatic after isolated surgical lateral ankle stabilization [41, 42].

1.3 The Ligaments of the Tibiofibular Syndesmosis

1.3.1 Importance of the Syndesmosis and the Tibiofibular Articulation

The distal tibiofibular syndesmosis is a ligamentous complex that provides stability to this joint. The anterior tibiofibular ligament (ATiFL) and posterior tibiofibular ligament (PTiFL) together with the interosseous tibiofibular ligament (ITiFL) form the syndesmosis. The inferior transverse tibiofibular ligament is sometimes considered a fourth ligament but should be seen as a continuation of the posterior tibiofibular ligament.

In 1–11% of the soft tissue injuries of the ankle, the syndesmosis is reported to be affected [44, 45]. Injury to the syndesmosis occurs through rupture or bony avulsion of the syndesmotic ligament complex [11]. These injuries are mostly the result of external rotation trauma [46]. Other trauma mechanisms that have been recognized to cause syndesmotic injury are abduction, dorsiflexion, and inversion. During external rotation of the foot, the fibula is translated posteriorly and rotated externally. This results in tensioning of the ATiFL and could be the main cause of isolated rupture of the ATiFL.

The distal tibiofibular articulation is a syndesmosis. This articulation permits vague mobility thus allowing the talus to enter the talar mortise during the dorsal flexion. This mobility consists of a minimal increase of the articular space followed by a medial rotation and small ascension of the fibula. On the other hand, in plantar flexion, the articular space narrows and the fibula rotates laterally and descends.

1.3.2 Contact Surfaces

At the base of the syndesmosis, there is a small area where the tibia and fibula are in direct contact. This area is called the tibiofibular contact zone. In this area, there is a small strip of hyaline cartilage which is a continuation of the cartilage of the tibial plafond and articular facet of the lateral malleolus. Between the distal fibula and tibia there is a synovial recess [21]. The superior part of this recess is limited by the interosseous ligament. The posterior part of this recess is often occupied by a reddish synovial fringe (Fig. 1.11). This tissue ascends when during dorsiflexion and descends during plantar flexion of the ankle. It has been reported to be responsible for impingement and chronic pain after ankle trauma.

1.3.3 Ligament Layers

1.3.3.1 Anterior Tibiofibular Ligament

The ligament originates in the anterior tubercle of the tibia (Chaput Tillaux tubercule), 5 mm on average above the articular surface, and its fibers extend in a distal and lateral direction to insert in the anterior margin of the lateral malleolus (Wagstaffe tubercle). The branches of the peroneal artery penetrate through the fascicles of this ligament (Fig. 1.12).

The most distal fascicle of the ATiFL appears to be independent of the rest of the structure. It is separated from the main part by a septum of fibroadipose tissue and it is located slightly deeper.

Nicolopoulus named this ligament accessory anteroinferior tibiofibular ligament [47]. After an anatomical study, Basset renamed it to distal fascicle of the anteroinferior tibiofibular ligament [48]. This fascicule reaches the lateral ridge of the talus. In dorsal flexion, this may lead to an impingement and cartilage erosion of the lateral talar ridge, especially if the ridge is widened (Fig. 1.12). This clinical symptomatic impingement appears frequently after a lateral ankle ligament injury.

1.3.3.2 Posterior Tibiofibular Ligament

The PiTFL consists of two different ligaments (Fig. 1.13) [19, 49]. The superficial component originates at the posterior edge of the lateral mal-

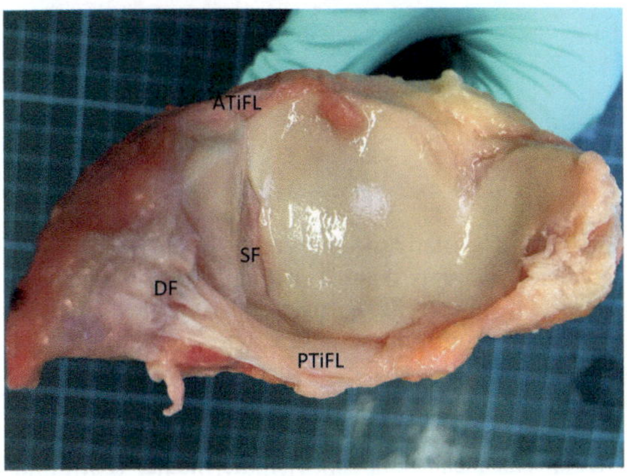

Fig. 1.11 Distal view of tibiofibular joint with synovial fringe (SF), digital fossa (DF)

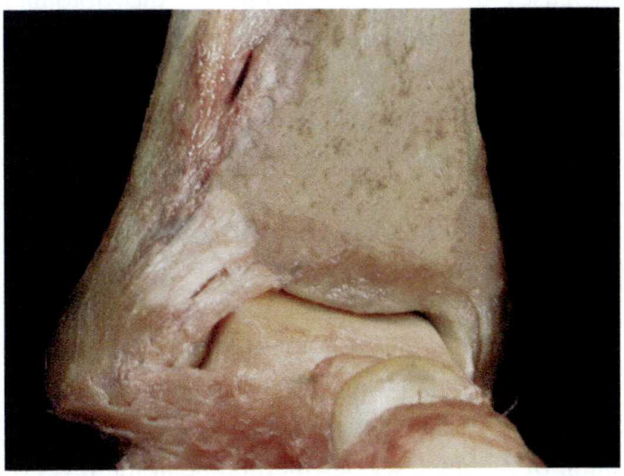

Fig. 1.12 Distal fascicle of the anteroinferior tibiofibular ligament

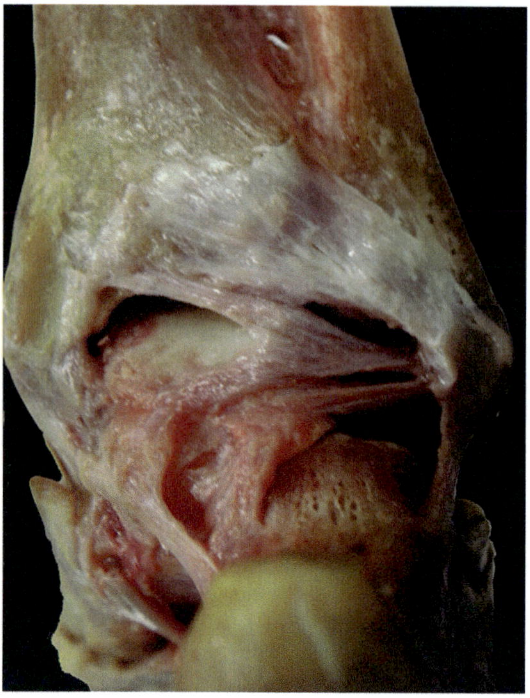

Fig. 1.13 Posterior tibiofibular ligament

leolus and runs proximally and medially to insert in the posterior tibial tubercle, the Volkmann crest. This component would be homologous to the anterior tibiofibular ligament. The profound component is the inferior transverse ligament (ITL), which is the most distal part of the PiTFL (Fig. 1.13). The ITL increases the amount of articular surface of the posterior part of the tibia playing the same role as the labrum in the shoulder. Biomechanically, it increases the articular stability of the tibiotalar articulation by avoiding the posterior displacement of the talus. Its origin is located in the proximal region of the malleolar fossa and its insertion is found in the posterior ridge of the tibia.

1.3.3.3 Interosseus Tibiofibular Ligament

The ITiFL is a dense mass of short fibers, which, together with adipose tissue and small branching vessels from the peroneal artery, span the tibia to the fibula. It can be considered as a distal continuation of the interosseous membrane at the level of the tibiofibular syndesmosis [8, 21]. Some investigators have suggested that the interosseous ligament is mechanically insignificant, whereas others consider it the primary band between the tibia and fibula. Nevertheless, the ITiFL is not consistently considered by all the authors as a part of the tibiofibular syndesmosis, suggesting that it may play an important role in the stability of the ankle.

1.4 The Subtalar Ligaments

1.4.1 The Different Layers

Multiple ligamentous structures have their origin in the tarsal sinus and canal. The anatomy of these structures is rather complex (Fig. 1.14).

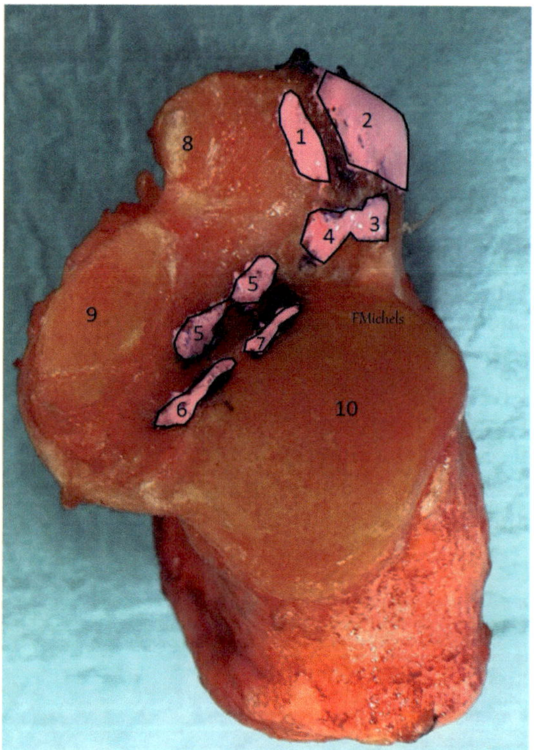

Fig. 1.14 Cavaderic specimen of the right calcaneus with ligament footprints painted in pink. Superior view. (1) Cervical ligament. (2) Extensor digitorum brevis muscle. (3) Lateral root of the inferior extensor retinaculum. (4) Confluent insertion of the intermediate root of the inferior extensor retinaculum and lateral calcaneal component of the medial root of the inferior extensor retinaculum. (5) Medial calcaneal component of the medial root of the inferior extensor retinaculum. (6) Interosseous ligament. (7) Anterior capsular ligament. (8) Anterior calcaneal articular surface. (9) Middle calcaneal articular surface. (10) Posterior calcaneal articular surface

Harper categorized these structures into three groups from superficial to deep: a superficial layer, an intermediate layer, and a deep layer (Fact Box 3) [37]. We added the anterior capsular ligament to the deep layer.

More recently, Yamaguchi et al. examined the anatomical relationship between the fibrous tissues of the tarsal canal and sinus and the articular capsules of the subtalar joint [50]. They distinguished three layered structures from posterior to anterior: the anterior capsule of the posterior talocalcaneal joint, including the ACaL; the ITCL and IER layers; and the posterior capsule of the talocalcaneonavicular joint, including the CL.

Fact Box 3 Lateral Ligamentous Structures of the Subtalar Joint

1. superficial layer:
   - lateral root of the inferior retinaculum
   - lateral talocalcaneal ligament
   - calcaneofibular ligament
2. intermediate layer:
   - intermediate root of the retinaculum
   - cervical ligament
3. deep layer:
   - anterior capsular ligament
   - medial root of the retinaculum
   - interosseus talocalcaneal ligament.

1.4.2 The Interosseous Talocalcaneal Ligament

The interosseous talocalcaneal ligament, or ligament of the tarsal canal, is medially located in the tarsal canal. The ITCL blends with the fibers of the medial root of the inferior extensor retinaculum at the origin of the calcaneus, which forms a V-shape. The ITCL has a length of 10 mm and a width of 8.5 mm.

We can distinguish three types according to its shape: the band type, the fan type, and a multiple type [51].

- The **band type** is the most common one. It is a flat, thick, band-like ligament.
- The **fan type** originates from a broad area of the tarsal canal and runs obliquely towards the calcaneus. It decreases in width and inserts on the tarsal canal of the calcaneus.
- The **multiple type** consists of three distinct bands and is rather uncommon.

Historically, the ITCL has been described as a stabilizer of the subtalar joint. However, more recent studies question the importance of this ligament [50, 52].

1.4.3 The Anterior Capsular Ligament

The anterior capsular ligament (ACaL) is a flat and thin ligament defined as the thickened segment of the anterior aspect of the joint capsule of the posterior talocalcaneal facet [51, 53, 54]. Jotoku et al. found the ACaL in 95% of the examined feet (38/40) [51]. The ACaL originates at the anterior border of the posterior facet of the talus and runs vertically across the subtalar joint before attaching to the calcaneus. The ITCL and the ACaL are two distinct structures (Fig. 1.15) [50, 51, 53, 54]. The ACaL has a length of 8.3 mm, a width of 8.3 mm, and a thickness of 1.4 mm [51]. This ligament plays a major role in subtalar stability in all positions [50, 54, 55] and ACaL injuries have been related to subtalar instability [56, 57].

1.4.4 The Cervical Ligament

The cervical ligament (CL)(or external talocalcaneal ligament, anterolateral talocalcaneal ligament) is the strongest ligament connecting the talus to the calcaneus. This ligament is located in the sinus tarsi. It originates from the anterior tubercle on the calcaneus and runs anteriorly and medially to the inferior aspect of the talar neck (Figs. 1.15 and 1.16).

The CL is a broad bundle of fibers with a length between 8.3 and 20 mm, a width of

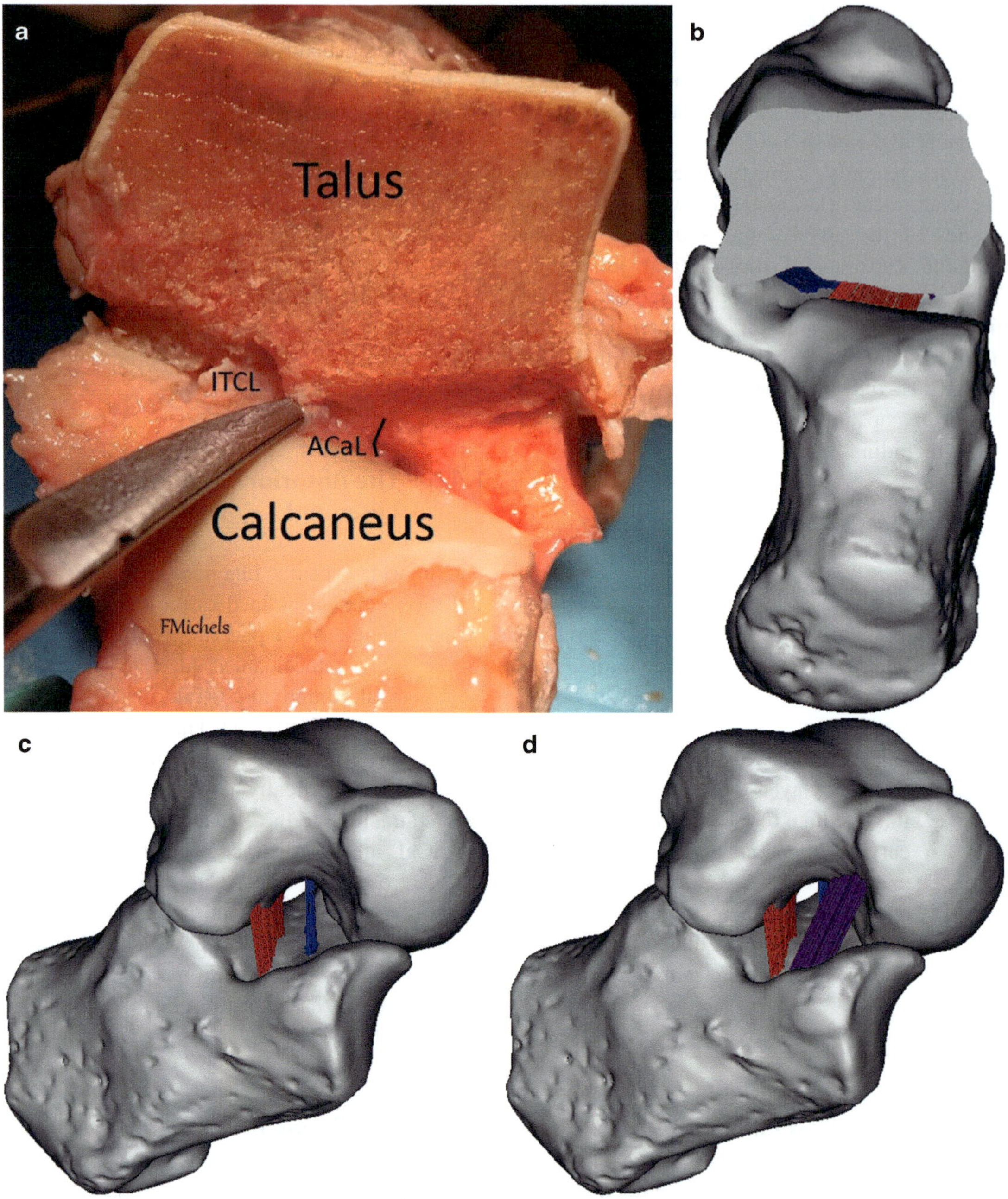

Fig. 1.15 View of the ACaL and ITCL. (a) Cadaveric specimen with osteotomized talus. Scissors behind anterior capsular ligament and in front of ITCL. (b) 3D image with a similar view. (c) 3D image with sinus tarsi view. (d) 3D image with sinus tarsi view and CL. ACaL (red), ITCL (blue), CL (purple)

11.6 mm, and a thickness of 2.8 mm [58, 59]. In a recent study of Li, the CL consisted usually of multiple bands in the same plane or inferiorly to the main bunch [52].

Clanton described footprint center distances [60]. On average, its attachment site on the calcaneus was 23.4 mm anterior to the articular surface of the calcaneus, 9.0 mm posterior to the

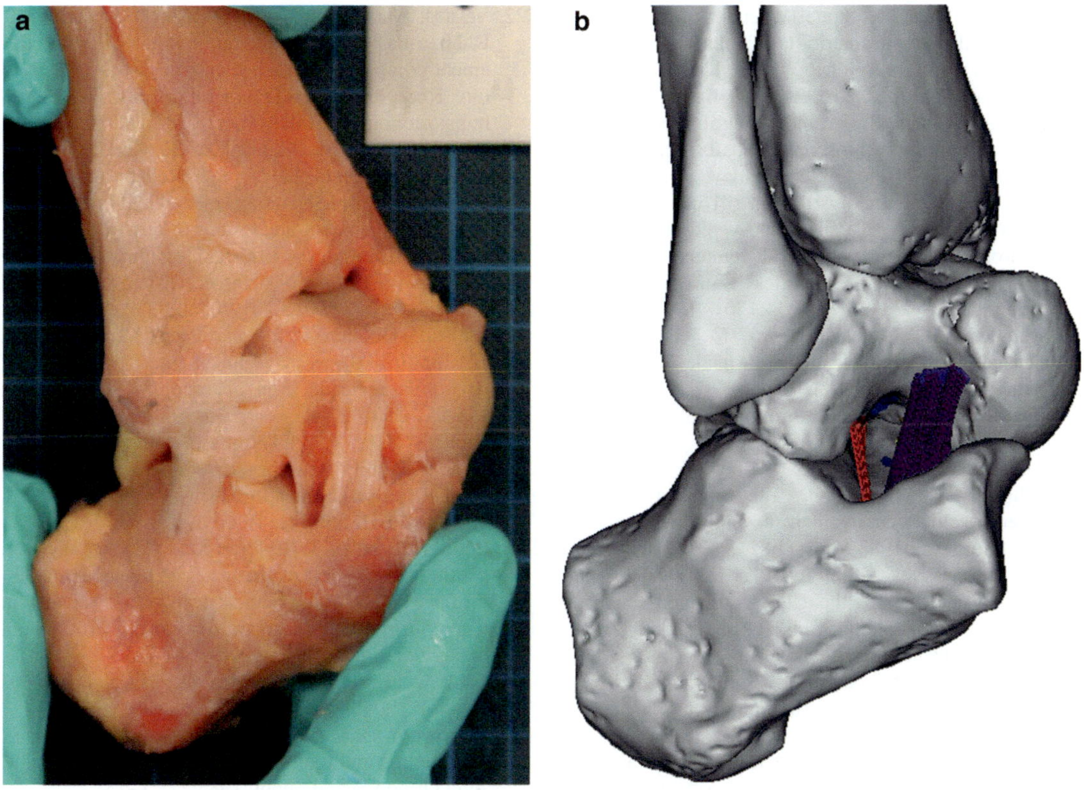

Fig. 1.16 Cadaveric specimen and 3D image with the cervical ligament (purple) and anterior capsular ligament (red)

calcaneocuboid joint line along the calcaneal lateral ridge of the sinus tarsi, and 7.2 mm perpendicular to the calcaneal lateral ridge of the sinus tarsi. Its talar attachment site was an average of 8.0 mm anterior to the proximal point of the talar neck adjacent to the anterior border of the trochlea, 7.0 mm posterior to the distal point of the talar neck at the talonavicular joint line, and 12.8 mm perpendicular to the line connecting the proximal and distal points of the talar neck [60]. The long axis of the ligament makes an angle of 45°–50° with the long axis of the calcaneus in the sagittal plane and nearly parallels the average direction of the CFL. In valgus, the cervical ligament is more horizontal. In varus, the CL is more vertical. The CL probably plays a major role in subtalar stability [54, 55, 61].

Acknowledgments We thank Dr. Diego A. Quintero from the Department of Applied Anatomy, Faculty of Medical Sciences, National University of Rosario (FCM UNR), Argentina for the contribution to some of the images of the lateral ligaments.

References

1. Golanó P, Vega J, de Leeuw P, et al. Anatomy of the ankle ligaments: a pictorial essay. Knee Surg Sports Traumatol Arthrosc. 2010;18(5):557–69.
2. Guillo S, Archbold P, Perera A, et al. Arthroscopic anatomic reconstruction of the lateral ligaments of the ankle with gracilis autograft. Arthrosc Tech. 2014;3:e593–8.
3. Michels F, Cordier G, Burssens A, et al. Endoscopic reconstruction of CFL and the ATFL with a gracilis graft: a cadaveric study. Knee Surg Sports Traumatol Arthrosc. 2016;24:1007–14.

4. Takao M, Matsui K, Stone JW, et al. Ankle instability group arthroscopic anterior talofibular ligament repair for lateral instability of the ankle. Knee Surg Sports Traumatol Arthrosc. 2016;24:1003–6.
5. Thès A, Klouche S, Ferrand M, et al. Assessment of the feasibility of arthroscopic visualization of the lateral ligament of the ankle: a cadaveric study. Knee Surg Sports Traumatol Arthrosc. 2016;24:985–99.
6. Vega J, Golanó P, Pellegrino A, et al. All-inside arthroscopic lateral collateral ligament repair for ankle instability with a knotless suture anchor technique. Foot Ankle Int. 2013;34:1701–9.
7. Rouviere H, Canela Lazaro M. Le ligament Peroneo-Astragalo-Calcaneen. Annales d'anatomie pathologique. 1932;7(IX):745–50.
8. Testut L. Tratado de anatomía humana. Barcelona: Salvat Editores S.A.; 1987. p. 704–19. [in Spanish].
9. Johnson EE, Markolf KL. The contribution of the anterior talofibular ligament to ankle laxity. J Bone Joint Surg Am. 1983;65-A(1):81–8.
10. Shibata Y, Nishi G, Masegi A, et al. Stress test and anatomical study of the lateral collateral ligaments of the ankle. Nihon Seikeigeka Gakkai Zasshi. 1986;60(6):611–22. [in Japanese].
11. Broström L. Sprained ankles V. treatment and prognosis in recent ligament ruptures. Acta Chir Scand. 1966;132:537–50.
12. Colville MR, Marder RA, Boyle JJ, et al. Strain measurement in lateral ankle ligaments. Am J Sports Med. 1990;18:196–200.
13. Kannus P, Renstrom P. Treatment for acute tears of the lateral ligaments of the ankle. Operation, cast, or early controlled mobilization. J Bone Joint Surg Am. 1991;73:305–12.
14. Renstrom P, Wertz M, Incavo S, et al. Strain in the lateral ligaments of the ankle. Foot Ankle. 1988;9(2):59–63.
15. Van Den Bekerom MPJ, Oostra RJ, Golano P et al. (2008) The anatomy in relation to injury of the lateral collateral ligaments of the ankle: a current concepts review. Clin Anat 21:619–626.
16. Burks RT, Morgan J. Anatomy of the lateral ankle ligaments. Am J Sports Med. 1994;22:72–7.
17. Golanó P, Dalmau-Pastor M, Vega J, et al. Anatomy of the ankle. In: d'Hooghe P, Kerkhoffs G, editors. The ankle in football. France: Springer; 2014. p. 1–24.
18. Golano P, Mariani PP, Rodriguez-Niedenfuhr M, et al. Arthroscopic anatomy of the posterior ankle ligaments. Arthroscopy. 2002;18:353–8.
19. Golanó P, Vega J, de Leeuw P, et al. Anatomy of the ankle ligaments: a pictorial essay. Knee Surg Sports Traumatol Arthrosc. 2016;24(4):944–56.
20. Golanó P, Vega J, Pérez-Carro L, et al. Ankle anatomy for the arthroscopist. Part I: the portals. Foot Ankle Clin. 2006;11(2):275–96.
21. Sarrafian SK. Anatomy of the foot and ankle. descriptive, topographic, functional. 2nd ed. Philadelphia: J.B. Lippincott; 1993. p. 159–217.
22. Vega J, Malagelada F, Manzanares Céspedes MC, Dalmau-Pastor M. The lateral fibulotalocalcaneal ligament complex: an ankle stabilizing isometric structure. Knee Surg Sports Traumatol Arthrosc. 2018;28:8. https://doi.org/10.1007/s00167-018-5188-8.
23. Dalmau-Pastor M, Malagelada F, Kerkhoffs GM, Karlsson J, Guelfi M, Vega J. Redefining anterior ankle arthroscopic anatomy: medial and lateral ankle collateral ligaments are visible through dorsiflexion and non-distraction anterior ankle arthroscopy. Knee Surg Sports Traumatol Arthrosc. 2019;28:18. https://doi.org/10.1007/s00167-019-05603-2.
24. Batista J, Quintero D, Dalmau-Pastor M. Artroscopia de tobillo. Bases y Fundamentos. Capítulo 3: Anatomía aplicada a la artroscopía; 2017. ISBN: 978-987-3979-22-4.
25. Guillo S, Bauer T, Lee JW, et al. Consensus in chronic ankle instability: aetiology, assessment, surgical indications and place for arthroscopy. Orthop Traumatol Surg Res. 2013;99:S411–9.
26. Lopes R, Noailles T, Brulefert K, et al. Anatomic validation of the lateral malleolus as a cutaneous marker for the distal insertion of the calcaneofibular ligament. Knee Surg Sports Traumatol Arthrosc. 2016;26:869. https://doi.org/10.1007/s00167-016-4250-7.
27. Laidlaw PL. The varieties of the os calcis. J Anat Physiol. 1904;38:133–43.
28. Rasmussen O. Stability of the ankle joint analysis of the function and traumatology of the ankle ligaments. Acta Orthop Scand Suppl. 1985;211:1–75.
29. Ruth CJ. The surgical treatment of injuries of the fibular collateral ligaments of the ankle. J Bone Joint Surg Am. 1961;43-A:229–39.
30. Trouilloud P, Dia A, Grammont P, et al. Variations in the calcaneo-fibular ligament (lig. Calcaneofibulare). Application to the kinematics of the ankle. Bull Assoc des Anat. 1988;72:31–5.
31. Savage-Elliott I, Murawski CD. The deltoid ligament: an in-depth review of anatomy, function, and treatment strategies. Knee Surg Sports Traumatol Arthrosc. 2013;21:1316–27.
32. Yammine K. The morphology and prevalence of the deltoid complex ligament of the ankle. Foot Ankle Spec. 2017;10:55–62.
33. Boss AP, Hintermann B. Anatomical study of the medial ankle ligament complex. Foot Ankle Int. 2002;23:547–53.
34. Campbell KJ, Michalski MP. The ligament anatomy of the deltoid complex of the ankle: a qualitative and quantitative anatomical study. J Bone Joint Surg Am. 2014;96(8):e62.
35. Milner CE, Soames RW. Anatomy of the collateral ligaments of the human ankle joint. Foot Ankle Int. 1998;19:757–60.
36. Hintermann B, Knupp M. Deltoid ligament injuries: diagnosis and management. Foot Ankle Clin. 2006;11:625–37.
37. Harper MC. The lateral ligamentous support of the subtalar joint. Foot Ankle. 1991;11(6):354–8.

38. Michelson JD, Hamel AJ, Buczek FL, et al. The effect of ankle injury on subtalar motion. Foot Ankle Int. 2004;25(9):639–46.
39. Hintermann B, Sommer C. Influence of ligament transection on tibial and calcaneal rotation with loading and dorsi-plantarflexion. Foot Ankle Int. 1995;16:567–71.
40. Xu C, Zhang MY. Biomechanical evaluation of tenodesis reconstruction in ankle with deltoid ligament deficiency: a finite element analysis. Knee Surg Sports Traumatol Arthrosc. 2012;20:1854–62.
41. Crim JR, Beals TC. Deltoid ligament abnormalities in chronic lateral ankle instability. Foot Ankle Int. 2011;32:873–8.
42. Hintermann B, Valderrabano V. Medial ankle instability: an exploratory, prospective study of fifty-two cases. Am J Sports Med. 2004;32:183–90.
43. Schäfer D, Hintermann B. Arthroscopic assessment of the chronic unstable ankle joint. Knee Surg Sports Traumatol Arthrosc. 1996;4:48–52.
44. Hopkinson W, Pierre PS, Ryan J, et al. Syndesmosis sprains of the ankle. Foot Ankle. 1990;10:325–30.
45. Ogilvie-Harris DJ, Reed SC, Hedman TP. Disruption of the ankle syndesmosis: biomechanical study of the ligamentous restraints. Arthroscopy. 1994;10:558–60.
46. Beumer A, Hemert WV, Swierstra B, et al. A biomechanical evaluation of the tibiofibular and tibiotalar ligaments of the ankle. Foot Ankle Int. 2003;24:426–9.
47. Nikolopoulos CE. Anterolateral instability of the ankle joint. An anatomical, experimental and clinical study. Thesis, University of Athens, Athens, Greece; 1982.
48. Bassett FH, Gates HS, Billys JB, et al. Talar impingement by the anteroinferior tibiofibular ligament. A cause of chronic pain in the ankle after inversion sprain. J Bone Joint Surg Am. 1990;72(1):55–9.
49. Lee SH, Jacobson J, Trudell D, et al. Ligaments of the ankle: normal anatomy with MR arthrography. J Comput Assist Tomogr. 1998;22:807–13.
50. Yamaguchi R, Nimura A, Amaha K, Yamaguchi K, Segawa Y, Okawa A, et al. Anatomy of the Tarsal Canal and sinus in relation to the subtalar joint capsule. Foot Ankle Int. 2018;27:1071100718788038. https://doi.org/10.1177/1071100718788038.
51. Jotoku T, Kinoshita M, Okuda R, et al. Anatomy of ligamentous structures in the tarsal sinus and canal. Foot Ankle Int. 2006;27(7):533–8.
52. Li SY, Hou ZD, Zhang P, et al. Ligament structures in the tarsal sinus and canal. Foot Ankle Int. 2013;34(12):1729–36.
53. Kelian A. Sarafian's anatomy of the foot and ankle: descriptive topographical, functional. 3rd ed. Philadelphia: Lippincott Williams & Wilkins; 2011. p. 163–222.
54. Stephens MM, Sammarco GJ. The stabilizing role of the lateral ligament complex around the ankle and subtalar joints. Foot Ankle. 1992;13(3):130–6.
55. Michels F, Clockaerts S, Van Der Bauwhede J, Stockmans F, Matricali G. Does subtalar instability really exist? A systematic review. J Foot Ankle Surg. 2019;26:119. https://doi.org/10.1016/j.fas.2019.02.001.
56. Kim TH, Moon SG, Jung HG, Kim NR. Subtalar instability: imaging features of subtalar ligaments on 3D isotropic ankle MRI. BMC Musculoskelet Disord. 2017;18(1):475. https://doi.org/10.1186/s12891-017-1841-5.
57. Yoon DY, Moon SG, Jung HG, Kim NR. Differences between subtalar instability and lateral ankle instability focusing on subtalar ligaments based on three dimensional isotropic magnetic resonance imaging. J Comput Assist Tomogr. 2018;42:566. https://doi.org/10.1097/RCT.0000000000000717.
58. Cahill DR. The anatomy and function of the contents of the human tarsal sinus and canal. Anat Rec. 1965;153:1–18.
59. Poonja AJ, Hirano M, Khakimov D, Ojumah N, Tubbs RS, Loukas M, et al. Anatomical study of the cervical and interosseous talocalcaneal ligaments of the foot with surgical relevance. Cureus. 2017;9(6):e1382. https://doi.org/10.7759/cureus.1382.
60. Clanton TO, Campbell KJ, Wilson, et al. Qualitative and quantitative anatomic investigation of the lateral ankle ligaments for surgical reconstruction procedures. J Bone Joint Surg Am. 2014;96(12):e98.
61. Michels F, Matricali G, Vereecke E, et al. The intrinsic subtalar ligaments have a consistent presence, location and morphology. Foot Ankle Surg. 2020;6:S1268–7731(20)30040-0. https://doi.org/10.1016/j.fas.2020.03.002.

2 Anatomic Perspective on the Role of Inferior Extensor Retinaculum in Lateral Ankle Ligament Reconstruction

M. Dalmau-Pastor, G. M. M. J. Kerkhoffs, J. G. Kennedy, Jón Karlsson, F. Michels, and J. Vega

2.1 Introduction

The extensor retinaculum is an aponeurotic structure that reinforces the anterior crural fascia at the level of the distal leg, ankle, and tarsus. It is commonly divided into the superior extensor retinaculum and inferior extensor retinaculum, and both structures are continuous with the anterior fascia of the leg. As any retinacula, its main function is to maintain tendons in their right position and prevent them from bowstringing or subluxation. In this case, it acts on the tendons of the anterior compartment of the leg (from medial to lateral: tibialis anterior, extensor hallucis longus, extensor digitorum longus, and peroneus tertius). The superior extensor retinaculum is found at the distal part of the leg as a transverse aponeurotic band, but it does not carry a significant clinical interest.

The inferior extensor retinaculum (IER) is located on the anterior aspect of the ankle and tarsus [1]. The proximity of the IER to the anterior talofibular ligament (ATFL) induced the description of a technique in which it was used to

M. Dalmau-Pastor (✉)
Human Anatomy Unit, Department of Pathology and Experimental Therapeutics, School of Medicine, University of Barcelona, Barcelona, Spain

GRECMIP—MIFAS (Groupe de Recherche et d'Etude en Chirurgie Mini-Invasive du Pied—Minimally Invasive Foot and Ankle Society), Merignac, France
e-mail: mikeldalmau@ub.edu

G. M. M. J. Kerkhoffs
Department of Orthopedic Surgery, Academic Medical Center, University of Amsterdam, Amsterdam, The Netherlands

Academic Center for Evidence Based Sports Medicine (ACES), Amsterdam, The Netherlands

Amsterdam Collaboration for Health and Safety in Sports (ACHSS), AMC/VUmc IOC Research Center, Amsterdam, The Netherlands

J. G. Kennedy
Department of Orthopedic surgery, Division Foot and Ankle Surgery, New York University, New York, USA
e-mail: john.kennedy@nyulangone.org

J. Karlsson
GRECMIP—MIFAS (Groupe de Recherche et d'Etude en Chirurgie Mini-Invasive du Pied—Minimally Invasive Foot and Ankle Society), Merignac, France

Department of Orthopaedics, Sahlgrenska University Hospital, Sahlgrenska Academy, Gothenburg University, Gothenburg, Sweden
e-mail: jon.karlsson@telia.com

F. Michels
Orthopaedic Department, AZ Groeninge, Kortrijk, Belgium

J. Vega
GRECMIP—MIFAS (Groupe de Recherche et d'Etude en Chirurgie Mini-Invasive du Pied—Minimally Invasive Foot and Ankle Society), Merignac, France

Foot and Ankle Unit, iMove MiTres Torres, Barcelona, Spain

H. Pereira et al. (eds.), *Lateral Ankle Instability*, https://doi.org/10.1007/978-3-662-62763-1_2

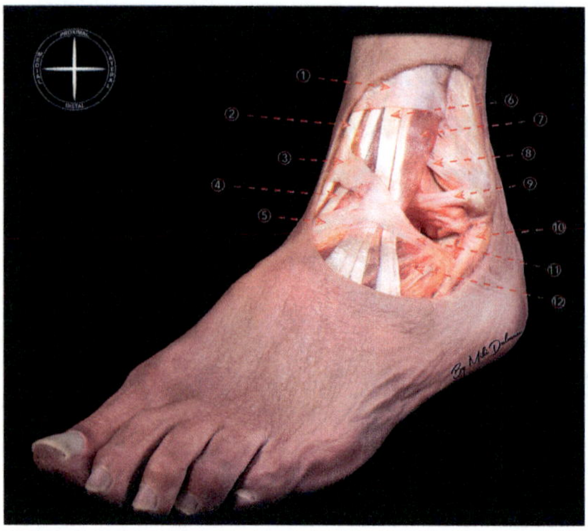

Fig. 2.1 Anterolateral view of a dissection of a left ankle showing the morphology of the inferior extensor retinaculum and its relation with the anterior talofibular ligament. (1) Superior extensor retinaculum. (2) Tibialis anterior tendon. (3) Oblique superomedial band of the inferior extensor retinaculum. (4) Extensor hallucis longus tendon. (5) Oblique inferomedial band of the inferior extensor retinaculum. (6) Extensor digitorum longus tendon. (7) Peroneus tertius muscle. (8) Distal fascicle of the anterior tibiofibular ligament (partially covered by peroneus tertius muscle). (9) Anterior talofibular ligament. (10) Peroneus brevis tendon. (11) Stem or frondiform ligament (lateral part of the inferior extensor retinaculum). (12) Extensor digitorum brevis muscle. (Figure reproduced with permission from Dalmau-Pastor, M., Yasui, Y., Calder, J.D., Karlsson, J. Anatomy of the inferior extensor retinaculum and its role in lateral ankle ligament reconstruction: a pictorial essay. Knee Surgery, Sport Traumatol Arthrosc. 1–6, https://doi.org/10.1007/s00167-016-4082-5 (2016)

reinforce a repair of that ligament [2] (Fig. 2.1). Since its original description in 1980, the Bröstrom-Gould technique has been widely used for the treatment of chronic ankle instability [3–9]. However, it is usually not specified in the literature which band of the IER is used during this procedure [2, 3, 7–9], and some references just mention that its "lateral aspect" is used to reinforce the ATFL repair/reconstruction [4–6].

2.2 Anatomic Details

Descriptions of the IER both as Y-shaped [10–12] and X-shaped structure [13–17] exist in the scientific literature. When presented as a Y-shaped structure it is reported to be formed by the stem ligament, oblique superomedial, and oblique inferomedial bands. On the other hand, when it is presented as an X-shaped structure, it is reported as a variable structure, due to the presence of an additional and nonconstant oblique superolateral band.

The anatomy of the three constant parts of the IER is well known [1]:

- Stem ligament; is the lateral part of the IER, which maintains the tendons of peroneus tertius and extensor digitorum longus against talus and calcaneus. It has its origin in the sinus tarsi through three roots, one lateral, one intermediary, and one medial [1, 18]. Approximately at the level of the talar neck, the three roots forming the stem ligament are continued by the two medial bands of the IER.
- Oblique superomedial band; this band, continuing in the direction of the stem ligament, directs towards the medial malleolus, where it inserts. It passes over the tendon of the extensor hallucis longus, but under the tibialis anterior tendon. This explains why the tibialis anterior tendon is the most prominent tendon on the anterior aspect of the ankle when its muscle contracts, as it has no fixation.
- Oblique inferomedial band; this band arises from the stem ligament and is directed inferomedially towards the medial side of the foot. During its course, its fibers pass over the extensor hallucis longus tendon and the anterior neurovascular bundle (deep peroneal nerve, dorsalis pedis artery, and accompanying vessels). When arriving at the tibialis anterior tendon, its fibers are divide into a superficial (passing over the tendon) and a deep component (passing under the tendon). This creates a partial fixation of anterior tibialis tendon. The superficial fibers continue medially and contribute to the formation of the abductor hallucis muscle fascia, while the deep fibers insert on the navicular and medial cuneiform bones.

These three components (stem ligament, oblique superomedial, and oblique inferomedial bands) contribute to the IER a Y-shaped morphology (Fig. 1 (2016 paper)). However, in a percentage that varies between 25% and 81% [1, 13, 14, 16, 17] an additional band is present: the oblique superolateral band. This band arises from the stem ligament and, directing proximally and laterally, becomes continuous with those of the peroneal retinacula. In the cases where this band is present, the IER has an X-shaped morphology (Figs. 2.2 and 2.3) [17].

2.3 Clinical Implications

As explained before, in studies describing the use of the IER as reinforcement of an ATFL repair, it is not specified which part of it is used [2–9]. It is possible that due to the limited visibility in the surgical field and the fact that fascial and aponeurotic structures can be easily confused even during anatomical dissection, the real use of IER as reinforcement of an ATFL repair can be questioned, as it could be possible that the fascia is used as reinforcement, and not true IER tissue. In fact, Jeong et al. performed a study [19] to ascertain the feasibility of performing a Broström-Gould reconstruction in cadaveric ankle specimens. They found that in 24% of the ankles, reinforcement using IER was not possible due to anatomical variations. In addition, clinical and radiological outcomes were compared between those cases where IER reinforcement was possible and those where it was not, and no differences were found. According to the authors, those findings suggested that a simple ATFL repair without IER reinforcement can be sufficient to restore ankle laxity.

Another study compared the biomechanical restoration of ankle laxity of a simple Broström with a Broström-Gould reconstruction in cadaveric ankle specimens [20]. Their conclusion was that the inclusion of IER reinforcement had no additional effect on the restoration of ankle laxity.

A study comparing ligament reconstruction with and without IER reinforcements in real patients was published by Karlsson et al. [5]. No statistical significance in ankle stability was found between the two groups of patients, and it was concluded that both methods were equally good in restoring ankle laxity. However, an interesting point was found in this publication when stating that intraoperative nerve injuries were more common in the IER reinforcement group.

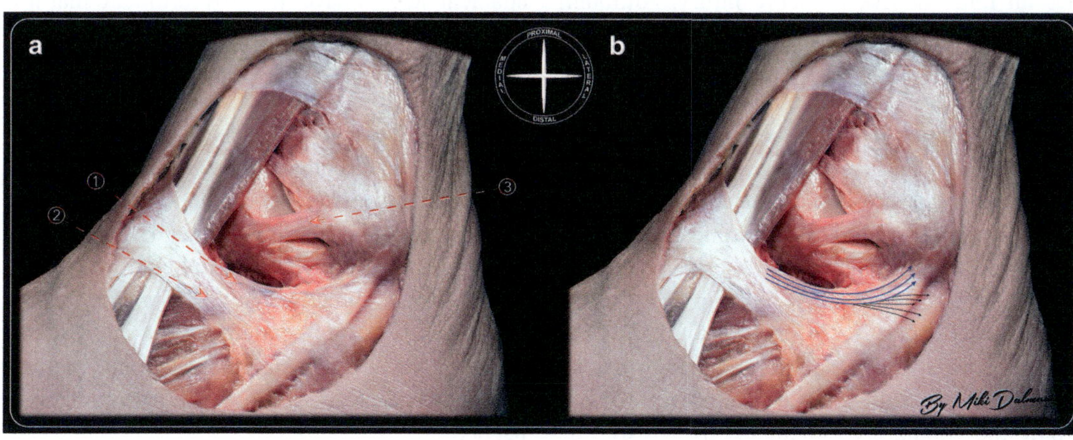

Fig. 2.2 Anterolateral view of a dissected ankle showing an inferior extensor retinaculum with an oblique superolateral band. (**a**) (1) Oblique superolateral band. (2) Stem of frondiform ligament. (3) Anterior talofibular ligament. (**b**) Oblique superolateral band has been highlighted. Its fibers are directed towards the anterior part of the lateral malleolus (blue arrows), and some of its fibers are continuous with the superior peroneal retinaculum (black arrows). (Figure reproduced with permission from Dalmau-Pastor, M., Malagelada, F., Kerkhoffs, G.M.M.J., Manzanares, M.C., Vega, J. X-shaped inferior extensor retinaculum and its doubtful use in the Bröstrom–Gould procedure. Knee Surgery, Sport Traumatol Arthrosc. 1–6, https://doi.org/10.1007/s00167-017-4647-y (2017)

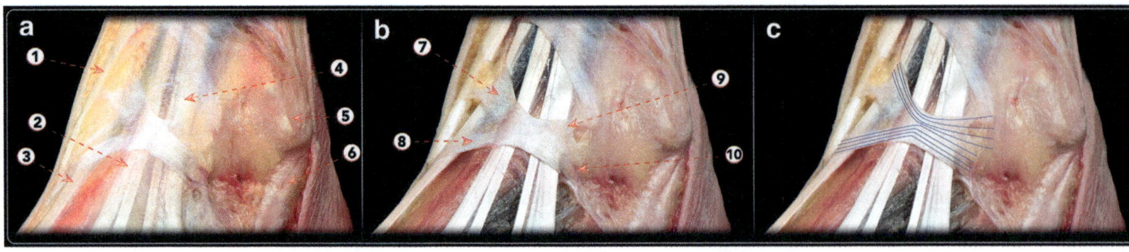

Fig. 2.3 Anatomic dissection of the anterior area of the ankle. (**a**) Crural fascia continuous with inferior extensor retinaculum. (**b**) Crural fascia has been removed and X-shaped inferior extensor retinaculum is shown. (**c**) X-shaped inferior extensor retinaculum is highlighted. (1) Tibialis anterior tendon. (2) Extensor digitorum longus tendons. (3) Extensor hallucis longus tendon. (4) Peroneus tertius tendon. (5) Fibular malleolus. (6) Peroneal tendons. (7) Oblique superomedial band of the inferior extensor retinaculum. (8) Oblique inferomedial band of the inferior extensor retinaculum. (9) Oblique superolateral band of the inferior extensor retinaculum. (10) Stem or frondiform ligament of the inferior extensor retinaculum. (Figure reproduced with permission from Dalmau-Pastor, M., Malagelada, F., Kerkhoffs, G.M.M.J., Manzanares, M.C., Vega, J. X-shaped inferior extensor retinaculum and its doubtful use in the Bröstrom–Gould procedure. Knee Surgery, Sport Traumatol Arthrosc. 1–6, https://doi.org/10.1007/s00167-017-4647-y (2017)

In previous anatomical studies [16, 17] the relationship between the IER and the superficial peroneal and sural nerve was assessed. It was found that the intermediate dorsal cutaneous nerve (branch of the superficial peroneal nerve) crosses the stem ligament and the oblique superolateral band (when present) in every case (Fig. 2.3). Consequently, when reinforcement for an ATFL repair has to be made using the IER, the intermediate dorsal cutaneous nerve has to be dissected off the IER. This surgical approach carries an inherent risk of nerve injury. Although some Broström-Gould case series do not, surprisingly, report any kind of nerve-related complications [3, 4, 6, 7, 9, 21, 22], other series report it as a frequent complication, ranging from 4.54% [23] to 13.3% [5].

Recently, arthroscopic-assisted techniques have been developed to treat chronic ankle instability. Some of the techniques describe a percutaneous step to grasp the IER in order to reinforce the ligament repair [8, 24, 25]. In a related anatomical study [26], the authors conclude that in neutral ankle dorsiflexion, a distance of 15 mm from the fibula is adequate to grasp the IER. However, in 10% of the cases no IER was grasped, and when grasped percutaneously, only 7 ± 3 mm of the IER was obtained. The researchers assert that this variability was due to anatomic variability of the IER as well as small variations in the technique.

In addition, anatomical studies about the IER and specifically about the oblique superolateral band state that this band is very weak, and put in doubt that a reinforcement using this band could provide additional ankle stability [16, 17].

It could be argued that if a high index of failure of ATFL repairs was observed in the literature, reinforcement is necessary. In that case, an augmentation using the IER could have the benefits of being a biological augmentation, in contrast with artificial augmentations. However, biomechanical studies have not proved to date that it is beneficial to use the IER as reinforcement.

Another possible issue that could support the use of the IER as reinforcement is that of subtalar instability. Because of its insertions on the calcaneus, IER reinforcement of an ATFL repair would hypothetically restore ankle and subtalar laxity. In that case, the slightly higher risk of nerve-related complications would not be important, as an additional joint is treated. However, before this can be recommended additional research proving that IER reinforcement produces significant differences in ankle or subtalar stability is needed.

Take-Home Message

There is relevant anatomic variation in IER and it is composed of at least three constant parts.

Given the limited visibility during surgical procedures, it is not easy to be sure which structures are being used when augmentation of anterolateral instability repair is intended by means of using the IER.

One should keep in mind that the use of IER has an inherent risk of nerve injury.

The oblique superolateral band has poor biomechanical properties.

Despite its widespread use and published favorable outcomes of several series, there is no biomechanical evidence, so far, proving the advantage of using the IER as reinforcement.

Fact Box 1 Key Messages About Inferior Extensor Retinaculum (IER)

- There is frequent anatomic variation
- It has been described as either Y-shaped or X-shaped structure
- Limitations in visualization during surgeries make it difficult to identify and not always reliable to know which structure is being used for augmentation of ankle anterolateral ligaments' repair
- Some risk of nerve lesion should be taken into account when using IER
- IER might play a role in ankle anterolateral instability; however, there is no evidence-based support from biomechanical studies
- IER might play a role in addressing subtalar instability

References

1. Sarrafian SK. Anatomy of the foot and ankle. Descriptive, topographic, functional. Philadelphia: J.B. Lippincott Co; 1983.
2. Gould N, Seligson D, Gassman J. Early and late repair of lateral ligament of the ankle. Foot Ankle. 1980;1(2):84–9.
3. Brodsky AR, O'Malley MJ, Bohne WH, Deland JA, Kennedy JG. An analysis of outcome measures following the Broström-Gould procedure for chronic lateral ankle instability. Foot Ankle Int. 2005;26(10):816–9.
4. Hamilton WG, Thompson FM, Snow SW. The modified Brostrom procedure for lateral ankle instability. Foot Ankle. 1993;14(1):1–7. https://doi.org/10.1177/107110079301400101.
5. Karlsson J, Eriksson BI, Bergsten T, Rudholm O, Sward L. Comparison of two anatomic reconstructions for chronic lateral instability of the ankle joint. Am J Sports Med. 1997;25(1):48–53. https://doi.org/10.1177/036354659702500109.
6. Keller M, Grossman J, Caron M, Mendicino RW. Lateral ankle instability and the Brostrom-Gould procedure. J Foot Ankle Surg. 1996;35(6):513–20. https://doi.org/10.1016/S1067-2516(96)80123-2.
7. Molloy AP, Ajis A, Kazi H. The modified Broström-Gould procedure—early results using a newly described surgical technique. Foot Ankle Surg. 2014;20(3):224–8. https://doi.org/10.1016/j.fas.2014.01.002.
8. Nery C, Raduan F, Del Buono A, Asaumi ID, Cohen M, Maffulli N. Arthroscopic-assisted Brostrom-Gould for chronic ankle instability: a long-term follow-up. Am J Sports Med. 2011;39(11):2381–8. https://doi.org/10.1177/0363546511416069.
9. Ng ZD, Das De S. Modified Brostrom-Evans-Gould technique for recurrent lateral ankle ligament instability. J Orthop Surg (Hong Kong). 2007;15(3):306–10, at <http://www.ncbi.nlm.nih.gov/pubmed/18162676>.
10. Rouviere H, Delmas A. Anatomía humana. Barcelona: Masson; 2002.
11. Testut L, Latarjet A. Anatomía humana. Barcelona: Salvat Editores; 1981.
12. Williams P, Warwick R. Gray anatomía. Madrid: Churchill Livingstone/Elsevier; 1992.
13. Abu-hijleh MF, Harris PF. Deep fascia on the dorsum of the ankle and foot: extensor retinacula revisited. Clin Anat. 2007;20(2):186–95. https://doi.org/10.1002/ca.20298.
14. Meyer P. La morphologie du ligament annulaire anterieur du cou-de-pied chez l'homme. Comptes-Rendus Assoc Anat. 1955;84:286.
15. Wood Jones F. Structure and function as seen in the foot. London: Baillière, Tindall and Cox; 1949.
16. Dalmau-Pastor M, Yasui Y, Calder JD, Karlsson J. Anatomy of the inferior extensor retinaculum and its role in lateral ankle ligament reconstruction: a pictorial essay. Knee Surg Sports Traumatol Arthrosc. 2016;24:957–62. https://doi.org/10.1007/s00167-016-4082-5.
17. Dalmau-Pastor M, Malagelada F, Kerkhoffs GMMJ, Manzanares MC, Vega J. X-shaped inferior extensor retinaculum and its doubtful use in the Bröstrom–Gould procedure. Knee Surg Sports Traumatol Arthrosc. 2017;26:2171–6. https://doi.org/10.1007/s00167-017-4647-y.
18. Li S-Y, Hou Z-D, Zhang P, Li H-L, Ding Z-H, Liu Y-J. Ligament structures in the tarsal sinus and canal. Foot Ankle Int. 2013;34(12):1729–36. https://doi.org/10.1177/1071100713500653.
19. Jeong BO, Kim MS, Song WJ, Soohoo NF. Feasibility and outcome of inferior extensor retinaculum reinforcement in modified Broström procedures. Foot Ankle Int. 2016;35:1137–42. https://doi.org/10.1177/1071100714543645.

20. Behrens SB, et al. Biomechanical analysis of brostrom versus Brostrom-Gould lateral ankle instability repairs. Foot Ankle Int. 2013;34(4):587–92. https://doi.org/10.1177/1071100713477622.
21. Aydogan U, Glisson RR, Nunley JA. Extensor retinaculum augmentation reinforces anterior talofibular ligament repair. Clin Orthop Relat Res. 2006;442:210–5. https://doi.org/10.1097/01.blo.0000183737.43245.26.
22. Bell SJ, Mologne TS, Sitler DF, Cox JS. Twenty-six-year results after Broström procedure for chronic lateral ankle instability. Am J Sports Med. 2006;34(6):975–8. https://doi.org/10.1177/0363546505282616.
23. Messer TM, Cummins CA, Ahn J, Kelikian AS. Outcome of the modified Brostrom procedure for chronic lateral ankle instability using suture anchors. Foot Ankle Int. 2000;21(12):996–1003.
24. Corte-Real NM, Moreira RM. Arthroscopic repair of chronic lateral ankle instability. Foot Ankle Int. 2009;30(3):213–7. https://doi.org/10.3113/FAI.2009.0213.
25. Acevedo J, Mangone P. Arthroscopic brostrom technique. Foot Ankle Int. 2015;36(4):465–73. https://doi.org/10.1177/1071100715576107.
26. Acevedo J, Ortiz C, Golano P. Arthrobrostrom lateral ankle stabilization technique: an anatomical study. Arthrosc J Arthrosc Relat Surg. 2014;30(6):e28. https://doi.org/10.1016/j.arthro.2014.04.062.

Biomechanics of the Ankle

3

Kenneth J. Hunt, Todd Baldin, Pieter D'Hooghe, and Hélder Pereira

3.1 Introduction

The biomechanical behavior of the ankle joint is not one of simple dorsiflexion and plantarflexion movement within one degree of freedom. The mechanical role of the ankle in gait is to transfer all forces occurring during gait, including body weight and directional forces, to the entire foot and to distribute a system of vertical stresses to a horizontally moving system that can rapidly change directions. There is a clear interdependence between the ankle joint and the subtalar joint [1], with the subtalar joint having a preferential rotation mobility allowing the foot to adapt to the ground. This chapter explores basic ankle biomechanics as it relates to ankle instability conditions, including gait and joint mechanics, ligament function, the impact of intrinsic and extrinsic risk factors, and the biomechanical basis of current treatment strategies.

K. J. Hunt (✉) · T. Baldin
Department of Orthopaedic Surgery, University of Colorado School of Medicine, Aurora, CO, USA
e-mail: kenneth.j.hunt@ucdenver.edu; Todd.Baldini@ucdenver.edu

P. D'Hooghe
Department of Orthopaedic Surgery, Aspetar Orthopaedic and Sports Medicine Hospital, Aspire Zone, Doha, Qatar
e-mail: pieter.dhooghe@aspetar.com

H. Pereira
Orthopedic Department of Póvoa de Varzim, Vila do Conde Hospital Centre, Póvoa de Varzim, Portugal

Ripoll y De Prado Sports Clinic: Murcia-Madrid FIFA Medical Centre of Excellence, Murcia, Spain

International Centre of Sports Traumatology of the Ave, Taipas, Portugal

ICVS/3B's—PT Government Associated Laboratory, University of Minho, Braga-Guimarães, Portugal

3.2 Bone and Ligament Anatomy of the Ankle

The ankle joint is a hinge-type synovial joint that primarily allows for plantar flexion and dorsiflexion. This section will only describe the ankle joint as being comprised of three bones, the tibia, fibula, and talus that form a mortise. Some literature will also include the calcaneus as part of the ankle. The joint formed by the talus and calcaneus, the subtalar joint, will be described in a later section. The tibia is on the medial side and the fibula is on the lateral side. The distal medial side of the fibula is connected to the distal lateral side of the tibia at the distal tibiofibular syndesmosis, a slightly moveable fibrous joint. The distal end of the tibia that articulates with the superior surface of the talus is the plafond. In the anterior/posterior view, the plafond is generally horizontal with a slight convexity. In the medial/lateral view the plafond is concave. The distal medial process of the tibia that protrudes below the plafond and articulates with the medial talus

H. Pereira et al. (eds.), *Lateral Ankle Instability*, https://doi.org/10.1007/978-3-662-62763-1_3

is the medial malleolus. On the lateral side, the fibula articulates with the superior lateral surface of the talus. The distal lateral fibula also has a bony process that extends below the plafond and articulates with the lateral talus. This is the lateral malleolus. The distance between the talus and the plafond, lateral malleolus, and medial malleolus is approximately 2 mm [2]. The medial and lateral malleolus limit the medial/lateral translation and inversion/eversion of the talus (Fig. 3.1).

The talus (Fig. 3.2) is a complex bony structure that is comprised of three main parts; the body, neck, and head. Only the body is part of the ankle joint that articulates with the tibia and fibula. The superior surface is covered with articular cartilage which is known as the trochlea tali and articulates with the plafond of the tibia. In the anterior/posterior view, the superior talus is predominately horizontal with a slight concavity. In the medial/lateral view the superior talus is convex. The medial and lateral sides of the body of the talus have cartilage facets that articulate with the medial and lateral malleolus. Anteriorly the talus body narrows to form the neck, then expands to form the head. The anterior surface of the talus head articulates with the navicular bone. The inferior surface of the talus articulates with the calcaneus.

There are several ligaments that stabilize the ankle joint. On the lateral side (Fig. 3.3) are the anterior talofibular ligament (ATFL), the calcaneofibular ligament (CFL), and the posterior talofibular ligament. The ATFL runs anteriorly and medially from the anterior aspect of the distal fibula malleolus to the superior lateral surface of the talus, in front of its lateral articular facet. The CFL originates at the anterior border of the distal fibula below the origin of the ATFL. The ligament extends inferiorly and slightly posteriorly where it attaches to a tubercle on the lateral surface the calcaneus. The CFL has approximately 2.5 times greater ultimate strength (345 N) than the ATFL (138 N) [3]. The posterior talofibular ligament runs posteriorly, almost horizontal, from the lateral malleolus of the fibula to a prominent tubercle on the posterior surface of the talus.

The medial side of the ankle is supported by the deltoid ligament, also known as the medial collateral ligament of the ankle. The deltoid ligament is a complex triangular band that originates at the distal tip of the medial malleolus and fans out to connect to the talus, calcaneus, and navicular bones. The deltoid ligament has a superficial and a deep layer. The superficial layer consists of the superficial posterior tibiotalar, tibionavicular,

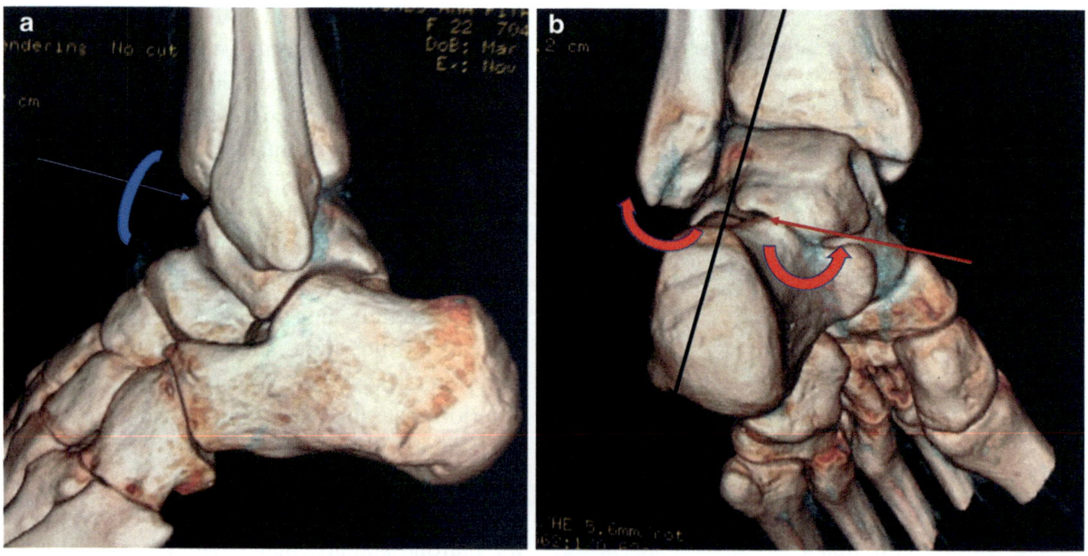

Fig. 3.1 Bones of the Ankle (**a**) and Subtalar Joint (**b**). Dorsiflexion-plantarflexion mainly in the tibiotalar ("true ankle") joint (blue arrows); Pronation-supination mainly in the subtalar joint (red arrows)

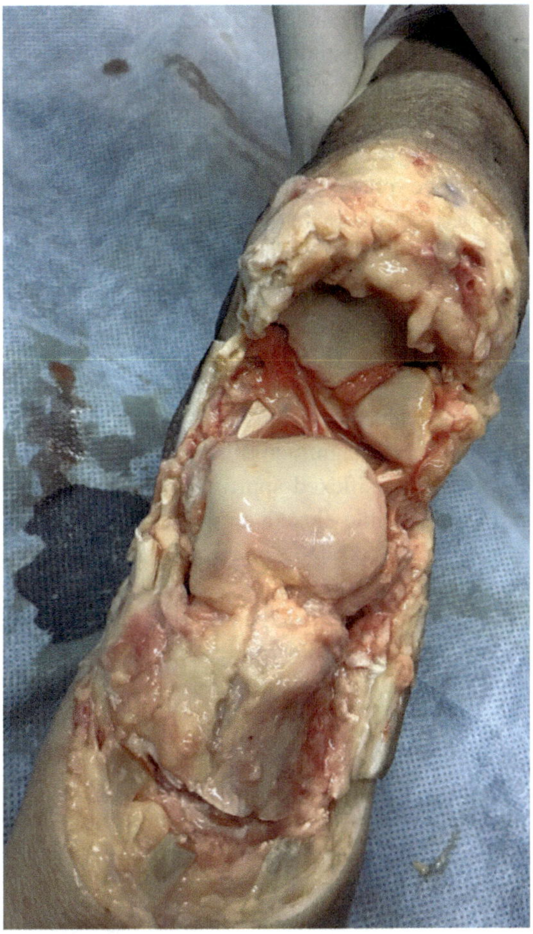

Fig. 3.2 The Talus is exposed in a superior view after lifting the distal tibia and fibula. The talar dome and its relations with the other bones is visible

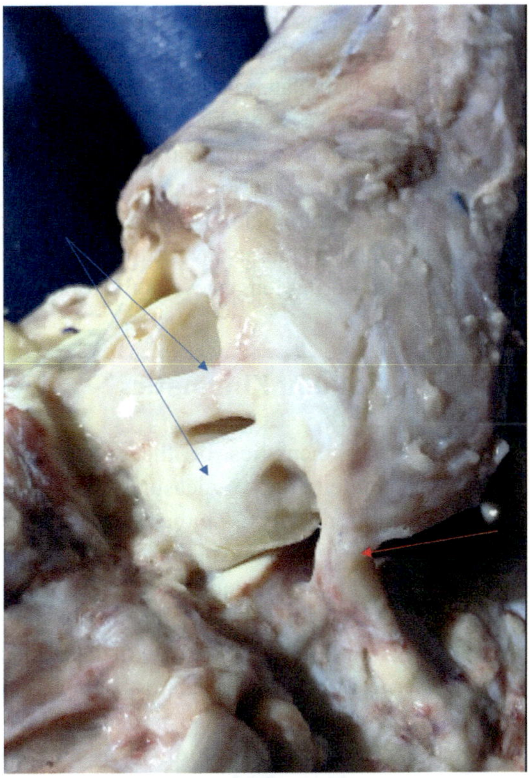

Fig. 3.3 The anterior talofibular ligament (ATFL) with its frequent superior and inferior parts (blue arrows) and the calcaneofibular ligament (CFL—red arrow), are shown in this dissection

and tibiocalcaneal ligaments. The posterior tibiotalar ligament runs posterior and laterally to connect to a prominent tubercle on the posterior surface of the talus. The tibionavicular ligament runs anteriorly to the tuberosity of the navicular bone. The tibiocalcaneal ligament runs inferiorly to the calcaneus. The deep layer consists of the deep posterior tibiotalar ligament and the deep anterior tibiotalar ligament. The posterior tibiotalar ligament connects to the posterior surface of the talus. The anterior tibiotalar ligament runs anteriorly and attaches to the neck of the talus.

The distal tibiofibular syndesmosis is made up of three separate soft tissue structures, the anterior inferior tibiofibular and posterior inferior tibiofibular ligament of the lateral malleolus, and the interosseous membrane. The anterior inferior ligament of the lateral malleolus runs transversely and inferiorly from the anterior tibia to the anterior fibula. The posterior inferior ligament of the lateral malleolus runs transversely and inferiorly from the posterior tibia to the posterior fibula. The interosseous membrane is a thin lamina of fibers that run laterally and inferiorly from the tibia to the fibula along the length of both bones.

Although there are no tendons that insert directly into the talus, there are several important muscle/tendon complexes that control the motion and aid in stabilizing the ankle joint that must be discussed. The gastrocnemius and soleus muscles connect to the Achilles tendon which inserts into the posterior calcaneus and predominantly plantarflexes the ankle. The peroneus longus and peroneus brevis lie on the lateral side of the ankle and evert and plantarflex the foot. The peroneus tertius is also on the lateral side of the ankle and everts and dorsiflexes the foot. The tibialis anterior, extensor digitorum longus, and extensor hallucis longus are in the anterior compartment of the leg and dorsiflex the ankle. The tibialis anterior and extensor hallucis longus inverts the foot while the extensor digitorum longus everts the foot.

3.3 Ankle Joint Kinematics

Measuring the kinematics of the ankle joint in vivo is challenging to measure because a majority of motion analysis studies use reflective markers attached to the skin or footwear and there is no way to independently track the motion of the talus. The result is the kinematics of both the ankle joint and subtalar joint are measured as one joint. One technique that is now being used to measure only the ankle joint is dual fluoroscopy (DF). Wang et al. showed this technique to be accurate within 0.30 ± 0.35 mm and 0.25 ± 0.81° [4]. There are limits to this technique because the dual fluoroscopy system is stationary and can only measure subjects on a treadmill or performing stationary activities. The first part of this section will report on ankle kinematics during barefoot walking on a treadmill. The second part will report ankle kinematics during running barefoot or shod on a treadmill.

During contact with the ground gait is broken into four stages, heel strike, early midstance, late midstance, and toe-off. Three studies that used DF to measure ankle joint mechanics during barefoot walking on a treadmill showed similar trends during the stance phase but their magnitudes varied considerably [4–6]. At heel strike, Wang et al. showed the ankle in greater than 20° dorsiflexion, Nichols et al. showed the ankle at 0°, and Koo et al. showed the ankle plantarflexed close to 10°. In all three studies, the ankle flexed approximately 5° from heel strike to early midstance. All three studies were unable to track the ankle from early midstance to late midstance. From late midstance to toe-off the ankle extended and was dorsiflexed at toe-off. The magnitude at toe-off varied from 5° to 20° of dorsiflexion. Only two of the studies reported on ankle inversion and ankle rotation [5, 6]. Not surprisingly both studies showed constant inversion and axial rotation angles with minimal changes throughout the stance phase [5, 6]. None of the studies reported translations of the talus.

Peltz et al. studied runners on a treadmill [7]. All subjects were tested in three different conditions, barefoot, wearing minimalist running shoes, and wearing motion control running shoes. The shod runners showed similar trends to the barefoot walkers described in the previous section but their magnitude differed. The shod runners were dorsiflexed approximately 17° at heel strike, the ankle flexed approximately 5° until early midstance, then started to extend and were dorsiflexed approximately 25° at toe-off. The barefoot runners showed a different ankle flexion pattern than the shod runners and the barefoot walkers. The barefoot runners were dorsiflexed approximately 2° at heel strike then extended throughout the gait cycle to toe-off in approximately 2° more dorsiflexion than the shod runners. The barefoot runners did not exhibit the same ankle flexion pattern after heel strike as the shod runners or barefoot walkers.

The barefoot runners showed significantly less ankle eversion than the shod runners at heel strike but were not significantly different throughout the rest of the gait cycle. The runners showed a similar trend to the walkers with the eversion angle remaining relatively constant during the stance phase. The barefoot runners were significantly more internally rotated than the shod runners during the first 40% of the stance phase but were not significantly different throughout the rest of the stance phase. The runners showed more internal rotation, between 10° and 15°, than the walkers, less than 5° [5–7].

3.4 Subtalar Joint Mechanics

While the CFL also stabilizes the subtalar joint (STJ), the STJ has its own ligament system. The talus and the calcaneus articulate through two completely distinct joints, a posterior facet, and an anterior articulation made up of a middle and anterior facet. These two articulations are separated by a groove called the sinus tarsi. The interosseous talocalcaneal ligament occupies this space with both vertical and diagonal bands. This ligamentous complex is the central pivot of rotatory stability, similar to the cruciates of the knee. Also conferring stability on the subtalar joint are collateral ligaments, including medial, posterior, lateral talocalcaneal, and anterolateral talocalcaneal ligament (ATCL). The ATCL corresponds to the cervical ligament joining the neck of the talus with the lateral edge of the calcaneus and is the first anterolateral stabilizer of the subtalar joint. It is interlinked laterally with the extensor retinaculum.

The STJ is a single-axis joint that acts as a mitered hinge connecting the talus and the calcaneus [8]. When the STJ axis is inclined at 45° from transverse, rotation of the vertical component is coupled to equal rotation of the horizontal component. A vertically aligned STJ axis at greater than 45°, as occurs in a cavus foot, results in greater rotational forces on the vertical component causes less rotation of the horizontal segment for a given rotation of the vertical one [9]. A more horizontally aligned axis, such as occurs in pes planovalgus, causes a greater rotation of the horizontal member for a given rotation of the vertical member. Thus, individuals with a flatfoot deformity show greater supination/pronation (Fig. 3.4) for a given external/internal rotation of the vertical segment. Isman and Inman pointed out the variability in STJ axis alignment. Their study on 46 cadaveric legs found that, in the transverse plane, the axis deviated 23° medial to the long axis of the foot with a range of 4°–47°, whereas in the sagittal plane, the axis was close to 41°, with a range of 21°–69° [10].

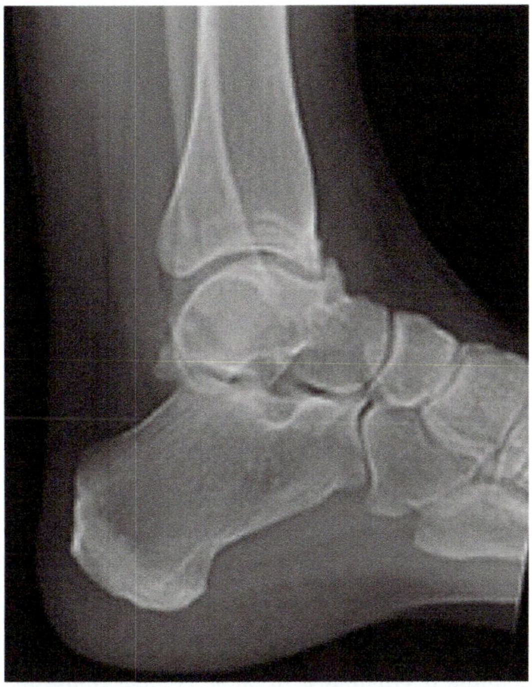

Fig. 3.4 Bony ankle impingement lesion, X-ray lateral view

3.5 Pathomechanics of Ankle Ligament Injury

By far, the most common mechanism of ankle sprain is the inversion injury with the ankle in plantarflexion [11, 12]. This typically causes injury first to the cervical ligament (lateral talocalcaneal ligament) and the anterior talofibular ligament (ATFL), and sometimes the bifurcate ligament when there is significant torsion [13]. Associated lesions such as overstretching of the sensory nerves (usually branches of the sural and superficial peroneal nerves that participate in capsular innervation) or peroneal tendons can occur [14]. Traditionally, the calcaneofibular ligament will be injured during inversion with a varus moment in the hindfoot and the ankle in a neutral or dorsiflexed position. Forced plantarflexion of the ankle due to catching the forefoot typically injures the anterior fibers of the lateral and medial collateral ligaments as well as the anterior joint capsule. Thus, a careful history and clinical and imaging examinations to analyze all the ligament structures of the ankle is critical for proper treatment decisions.

3.6 Ankle Instability

Ankle ligament injuries, particular higher grade and repeat injuries can lead to instability. In fact, a very high percentage of patients with high-grade ankle ligament injury can go on to experience recurrent injury or chronic ankle instability [15]. There are two general categories of instability: *mechanical instability*, which is related to anatomic abnormalities of the ankle that can be detected on physical examination and *functional instability*, which is usually related to a proprioceptive deficit that results in the subjecting feeling of the ankle giving way [16, 17].

3.6.1 Mechanical Instability

Mechanical instability of the ankle joint can be related to abnormalities of bone structure or alignment, underlying ligament laxity, or impairment of dorsiflexion range of motion of the ankle joint related to impingement. Ankle instability does not always result exclusively from injury. Constitutional hyperlaxity also exists, with or without the diagnosis of an associated syndrome (e.g., Marfan or Ehlers-Danlos) [18]. In addition, the configuration of the talus within the mortise (i.e., wider in the front) creates a more stable environment with the ankle in dorsiflexion. When an impingement lesion exists from osteophytes or excessive synovial hypertrophy or fibrous scarring, full dorsiflexion is prevented and the ankle can be in a less biomechanically stable position during the injury moment, increasing risk. (Fig. 3.5) Finally, gastrocnemius tightness can contribute to ankle instability [19]. All factors that can contribute to instability should be evaluated as this may impact the ultimate treatment strategy to optimize outcomes.

3.6.2 Functional Instability

Functional stabilization of the ankle joint is produced by muscle and tendon structures, which are an integral part of a much more complex postural control system of proprioception. Proprioception is the brain's conscious or unconscious perception of body parts' position relative to one another and involves receptors, pathways, and nerve centers. Four types of receptors exist around the ankle joint: neuromuscular spindles, Golgi tendon organs, Ruffini joint mechanoreceptors, and the plantar cutaneous mechanoreceptors [20]. These receptors induce reflexes in the muscular system controlling the ankle through both suprasegmental unconscious pathways and conscious, cortical pathways to control movement. At the same time, the reflex will stimulate or relax antagonist muscles. For example, during a forced inversion mechanism, the peroneal muscles and extensors of the toes are stretched, inducing reflexive firing of these muscles and relaxation of posterior tibial muscles and toe flexors. The Golgi tendon organs, which are located at the muscle-tendon junction, protect the tendons from overstretching. The joint mechanoreceptors, which are sensitive to speed, direction, and range of motion, are stimulated during extreme movements making them essential to protecting joints. There is a muscle preactivation that occurs during dynamic movement just before landing which reduces the lag in peroneal muscle activation and reduces injury risk. [21] Disruption in the proprioceptive response can put the ankle at higher risk of injury and potentially more severe injury. Repeated hopping on one foot is a reliable examination finding since it relies upon preactivation of the ankle's stabilizing muscles (peroneals, tibialis posterior, gastroc/soleus) [22].

A delay in muscle reaction to protect the ankle joint from inversion injury can be caused by a neurologic deficit or a mechanical muscle defect (e.g., peroneal tenosynovitis or subluxation). Morrison and Kaminski [23] identified gait factors that impact ankle stability, which include an increase in ground contact time, lateralization of pressure of the lateral edge of the midfoot and the forefoot, increased dorsiflexion of the first metatarsophalangeal joint, and increased foot supination. It is known that a hindfoot varus alignment (Fig. 3.6) can contribute to inversion injury risk and is a risk factor for ankle instability [24]. Varus results in excessive pressure on the lateral edge of the foot and postural imbalance during gait progression. It can also lead to excessive tension of the peroneal musculature and loss of protective reflexes. Other postural issues that can lead to excessive pressure on the lateral edge of the foot include unequal length of the lower limbs where the shorter limb tends to position itself in

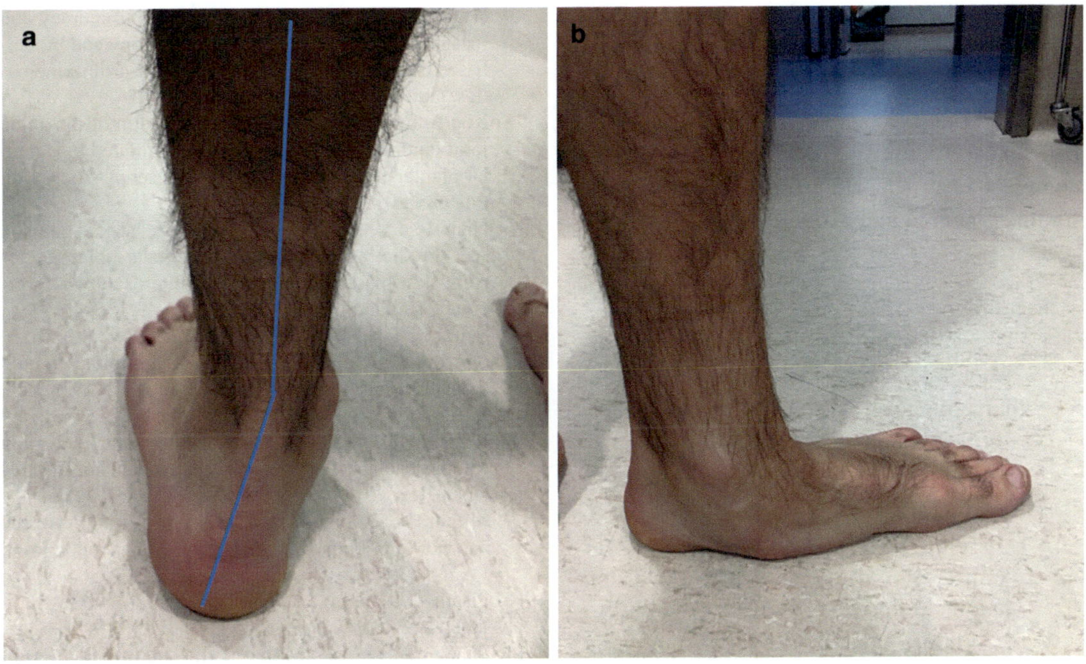

Fig. 3.5 (**a**) Posterior and (**b**) Medial photographs of flatfoot deformity with greater supination/pronation motion

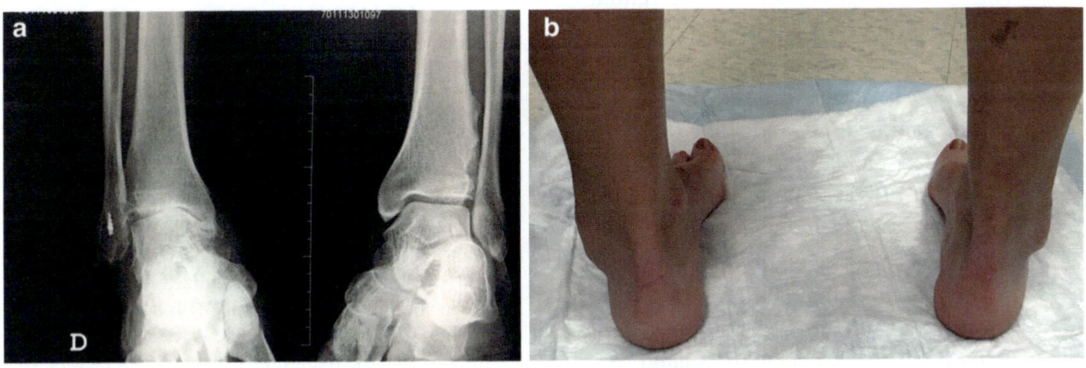

Fig. 3.6 Hindfoot varus alignment have higher risk of an inversion injury risk. On the x-ray (**a**) an anchor related to previous lateral instability repair is visible. Varus malalignment of the hindfoot (**b**) is a risk factor for ankle instability

varus, causing an unstable dynamic supination movement during weight-bearing.

3.7 Conclusion

The ankle is a dynamic and joint complex with interrelated mechanical, postural, anatomical, neurologic, and functional factors that impact ankle stability. Many of these factors are difficult to assess with current diagnostic technologies. Recurrent sprains and ligament repair failures are typically related to an unaddressed deficit in one of these elements. A clear understanding of these issues and a thorough history and examination of these patients is critical to optimize treatment selection and the outcome of any treatment strategy. As we treat patients with chronic instability, it is important to consider that restoring ligaments to appropriate tension is only a part of restoring full function and mitigating the risk of recurrent injury or treatment failure. Restoration of ankle mechanics, proprioception, strength, postural balance, and muscle conditioning is also critical. Ongoing advances in technology present an opportunity to more readily assess these patients and identify risk factors so that more complete treatment algorithms might be created for this common and expensive condition.

Fact Box

- The ankle joint enrolls a complex set of articulations that are critical to athletic performance in several sports, and are frequently subject of injury.
- Varus malalignment of the hindfoot is a risk factor for ankle instability.
- The mechanical role of the ankle in gait is to transfer all forces occurring during gait, including body weight and multidirectional forces, in a dynamic moving system which might quickly change directions.
- The subtalar joint has a preferential rotation mobility permitting the foot to adapt to the ground.
- There are several ligaments that stabilize the ankle joint and knowledge of anatomy is mandatory (see Chap. 1).
- There are two general categories of instability: *mechanical instability,* which is related to anatomic abnormalities of the ankle that can be detected on physical examination and *functional instability*, which is usually related to a proprioceptive deficit that results in the subjecting feeling of the ankle giving way.

References

1. Hintermann B, Knupp M, Barg A. Peritalar instability. Foot Ankle Int. 2012;33(5):450–4.
2. Imai K, Ikoma K, Kido M, et al. Joint space width of the tibiotalar joint in the healthy foot. J Foot Ankle Res. 2015;8:26.
3. Attarian DE, McCrackin HJ, DeVito DP, McElhaney JH, Garrett WE Jr. Biomechanical characteristics of human ankle ligaments. Foot Ankle. 1985;6(2):54–8.
4. Wang B, Roach KE, Kapron AL, et al. Accuracy and feasibility of high-speed dual fluoroscopy and model-based tracking to measure in vivo ankle arthrokinematics. Gait Posture. 2015;41(4):888–93.
5. Koo S, Lee KM, Cha YJ. Plantar-flexion of the ankle joint complex in terminal stance is initiated by subtalar plantar-flexion: a bi-planar fluoroscopy study. Gait Posture. 2015;42(4):424–9.
6. Nichols JA, Roach KE, Fiorentino NM, Anderson AE. Predicting tibiotalar and subtalar joint angles from skin-marker data with dual-fluoroscopy as a reference standard. Gait Posture. 2016;49:136–43.
7. Peltz CD, Haladik JA, Hoffman SE, et al. Effects of footwear on three-dimensional tibiotalar and subtalar joint motion during running. J Biomech. 2014;47(11):2647–53.
8. Krahenbuhl N, Horn-Lang T, Hintermann B, Knupp M. The subtalar joint: a complex mechanism. EFORT Open Rev. 2017;2(7):309–16.
9. Milner CE, Soames RW. Anatomical variations of the anterior talofibular ligament of the human ankle joint. J Anat. 1997;191(Pt 3):457–8.
10. Pisani G. The coxa pedis. Eur J Foot Ankle Surg. 1994;1:67–74.
11. Panagiotakis E, Mok KM, Fong DT, Bull AMJ. Biomechanical analysis of ankle ligamentous sprain injury cases from televised basketball games: understanding when, how and why ligament failure occurs. J Sci Med Sport. 2017;20(12):1057–61.
12. Fong DT, Ha SC, Mok KM, Chan CW, Chan KM. Kinematics analysis of ankle inversion ligamentous sprain injuries in sports: five cases from televised tennis competitions. Am J Sports Med. 2012;40(11):2627–32.
13. Leland RH, Marymont JV, Trevino SG, Varner KE, Noble PC. Calcaneocuboid stability: a clinical and anatomic study. Foot Ankle Int. 2001;22(11):880–4.
14. Hunt G. Injuries of peripheral nerves of the leg, foot and ankle: an often unrecognized consequence of ankle sprains. Foot. 2003;13(1):14–8.
15. McKay GD, Goldie PA, Payne WR, Oakes BW. Ankle injuries in basketball: injury rate and risk factors. Br J Sports Med. 2001;35(2):103–8.
16. Hertel J. Functional anatomy, pathomechanics, and pathophysiology of lateral ankle instability. J Athl Train. 2002;37(4):364–75.
17. Beynnon BD, Murphy DF, Alosa DM. Predictive factors for lateral ankle sprains: a literature review. J Athl Train. 2002;37(4):376–80.
18. Wolf JM, Cameron KL, Owens BD. Impact of joint laxity and hypermobility on the musculoskeletal system. J Am Acad Orthop Surg. 2011;19(8):463–71.
19. Riemann BL, DeMont RG, Ryu K, Lephart SM. The effects of sex, joint angle, and the gastrocnemius muscle on passive ankle joint complex stiffness. J Athl Train. 2001;36(4):369–75.
20. Michelson JD, Hutchins C. Mechanoreceptors in human ankle ligaments. J Bone Joint Surg Br. 1995;77(2):219–24.

21. Vaes P, Duquet W, Van Gheluwe B. Peroneal reaction times and eversion motor response in healthy and unstable ankles. J Athl Train. 2002;37(4):475–80.
22. Jerosch J, Bischof M. Proprioceptive capabilities of the ankle in stable and unstable joints. Sports Exerc Inj. 1996;2:167–71.
23. Morrison KE, Kaminski TW. Foot characteristics in association with inversion ankle injury. J Athl Train. 2007;42(1):135–42.
24. Klammer G, Benninger E, Espinosa N. The varus ankle and instability. Foot Ankle Clin. 2012;17(1):57–82.

History and Clinical Examination of Lateral Ankle Instability

4

David Miller, James Stone, and James Calder

4.1 Introduction

Ligamentous injuries to the ankle are common. Approximately 75% of all injuries to the ankle are sprains and of these, the majority are inversion injuries [1]. This pattern of injury commonly leads to damage to the lateral ankle ligamentous restraints, specifically the anterior talofibular ligament (ATFL) and the calcaneofibular ligament (CFL) [2]. Most injuries can be treated conservatively with appropriate immobilization, rehabilitation, and targeted physiotherapy. Approximately 20–40% of patients continue to suffer episodes of recurrent instability and develop chronic lateral ankle instability despite conservative treatment [3, 4]. An accurate history and physical examination are critical in the assessment and diagnosis of lateral ankle instability. A properly performed physical examination has the potential to diagnose over 90% of lateral ligament injuries allowing prompt treatment and minimizing the risk of long-term joint sequelae [5].

D. Miller (✉) · J. Calder
Fortius Clinic, London, UK
e-mail: James.Calder@fortiusclinic.com

J. Stone
Orthopedic Surgery, Medical College of Wisconsin, Milwaukee, WI, USA

4.2 History

A detailed and targeted history is vital in the assessment of patients with lateral ankle instability. The fundamental principle in ankle ligament injuries is that the position of the ankle at the time of the injury and the applied force will generally determine which structures of the ankle are injured. It is important to distinguish those patients presenting with acute ligament injury due to an ankle sprain from those with a history of chronic ankle instability early in the evaluation process, and a precise history is crucial in making this determination.

4.2.1 Acute Ligament Injury

In acute ankle injury, history should focus on establishing the exact mechanism of the initial trauma. The patient usually describes "rolling the ankle over" in a combination of inversion and plantarflexion. There is an immediate onset of pain and rapid development of swelling with impairment of the ability to weight bear. If injured during a sporting event, the patient is often unable to continue playing. The swelling often takes a number of days to resolve and is replaced by a hematoma with subsequent ecchymosis (Fig. 4.1) over the following days [6]. Although patients will frequently describe a popping or tearing sensation, an audible noise, or the

H. Pereira et al. (eds.), *Lateral Ankle Instability*, https://doi.org/10.1007/978-3-662-62763-1_4

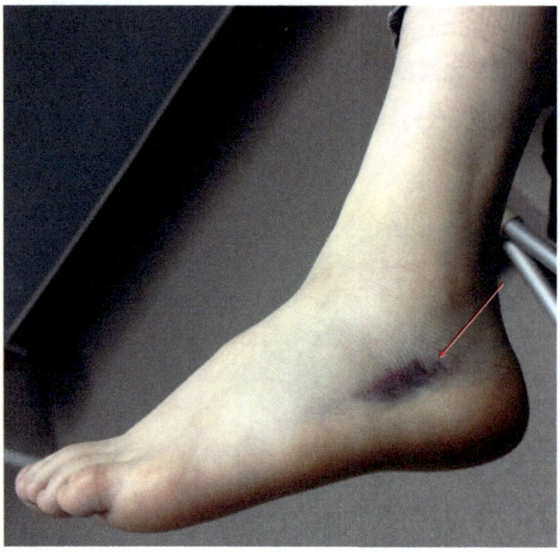

Fig. 4.1 Typical ecchymosis (red arrow) connected to the hematoma some days after an acute sprain

sensation of immediate swelling, the value of these symptoms in predicting the anatomy of the injury is poor [7].

It is important to establish if the injury occurred in a sporting event and if so the type and level played. The prognosis and expected level of recovery will differ from an elite professional athlete to a recreational sportsman. Additionally, the type of sport is very important, as certain sporting activities such as basketball and netball have been shown to have high rates of lateral ankle ligamentous injuries [8, 9]. Additionally, among football (soccer) players, artificial grass seems to put players at a slightly increased risk of lateral ligament injuries [10].

4.2.2 Chronic Instability

Patients with chronic ankle instability usually complain of recurrent sprains, the sensation of giving way, and persistent pain [11]. They often describe a previous, initial traumatic event with subsequent multiple further episodes of instability which may occur with little to no precipitating force [12]. There is frequent apprehension and difficulty walking on uneven surfaces, such as sand or cobblestone roads. It is common for each episode of recurrent instability to be followed by a relatively shorter period of dysfunction compared to the initial injury [12].

It is important to establish whether the patient has had any previous physiotherapy. The literature supports the use of targeted functional rehabilitation in the treatment of ankle instability [13]. It is important to determine the type, frequency, and intensity of these sessions as well as patient compliance with the rehabilitation program to gauge their success in decreasing symptoms of instability. Additionally, the previous use of ankle braces or taping should be explored along with their success in improving the patient's symptoms of ankle instability.

In both acute and chronic instability, it is important to identify any possible underlying risk factors or associated injuries. The greatest risk factor is a previous sprain [14]. Other risk factors include males between the age of 15–25 and females between 30 and 39 years old [14]. Several studies have shown a relatively high incidence of 3–19% of talus osteochondral defects in patients with lateral ankle instability [1, 12]. Often these patients describe deep-seated chronic anterior ankle joint pain. If the OCD is located medially then the pain is frequently located posteromedially. Additionally, an incidence of 3–24% of loose bodies has been reported in patients with instability. Patients with loose bodies often describe true locking of the ankle as opposed to those with pure instability who complain of giving way and pain associated with the giving way episodes. Anterior ankle impingement may occur in up to 14% of patients with ankle instability and may frequently have associated distal tibial osteophytes leading to medial bone impingement or soft-tissue hypertrophy causing anterolateral impingement. Often patients describe limited ankle dorsiflexion and pain on forced dorsiflexion maneuvers such as squatting and lunging [1].

As with all ankle injuries, it is important to exclude relevant medical comorbidities that might influence treatment and prognosis. These include diabetes, immunosuppressive disorders, current or past cigarette smoking, previous deep vein thrombosis, or pulmonary embolism. With the last, it is also important to note that female patients who are obese and/or who are taking oral contraceptive medications are at increased risk of thromboembolic events.

4.3 Examination

Physical examination of the unstable ankle has been shown to be potentially very accurate in the diagnosis of lateral ankle ligament injury and ankle laxity. Several studies have shown that a properly performed physical examination will accurately diagnose 91–95% of lateral ligament injuries [5, 6, 15]. An understanding of the expected time frame of physical findings and the anatomical basis of special tests is essential.

A careful evaluation of gait and shoe wear is important when assessing chronic ankle instability. Shoe type, wear, and the use of orthotics can provide important information on foot and ankle alignment and mechanics. For example, a varus hindfoot will cause more lateral wear on the sole of the shoe. Use of a medial heel wedge orthotic acts to increase hindfoot varus and may exacerbate lateral ankle symptoms. Additionally, patients with chronic lateral instability often use lace-up boots or trainers which provide more ankle support than high-heel or flexible shoes. The use of ankle braces during sport or daily activity should be noted as it may indicate a chronic ankle instability issue of significant severity. Gait evaluation should focus on factors which may predispose to ankle instability, such as hindfoot varus and calf or foot muscle atrophy. If hindfoot varus is suspected from clinical examination then radiographic evaluation of hindfoot alignment should be performed (Fig. 4.2).

Marked lateral swelling, pain on palpation, and pain with weight-bearing are cardinal features in an acute lateral ligament injury. Although lateral swelling is a common finding with lateral ligament injury, it is not diagnostic. Van Dijk et al. demonstrated that while lateral swelling was present in 78% of ankles with ligament injury, it was still present in 55% of those who did not have ligamentous injury [5]. Additionally, Funder et al. showed in their series that 70% of the patients with ruptured lateral ligaments had swelling lateral and anterior to the lateral malleolus ≥4 cm [15].

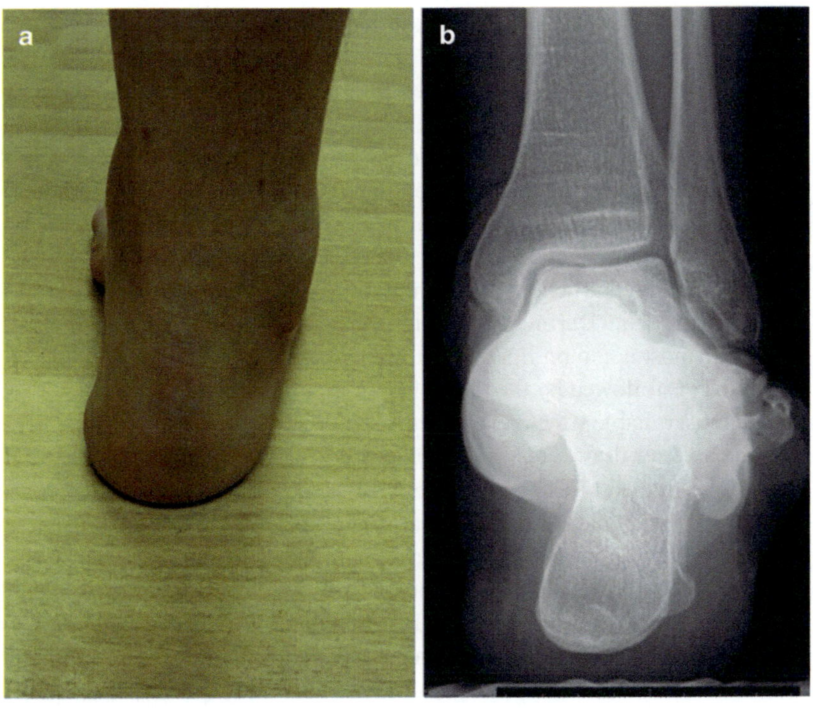

Fig. 4.2 Hindfoot varus—weight-bearing view (**a**) and corresponding hindfoot alignment radiograph (**b**)

The diagnostic accuracy in acute lateral ligament injury is significantly improved by reexamining the patient 5–7 days after injury. The series by Van Dijk examined 160 people with lateral ligament injuries. They demonstrated that a delayed physical examination had a diagnostic sensitivity of 96% and specificity of 84%. A delayed examination allows the swelling and pain to subside allowing a more detailed examination. They found that an absence of swelling at a delayed examination suggests that there is no ligament injury (predictive value 58%) but if extensive swelling is still present then it has a predictive value of 87%. Moreover, they showed that the single most reliable test was the presence of skin discoloration from a hematoma around the lateral ligaments. This feature had a predictive value of 92% for ligament injury [5, 6].

4.3.1 Mechanical Ankle Instability

Traditionally, chronic ankle instability has been attributed to both functional and mechanical causes. Knowledge of the interplay between these two is integral in the physical examination of a patient with ankle instability [8].

Mechanical instability of the ankle refers to pathologic laxity of the ankle after an injury to the supporting ligaments. It is caused by plastic deformation of the supportive ligaments by either secondary to an acute injury or recurrent sprains resulting in frank rupture or permanent lengthening. It can also be caused by degenerative changes that alter the congruency of the articular joint or synovial changes such as inflammation or impingement [8]. During an ankle inversion injury, the most common ligaments to be injured are the ATFL followed by the CFL [14].

The most reliable way to examine the ATFL is with the anterior drawer test (ADT) and the CFL with a talar tilt test (TTT). While the ADT is the most common clinical test for examining for ankle joint laxity, its accuracy is dependent on the clinician's sensitivity and experience [16]. To perform the ADT the examiner stabilizes the tibia and then grasps the heel and applies a posterior to anterior force (Fig. 4.2). Laxity of the ATFL allows the foot to subluxate anteriorly [17]. The lateral ankle ligaments are not isometric. During ankle plantarflexion, the anterior talofibular ligament lengthens becoming tighter. In addition, in this position the narrower portion of the posterior talus is engaged in the mortise. The anterior drawer test should therefore be performed with the joint in plantarflexion and comparison should be made with the normal opposite joint. Gould et al. showed when a force is applied to the ankle which results in ATFL elongation of 4 mm or 20% of its resting length, the ligament will fail and cause the patient to have a positive ADT [18]. A "sulcus" sign may be seen whereby the lateral soft-tissues indent overlying the ATFL rupture when there is profound laxity (Fig. 4.3).

To perform the TTT, the examiner stabilizes the tibia with one hand while the other hand applies an inversion/adduction force to the talus [4, 19]. The difficulty with this test is isolating the talus and distinguishing between an abnormal pathologic lateral tilt of the talus and a normal or pathologic movement of the subtalar joint [4]. As the CFL is at its greatest length with the ankle at neutral position, the TTT should be performed in this position rather than in plantarflexion. To our knowledge, there has been no validated method to accurately assess the degree of CFL instability although fluoroscopically assisted examination may be helpful.

Traditionally, the ADT is performed by applying a posterior to anterior vector. However, when the talus subluxates in the mortise it pivots off the intact deltoid ligament [20]. This results in the talus moving not only in a posterior to anterior ankle direction but in a multidirectional manner—moving anteriorly and internally rotating.

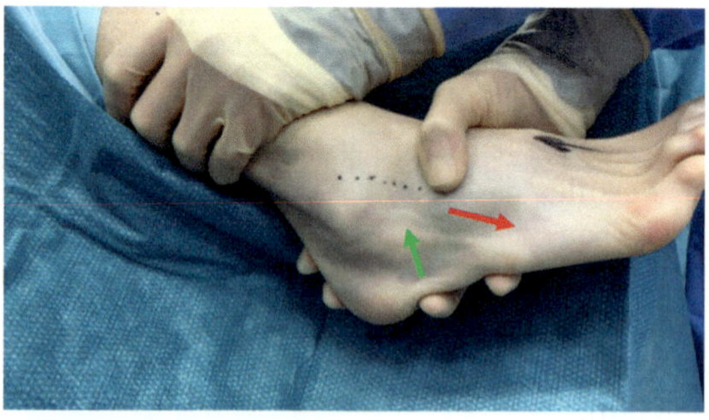

Fig. 4.3 Anterior drawer performed in 20° plantarflexion (direction of red arrow) and sulcus sign (green arrow)

Several studies have suggested that the ADT should be performed not as a direct AP vector but as an anterolateral drawer test. Miller et al. performed a cadaveric study examining the difference between a purely anterior-posterior drawer test and an anterolateral drawer test. They found that an anterolateral drawer test caused almost twice the talar displacement compared to a direct anterior drawer test. They concluded that allowing rotational freedom of the ankle while performing an ADT may allow the examiner to detect more subtle degrees of ankle instability [20].

There is currently no consensus in the literature regarding the most appropriate degree of ankle flexion to perform the ADT. Anatomically, the ATFL originates from the anterior border of the fibula and inserts anteromedially on the talus. It usually consists of two bands (inferior and superior) but it has been documented to range from one to three. Golano et al. showed that in plantarflexion the inferior band of the ligament is taut and the upper band is relaxed whereas in dorsiflexion the upper band is taught and the inferior band is relaxed. The CFL has been shown to be most taut in dorsiflexion [21].

Several cadaveric studies have looked at the effect of sectioning of the ATFL and CFL on ankle instability at varying degrees of flexion. Kjaesgaard-Anderson et al. showed that isolated ATFL injuries caused significant anterior-posterior laxity of the ankle joint through the entire range of flexion but were most pronounced in neutral position [22]. Additionally, Hollis et al. found a similar result [23]. In contrast, however, Bahr et al. and Tahyama et al. showed in their series that ATFL resection caused maximal talar translation in plantarflexion [24, 25]. In most series, however, sectioning of the CFL in addition to the ATFL causes an increase in laxity as assessed by the ADT, particularly with the ankle in dorsiflexion. Several studies have suggested that when there is an isolated ATFL injury there is increased laxity in plantarflexion to neutral but when there is a combined ATFL and CFL injury then there is increased laxity in slight dorsiflexion [26].

Some studies have questioned the accuracy of the ADT in diagnosing lateral ligament injury. Croy et al. showed in their series of 66 subjects with a history of lateral ankle sprain that the ADT had a sensitivity of 74–83% but a specificity of only 38–40%, as measured by the degree of anterior translation [17]. Additionally, Lahde et al. found that 28% of ATFL injuries and 38% of combined ATFL and CFL ligament injuries were not detected using the ADT [27]. Seligson et al. examined the reproducibility and normal range of the ADT and TTT in 25 functionally normal ankles. They showed that that the ADT had a very small range of <3 mm in functionally normal ankles with good reproducibility in their series. The TTT, however, had a wide range in the normal ankles of 0–18° and was less reliable. They concluded that the ADT evaluates the lateral ligament integrity of the ankle more critically than the TTT [28]. It may be difficult to describe the degree of ankle laxity of the anterior drawer test between examiners and therefore a simple description of stable, unstable, or unstable with sulcus sign may be preferred [29].

Injuries of the ATFL and CFL also cause significant laxity with ankle inversion and rotation. Several studies have shown that the rupture of the CFL causes a significant increase in hindfoot inversion and ankle joint external rotation [19]. Although the TTT is difficult to perform and interpret, it should be expected that when the CFL is ruptured or is not competent there is increased hindfoot inversion. This has been shown to be maximum in dorsiflexion [19].

Despite the variability in the literature regarding the accuracy of the ADT and TTT, they still remain an integral component in the physical examination in a patient with lateral ankle instability. The ADT is the most common examination for ankle instability and has been shown to be more accurate than the TTT. It is important for the examiner to recognize that the laxity is multidirectional and multi-planar. An ADT should allow internal rotation of the talus in the mortise and should be performed through plantarflexion to dorsiflexion. If there is increased instability in dorsiflexion a combined ATFL and CFL should be suspected. The TTT should be tested in dorsiflexion and an attempt should be made to try to isolate pathologic talar tilt from normal or pathologic subtalar motion by identifying the lateral talar process with a finger and assessing its separation from the tip of the fibula during stress-testing. A comparison with the contralateral side is vital in this assessment.

When considering the timing of examination, Van Dijk et al. showed that in the acute period (within 48 h of injury) the ADT had very poor diagnostic accuracy with a sensitivity of only 71% and a specificity of 33%. The accuracy was substantially increased by repeating the examination 5 days after the injury when the specificity increased to 74% and sensitivity to 86%. They attributed the poor initial sensitivity and specificity to be due to the acute pain and swelling around the ankle which resulted in guarding which limited the accuracy of the initial examination. Reexamination of the ankle 5 days later allowed the swelling and pain to subside and a more accurate examination could then be performed [5, 6].

The most reliable time to examine the ankle is approximately 5 days post injury. The single most reliable finding to indicate ligament injury has been shown to be the presence of a hematoma 5 days post injury (predictive value 92%). The combination of lateral hematoma, a positive anterior drawer, and pain on palpation of the ATFL has a predictive value of 95% for a lateral ligament injury. Additionally, Funder et al. found in their series that 91% of their patients with lateral ligament injury had the combination of tenderness over the ATFL or CFL, pain on supination and inversion of the foot, and swelling ≥4 cm. Interestingly, in their series more patients with lateral ligamentous injuries had tenderness over the CFL than the ATFL [15]. In the series by Van Dijk et al. a negative anterior drawer test and absence of discoloration always indicated an intact lateral ligament complex [6].

4.3.2 Functional Ankle Instability

Functional instability was first described by Freeman et al. in 1965 [30]. He described the condition in which the patient complained of ankle instability which was due to an insufficiency of proprioception, neuromuscular control, postural control, or strength in contrast to patients with mechanical instability due to ligament injury. Damage to the mechanoreceptors in the ligaments and impaired neuromuscular control was proposed to contribute to a deficiency in the defense mechanisms that prevent hypersupination of the foot [8]. Examination is based upon the assessment of the above functions. A simple method to test proprioception is with a Rhomberg test. The patient is asked to perform a single leg stance on the affected leg initially with their eyes open and then with them closed. The test is positive when the patient is unable to stand on the affected leg with the eyes closed [31]. The test should always be compared to the contralateral leg. Tropp et al. used a stability instrument to assess 15 sportsmen with unilateral functional instability. The results of their study showed that patients with functional instability had a defective proprioceptive mechanism [32]. Additionally, Friden et al. (1989) similarly demonstrated poor proprioceptive control in patients with functional instability [33].

Functional instability can also be examined by testing the strength of the major muscle groups crossing the ankle. In particular, the peroneal muscles are important in ankle stability and control. Peroneal weakness is commonly seen in functional ankle instability. Weakness can lead to a diminished ability for the ankle to compensate and prevent sudden hindfoot inversion/supination [31, 33–35]. Konradsen et al. showed with EMG monitoring that the peroneal muscle reaction time is also delayed in ankle instability, potentiating any inherent weakness [33].

4.3.3 Other

While an inversion injury can result in rupture of the lateral ligaments, other intra-articular and extra-articular injuries may occur, and, if missed, they can lead to significant long-term morbidity. Therefore, it is important that these associated injuries be examined and excluded. DiGiovanni et al. published one of the earliest reports of associated injuries in ankle instability. In their series, no patients were found to have an isolated lateral ligament injury at the time of surgery. The most common associated pathologies included synovitis (100%), talar fibrillation (25%), talar chondral defect (14%), anterolateral impingement (14%), distal tibial osteophyte (14%), and loose bodies (11%) [12]. The physical examination should include palpation and testing for all of these injuries, especially the presence of intra-articular pathologies such as loose bodies or osteochondral lesions. Finally, predisposing or risk factors should always be assessed. These include increased BMI, presence of hindfoot or midfoot malalignment, poor neuromuscular control (as described above), and generalized ligamentous laxity. Deformities that can predispose include hindfoot varus, first ray plantarflexion, and midfoot cavus [14].

Take-Home Message

A thorough and targeted history and physical examination have been shown to be able to diagnose greater than 90% of ankle lateral ligament injuries. History should be focused on identifying those with acute ligament injury or chronic ankle instability. In the acute setting, the mechanism of injury and the type and level of sporting activity are important to establish. In the chronic setting, history should be more focused on the severity of instability, predisposing factors, and excluding associated injuries.

The examination should address both mechanical and functional causes of instability. The most reliable physical examination test for ankle joint laxity is the ADT. It should be performed through multiple ranges of ankle flexion and should include both a posterior to anterior directed force as well as internal rotation. The TTT is more difficult to perform accurately and to interpret. It should be performed with the ankle in neutral to dorsiflexion. A positive TTT characterized by increased talar tilt on inversion stress indicates an injury to the CFL. Examination 5 days after the injury appears to have the highest sensitivity and specificity for diagnosing a lateral ligament injury. The combination of lateral hematoma, a positive anterior drawer, and tenderness on palpation of the ATFL are the cardinal signs and have a positive predictive value of 95% for lateral ligament injury.

Fact Box

- The position of the ankle at the time of injury and applied force will generally determine which ligamentous structures of the ankle are injured.
- Acute injuries present with instant pain, swelling, and an inability to weight bear.
- A description of swelling, popping, or a tearing sensation or audible noise has a poor predictive value in diagnosing lateral ligament injury.
- Patients with chronic instability usually complain of intermittent episodes of instability, recurrent sprains, and persistent pain.
- Examination in the acute period (<48 h) has poor diagnostic accuracy.
- The ATFL is examined by performing an anterior drawer test.
- Elongation of the ATFL of 4 mm or 20% will cause it to fail.
- The CFL is examined by performing a talar tilt test.
- An anterior drawer test acutely has a sensitivity of 71% and specificity of 33%.
- Delayed examination at 5 days post injury has an increased specificity of 74% and sensitivity of 86%.
- The combination of a lateral hematoma, positive anterior drawer test, and pain on palpation of the ATFL has a positive predictive value of 95% for a lateral ligament injury.
- Ninety-one percent of patients with a lateral ligament injury will generally have tenderness over the ATFL or CFL, pain on supination and inversion of the foot, and lateral swelling ≥4 cm.

References

1. Lee J, Hamilton G, Ford L. Associated intra-articular ankle pathologies in patients with chronic lateral ankle instability: arthroscopic findings at the time of lateral ankle reconstruction. Foot Ankle Spec. 2011;4(5):284–9.

2. Strauss J, Forsberg J, Lippert F. Chronic lateral ankle instability and associated conditions: a rationale for treatment. Foot Ankle Int. 2007;28(10):1041–4.
3. Bischof J, Spritzer C, Caputo A, Easley M, DeOrio J, Nunley J, DeFrate L. In vivo cartilage contact strains in patients with lateral ankle instability. J Biomech. 2010;43:2561–6.
4. Chan K, Ding B, Mroczek K. Acute and chronic lateral ankle instability in the athlete. Bull NYU Hosp Jt Dis. 2011;69(1):17–26.
5. Van Dijk C, Lim L, Bossuyt P, Marti R. Physical examination is sufficient for the diagnosis of sprained ankles. J Bone Joint Surg Br. 1996;78-B:958–62.
6. Van Dijk C, Mol B, Lim L, Marti R, Bossuyt P. Diagnosis of ligament rupture of the ankle joint: physical examination, arthrography, stress radiography and sonography compared in 160 patients after inversion trauma. Acta Orthop Scand. 1996;67(6):566–70.
7. Pijnenburg A, Bogaard K, Krips R, Marti R, Bossuyt P, van Dijk C. Operative and functional treatment of rupture of the lateral ligament of the ankle. J Bone Joint Surg Br. 2003;85-B(4):525–30.
8. Hertel J. Functional anatomy, pathomechanics and pathophysiology of lateral ankle instability. J Athl Train. 2002;37(4):364–75.
9. McKay G, Goldie P, Payne W, Oakes B. Ankle injuries in basketball: injury rate and risk factors. Br J Sports Med. 2001;35:103–8.
10. Ekstrand J, Timpka T, Hagglund M. Risk of injury in elite football played on artificial turf versus natural grass: a prospective two-cohort study. Br J Sports Med. 2006;40:975–80.
11. Wright C, Arnol B, Rose S, Ketchum J, Ericksen J, Pidcoe P. Clinical examination results in individuals with functional ankle instability and ankle-sprain copers. J Athl Train. 2013;49(5):581–9.
12. DiGiovanni B, Fraga C, Cohen B, Shereff M. Associated injuries found in chronic lateral ankle instability. Foot Ankle Int. 2000;21(10):809–15.
13. Kerkhoffs G, Ban den Bekerom M, Elders L, et al. Diagnosis, treatment and prevention of ankle sprains: an evidence based clinical guidelines. Br J Sports Med. 2012;46:854–60.
14. Shakked R, Sheskier S. Acute and chronic lateral ankle instability: diagnosis, management and new concepts. Bull Hosp Jt Dis. 2017;75(1):71–80.
15. Funder V, Jorgensen J, Andersen A, Bryde Anderson S, Lindholmer E, Niedermann B, Vuust M. Ruptures of the lateral ligaments of the ankle: clinical diagnosis. Acta Orthop Scand. 1982;53:997–1000.
16. Kerkhoff G, Blankevoort L, van Poll D, Marti R, van Dijk C. Anterior lateral ankle ligament damage and anterior talo-crural-joint laxity: an overview of the in vitro reports in literature. Clin Biomech. 2001;16:635–43.
17. Croy T, Koppenhaver S, Saliba S, Hertel J. Anterior talocrural joint laxity: diagnostic accuracy of the anterior drawer test of the ankle. J Orthop Sports Phys Ther. 2013;43(12):911–9.
18. Gould N, Seligson D, Gassman J. Early and late repair of lateral ligament of the ankle. Foot Ankle. 1980;1(2):84–9.
19. Kjoersgaard-Anderson P, Wethelund J, Helmin P, et al. Effect of the calcaneofibular ligament on hindfoot rotation in amputation specimens. Acta Orthop Scand. 1987;58:135–8.
20. Miller A, Myers S, Parks B, Guyton G. Anterolateral drawer versus anterior drawer test for ankle instability: a biomechanical model. Foot Ankle Int. 2016;37(4):407–10.
21. Golano P, Vega J, deLeeuw P, et al. Anatomy of the ankle ligaments: a pictorial essay. Knee Surg Sports Traumatol Arthrosc. 2010;18:557–69.
22. Kjaersgaard-Anderson P, Frich L, Madsen F, et al. Instability of the hindfoot after lesion of the lateral ankle ligaments: investigations of the anterior drawer and adduction maneuvers in autopsy specimens. Clin Orthop Relat Res. 1991;266:170–9.
23. Hollis J, Blasier D, Flahiff C. Simulated lateral ankle ligamentous injury. Am J Sports Med. 1995;23(6):672–7.
24. Bahr R, Pena F, Shine J, Lew W, Lindquist C, Tyrdal S, Engebretsen L. Mechanics of the anterior draw and talar tilt tests: a cadaver study of lateral ligament injuries of the ankle. Acta Orthop Scand. 1997;68(5):435–41.
25. Tohyama H, Beynnon B, Renstrom P, et al. Biomechanical analysis of the ankle anterior drawer and talar tilt tests. J Orthop Res. 1995;13:609–14.
26. Rasmussen O, Tovborg-Jensen I. Anterolateral rotational instability of the ankle joint: an experimental study of anterolateral rotational instability, talar tilt, and anterior drawer sign in relation to injuries to the lateral ligament. Act Orthop Scand. 1981;52:99–102.
27. Lahde S, Putkonen M, Puranen J, et al. Examination of the sprained ankle: anterior drawer test or arthrography? Eur J Radiol. 1998;8:255–7.
28. Seligson D, Gassman J, Pope M. Ankle instability: evaluation of the lateral ligaments. Am J Sports Med. 1980;8(1):39–42.
29. Guillo S, Bauer T, Lee J, et al. Consensus in chronic ankle instability: aetiology, assessment, surgical indications and place for arthroscopy. Orthop Traumatol Surg Res. 2013;99(8 Suppl):S411–9.
30. Freeman M, Dean M, Hanham I. The etiology and prevention of functional instability of the foot. J Bone Joint Surg. 1965;47B(4):678–85.
31. Ryan L. Mechanical stability, muscle strength and proprioception in the functionally unstable ankle. Aust J Physiother. 1994;40(1):41–7.
32. Tropp H, Ekstrand J, Gillqurist J. Stabilometry in functional instability of the ankle and its value in predicting injury. Med Sci Sports Exerc. 1984;16:128–36.

33. Friden T, Zatterstrom R, Lindstrand A, et al. A stabilometric technique for evaluation of lower limb instabilities. Am J Sports Med. 1989;17:118–22.
34. Konradsen L, Ravn J. Ankle instability caused by prolonged peroneal reaction time. Acta Orthop Scand. 1990;61:388–90.
35. Willems T, Witvrouw E, Verstuyft J, Ves P, DeClercq D. Proprioception and muscle strength in subjects with a history of ankle sprains and chronic instability. J Athl Train. 2002;37(4):487–93.

Lateral Ankle Instability Imaging

5

Justin C. Lee, Adam W. M. Mitchell,
and Lionel Pesquer

5.1 Introduction

Inversion injuries of the ankle are common in athletes and the general public accounting for up to 10% of visits to the emergency department [1]. Overall incidence is in the region of 1:10,000 persons per day and lateral ankle ligament injuries in athletes account for up to 45% of injuries in high-risk sports such as soccer and baseball [2, 3].

The severity of the ligamentous injuries depends on the force of the trauma, the degree of internal rotation, and inversion of the tibiotalar joint [4]. Injuries occur with the ankle in plantarflexion and the ATFL is the first ligament to tear [5]. Although most lateral ligament injuries heal well with conservative management, a significant proportion of these injuries are associated with chronic symptoms of pain, swelling, and recurrent sprains [6].

Diagnostic imaging of lateral ankle injuries has two primary goals:

1. Assessment of ligament integrity.
2. Identification of associated injuries.

J. C. Lee (✉) · A. W. M. Mitchell
Fortius Clinic, London, UK
e-mail: Justin.lee@fortiusclinic.com;
adam.mitchell@fortiusclinic.com

L. Pesquer
Msk Imaging Department, Clinique du Sport de Bordeaux, Rue Georges Negrevergne, Merignac, France

The imaging modality of choice depends on the clinical presentation and time post-injury. In the acute setting, the patient may require plain radiographs to exclude bony injury according to the Ottawa rules (see below). If bony injury is not suspected, no imaging is required at the time of initial injury [7].

If the patient presents several weeks after initial injury, then the following investigations are indicated:

1. Plain radiography (X-ray).
2. Magnetic resonance imaging (MRI).
3. Ultrasound (US).
4. Computed tomography.

In this chapter, we will define the role of each imaging modality in both the acute and chronic presentation of lateral ankle instability.

5.2 Plain Radiography

In the acute setting, an X-ray of the ankle is indicated if there is a pain in the region of the malleoli and any one of the following:

1. Bone tenderness along the distal 6 cm of the posterior edge of the tibia or tip of the medial malleolus.
2. Bone tenderness along the distal 6 cm of the posterior edge of the fibula or tip of the lateral malleolus.

H. Pereira et al. (eds.), *Lateral Ankle Instability*, https://doi.org/10.1007/978-3-662-62763-1_5

3. An inability to bear weight both immediately and in the emergency department for at least four steps.

An X-ray of the foot is indicated if there is a pain in the midfoot region and any of the following:

1. Bone tenderness at the base of the fifth metatarsal.
2. Bone tenderness at the navicular bone.
3. An inability to bear weight both immediately and in the emergency department for four steps.

Applying these "Ottawa rules" has been shown to reduce the number of unnecessary radiographs and reduce attendance time within the emergency department [8].

In the chronic setting, plain radiographs are indicated to exclude missed fracture, assess ankle alignment, and to detect osteochondral lesions of the talus (OLTs). It should be noted that up to 50% of OLTs will be missed on plain radiographs [9].

Dynamic stress radiographs may also be used to assess laxity and instability of the hindfoot joints. The stress views can be performed manually or mechanically using a Telos device. In the chronic instability setting, the muscular defense reactions are not significantly inhibitory to affect the results [10]. Faure et al. demonstrated high specificity for the identification of deficient ATFL using equinovarus lateral opening of more than 10° degrees on the AP view and anterior talar drawer of more than 8 mm on the lateral view. The sensitivities were lower for each measurement (65% for AP talar tilt, 52% for anterior drawer, and 74% for both combined). The value of stress radiographs, therefore, is only appreciated when they are positive [11].

Fact Box 1

1. Plain film assessment of the ankle is not mandatory in the initial stage of injury management.
2. "Ottawa Rules" should be used to decide of early X-ray is needed and may avoid unnecessary advanced imaging if a fracture is detected.
3. Stress radiographs may be useful, particularly when positive.

5.3 Magnetic Resonance Imaging (MRI)

MRI is a noninvasive imaging modality that provides an accurate assessment of the soft-tissue and bony pathologies associated with lateral ankle instability [12]. The images acquired provide a global overview of the ankle which enhances image interpretation and understanding for the referring clinician. As mentioned above, the goal of imaging in both the acute and chronic setting is to identify injuries to the lateral/fibular collateral ligaments of the ankle and to detect associated chondral, osteochondral, and tendon injuries. In the acute setting, MRI is rarely indicated. However, in the elite athlete MRI should be performed early to determine injury severity with a view to guiding prognosis and anticipated return to play.

Although protocols vary across imaging centers, all studies should be able to answer the primary questions of ligament status and detection of associated injuries. Therefore, it is important that at least one fluid-sensitive sequence is acquired, i.e., Short Tau Inversion Recovery (STIR), fat-saturated T2 (FST2), or fat-saturated proton density (FSPD) weighted sequence [13]. Most centers will now acquire fluid-sensitive sequences in three orthogonal planes (axial, sagittal, and coronal) and it is advised that at least one T1-weighted series is acquired as this sequence is optimal for fracture detection. Finally, at least one cartilage-*sensitive* sequence should also be included. Cartilage-sensitive sequences include proton density (PD) and FSPD series while cartilage-*specific* sequences, which typically employ some variant of gradient echo acquisition, may also be used but these have generally lost favor as PD and FSPD images are not only able to assess the cartilage but also the ligaments and tendons at the same time [14]. A suggested MRI protocol for ankle imaging is given in Table 5.1.

Table 5.1 Appropriate ankle protocol at 1.5 T MRI

Sequence	FOV	Matrix	Slice thickness/interval	TR	TE	TI
Sagittal T1 SE	16–18	384×384	3 mm/1 mm	400–800	16	
Sagittal STIR	16–18	256×192	3 mm/1 mm	>1500	40	120
Axial PD TSE	14–16	384×384	3 mm/1 mm	3000	32	
Axial FSPD TSE	14–6	256×256	3 mm/1 mm	4000	33	
Coronal FSPD TSE	14	256×256	3 mm/1 mm	3400	37	

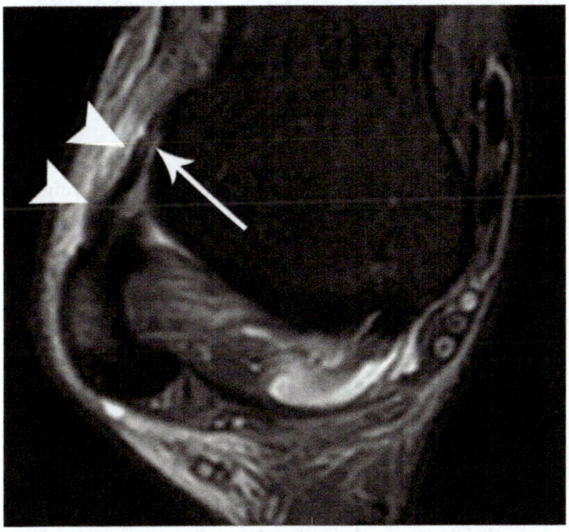

Fig. 5.1 Axial fat-saturated proton density-weighted MRI of the ankle. There is a partial tear of the talar attachment of the anterior talofibular ligament (arrow). The white arrowheads point out the typical edema pattern on the superficial surface of the ligament

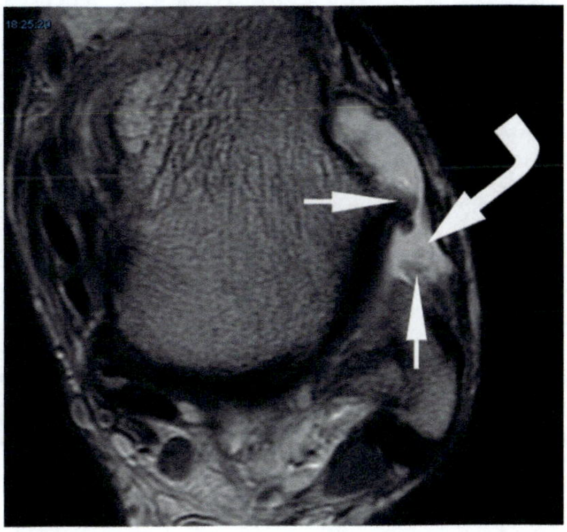

Fig. 5.2 Axial proton density-weighted MRI of the ankle. There is complete discontinuity of the anterior talofibular ligament (curved arrow). Small arrows delineate the retracted torn ligament ends

5.4 Primary Ligament Injury Findings on MRI

MRI has been shown to be a reliable tool in identifying and grading injuries to the lateral collateral ligaments of the ankle following acute inversion injury [15–17].

The diagnostic criteria for ligament injury on MRI include the following:

1. Increased ligament signal on fluid-sensitive sequences (FSPD, FST2, or STIR).
2. Complete or partial ligament discontinuity.
3. Irregularity or waviness of the ligament.

Grading of the lateral collateral ligament injuries is somewhat arbitrary but generally follows a three point system as follows [17]:

1. Grade 1: Increased signal within or surrounding the ligament on fluid-sensitive sequences.
2. Grade 2: As for grade 1 but the ligament also demonstrates partial discontinuity (Fig. 5.1).
3. Grade 3: As for grade 1 but the ligament also demonstrates complete discontinuity (Fig. 5.2).

In the chronic setting, the lateral collateral ligament complex follows the same diagnostic criteria as above but ligament size may be altered after healing. The ligament may become small by the process of cicatrization or, more commonly, heal by hypertrophic fibrosis producing a thickened cord-like appearance to the ligament (Fig. 5.3) [15]. Injuries to the ATFL are more accurately assessed on MRI than injuries to the CFL. Although studies have shown 100% specificity for the diagnosis of ATFL and CFL tears on

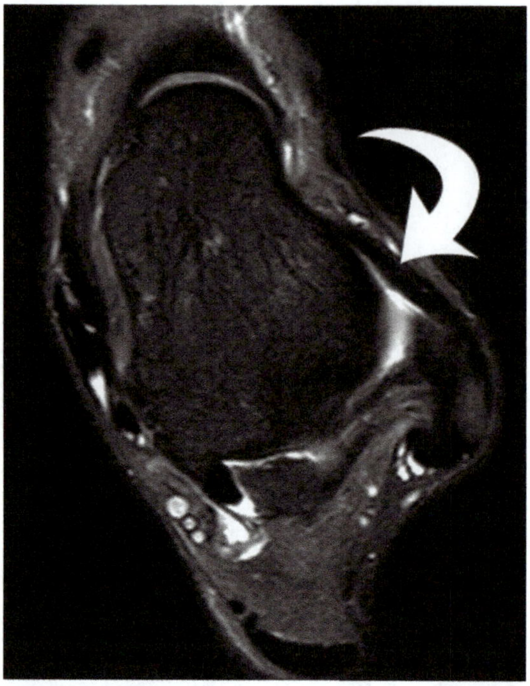

Fig. 5.3 Axial fat-saturated proton density-weighted MRI of the ankle. There is hypertrophic scarring of the anterior talofibular ligament (curved arrow). This is a common finding following previous injury

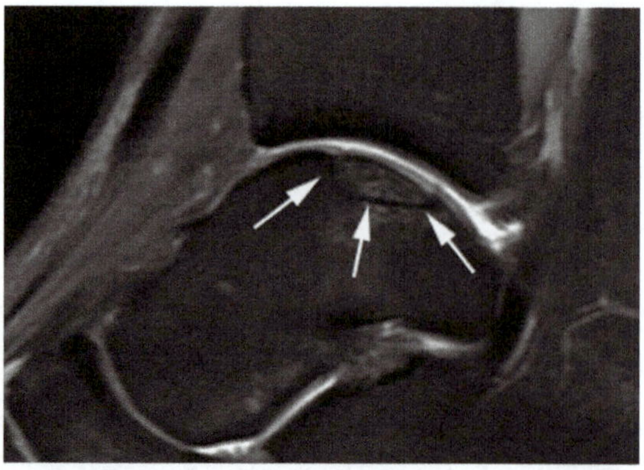

Fig. 5.4 Sagittal fat-saturated proton density-weighted MRI of the ankle. There is an osteochondral lesion of the talar dome (short arrows). The lack of fluid signal on the deep surface of the lesion indicates that this is a stable lesion

MRI compared to arthroscopy, the sensitivities are lower, particularly for CFL injuries with overall accuracy on MRI in detecting ATFL tears of 91.7% and CFL tears of 87.5% [18].

5.5 Secondary Lesions on MRI

MRI has been shown to be a useful tool in the preoperative setting in cases of chronic ankle instability [19]. Due to altered biomechanics within the joint, chronic lateral instability is associated with several other pathologies within the ankle including chondral and osteochondral lesions, loose bodies, anterolateral impingement, concomitant ligamentous injuries, and peroneal tendon pathology. Published data suggests that the specificity of MRI in detecting the majority of these lesions is high but the sensitivity is low and negative MRI in cases of chronic ankle instability should be viewed with caution by the referring clinician [20]. O'Neill et al. demonstrated an overall sensitivity for detecting lesions was 45% with chondral lesions identified preoperatively in 39% only (Fig. 5.4). Despite using high-field strength 3 T MRI, Staats et al. similarly demonstrated high specificity in the detection of secondary lesions but low sensitivity for additional ligamentous lesions, loose bodies, and chondral injuries [21].

Fact Box 2

1. MRI provides an accurate global overview of the ankle.
2. Sequence selection is key to answer the clinical question and should always include at least one fluid-sensitive sequence.
3. MRI can accurately detect injuries to the lateral collateral ligament complex both in the acute and chronic setting.
4. MRI is the optimal imaging tool to assess the secondary injuries associated with lateral ankle instability.
5. MRI is indicated early in the management of the elite athlete to assess injury severity, guide prognosis, and assist with an estimated return to play.

5.6 Computed Tomography (CT)

CT of the ankle following acute trauma is indicated for the following:

1. To delineate fracture configuration if the fracture appears complex on plain radiographs.
2. To provide an axial assessment of the inferior tibiofibular congruity in cases of syndesmosis injury.

In the chronic ankle instability setting, CT is indicated for the following:

1. Identification of marginal bone spurs.
2. Identification of intra-articular loose bodies.
3. To assess hindfoot alignment.
4. To assess the size of an OLT prior to surgery.
5. When combined with arthrography, the identification of chondral injuries and grading of osteochondral lesions (Fig. 5.5).

Dynamic stress CT of the ankle has also been shown to be useful in chronic ankle instability with some advantages over stress radiography including the identification of joint space narrowing, irregular and hypertrophic new bone formation at the middle subtalar joint. Furthermore, stress radiographs may artificially overestimate the degree of subtalar tilt due to changes in translatory and rotatory movements rather than true opening [22].

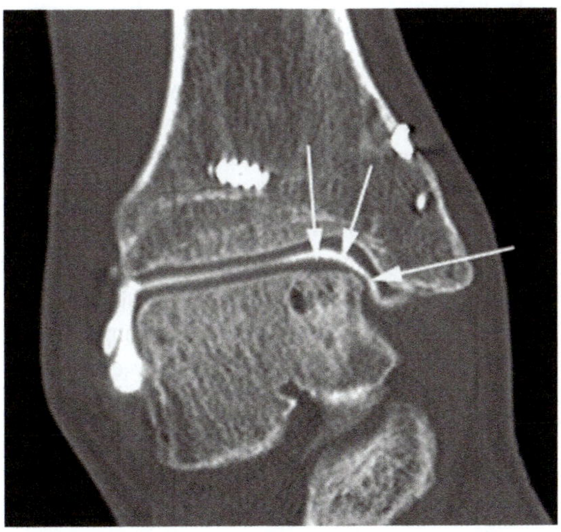

Fig. 5.5 Coronal reconstruction CT arthrogram. The intra-articular contrast is confined to the joint cavity and does not penetrate the articular cartilage indication stable osteochondral lesion

CT arthrography (CTA) can directly identify injuries to the ATFL by non-visualization and can indirectly assess injuries to the calcaneofibular ligament by distension of the peroneal tendon sheath with extravasation of intra-articular contrast [11]. CTA may also identify capsular adhesions, loose bodies, and occult bone injuries.

5.7 Ultrasound (US)

US is a noninvasive, cheap, widely available imaging modality which can be readily performed after acute trauma and physical examination [4]. US has excellent temporal and spatial resolution allowing accurate assessment of superficial structures [23]. US is the only modality which can provide dynamic imaging assessment for the distinction between partial and full-thickness tears and tendinous snapping [24].

The goal of US is to assess the ankle ligaments, especially the anterior talofibular ligament (ATFL) and the calcaneofibular (CFL) ligaments [5]. The posterior talofibular ligament is rarely torn and is more difficult to assess with US [25]. Associated injuries such as joint effusion and tendinitis may also be detected readily in US [26]. The study is performed with the patient lying on a bed in a supine position, with the knee of the relevant leg flexed 90° and with the foot sightly internally rotated using a high-frequency (15–20 MHz) superficial probe [2, 5, 6]. The use of a standardized method may help reduce the operator dependence of US [23, 26].

5.7.1 Anterior Talofibular Ligament

The ATFL is assessed with axial and sagittal slices. The ankle must be positioned with a maximal degree of inversion and internal rotation in order to stretch the ligament (Fig. 5.6). The ATFL

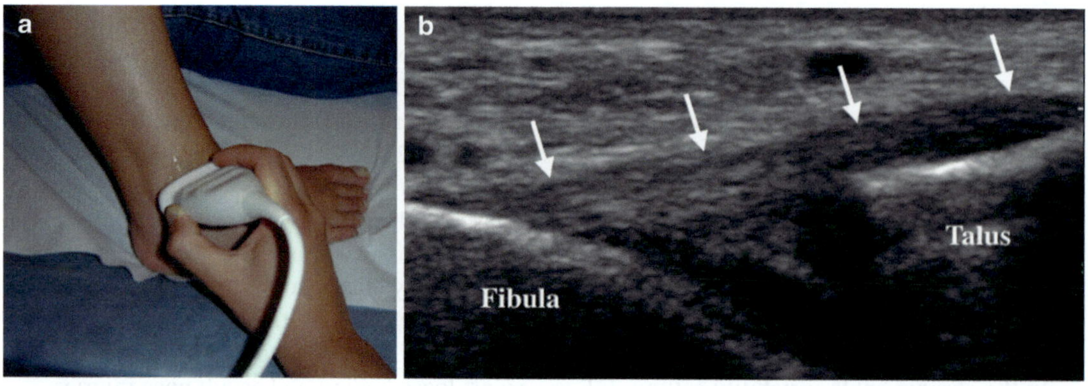

Fig. 5.6 Normal appearance of the ATFL. Probe position (**a**) and normal fibrillar aspect of the ATFL (arrows) in an asymptomatic athlete (**b**)

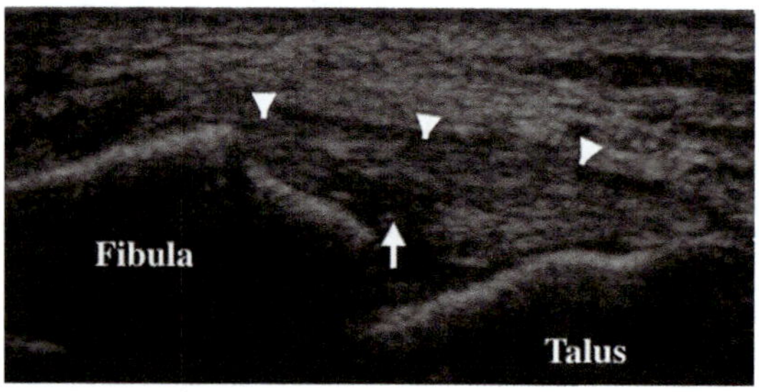

Fig. 5.7 Partial tear of the ATFL. US axial image shows normal continuity of the ligament (arrowheads) with partial-thickness tear at the proximal and deep aspect of the ligament (arrow)

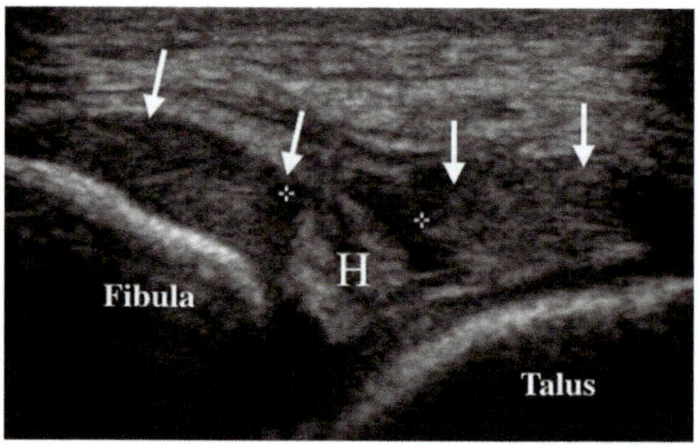

Fig. 5.8 Complete tear of the ATFL. US axial image reveals that the ligament (arrows) appears thickened with discontinuity and hematoma (H) of the middle-third

is a fibrillar structure which runs from the anterolateral border of the tip of the fibula until the lateral side of the talus [27]. On its superficial aspect, a small artery and vein may be identified whereas on its deep aspect lies the anterolateral gutter where a small amount of fluid may be present [25]. After acute inversion injury, an isolated ATFL tear is encountered in 70% of the patients, with combined tears of ATFL and CFL occurring in 30% of cases [26]. Axial slices are more useful than sagittal slices. In case of ligamentous stretching, the ligament appears thickened and hypoechoic but its continuity remains intact (Fig. 5.7). Hyperemia on color Doppler ultrasound is usually observed. If the tear is recent, the free edges of the ligament are separated by a heterogeneous area which consists of an accumulation of joint fluid mixed with blood (Fig. 5.8). When the tear is not obvious, dynamic maneuvers can be performed in order to increase the size of the tear and to ensure the diagnosis of a full-thickness tear [5, 23, 26]. Dynamic maneuvers must be performed carefully to avoid the onset of pain and a muscular contraction that would limit the range of motion. To stress the ATFL, the examiner may use the anterior drawer test: the patient must lie on the examination bed in a prone position and the ankle must be slowly positioned at a maximal degree of plantarflexion and internal rotation [26]. In a study comparing the accuracy of imaging versus arthroscopy, US and MRI showed an accuracy of 91 and 97% [28]. Superficial hematoma communicating with the tibiotalar joint may be observed in case of capsular tear. Avulsion fracture is not rare and may involve periosteum or cortical bone. According to the study of Haraguchi, it was diagnosed in 26% of the 169 patients and was most common among children and patients over 40 years of age [29].

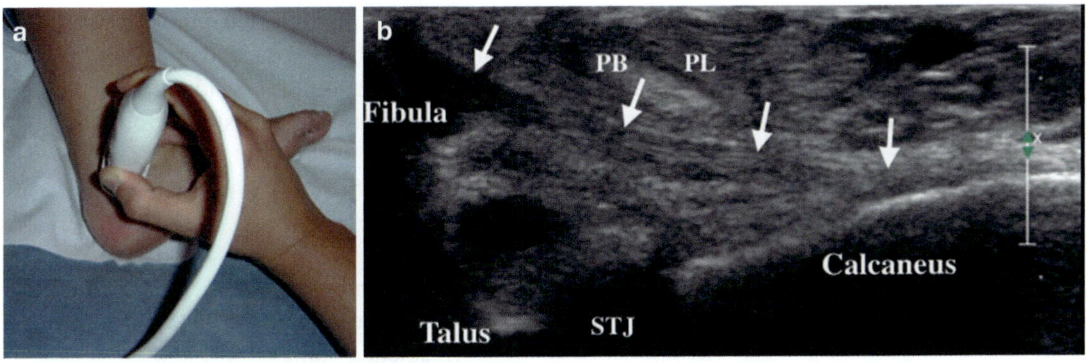

Fig. 5.9 Normal appearance of the CFL. Probe position (**a**) and normal fibrillar aspect of the CFL (arrows) in an asymptomatic athlete (**b**). *PB* Peroneus brevis, *PL* Peroneus longus, *STJ* Subtalar joint

5.7.2 Calcaneofibular Ligament

The CFL is assessed with axial and longitudinal slices when putting the ankle in forced dorsiflexion [23]. It is a fibrillar structure which runs between the distal tip of the fibula and the lateral side of the calcaneus and crosses both the talocrural and talocalcaneal joints [27]. It has an oblique course and is slightly concave (Fig. 5.9). Peroneal tendons lie on its surface at their inframalleolar course [23]. Deep to the ligament, the posterior subtalar joint can be observed and joint effusion may be noted. It is important to avoid anisotropy artifact caused by the spontaneous concave course of ligament and/or a prominent lateral malleolus which may suggest that a tear is present due to loss of reflectivity within the curved ligament [23, 25]. In that case, care should be taken that dorsiflexion is sufficient and the examiner should use more gel in order to place the beam in a parallel position to the ligament. Tears occur mainly at the proximal or middle third of the ligament and are usually hypoechoic (Fig. 5.10) [26]. The distinction between a partial and a full-thickness tear may be difficult and the use of dynamic maneuvers is sometimes useful to provide a correct diagnosis. Dorsiflexion of the ankle displaces and rotates the peroneal tendons when the CFL is normal. The lack of peroneal tendon displacement is an indirect sign of tear [25]. The presence of fluid within the sheath of the peroneal tendons is often associated with a full-thickness tear of the ligament. Sometimes, the tear extends until the superior peroneal retinaculum and may contribute to the onset of a peroneal tendon snapping [24]. Periosteal or cortical avulsions are common and occur mainly at the proximal insertion [29].

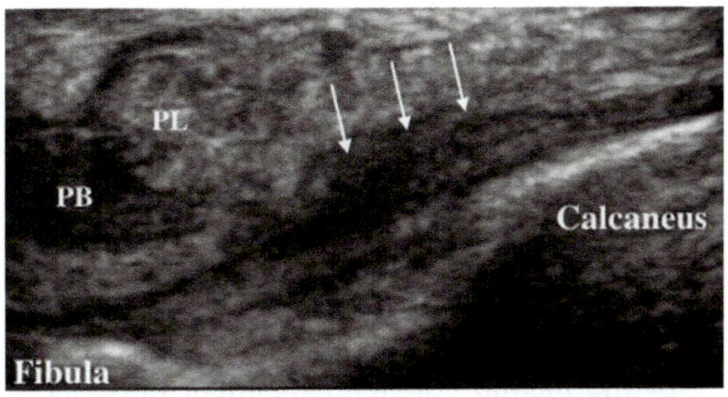

Fig. 5.10 Partial tear of the CFL. US longitudinal image shows a hypoechoic thickening of the distal third of the ligament (arrows)

5.7.3 Chronic Ligamentous Tears

Repeated injuries may lead to progressive thinning of the ligament or insufficient healing and progressive instability. Sometimes, calcifications and ossifications may involve the ligaments or the capsule and can represent a pitfall for the radiologist [26]. Color Doppler may help to rule out synovitis due to an incomplete healing or an anterolateral impingement [30]. CFL is sometimes thinned or stretched and its failure may lead to instability, especially at the subtalar joint. Dynamic examination consists in assess the CFL in dorsiflexion to see if it lifts the peroneal tendons or not.

5.7.4 Injury Classification

Martinoli described a 4-grade injury classification using ultrasound [26]:

1. Grade 1: stretching or partial tear of the ATFL.
2. Grade 2: complete tear of the ATFL.
3. Grade 3: complete tear of the ATFL with a partial tear of the CFL.
4. Grade 4: complete tear of the ATFL and CFL.

Grade 1 and 2 injuries usually heal after conservative treatment including rest, cast, and physiotherapy for 4–6 weeks. Grade 3 and 4 injuries may lead to tibiotalar instability and may require surgical treatment [26].

5.7.5 Associated Injuries Assessable on US

- Medial collateral ligament strain: After lateral ankle ligament injury, contrecoup contusion of the medial collateral ligament may occur. US may show a loss of the fibrillar aspect of the ligament and hyperemia on color Doppler which is usually located at the anterior tibiotalar fascicle [30].
- Anterior inferior tibiofibular ligament (AiTFL): Part of the tibiofibular syndesmosis but requires a different mechanism by eversion and external rotation to be torn [31]. The ligament is optimally assessed by tilting the probe 70° from the horizontal plane.
- Dorsal lateral ligaments of the midfoot: The calcaneocuboid ligament and dorsal talonavicular ligament can be easily assessed by US [25].
- Tibiotalar and subtalar joint: Effusions can be seen in US especially in presence of loose bodies or if bone marrow edema is detected on the correlation MRI [25].

5.8 Conclusion

In conclusion, US provides a detailed depiction of normal anatomic structures and is effective for evaluating ligament injuries. US is the only tool to allow us to perform dynamic maneuvers. Its accuracy is high but is dependent on the operator experience. The use of a standardized method is required to improve diagnostic performance.

Fact Box 3

1. Ultrasound is the only truly dynamic way of assessing the lateral collateral ligament complex of the ankle.
2. Although operator dependency and experience are important, a standardized approach may minimize error.
3. Patient positioning is key to accurate ultrasound assessment.
4. US can be used to grade the injury severity and guide prognosis.
5. US can be used to detect secondary injuries associated with lateral ankle instability but cannot assess the articular cartilage of the ankle.

Take-Home Messages

1. Inversion injuries are common in both the elite athlete and the general population.
2. Although not all ankle injuries require urgent imaging, there are clearly defined criteria in the form of the "Ottawa Rules" for those who require X-ray in the initial stages of injury management.
3. Advanced imaging is indicated in the elite athlete in the early stage to guide prognosis.
4. MRI and CT scan provide accurate global assessment of the internal and external structures of the ankle.
5. Ultrasound (US) provides an accurate dynamic assessment of the ligamentous stabilizers of the ankle.

References

1. Campbell SE, Warner M. MR imaging of ankle inversion injuries. Magn Reson Imaging Clin N Am. 2008;16:1–18.

2. Garrick JG, Requa RK. The epidemiology of foot and ankle injuries in sports. Clin Podiatr Med Surg. 1989;6:629–37.
3. Yeung MS, Chan KM, So CH, et al. An epidemiological survey on ankle sprain. Br J Sports Med. 1994;28:112–6.
4. van Dijk CN, Mol BW, Lim LS, Marti RK, Bossuyt PM. Diagnosis of ligament rupture of the ankle joint. Physical examination, arthrography, stress radiography and sonography compared in 160 patients after inversion trauma. Acta Orthop Scand. 1996;67(6):566–70.
5. Golanó P, Vega J, de Leeuw PA, Malagelada F, Manzanares MC, Götzens V, van Dijk CN. Anatomy of the ankle ligaments: a pictorial essay. Knee Surg Sports Traumatol Arthrosc. 2016;24:944–56.
6. Konradsen L, Bech L, Ehrenbjerg M, et al. Seven years follow-up after ankle inversion trauma. Scand J Med Sci Sports. 2002;12:129–35.
7. Stiell IG, Greenberg GH, McKnight RD, Nair RC, McDowell I, Worthington JR. A study to develop clinical decision rules for the use of radiography in acute ankle injuries. Ann Emerg Med. 1992;21(4):384–90.
8. Stiell I, Wells G, Laupacis A, et al. Multicentre trial to introduce the Ottawa ankle rules for use of radiography in acute ankle injuries. Multicentre Ankle Rule Study Group. BMJ. 1995;311:594–7.
9. Loomer R, Fisher C, Lloyd-Smith R, Sisler J, Cooney T. Osteochondral lesions of the talus. Am J Sports Med. 1993;21:13–9.
10. Frost SC, Amendola A. Is stress radiography necessary in the diagnosis of acute or chronic ankle instability? Clin J Sport Med. 1999;9:40–5.
11. Faure C, Deplus F, Besse JL, Moyen B, Bochu M. Instabilités chroniques externes de la cheville. Apport des radiographies dynamiques, de la tomodensitométrie et de l'arthro-tomodensitométrie. J Radiol. 1997;78:629–34.
12. Watson AD. Ankle instability and impingement. Foot Ankle Clin. 2007;12:177–95.
13. Sofka CM. Technical considerations: best practices for MR imaging of the foot and ankle. Magn Reson Imaging Clin N Am. 2017;25:1–10.
14. Siriwanarangsun P, Bae WC, Statum S, Chung VB. Advanced MRI techniques for the ankle. AJR Am J Roentgenol. 2017;209:511–24.
15. Erickson SJ, Smith JW, Ruiz ME, Fitzgerald SW, Kneeland JB, Johnson JE, et al. MR imaging of the lateral collateral ligament of the ankle. AJR Am J Roentgenol. 1991;156:131–6.
16. Kreitner KF, Ferber A, Grebe P, Runkel M, Berger S, Thelen M. Injuries of the lateral collateral ligaments of the ankle: assessment with MR imaging. Eur Radiol. 1999;9:519–24.
17. Cardone BW, Erickson SJ, Den Hartog BD, Carrera GF. MRI of injury to the lateral collateral ligamentous complex of the ankle. J Comput Assist Tomogr. 1993;17(1):102–7.
18. Joshy S, Abdulkadir U, Chaganti S, Sullivan B, Hariharan K. Accuracy of MRI scan in the diagnosis of ligamentous and chondral pathology in the ankle. Foot Ankle Surg. 2010;16:78–80.
19. O'Neill PJ, Van Aman SE, Guyton GP. Is MRI adequate to detect lesions in patients with ankle instability. Clin Orthop Relat Res. 2009;468:1115–9.
20. Cha SD, Kim HS, Chung ST, Yoo JH, Park JH, Kim JH, Hyung JW. Intra-articular lesions in chronic lateral ankle instability: comparison of arthroscopy with magnetic resonance imaging findings. Clin Orthop Surg. 2012;4:293–9.
21. Staats K, Sabeti-Aschraf M, Apprich S, et al. Preoperative MRI is helpful but not sufficient to detect associated lesions in patients with chronic ankle instability. Knee Surg Sports Traumatol Arthrosc. 2017;26:2103. https://doi.org/10.1007/s00167-017-4567-x.
22. Van Hellemondt FJ, Louwerens JW, Sijbrandij ES, van Gils AP. Stress radiography and stress examination of the talocrural and subtalar joint on helical computed tomography. Foot Ankle Int. 1997;18:482–8.
23. Peetrons P, Creteur V, Bacq C. Sonography of ankle ligaments. J Clin Ultrasound. 2004;32:491–9.
24. Pesquer L, Guillo S, Poussange N, Pele E, Meyer P, Dallaudière B. Dynamic ultrasound of peroneal tendon instability. Br J Radiol. 2016 Jul;89(1063):20150958. https://doi.org/10.1259/bjr.20150958.
25. Sconfienza LM, Orlandi D, Lacelli F, Serafini G, Silvestri E. Dynamic high-resolution US of ankle and midfoot ligaments: normal anatomic structure and imaging technique. Radiographics. 2015;35(1):164–78. https://doi.org/10.1148/rg.351130139.
26. Martinoli C, Bianchi S. Ankle. In: Bianchi S, Martinoli C, editors. Ultrasound of the musculoskeletal system. Milan, Italy: Springer; 2099. p. 773–834.
27. De Maeseneer M, Marcelis S, Jager T, et al. Sonography of the normal ankle: a target approach using skeletal reference points. AJR Am J Roentgenol. 2009;192(2):487–95.
28. Oae K, Takao M, Uchio Y, Ochi M. Evaluation of anterior talofibular ligament injury with stress radiography, ultrasonography and MR imaging. Skelet Radiol. 2010 Jan;39(1):41–7. https://doi.org/10.1007/s00256-009-0767-x.
29. Haraguchi N, Toga H, Shiba N, et al. Avulsion fracture of the lateral ankle ligament complex in severe inversion injury: incidence and clinical outcome. Am J Sports Med. 2007;35(7):1144–52. https://doi.org/10.1177/0363546507299531.
30. Pesquer L, Guillo S, Meyer P, Hauger O. US in ankle impingement syndrome. J Ultrasound. 2013;17(2):89–97. https://doi.org/10.1007/s40477-013-0054-5.
31. Clanton TO, Paul P. Syndesmosis injuries in athletes. Foot Ankle Clin. 2002;7(3):529–49.

Microinstability of the Ankle

6

Jordi Vega, Erik Montesinos, Francesc Malagelada, Matteo Guelfi, Albert Baduell, and Miki Dalmau-Pastor

6.1 Introduction

Microinstability, although a common diagnosis in other joints, is an emerging concept among the potential causes of ankle pain and disability.

Microinstability of the ankle may result from an injury to the superior fascicle of the anterior talofibular ligament (ATFL) [1–3]. During an ankle supination-inversion injury, the superior fascicle of the ATFL is injured first and it is often in isolation. With poor healing of the ligament, a minor restraining deficit of the ligament is produced, with microinstability of the ankle as a consequence.

A tear of ATFL's superior fascicle results in an increased movement of the talus with respect to the tibia. A subtle talar anterior translation in combination with internal rotation may be observed with ankle intra-articular damage as a secondary consequence. The presence of bone and soft-tissue impingement syndromes, lesions of the talar cartilage, deltoid ligament symptoms, or a combination of them all together with a history of ankle inversion sprains should raise the suspicion of ankle microinstability.

Classically, two types of ankle instability have been described: functional and mechanical. Functional instability has been defined as the subjective feeling of ankle instability, recurrent symptomatic ankle sprains or both, without evidence of a ligament injury [4]. Mechanical instability is defined as ankle movement beyond the normal physiologic limit of the ankle's range of

J. Vega (✉)
Foot and Ankle Unit, iMove-Tres Torres and Hospital Quirón Barcelona, Barcelona, Spain

Laboratory of Arthroscopic and Surgical Anatomy, Department of Pathology and Experimental Therapeutics (Human Anatomy Unit), University of Barcelona, Barcelona, Spain

Groupe de Recherche et d'Etude en Chirurgie Mini-Invasive du Pied (GRECMIP), Merignac, France
e-mail: jordivega@hotmail.com

E. Montesinos
Orthopaedic and Trauma Surgery, Clinique CIC Riviera, Clarens, Vaud, Switzerland

F. Malagelada
Foot and Ankle Unit, Department of Trauma and Orthopaedic Surgery, Royal London Hospital, Barts Health NHS Trust, London, UK

M. Guelfi
Casa di Cura Villa Montallegro, Genoa, Italy

Department of Orthopaedic Surgery "Gruppo Policlinico di Monza", Clinica Salus, Alessandria, Italy

A. Baduell
Orthopaedic and Trauma Surgery, Hospital Clinic, Barcelona, Spain

M. Dalmau-Pastor
Laboratory of Arthroscopic and Surgical Anatomy, Department of Pathology and Experimental Therapeutics (Human Anatomy Unit), University of Barcelona, Barcelona, Spain

Groupe de Recherche et d'Etude en Chirurgie Mini-Invasive du Pied (GRECMIP), Merignac, France

H. Pereira et al. (eds.), *Lateral Ankle Instability*, https://doi.org/10.1007/978-3-662-62763-1_6

motion. It is usually the result of a ligament injury affecting the lateral collateral ligament, and the instability is easily demonstrable during clinical examination. Microinstability of the ankle is considered as a subtle degree of mechanical ankle instability. Because of the similarities in clinical presentation, it is possible that some patients with functional instability have a component of microinstability. Our hypothesis is that in these cases the ligament injury is not observed in imaging studies, because present-day imaging techniques are not sensitive enough to detect such a subtle tear of ATFL's superior fascicle although it may be observed intraoperatively.

6.2 Pathomechanism

The currently proposed pathomechanism of ankle microinstability is a partial tear of the ATFL as the result of an ankle sprain [1–3].

Ankle sprains are one of the most common injuries and frequently occurs during sports [5–7]. With ankle supination-inversion [8], the ATFL is the first ligament, and in some instances the only one to suffer an injury. During this injury, the rupture of the superior fascicle of the ATFL is followed by damage to the inferior ATFL fascicle and to the calcaneofibular ligament (CFL), with the posterior talofibular ligament rarely being affected [9, 10]. Rupture of a branch of the peroneal artery located between the superior and inferior fascicles of the ATFL indicates a complete rupture of the superior fascicle. Rupture of this artery causes the lateral hematoma observed during the physical examination and this indicates that there is not just a "simple ankle sprain" but there is a significant ankle ligament rupture which requires appropriate treatment.

The ATFL is the weakest component of the lateral collateral ligament of the ankle, and the superior fascicle is its weakest point [11, 12]. The superior fascicle of the ATFL restricts anterior translation and internal rotation of the talus when the ankle is in plantar flexion. Therefore, with a deficit of this ligament, an anterior translation in addition to an internal talar rotation may be observed with the plantarflexed ankle without symptomatic giving way of the ankle joint.

6.3 Symptomatology

Ankle microinstability is poorly defined as a clinical entity. The lack of consistent objective findings on clinical examination contributes to its poor definition.

Although a partial tear of the ATFL can be observed in most of the patients after an ankle sprain, microinstability of the ankle is usually symptomatic only in patients with a moderate or high level of physical activity. When patients become symptomatic, they describe a subjective feeling of ankle instability, recurrent symptomatic ankle sprains, chronic anterolateral pain, or a combination of them all.

Chronic anterolateral ankle symptoms such as soft-tissue impingement and mechanical instability are a frequent scenario after an ankle supination-inversion sprain [7, 13–15]. At least two-thirds of the patients with the diagnosis of anterolateral soft-tissue impingement syndrome have a partial tear of the ATFL. However, half of the patients with anterolateral ankle pain after an ankle sprain do not have any soft-tissue mass on the lateral recess that could explain this pain and microinstability resulting from the partial tear of the ATFL may explain their complaints [1–3].

Although patients may give a clear history of a feeling of ankle insecurity and repeated ankle sprains, the ATLF injury may not be severe enough to enable clinical detection of instability with a positive anterior draw sign. There may be a subtle laxity of the ankle during ankle plantarflexion which may be compared to the contralateral side. Because of this characteristic subtle instability in plantarflexion, the wearing of high-heel shoes as well as walking on tiptoes are frequently not well tolerated.

6.4 Diagnosis

Diagnosis of ankle microinstability is based mainly on a thorough patient history and physical examination to rule out the presence of traditional instability. The magnitude of the displacement during ankle examination (anterior ankle drawer test, talar tilt test, and tibiotalar posterior drawer test) should be compared with the healthy contralateral side.

As the ATFL restricts anterior translation and the internal rotation of the talus when the ankle is in plantar flexion, a maneuver is proposed to evaluate patients with high suspicion of ankle microinstability (the tibiotalar posterior drawer test). With the patient lying on the examining table, the hip and the knee are flexed at 90° allowing the foot to fully rest on the table; thus, the ankle is plantarflexed, without any degree of rotation. In this position, the tibia is pushed posteriorly. If the tibia and fibula translate to posterior the test indicates a superior ATFL fascicle rupture. However, as the test can also be positive for patients with classical ankle instability, a second maneuver is performed. Without changing the patient positioning, the tibia and fibula are then pushed proximally intending to distract the tibiotalar joint. If the tibia separates from the talus the test indicates that the injury includes the inferior ATFL fascicle and also the CFL (Fig. 6.1a and b).

Stress radiographic evaluation will not show any signs of instability and is therefore not useful.

Conventional MRIs are rarely helpful for the diagnosis as they do not show the partially exposed footprint of ATFL attachment onto the fibula. A nonspecific abnormality of the ATFL may be observed but the main objective of MRI in microinstablity is to indentify concomitant injuries and indirect sings to support the diagnosis. Since the patient is lying supine with the heel on the table during an MRI examination, anterior translation of the lateral area of the talus, with no translation of its medial area, indicates ankle microinstability due to an injury to the superior fascicle of the ATFL (Fig. 6.2). Some unstable ankles present with rupture of the posterior tibiotalar capsule, allowing synovial fluid to access the synovial sheath of the flexor hallucis longus tendon. When a large amount of synovial fluid exists, it may also allow for observation of the ligament detachment from the fibular malleolus (Fig. 6.3).

If there is a strong suspicion of ankle microinstability and the MRI fails to demonstrate any ligament injury or signs of associated injuries seen in ankle instability, an MRI with intra-articular contrast is recommended. The contrast enables identification of ATFL ligament detachment or partial rupture.

The radiologist or evaluating surgeon needs to have a high level of suspicion to detect all these

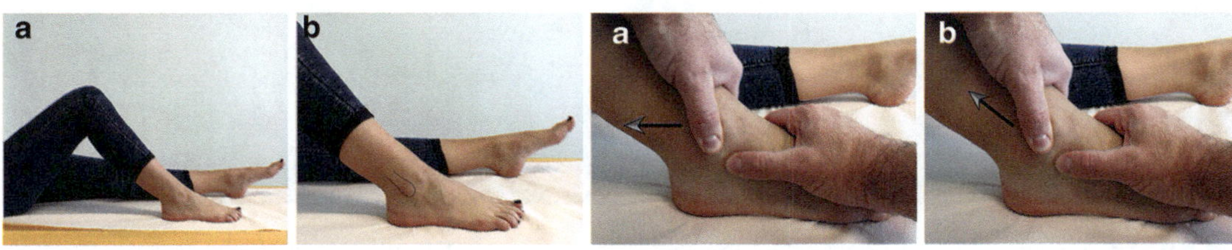

Fig. 6.1 The tibiotalar posterior drawer test. (**1a**) Positioning of the patient (**a**). Anterior distal tibia and fibula are recognized (**b**). (**1b**) One of the hands hold the foot and the other hand is positioned in the anterior area of the distal tibia and fibula. A posterior tibia translation indicates a superior ATFL fascicle rupture (**a**). If tibia separates from the talus the test indicates an injury including the inferior ATFL fascicle and the CFL (**b**)

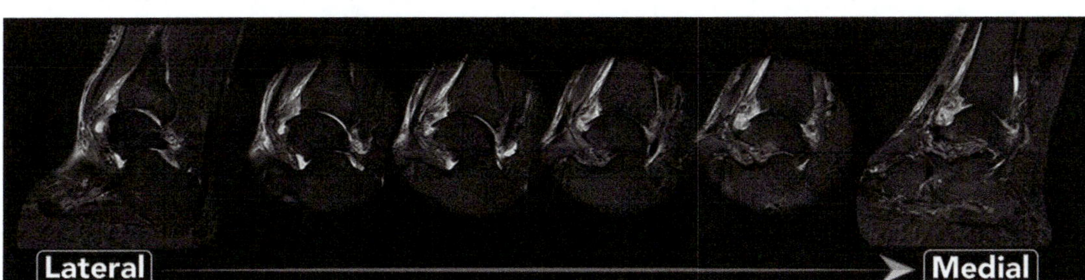

Fig. 6.2 Ankle MRI sequence in a patient with ankle microinstability, observing anterior translation of the lateral area of the talus, with no translation of its medial area

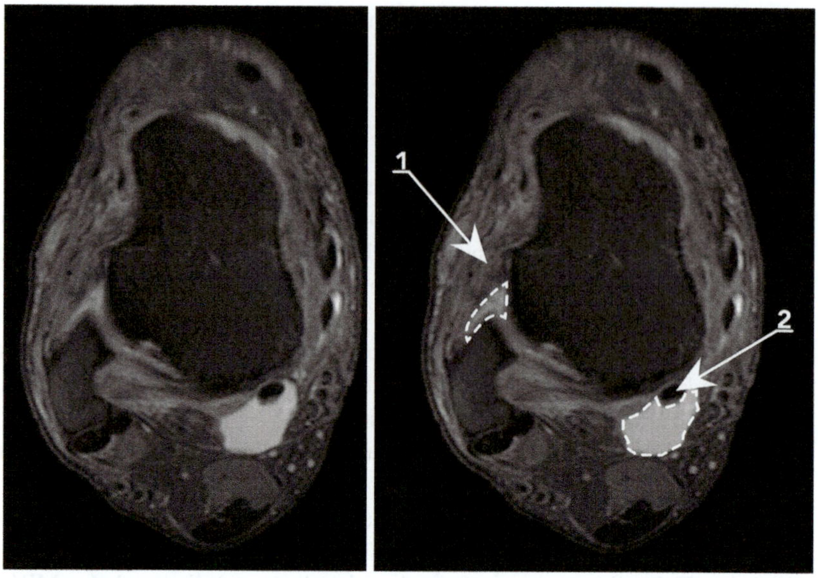

Fig. 6.3 Ankle MRI observing synovial fluid inside the synovial sheath of the flexor hallucis longus tendon, and accessing the superior ATFL fascicle detachment at the fibular malleolus. (1) Superior ATFL fascicle. (2) Flexor hallucis longus tendon

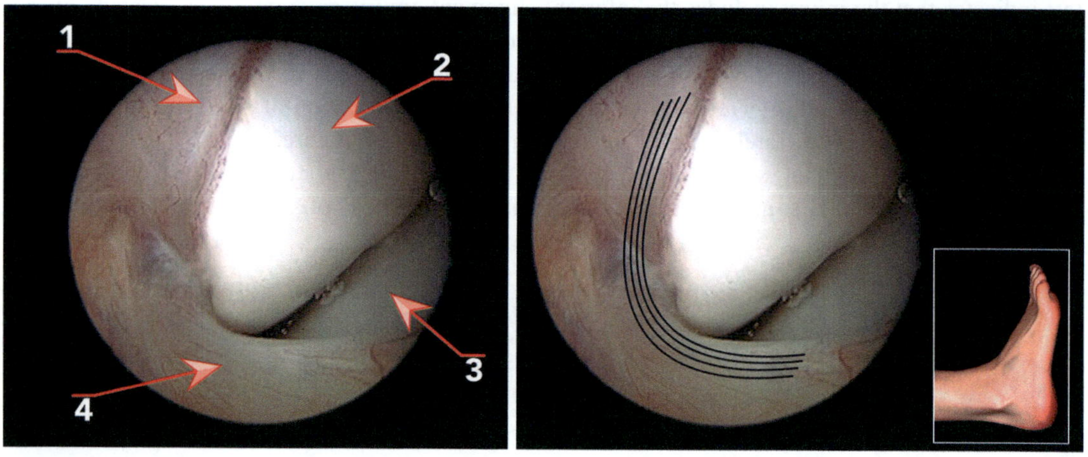

Fig. 6.4 Arthroscopic view in the right ankle. The ankle is dorsiflexed, and the scope is introduced through the anteromedial portal and directed to the lateral gutter. The fibular origin of the superior fascicle of the ATFL is seen in continuity of the distal fascicle of the anterior tibiofibular ligament. (1) Distal fascicle of the anterior tibiofibular ligament. (2) Lateral malleolus. (3) Lateral wall of the talus. (4) Superior ATFL fascicle

minor lesions. However, when ankle microinstability is suspected, and no imaging studies demonstrate the ligament tear, an arthroscopic evaluation can be useful.

A systematic arthroscopic examination of the ankle is mandatory for each ankle to ensure that no intra-articular pathology is missed. In cases with synovitis or adhesions in the lateral gutter, the occupying soft-tissue mass should be carefully debrided to visualize the ATFL without injuring the ligamentous structures. In the dorsiflexion and non-distraction arthroscopic technique, the superior fascicle of the ATFL lies as a hammock from the fibula to the talar neck occupying the floor of the lateral gutter. Its fibular origin has a close relationship with the fibular attachment of the distal fascicle of the anterior tibiofibular ligament which can be also observed during ankle arthroscopy (Fig. 6.4). Due to different anatomical characteristics of the ATFL in their insertional areas, the fibular attachment of the ligament is weaker than the talar [16]. Consequently, the fibular insertional area is the commonest location for ATFL injuries. Because of that, when the superior fascicle of the ATFL is injured, a gap or a denudated area in the anterior

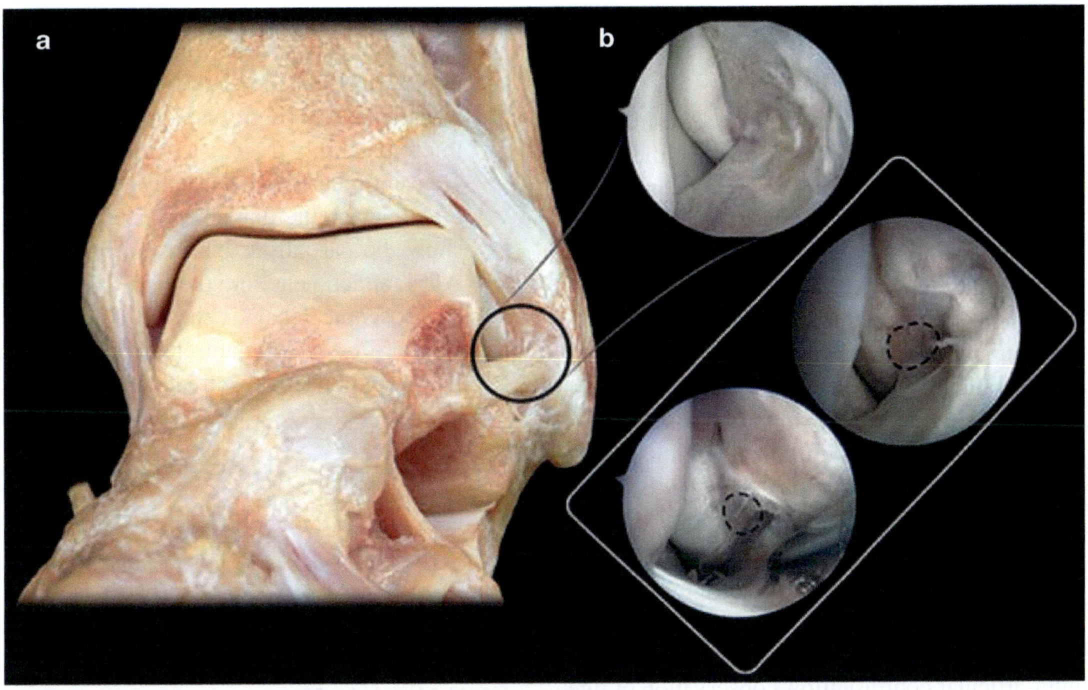

Fig. 6.5 A gap or a denudated area in the anterior part of the lateral malleolus is observed during ankle arthroscopy in patients with ankle microinstability. (**a**) Anatomic and arthroscopic view of the normal lateral gutter. (**b**) Arthroscopic view of two different patients with a partial detachment of the superior ATFL fascicle. A fibular bare area distal to the fibular insertion of the distal fascicle of the anterior tibiofibular ligament is observed and indicated with dotted line

part of the lateral malleolus is observed during ankle arthroscopy. Arthroscopic diagnosis of superior fascicle ATFL injury includes: discontinuity or avulsion of the ligament at its fibular insertion with or without fibrous tissue; observation of a fibular bare area distal to the fibular insertion of the distal fascicle of the anterior tibiofibular ligament that corresponds to the ligament footprint; an abnormal course of the ligament with a decrease in the ligament tension (Fig. 6.5).

6.5 Treatment

As in other joints, microinstability of the ankle should initially be treated with conservative measures, including proprioceptive training and strengthening of the muscles about the ankle. A minimum of 3 months of physiotherapy is recommended before assuming that conservative treatment has failed and surgical treatment should be proposed.

The surgical treatment of ankle microinstability should focus on addressing the underlying etiology (injury of ATFL superior fascicle), and associated intra-articular (chondral-osteochondral lesion, osteophytes, soft-tissue impingement, anterior deltoid ligament tear) and/or extra-articular pathology (intrasheath subluxation of the peroneal tendons, peroneal tendons tear, posterior impingement syndrome). Any associated pathology should be treated first. Finally, the ATFL tear is addressed. As in open techniques, several arthroscopic options to restore ankle stability have been proposed. Although other arthroscopic or open techniques would probably solve the problem, the anatomic all-inside repair of the ligament tear under direct arthroscopic visualization is preferred [3, 17–19]. The advantages of the arthroscopic all-inside repair include its minimally invasive approach and the possibility to treat concomitant intra-articular pathology through the same portals. In addition, the all-inside repair respects the original anatomy of the ligament and allows the surgeon to use the native ligamentous tissue, which ensures that the biomechanical properties of the ligament remain intact. This contrasts with the reconstruction techniques.

6.6 Conclusion—Take-Home Message

Microinstability of the ankle is the result of an injury affecting the superior fascicle of the ATFL, following an ankle sprain. A subtle talar anterior translation in combination with internal rotation when the ankle is in plantarflexion results from partial injury to the ATFL.

Patients with ankle microinstability can be asymptomatic, or describe a subjective feeling of ankle instability/insecurity, recurrent symptomatic ankle sprains, chronic anterolateral pain, or a combination of these symptoms. Eventually secondary ankle intra-articular damage occurs—impingement syndrome, talar chondral damage, or deltoid ligament injury.

The diagnosis of ankle microinstability is based mainly on obtaining a thorough patient history and careful clinical examination. MRI with intra-articular contrast allows observation of ligament detachment or partial rupture.

The arthroscopic all-inside repair of the ligament tear is the treatment of choice.

Current classical methods for diagnosing ankle instability fail to acknowledge microinstability. Thus, new ankle instability diagnosis criteria are needed to identify which symptomatic patients without objective signs of mechanical instability may have ankle microinstability.

Fact Box

- Microinstability is a developing concept among the possible causes of ankle pathology.
- Microinstability of the ankle may result from an injury to the superior fascicle of the anterior talofibular ligament (ATFL).
- It is possible that some patients with functional instability have a component of microinstability; however, limitations of current imaging techniques do not enable detection of small tears of ATFL's superior fascicle despite these may be confirmed intraoperatively.
- The tibiotalar posterior drawer test is a clinical test which should be performed in patients with high suspicion of ankle microinstability.
- Conventional MRIs usually are not effective for the diagnosis once do not show the partially exposed footprint of ATFL attachment onto the fibula.
- Arthroscopic repair is the treatment of choice in symptomatic patients after failure of conservative treatment.

References

1. Vega J, Rabat E. Innovations in chronic ankle instability. Rev Cir Pie. 2013;27(2):71–9.
2. Vega J, Peña F, Golanó P. Minor or occult ankle instability as a cause of anterolateral pain after ankle sprain. Knee Surg Sports Traumatol Arthrosc. 2016;24(4):1116–23.
3. Vega J, Dalmau M, Malagelada F, Fargues-Polo B, Peña F. Ankle arthroscopy: an update. J Bone Joint Surg Am. 2017;99:1395–407.
4. Hertel J. Functional instability following lateral ankle sprain. Sports Med. 2000;29:361–71.
5. Brooks SC, Potter BT, Rainey JB. Treatment for partial tears of the lateral ligament of the ankle: a prospective trial. Br Med J. 1981;282:606–7.
6. Ferran NA, Maffulli N. Epidemiology of sprains of the lateral ankle ligament complex. Foot Ankle Clin. 2006;11(3):659–62.
7. Ferran NA, Oliva F, Maffulli N. Ankle instability. Sports Med Arthrosc. 2009;17(2):139–45.
8. Renstrom FH, Lynch SA. Acute injuries of the ankle. Foot Ankle Clin. 1999;4:697–711.
9. Baumhauer JF, O'Brien T. Surgical considerations in the treatment of ankle instability. J Athl Train. 2002;37(4):458–62.
10. Broström L. Sprained ankles: V. Treatment and prognosis in recent ligament ruptures. Acta Chir Scand. 1966;132(5):537–50.
11. Golanó P, Vega J, de Leeuw PAJ, Malagelada F, Manzanares MC, Götzens V, van Dijk CN. Anatomy of the ankle ligaments: a pictorial essay. Knee Surg SportsTraumatol Arthrosc. 2010;18(5):557–69.
12. Golanó P, Dalmau-Pastor M, Vega J, Batista JP. Anatomy of the ankle. In: D'Hooghe PPRN, Kerkhoffs GMMJ, editors. The ankle in football, sports and traumatology. 1st ed. France: Springer; 2014. p. 1–24.
13. Ferkel RD, Karzel RP, Del Pizzo W, Friedman MJ, Fischer SP. Arthroscopic treatment of anterolat-

eral impingement of the ankle. Am J Sports Med. 1991;19(5):440–6.
14. Ferkel RD. Soft-tissue lesions of the ankle. In: Whipple TL, editor. Arthroscopic surgery: the foot and ankle. Philadelphia: Lippincott-Raven; 1996. p. 121–43.
15. Gerber JP, Williams GN, Scoville CR, Arciero RA, Taylor DC. Persistent disability associated with ankle sprains: a prospective examination of an athletic population. Foot Ankle Int. 1998;19(19):653–60.
16. Kumai T, Takakura Y, Rufai A, Milz S, Benjamin M. The functional anatomy of the human anterior talofibular ligament in relation to ankle sprains. J Anat. 2002;200:457–65.
17. Batista JP, del Vecchio JJ, Patthauer L, Ocampo M. Arthroscopic lateral ligament repair through two portals in chronic ankle instability. Open Orthop J. 2017;11:3–17.
18. Takao M, Matsui K, Stone JW, Glazebrook MA, Kennedy JG, Guillo S, Calder JD, Karlsson J, Ankle Instability Group. Arthroscopic anterior talofibular ligament repair for lateral instability of the ankle. Knee Surg Sports Traumatol Arthrosc. 2016;24(4):1003–6.
19. Vega J, Golanó P, Pellegrino A, Rabat E, Peña F. All-inside arthroscopic lateral collateral ligament repair for ankle instability with a knotless suture anchor technique. Foot Ankle Int. 2013;34(12):1701–9.

Assessment of Subtalar Instability

7

Frederick Michels, Satoru Ozeki, Siu Wah Kong, and Giovanni Matricali

7.1 Introduction

Subtalar instability can be defined as a problem causing chronic symptoms of hindfoot instability due to an abnormally increased motion of the subtalar joint [1].

Subtalar instability remains difficult to diagnose and is often overlooked [2–5]. Talocrural instability is often associated with subtalar instability (STI), and unrecognized STI is a possible cause of failure of its surgical treatment [6]. Unrecognized STI has also been seen as one of the causes of functional instability resistant to nonsurgical treatment [7, 8]. The exact incidence of STI remains unknown but has been estimated from 10 to 80% in patients suffering from chronic lateral ankle instability [6, 7, 9, 10].

A recent systematic review investigated the different diagnostic tools to assess subtalar instability [1]. Several of the included studies demonstrated the existence of a group with STI. In particular, seven studies [9, 11–16] indeed revealed an abnormal increased subtalar motion and six studies [14, 16–20] demonstrated abnormalities of the subtalar ligaments: CFL, CL, ITCL, and ACaL. This review did not find one specific ligament responsible for STI. The findings in different studies suggest the existence of different injury patterns and different degrees of STI [10, 13].

7.2 Biomechanical Aspects

The subtalar joint complex is formed by the posterior talocalcaneal joint and the acetabulum pedis nesting the talar head. The acetabulum pedis is formed by the middle and anterior calcaneal surfaces that are connected to the navicular articular surface by the inferior and superomedial calcaneonavicular ligaments. The motion of the subtalar complex is guided by the contour of the

F. Michels (✉)
Orthopaedic Department, AZ Groeninge, Kortrijk, Belgium

MIFAS by GRECMIP (Minimally Invasive Foot and Ankle Society), Merignac, France

S. Ozeki
First Dept. of Orthopaedic Surgery, Dokkyo Univ. Saitama Medical Center, Koshigaya, Japan

S. W. Kong
Foot and Ankle Surgery, Specialist in Orthopaedic and Traumatology, Asia Medical Specialists, Kowloon, Hong Kong

G. Matricali
Department of Development and Regeneration, KU Leuven, Leuven, Belgium

Department of Orthopaedics, Foot and Ankle Unit, University Hospitals Leuven, KU Leuven, Leuven, Belgium

Institute of Orthopaedic Research and Training, KU Leuven, Leuven, Belgium

H. Pereira et al. (eds.), *Lateral Ankle Instability*, https://doi.org/10.1007/978-3-662-62763-1_7

articular surfaces and the intrinsic and extrinsic ligaments [21].

In physiological conditions, three pairs of the talocalcaneal joint facets maintain contact with each other and the calcaneus rotates beneath the talus. Goto et al. analyzed three-dimensional in vivo kinematics of the subtalar joint during dorsi-plantarflexion (DPF) and inversion-eversion (IE) using MRI [22]. They reported that the axes of rotation of the calcaneus relative to the talus during DPF and IE had a very close spatial relationship, running obliquely from the antero-dorso-medial to postero-planto-lateral direction and through the talar neck. Anteriorly and medially relative to the z-axis of the coordinate system, the inclination of the axes of calcaneal rotation in DPF and IE had opening angles of 39° ± 8° and 40° ± 8°, respectively. Anteriorly and dorsally relative to the z-axis of the coordinate system, the inclination of the axes of rotation of the calcaneus in DPF and IE had opening angles of 46° ± 7° and 50° ± 8°, respectively (Fig. 7.1a, b). In addition, the authors determined the points on the subtalar surfaces of the talus and calcaneus through which the axes of rotation of the calcaneus passed; these were both found to be extremely close to the origin and insertion of the interosseous ligament [22].

The intrinsic ligaments are composed of the interosseous talocalcaneal ligament (ITCL) and the cervical ligament (CL). The ITCL exists between the middle and posterior talocalcaneal joint, and the CL connects the anterior part of the calcaneus and the talar neck. The extrinsic ligaments consist of the calcaneofibular ligament (CFL) and the tibiocalcaneal ligament. The CFL connects the fibula and the calcaneus beyond the talus.

To understand the function of these ligaments and to clarify the effects of the damages, several biomechanical sequential resection experiments have been performed. Kjaersgaard-Andersen et al. have reported that sectioning of the CL resulted in a 10% increase in rotation, and sectioning of the ITCL produced a 21% increase in rotation [23]. They also studied the role of the CFL and revealed a 77% increase in adduction at the talocalcaneal joint after sectioning the CFL, noting the significance of the CFL in maintaining lateral stability to the subtalar joint. Tochigi et al. studied the role of the ITCL in subtalar stability by sectioning the ITCL and applying multidirectional draw forces [24]. They found that the laxity for the 30° in inclination to the foot axis was significantly larger than all other directions in the intact condition, and after sectioning the ITCL, laxity for the same direction was significantly larger than all other directions; however, the flexibility was increased in the medial direction after sectioning (ITCL cut).

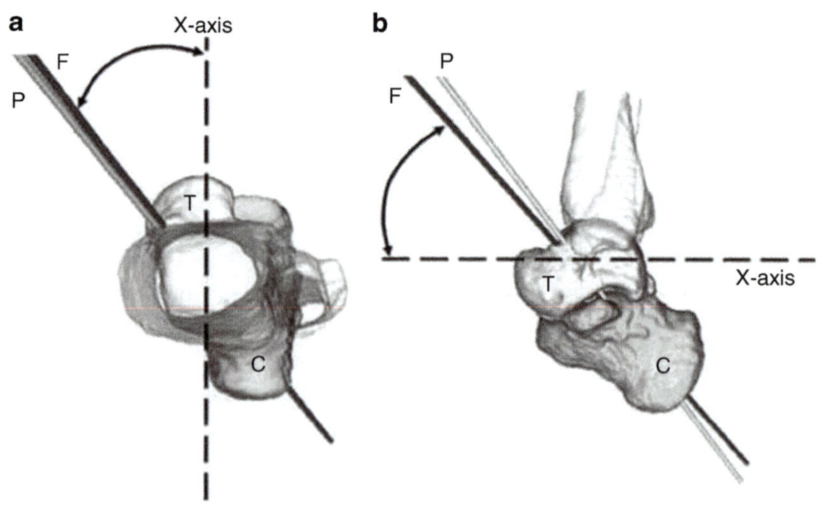

Fig. 7.1 Inclination of the axis of calcaneal rotation projected onto the transverse (**a**) and (**b**) planes. *T* Talus, *C* Calcaneus, *P* Axis of rotation during IE, *F* Axis of rotation during DPF. (Figure 4 in Foot Ankle Int. 30:432–8, 2009. Permission obtained)

Pellegrini et al. quantified subtalar joint motion in response to controlled inversion, eversion, internal rotation and external rotation moments, and multidirectional drawer forces [25]. Their results demonstrated that significant motion increases relative to the intact condition were unaffected by ligament-sectioning order and occurred only after transection of the CFL. Sectioning of this ligament produced increased inversion and external rotation, which was most evident with the foot dorsiflexed. They concluded that CFL disruption results in increases in subtalar inversion and external rotation that might be detectable during a manual examination [25].

Ozeki et al. measured CFL tension forces under circumferential weight loading at every 10° [26]. They observed that the largest force of the CFL was when the loading arm came to a posterolateral position (Fig. 7.2). At this point, the ankle was in plantarflexion, the foot was in a pronated and external rotated position, and the subtalar joint was firmly constrained. To draw a clinical equivalence, this foot position is similar to the position to which the foot presses strongly against the ground to accelerate in the opposite forward direction. The CFL (extrinsic ligament) has a significant role in stabilizing the subtalar joint. The tension of the CFL could be examined with palpation of the CFL in ankle plantarflexion by providing pronation and external stress. Insufficiency of the CFL is an important sign to suspect subtalar instability.

7.3 Assessment of Subtalar Instability

7.3.1 Introduction

Because subtalar instability is often associated with talocrural instability, diagnosis is very difficult. Among specialists, there is no consensus on which diagnostic test is recommended to assess this problem [5]. Stress radiographs have been described but there is still discussion about their reliability [1, 27–29]. Several other diagnostic tools have been published and are discussed in this section.

7.3.2 Clinical Examination

The clinical presentation of patients with subtalar instability is very similar to that of patients with chronic lateral ankle instability. Patients with subtalar instability have usually had a history of an acute ankle injury in the past. They may complain of lateral hindfoot pain and a recurrent feeling of instability of the ankle like "rolling over" or "giving way" [30]. The symptoms are worse when performing sports activities or walking on uneven ground [2, 31]. Lateral ankle swelling and stiffness may be present.

Clinically, it is virtually impossible to distinguish if the instability is originating from the tibiotalar or talocalcaneal portion of the ankle joint complex [3, 4]. However, some clinical signs and

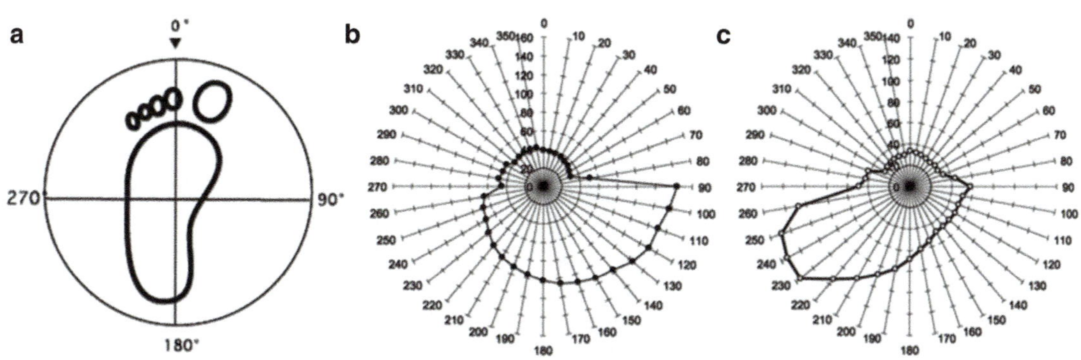

Fig. 7.2 Polar diagrams of ligament forces under 1 kg of loading. Mean ankle ligament forces are demonstrated. (**a**) Loading point, (**b**) ligament force of ATFL. (**c**) Ligament force of CFL. (Figure 3 in Foot and Ankle Int. 27:965–969, 2006. No permission needed)

tests have been described. Tenderness is often found in the sinus tarsi. Increased inversion is usually seen. An increase in internal rotation of the subtalar joint and an increase in forward translation of the calcaneus beneath the talus may be found [30, 32].

Zwipp described a **test for chronic anterolateral rotatory instability** of the subtalar joint [32, 33]. The examiner holds the heel and forefoot rigid with the foot in 10° of dorsiflexion while an inversion and internal rotation stress are applied to the heel. Then an adduction stress is applied to the forefoot (Fig. 7.3). A positive examination results in a medial shift (>5 mm) of the calcaneus under the talus, as well as an opening of the talocalcaneal angle (>5°). The accuracy of this clinical test was only tested in cadaveric specimens with Brodén stress views as a reference test.

Hertel described the **medial subtalar glide test**. The examiner holds the talus in subtalar neutral with one hand and glides the calcaneus medially on the fixed talus with the other hand [11]. Subtalar neutral was determined by manually maneuvering the foot between supination and pronation until the talar head could not be palpated or was felt equally medially and laterally. The results were compared with Brodén stress views. Good but no significant agreement was found.

An experienced clinician may be able to detect situations of major subtalar instability; however, clinical assessment remains very observer-dependent.

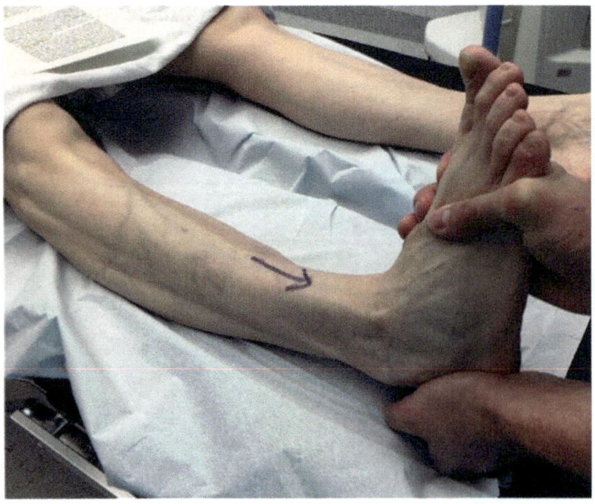

Fig. 7.3 Test for chronic anterolateral rotatory instability of the subtalar joint

7.3.3 Radiographs

Standard plain radiographs should include weight-bearing anteroposterior, lateral, and mortise views of the ankle and weight-bearing anteroposterior, lateral, and oblique views of the foot to rule out evidence of bone pathology. Alignment views are necessary because hindfoot malalignment can contribute to subtalar joint instability and dysfunction [34].

7.3.4 Stress Radiographs

7.3.4.1 Tomograms

The first stress radiographs were described by Rubin and Witten [35]. The authors used a hinged device to apply inversion stress to the ankle and foot. To assess the subtalar instability, tomograms were taken in the frontal plane. Actual cases of subtalar instability were not included in this study.

7.3.4.2 Brodén Stress Views

Laurin et al. used Brodén stress views in a cadaveric study and measured subtalar tilt [36, 37]. The patient's leg was internally rotated 40°, and forced inversion stress was applied (Fig. 7.4). The X-ray beam was tilted 20–40° and aimed at the sinus tarsi. Laurin stated that any loss of parallelism was diagnostic of subtalar instability. The initial Brodén views were used to assess fractures of the posterior facet of the calcaneus [36]. Zwipp found medial displacement and subtalar joint tilting in patients with injuries of the interosseous talocalcaneal ligament [16]. Harper found no correlation when comparing the lateral opening of the subtalar joint with stress X-rays between patients with symptoms of lateral ankle instability and an asymptomatic control group [27]. Heilman used Brodén stress views after selective sectioning of the calcaneofibular ligament, capsule, and interosseous ligaments [38]. Sectioning of the CFL alone produced a 5 mm opening of the subtalar joint. When combined with sectioning of the interosseous ligament, a 7 mm opening was produced. Karlsson defined subtalar instability when >2 mm separation of the

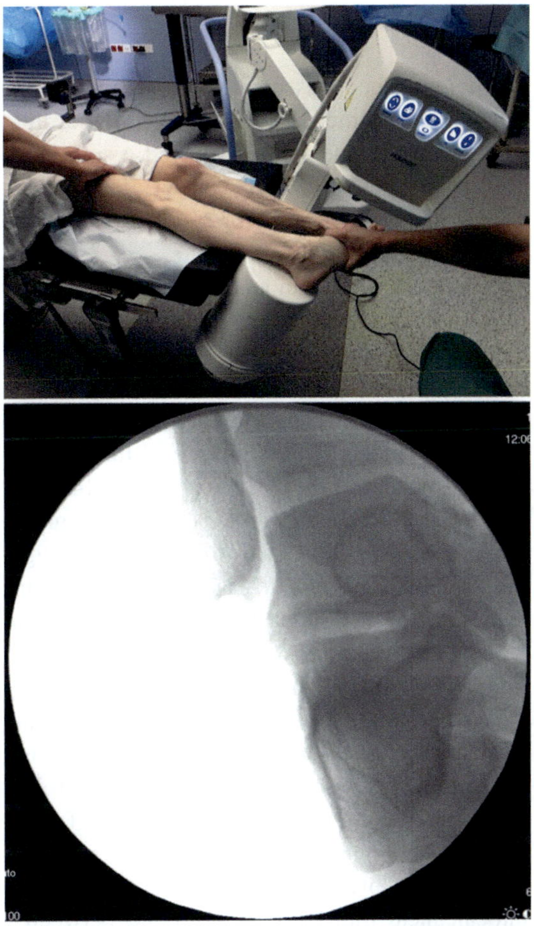

Fig. 7.4 Stress radiograph with ankle in internal rotation and fluoroscopy positioned obliquely

talocalcaneal surfaces in the anterior view was present compared to the contralateral side [31].

Yamamoto performed stress radiographs using Telos equipment and described an increased subtalar tilt angle in patients following acute and chronic lateral ligament injuries [15].

Louwerens found a wide range of subtalar displacement but no difference of talar tilt or shift between asymptomatic and asymptomatic feet [28]. Two studies of the same group compared stress radiographs with helical CT under stress [29, 39]. A variable amount of subtalar tilt was demonstrated in all cases on stress radiographs, without significant difference between the symptomatic and asymptomatic feet. However, contrary to the findings at the talocrural level, subtalar tilt was found in none of the patients using helical CT. Tilting was found on stress X-rays, but tilting within the subtalar joint was never found using CT-stress examination. The authors concluded that Brodén stress views may not be reliable for assessing subtalar instability. Stress radiographs assess mechanical instability in single planes while movement occurs in three dimensions. The authors doubt that the tilt seen during Brodén views is an accurate measure of true tilt [39]. Rather, the apparent tilt viewed on such radiographs is secondary to translation and rotation of the talus and calcaneus in relation to one another during inversion of the injured foot.

Because of the conflicting results, a recent systematic review gave a grade "I" recommendation, corresponding with insufficient or conflicting evidence, for or against the use of Brodén stress radiographs [1]. They should not be used as a reference test in other studies.

7.3.4.3 Other Stress Views

Kato described a stress radiograph when applying anterior stress on the calcaneus with a lateral and anteroposterior radiograph of the hindfoot [12]. He noted increased anterior displacement of the calcaneus on the talus in patients with instability of the subtalar joint. Ishii applied anterior drawer stress to the subtalar joint with the ankle in maximum supination and dorsiflexion [9]. The relative position of the lateral talar process relative to the subtalar joint was measured.

Recently, Lee published a new manual stress radiographic technique in comparison with MRI and surgical findings [13]. Under general anesthesia, the ankle joint was held in 10–15° plantarflexion. The foot was drawn anteriorly with maximal supination force and a lateral view was obtained with fluoroscopy. Then, the relative position of the talar inferior apex in the tarsal sinus was measured. Increased laxity was found in patients with injuries of ATFL and CFL along with cervical ligament insufficiency compared to patients with ATFL and CFL injuries with an intact cervical ligament.

A recent systematic review gave a grade B recommendation, corresponding to fair evidence, for the use of supination-anterior drawer stress radiographs [1].

7.3.5 Subtalar Arthrography

Meyer used arthrography to assess the degree of subtalar ligament injuries in the acute phase [10]. A lateral capsular leak corresponded with a lesion of the CFL, a sinus tarsi leak with a lesion of the interosseous talocalcaneal ligament. Subtalar arthrography in patients with an acute ankle sprain was found to be more accurate in diagnosing a CFL rupture than stress radiographs [19]. Subtalar arthrography was also found to be valuable in diagnosing injury to the CFL in patients with recurrent instability of the ankle [19].

7.3.6 Ultrasound

One study assessed subtalar instability using sonography by measurement of the fibula-trochlear angle [40]. The ratio between the angle measured in a neutral position and an inversion stress position was calculated. A ratio of greater than 1.6 was estimated as diagnostic for subtalar instability.

7.3.7 CT

CT scan offers the advantage of a three-dimensional view of the subtalar joint. Bony lesions such as avulsion fractures and early osteoarthritis can be seen. Teramoto used stress CT to assess the subtalar range of motion of healthy subjects [41]. Stress was applied using the Telos stress device and the angle between the posterior facet of the subtalar joint and the surface of the trochlea was measured in the coronal plane. Inversion and eversion range of motion of the subtalar joint was shown to be about 15° in healthy subjects. Colin used weight-bearing CT scans to assess the subtalar joint configuration in patients without ankle pathology [42]. Krähenbühl performed a cadaver study to investigate the use of weight-bearing CT scans to diagnose subtalar joint instability [43]. According to their findings, weight application negatively impacts the assessment of subtalar joint instability, while torque application exposes instability.

7.3.8 MRI

MRI allows the assessment of the ligaments and bone in three dimensions (Fig. 7.5). MRI evaluation in acute ankle sprains showed a significant correlation between ITCL or CL lesions and complaints of giving way or residual pain at follow-up of 6–28 months [24].

Mabit performed an anatomic and MRI study of the subtalar ligaments [44]. Coronal and coronal oblique planes were found the most useful for the assessment of the IER, CL, and ITCL. Several studies used MR imaging under stress in specimens, which significantly improved the sensitivity for the detection of abnormalities [44–46]. Lektrakul used reconstructed MR arthrograms along and perpendicular to the axes of the ligaments of the sinus tarsi to assess injury [47]. This technique offered improved visualization compared with conventional MRI. Lee compared MRI findings with subtalar arthroscopy [48]. Conventional MRI was found useful for detecting CL tears but inadequate for detecting ITCL tears.

Seebauer examined the use of MRI controlled ankle stress examination in the detection of instability [14]. Significant differences in talar tilt, subtalar tilt, anterior talar translation, and medial talocalcaneal translation were found between a group with instability compared with an asymptomatic control group. Although the results of this study are promising, further studies are necessary to confirm the reliability and determine thresholds using stress MRI.

Two studies of the same research group used 3D isotropic MRI to assess the ligament characteristics in patients with subtalar instability [18, 20]. First, they compared STI patients with an asymptomatic control group [18]. Second, they compared STI patients with a group with TTI [20]. Both studies demonstrated a significantly reduced thickness and width of the ACaL in patients with subtalar instability.

7.3.9 Subtalar Arthroscopy

Frey performed a retrospective review of 45 subtalar arthroscopies [49]. A tear of the ITCL was

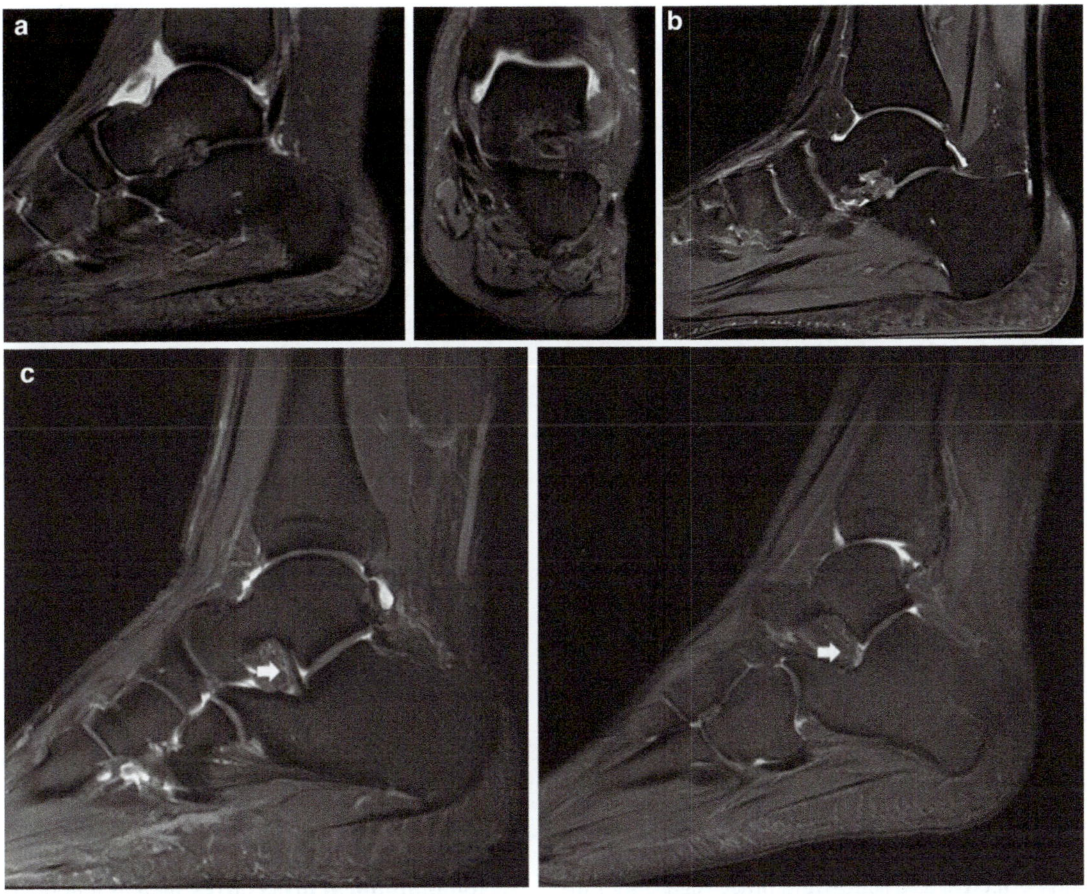

Fig. 7.5 (**a**) MRI showing an injury of the ITCL with bone edema. (**b**) MRI showing an avulsion of the cervical ligament insertion to the talus. (**c**) MRI showing a normal and absent anterior capsular ligament

associated with subtalar instability. In seven patients, subtalar instability was demonstrated arthroscopically as a medial glide of the calcaneus out from under the talus as the subtalar joint was stressed in varus. A partial (in six patients) or complete (in one patient) tear of the talocalcaneal interosseous ligament was found endoscopically. Using subtalar arthroscopy, Lee found 88% ITCL tears in patients with sinus tarsi syndrome [50].

7.3.10 Diagnostic Criteria

Recently, five diagnostic criteria were proposed to diagnose STI: recurrent ankle sprain, sinus tarsi pain and tenderness, hindfoot looseness or giving way, hindfoot instability on clinical examination, and positive Brodén stress radiographs [18, 20]. Four of the five criteria need to be fulfilled to confirm the diagnosis of STI. Because of the limited reliability of Brodén stress radiographs, it has been recommended to use anterior drawer-supination radiographs or MRI instead [1].

In patients with suspicion of subtalar instability and resistance to nonsurgical treatment, a surgical assessment of the different ligaments has been recommended [1, 51].

7.3.11 Conclusion

Many different diagnostic tools have been proposed to assess subtalar instability. The lack of a reliable diagnostic reference test makes assessment of the reliability of the published tests very difficult. The normal and abnormal biomechanics of the subtalar joint are complex, and therefore a reliable test must assess this joint in three dimensions. Ideally, the test should be noninvasive and easily available.

In clinical practice, in patients with persistent complaints of chronic hindfoot instability, the diagnosis of subtalar instability should be considered. A combination of different criteria can be used. Today anterior drawer-supination radiographs and MRI are the most useful imaging techniques. If surgery is needed, preoperative assessment is recommended.

7.4 Treatment of Subtalar Instability

7.4.1 Nonsurgical Treatment

The first approach in patients with subtalar instability is nonsurgical treatment. The treatment is similar to patients with talocrural instability and consists of bracing, appropriate shoe wear, and physiotherapy [2]. Choisne demonstrated the benefit of using a semi-rigid ankle brace following a subtalar ankle injury [52]. Taping appears similarly effective as a semi-rigid brace regarding limiting subtalar joint translation in chronic instability [53]. Lateral heel wedges may help to avoid hindfoot malpositioning [4]. Adequate rehabilitation should be supervised by a physiotherapist and consists of strengthening exercises of the active stabilizers of the ankle and proprioceptive training. Achilles tendon stretching and flexibility improves hindfoot positioning that could result from a tight gastrocnemius complex [3]. As in talocrural instability we recommend to continue nonsurgical treatment for at least 3–6 months [5].

7.4.2 Surgical Treatment

Surgical treatment can be considered in those who fail conservative management; however, the lack of a diagnostic reference standard complicates the preoperative assessment. Similar to talocrural ankle instability distinction may be made between repair and reconstruction.

7.4.2.1 Ligament Repair

A repair is defined as suturing of the torn lateral ligaments such as the classic Broström procedure in the treatment of talocrural ankle instability [54]. However, this is often associated with the Gould modification, an augmentation with a transfer of the extensor retinaculum [55]. As this extensor retinaculum has several insertion points to the calcaneus, this modification affects the subtalar mobility and subtalar joints after a subtalar joint injury. A biomechanical study of Choisne demonstrated the use of the Gould modification in reducing the instability of the talocrural and subtalar joint after an injury to the CFL, ITCL, and cervical ligament(CL) [56]. This is a very important finding because the use of an anatomical CFL and ATFL reconstruction in patients with combined talocrural and subtalar instability may not address the instability caused by injury of the ITCL and CL.

Karlsson published good results after repair of CFL, lateral talocalcaneal, and cervical ligaments [31].

7.4.2.2 Ligament Reconstruction

A reconstruction may be nonanatomical or anatomical.

Nonanatomical procedures such as tenodesis have been used in the surgical treatment of subtalar ankle instability. Chrisman and Snook published good results treating patients with subtalar ankle instability with a modified Elmslie peroneal tendon transfer [57]. The tendon was released proximally and threaded through the fibular bone tunnel in a retrograde fashion, then brought distally through a calcaneal tunnel antegrade. The remaining tendon end was sutured to the distal part. Larsen published satisfactory results in treating patients with isolated subtalar instability [58]. The peroneus brevis was rerouted from the fifth metatarsal base into the fibula and then back down into the calcaneus. An important disadvantage of a tenodesis procedure is the decrease of motion of the ankle or subtalar joints [59].

Anatomical Reconstruction attempts to reconstruct the injured ligaments similar to the normal anatomical situation. Commonly a graft is used. Controversy remains as to which ligaments require reconstruction.

The CFL, bridging both the tibiotalar and subtalar joint, is assumed to be an important stabilizer of both joints. In cases with suspicion of subtalar instability, it should be considered to reconstruct the CFL in addition to the ATFL [1, 5, 43, 60, 61]. Elmslie described a near-anatomic reconstruction of the ATFL and CFL using a fascia lata graft passed through curved bone tunnels [62]. The other techniques reconstructing the ATFL and CFL are discussed elsewhere in this book. Besides the ATFL and CFL, it is still not clear if other ligaments need to be reconstructed [1]. There are few publications about the surgical reconstruction of the interosseous talocalcaneal ligament or cervical ligament. Kato described a reconstruction of the interosseous talocalcaneal ligament using a partial Achilles tendon graft [12]. Schon described a triligamentous reconstruction attempting to reconstruct ATFL, CFL, and cervical ligament in a near-anatomic fashion [59]. The plantaris tendon or entire peroneus brevis tendon is passed through a lateral tunnel in the calcaneus, into the tarsal canal, through a curved tunnel in the talar neck, through the fibula, then into a posterior calcaneal tunnel. However, the peroneal tendons are important dynamic stabilizers of the hindfoot and harvesting these tendons for grafts or transfers may result in long-term weakness and loss of dynamic stabilization of the ankle and subtalar joints. In 1996, Mabit described ATFL reconstruction using the peroneus tertius tendon associated with reconstruction of the cervical ligament by inserting a flap of the extensor retinaculum in a talar tunnel [63]. Pisani described an open surgical technique to reconstruct the ITCL [64]. They used the anterior half of the peroneus brevis tendon as a graft. Liu used an arthroscopic approach for improved visualization for tunnel placement [65].

In these techniques, curved bone tunnels are frequently used. However, curved bone tunnels increase the risk of fixation failure by fracture of the bony bridge [66]. The need for two tunnels with entry points so close to each other compromises a correct anatomical reconstruction of the insertion sites. As in talocrural instability, the advent of newer fixation systems with straight bone tunnels and interference screws may improve surgical techniques when performing an anatomical reconstruction [60].

7.4.3 Conclusion

Several different techniques have been described treating patients with subtalar ankle instability with good result being reported. However, the questions concerning the reliability of the diagnostic tools raise questions with respect to patient selection, and therefore the results of the described surgical techniques should be interpreted with caution.

7.5 Acute Subtalar Dislocation

Although rare, acute subtalar dislocation can result in subtalar instability [2]. Subtalar dislocation (SD) is defined as simultaneous dislocation of the subtalar (talocalcaneal joint) and talonavicular joints [67] without the involvement of the calcaneocuboid or tibiotalar joints and without fracture of the neck of the talus [68]. It is also known as peritalar, talocalcaneonavicular, subastragaloid, or subastragalar dislocation [69–72].

7.5.1 Anatomy and Classification

Subtalar dislocation is frequently accompanied by fractures of the adjacent tarsal and metatarsal bones but also severe surrounding soft-tissue injury [67]. Subtalar dislocation can occur in any direction. The direction of subtalar dislocation has important prognostic effects and also affects the management plan.

Medial subtalar dislocations represent the majority of the cases in the literature (up to 85%) and occur about four times more frequently than lateral dislocations (17%); posterior (2.5%) and anterior (1%) dislocations occurrence are rare [68, 73–78]. In medial dislocation, the rest of the foot is displaced medially, the navicular is usually medial and sometimes dorsal to the talar head while the talar head is displaced in the dorsolateral aspect of the foot [79]. In a lateral dislocation, the rest of the foot is displaced lateral to the talus and the talar head is displaced medially. The navicular lies lateral to the talar neck. Rarely, subtalar dislocation is also reported to occur in a direct anterior or posterior direction [77, 80].

7.5.2 Mechanism of Injury

Subtalar dislocation is frequently caused by a fall from a height or during a motor vehicle accident (which accounts for 68% of subtalar dislocations) [81, 82]. In USA literature, a large number of patients suffer from medial subtalar dislocation when they jump and land incorrectly during basketball games; therefore, medial subtalar dislocation is also called "basketball foot" (low energy injury) [83, 84]. The severity of the initial injury affects the outcome and has a prognostic effect.

High-energy subtalar dislocations frequently have associated injuries. Bibbo reported that 88% of patients with subtalar dislocations had another foot and ankle injury to the talus, ankle, calcaneus, navicular, cuboid, cuneiform, or metatarsal [81]. In one large series, 45% of patients also have associated osteochondral lesions of the talus, the calcaneus, or the navicular [73–75].

Excessive inversion of the foot results in a medial subtalar dislocation, while eversion produces a lateral subtalar dislocation. When there is an excessive inversion or eversion force, the relative strong calcaneonavicular ligament resists disruption and force is dissipated through the weaker talonavicular and talocalcaneal ligaments; therefore, the calcaneus, navicular, and all distal bones of the foot are displaced as a unit either medially or laterally [79, 85].

7.5.3 Signs and Symptoms

Most of the subtalar dislocations have an obvious deformity. In medial dislocation, the foot deviates medially and looks like an acquired clubfoot (Fig. 7.6). The lateral dislocation may mimic an acquired flatfoot because the foot deviates to the lateral side [86]. Up to 40% of subtalar dislocations are open [87]. However, even with closed injuries, the skin is usually under considerable tension and may become necrotic due to pressure from the prominent head of the talus. Skin swelling may also mask the bone deformity. Prompt evaluation of skin condition and neurovascular impairment is important with timely reduction of the dislocation once it is confirmed in order to prevent soft tissue complications.

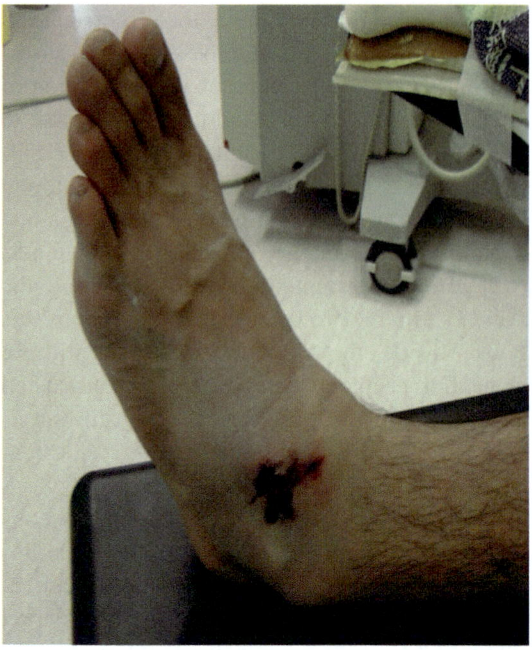

Fig. 7.6 Medial subtalar dislocation with prominence talar head at lateral side of foot, necrotic skin due to pressure from displaced talar head and adult acquired club foot deformity

7.5.4 Radiographic Findings

Severe soft tissue swelling and bone deformity may mean that obtaining true anteroposterior/lateral images plain radiographs of the foot is difficult and interpretation of the images complicated [88]. In a subtalar dislocation, ankle X-rays show a normal relationship of talus and distal tibia/fibula as the injury is distal to the ankle joint [88]. Therefore, identification of a talona-

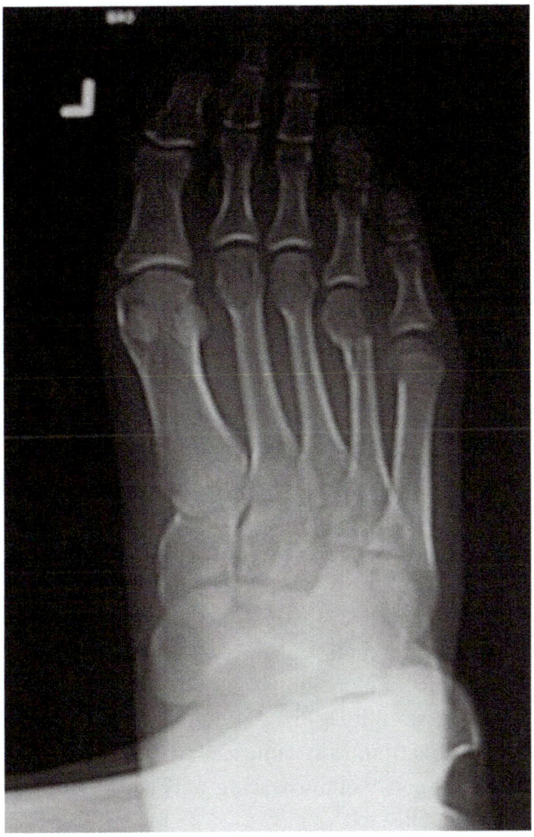

Fig. 7.7 Anteroposterior X-ray foot of the same patient in Fig. 7.6. Dislocation of talonavicular joint with talar head dislocated and pointing at lateral foot

vicular dislocation on an anteroposterior view of the foot shows is an important diagnostic key (Fig. 7.7). On lateral views, the head of the talus usually lies superior to the navicular and cuboid for a medial dislocation and may appear to be displaced inferiorly in a lateral dislocation.

Usually, careful interpretation of the plain radiographs provides adequate information to determine the direction of the dislocation and to facilitate an attempt of closed reduction. However, associated fractures may be missed on plain radiographs (Fig. 7.8), and post-reduction films may not be adequate in all cases to determine whether residual subluxation is present.

CT scanning (Fig. 7.9) therefore is very useful to determine whether associated fractures are present and to rule out talocalcaneal subluxation [81, 87, 89, 90].

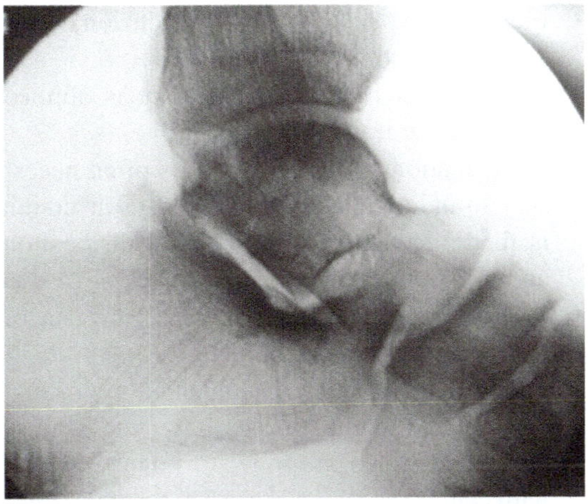

Fig. 7.8 Post-closed reduction X-ray, no obvious fracture seen and subtalar joint looks congruent

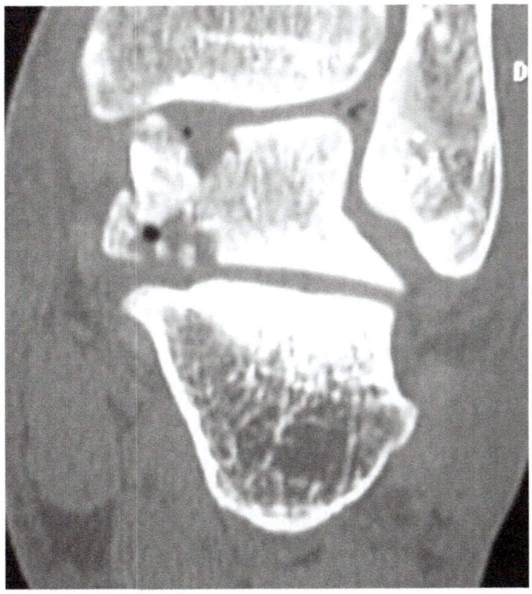

Fig. 7.9 Post-reduction CT scan shows a comminuted fracture of the talus not visible on plain X-rays

7.5.5 Treatment

7.5.5.1 Closed Reduction

All subtalar dislocations should have a gentle and timely reduction to reduce complications such as skin necrosis.

The principles of closed reduction [79]:

- Adequate relaxation, sedation, and pain control, either by general or local anesthesia.

- Flex the knee in order to reduce tension on the Achilles tendon.
- Longitudinal traction on the foot is applied with counter traction on the leg.
- Accentuation of the deformity is often necessary to unlock the calcaneum (e.g., inversion is therefore applied for a medial dislocation and eversion for a lateral dislocation).
- Once the calcaneus is unlocked, reversal of the deformity can be applied.
- Reduction is usually accompanied by a satisfying clunk. Digital pressure over the head of the talus can also be applied to aid in reduction with caution as it may cause further skin injury and potentially displace an osteochondral fracture.

The successful reduction should be confirmed by clinical examination and radiographs. The foot should be restored to normal alignment and range of motion of the subtalar/midtarsal joints. Plain radiographs should confirm the reduction and exclude associated fractures. If the dislocation is clinically stable, no internal fixation is necessary. The foot can then be immobilized in a short-leg cast for 4 weeks. Physical therapy is recommended to regain subtalar and midtarsal mobility [91]. In 10–32% of cases, both bone and soft tissue structures may be entrapped and cause failure of closed reduction and this may necessitate open reduction [75, 89, 92–94]. In medial dislocations, the talar head can become trapped by the capsule of the talonavicular joint, the extensor retinaculum, extensor tendons, the extensor digitorum brevis muscle, talonavicular impaction, impingement of the deep peroneal nerve, and dorsalis pedis branches [95]. In lateral dislocation, articular surface impaction, the posterior tibial tendon, and ruptured flexor retinaculum can all prevent talar head reduction [82].

7.5.5.2 Open Reduction

A longitudinal anteromedial skin incision is usually used for open reduction. This approach allows access to the structures that may be incarcerating the head of the talus and allows visualization of an interlocked impaction fracture of the talus and navicular. When there is associated impaction fracture, bone graft and internal fixation may be required. If the impaction fracture is small and suitable for repair this may be fixed with small screws or metal k-wires or the fragments may be excised to facilitate reduction. Osteochondral lesions may also be fixed or removed [79].

In lateral dislocation, the posterior tibial tendon when entrapped may present a substantial barrier to open reduction. We advocate making the anteromedial skin incision more medially located to facilitate manipulation of the posterior tibial tendon.

Following successful reduction, joint congruency and stability should be assessed. If there was only soft tissue interposition requiring open reduction, the joint is usually stable. However, if large or multiple bone fragments required removal, stability may be less than ideal. Internal fixation with metal k-wires across the subtalar and talonavicular joints may be necessary to maintain stability [96]. Following 4–6 weeks of immobilization, any internal fixation can be removed and weight-bearing and active physiotherapy can start.

7.5.6 Prognosis and Complications

Subtalar dislocations have a wide variance in prognosis and outcomes. Patients with concomitant soft tissue injury, extra-articular fracture, intra-articular fracture, open fractures, and osteonecrosis are associated with a worse outcome [76, 97]. The mechanism of injury is also an important factor in predicting long-term outcome with high-energy injury having a poor outcome [73].

The potential complications after subtalar dislocation include:

- Post-traumatic subtalar joint stiffness is common in most cases but may lead to a less significant functional deficit [58, 72, 74, 85].
- Osteonecrosis may develop after subtalar dislocation but fortunately it is uncommon, and is mostly associated with high-energy injury or open fracture. The incidence rate is from 12% to 33% [81, 98].

- Persistent subtalar instability is also uncommon [58, 99]; however, if the patient has persistent joint laxity [99] or insufficient immobilization [68], recurrent subluxation can occur. This may still be treated with repeated closed reduction and immobilization with good result reported [75].
- Post-traumatic arthritis is common with an incidence of 25–89% and normally follows those dislocations with a fracture or cartilage injury [68, 73, 75, 87, 89]. The arthritic change usually affects the subtalar joint but occasionally occurs in the ankle or midfoot joints.

Fact Box

- The calcaneofibular ligament is considered the most important stabilizer of the subtalar joint.
- Subtalar instability is still difficult to diagnose and is often unnoticed.
- The subtalar joint should always be assessed in patients with lateral ankle instability.
- Conservative treatment is usually the first approach in patients with subtalar instability.
- Upon failure of the former, surgical repair or reconstruction shall be considered.

References

1. Michels F, Clockaerts S, Van Der Bauwhede J, Stockmans F, Matricali G. Does subtalar instability really exist? A systematic review. J Foot Ankle Surg. 2019;26:119. https://doi.org/10.1016/j.fas.2019.02.001.
2. Aynardi M, Pedowitz D, Raikin SM. Subtalar instability. Foot Ankle Clin N Am. 2015;20:243–52.
3. Barg A, Tochigi Y, Amendola A, et al. Subtalar instability: diagnosis and treatment. Foot Ankle Int. 2012;33:151–60.
4. Clanton TO, Berson L. Subtalar joint athletic injuries. Foot Ankle Clin. 1999;4:729–43.
5. Michels F, Pereira H, Calder J, et al. Searching for consensus in the approach to patients with chronic lateral ankle instability: ask the expert. Knee Surg Sports Traumatol Arthrosc. 2017;26:2095. https://doi.org/10.1007/s00167-017-4556-0.
6. Brantigan J, Pedegana L, Lippert F. Instability of the subtalar joint. Diagnosis by stress tomography in three cases. J Bone Joint Surg Am. 1977;59(3):321–4.
7. Hertel J. Functional anatomy, pathomechanics, and pathophysiology of lateral ankle instability. J Athl Train. 2002;37:364–75.
8. Karlsson J, Eriksson BI, Renström PA. Subtalar ankle instability. A review. Sports Med. 1997;24:337–46.
9. Ishii T, Miyagawa S, Fukubayashi T, et al. Subtalar stress radiography using forced dorsiflexion and supination. J Bone Joint Surg Br. 1996;78(1):56–60.
10. Meyer JM, Garcia J, Hoffmeyer P. The subtalar sprain. A roentgenographic study. Clin Orthop Relat Res. 1988;226:169–73.
11. Hertel J, Denegar CR, Monroe MM, et al. Talocrural and subtalar joint instability after lateral ankle sprain. Med Sci Sports Exerc. 1999;31(11):1501–8.
12. Kato T. The diagnosis and treatment of instability of the subtalar joint. J Bone Joint Surg Br. 1995;77:400–6.
13. Lee BH, Choi KH, Seo DY, et al. Diagnostic validity of alternative manual stress radiographic technique detecting subtalar instability with concomitant ankle instability. Knee Surg Sports Traumatol Arthrosc. 2016;24:1029–39.
14. Seebauer JC, Bail HJ, Rump JC, Hamm B, et al. Ankle laxity: stress investigation under MRI control. Am J Roentgenol. 2013;201:496–504.
15. Yamamoto H, Yagishita K, Ogiuchi T, et al. Subtalar instability following lateral ligament injuries of the ankle. Injury. 1982;29:265–8.
16. Zwipp H, Tscherne H. Radiological diagnosis of instability of the subtalar joint. Unfallheilkunde. 1982;85:494–8.
17. Faure J, Deplus F, Besse JL, et al. Chronic external instability of the ankle. Contribution of dynamic radiographies, x-ray computed tomography and x-ray computed tomographic arthrography. J Radiol. 1997;78(9):629–34.
18. Kim TH, Moon SG, Jung HG, Kim NR. Subtalar instability: imaging features of subtalar ligaments on 3D isotropic ankle MRI. BMC Musculoskelet Disord. 2017;18(1):475.
19. Sugimoto K, Takakura Y, Samoto N, et al. Subtalar arthrography in recurrent instability of the ankle. Clin Orthop Relat Res. 2002;394:169–76.
20. Yoon DY, Moon SG, Jung HG, et al. Differences between subtalar instability and lateral ankle instability focusing on subtalar ligaments based on three dimensional isotropic magnetic resonance imaging. J Comput Assist Tomogr. 2018;42(4):566–73.
21. Sarrafian SK. Biomechanics of the subtalar joint complex. Clin Orthop Relat Res. 1993;290:17–26.
22. Goto A, Moritomo H, Itohara T, et al. Three-dimensional in vivo kinematics of the subtalar joint during dorsi-plantarflexion and inversion-eversion. Foot Ankle Int. 2009;30:432–8.
23. Kjaersgaard-Andersen P, Wethelund J, Nielsen S. Lateral talocalcaneal instability following section of the calcaneofibular ligament: a kinesiologic study. Foot Ankle. 1987;7:355–61.

24. Tochigi Y, Yoshinaga K, Wada Y, et al. Acute inversion injury of the ankle: magnetic resonance imaging and clinical outcomes. Foot Ankle Int. 1998;19(11):730–4.
25. Pellegrini MJ, Glisson RR, Wurm M, et al. Systematic quantification of stabilizing effects of subtalar joint soft tissue constraints in a novel cadaveric model. J Bone Joint Surg Am. 2016;98(10):842–8.
26. Ozeki S, Kitaoka H, Uchiyama E, et al. Ankle ligament tensile forces at the end points of passive circumferential rotating motion of the ankle and subtalar joint complex. Foot and Ankle Int. 2006;27:965–9.
27. Harper MC. Stress radiographs in the diagnosis of lateral instability of the ankle and hindfoot. Foot Ankle Int. 1993;13:435–8.
28. Louwerens JW, Ginai AZ, van Linge B, et al. Stress radiography of the talocrural and subtalar joints. Foot Ankle Int. 1995;16:148–55.
29. Sijbrandy ES, van Gils APG, van Hellemondt FJ, et al. Assessing the subtalar joint: the Brodén view revisited. Foot Ankle Int. 2001;22:329–34.
30. Keefe DT, Haddad SL. Subtalar instability. Etiology, diagnosis, and management. Foot Ankle Clin. 2002;7:577–609.
31. Karlsson J, Eriksson BI, Renström PA. Subtalar instability of the foot. A review and results after surgical treatment. Scand J Med Sci Sports. 1998;8:191–7.
32. Thermann H, Zwipp H, Tscherne H. Treatment algorithm of chronic ankle and subtalar instability. Foot Ankle Int. 1997;18:163–9.
33. Zwipp H, Krettek C. Diagnosis and therapy of acute and chronic ligament instability of the lower ankle joint. Orthopade. 1986;15:472–8.
34. Saltzman CL, el Khoury GY. The hindfoot alignment view. Foot Ankle Int. 1995;16:572–6.
35. Rubin G, Witten M. The subtalar joint and the symptoms of turning over on the ankle: a new method of evaluation utilizing tomography. Am J Orthop. 1962;4:16–9.
36. Brodén B. Roentgen examination of the subtalar joint in fractures of the calcaneus. Acta Radiol. 1949;31:85–91.
37. Laurin CA, Ouellet R, St-Jacques R. Talar and subtalar tilt: an experiment investigation. Can J Surg. 1968;11:270–9.
38. Heilman AE, Braly WG, Bishop JO, et al. An anatomic study of subtalar instability. Foot Ankle. 1990;10:224–8.
39. van Hellemondt FJ, Louwerens JW, Sijbrandij ES, et al. Stress radiography and stress examination of the talocrural and subtalar joint on helical computed tomography. Foot Ankle Int. 1997;18:482–8.
40. Waldecker U, Blatter G. Sonographic measurement of instability of the subtalar joint. Foot Ankle Int. 2001;22(1):42–6.
41. Teramoto A, Watanabe K, Takashima H, et al. Subtalar joint stress imaging with tomosynthesis. Foot Ankle Spec. 2014;7:182–4.
42. Colin F, Horn Lang T, Zwicky L, et al. Subtalar joint configuration on weightbearing CT scan. Foot Ankle Int. 2014;35(10):1057–62.
43. Krähenbühl N, Burssens A, Davidson NP, Allen CM, Henninger HB, Saltzman CL, Barg A. Can weightbearing computed tomography scans be used to diagnose subtalar joint instability? A cadaver study. J Orthop Res. 2019;37(11):2457–65. https://doi.org/10.1002/jor.24420.
44. Mabit C, Boncoeur-Martel MP, Chaudruc JM, et al. Anatomic and MRI study of the subtalar ligamentous support. Surg Radiol Anat. 1997;19:111–7.
45. Ringleb SI, Udupa JK, Siegler S, et al. The effect of ankle ligament damage and surgical reconstructions on the mechanics of the ankle and subtalar joints revealed by three-dimensional stress MRI. J Orthop Res. 2005;23:743–9.
46. Siegler S, Udupa JK, Ringleb SI, et al. Mechanics of the ankle and subtalar joints revealed through a 3D quasi-static stress MRI technique. J Biomech. 2005;38:567–78.
47. Lektrakul N, Chung CB, Ym L, et al. Tarsal sinus: arthrographic, MR imaging, MR arthrographic, and pathologic findings in cadavers and retrospective study data in patients with sinus tarsi syndrome. Radiology. 2001;219:802–10.
48. Lee KB, Bai LB, Park JG, et al. Efficacy of MRI versus arthroscopy for evaluation of sinus tarsi syndrome. Foot Ankle Int. 2008;29:1111–6.
49. Frey C, Feder KS, DiGiovanni C. Arthroscopic evaluation of the subtalar joint: does sinus tarsi syndrome exist? Foot Ankle Int. 1999;20:185–91.
50. Lee KB, Bai LB, Song EK, et al. Subtalar arthroscopy for sinus tarsi syndrome: arthroscopic findings and clinical outcomes of 33 consecutive cases. Arthroscopy. 2008;24:1130–4.
51. Mittlmeier T, Rammelt S. Update on subtalar joint instability. Foot Ankle Clin. 2018;23(3):397–413.
52. Choisne J, Hoch M, Bawab S, et al. The effects of a semi-rigid ankle brace on a simulated isolated subtalar joint instability. J Orthop Res. 2013;31:1869–75.
53. Kobayashi T, Saka M, Suzuki E, et al. The effects of a semi-rigid brace or taping on talocrural and subtalar kinematics in chronic ankle instability. Foot Ankle Spec. 2014;7:471–7.
54. Broström L. Sprained ankles. V. Treatment and prognosis in recent ligament ruptures. Acta Chir Scand. 1966;132:537–50.
55. Gould N, Seligson D, Gassman J. Early and late repair of lateral ligament of the ankle. Foot Ankle. 1980;1:84–9.
56. Choisne J, Hoch MC, Alexander I, et al. Effect of direct ligament repair and tenodesis reconstruction on simulated subtalar joint instability. Foot Ankle Int. 2017;38:324–30.
57. Chrisman OD, Snook G. Reconstruction of lateral ligament tears of the ankle: an experimental study and clinical evaluation of seven patients treated by a new modification of the Elmslie procedure. J Bone Joint Surg. 1969;51:904–12.

58. Larsen. Tendon transfer for lateral ankle and subtalar joint instability. Acta Orthop Scand. 1988;59:168–72.
59. Schon LC, Clanton TO, Baxter DE, et al. Reconstruction for subtalar instability: a review. Foot Ankle. 1991;11:319–25.
60. Michels F, Guillo S, Vanrietvelde F, et al. How to drill the talar tunnel in ATFL reconstruction? Knee Surg Sports Traumatol Arthrosc. 2016;24: 991–7.
61. Michels F, Matricali G, Guillo S, Vanrietvelde F, Pottel H, Stockmans F. An oblique fibular tunnel is recommended when reconstructing the ATFL and CFL. Knee Surg Sports Traumatol Arthrosc. 2019;28:124–31. https://doi.org/10.1007/s00167-019-05583-3.
62. Elmslie RC. Recurrent subluxation of the ankle-joint. Ann Surg. 1934;100:364–7.
63. Mabit C, Pecout C, Arnaud JP. La ligamentoplastie au troisième fibulaire(peroneus tertius) dans les laxités latérales de la cheville. Rev Chir Orthop. 1996;82:70–5.
64. Pisani G. Chronic laxity of the subtalar joint. Orthopedics. 1996;19:431–7.
65. Liu C, Jiao C, Hu Y, et al. Interosseous talocalcaneal ligament reconstruction with hamstrings autograft under subtalar arthroscopy: case report. Foot Ankle Int. 2011;32:1089–94.
66. Li HY, Hua YH, Wu ZY, et al. Strength of suture anchor versus transosseous tunnel in anatomic reconstruction of the ankle lateral ligaments: a biomechanical study. Arthroscopy. 2013;29:1817–25.
67. Hoexum F, Heetveld MJ. Subtalar dislocation: two cases requiring surgery and a literature review of the last 25 years. Arch OrthopTrauma Surg. 2014;134:1237–49.
68. Zimmer TJ, Johnson KA. Subtalar dislocations. Clin Orthop. 1989;238:190–4.
69. Barber JR, Bricker JD, Haliburton RA. Peritalar dislocation of the foot. Can J Surg. 1961;4:205–9.
70. Fahey JJ, Murphy JL. Dislocations and fractures of the talus. Surg Clin North Am. 1965;45:79–82.
71. Shand AR Jr. The incidence of subastragaloid dislocation of the foot with a report of one case of the inward type. J Bone Joint Surg. 1928;10:306.
72. Smith H. Subastragalar dislocation. J Bone Joint Surg Am. 1937;37:373.
73. De Lee JC, Curts R. Subtalar dislocations of the foot. J Bone Joint Surg Am. 1982;64:433–7.
74. Grantham SA. Medial subtalar dislocation: five cases with a common etiology. J Trauma. 1964;4:845–9.
75. Heppenstall RB, Farahvar H, Balderston R, et al. Evaluation and management of subtalar dislocations. J Trauma. 1980;20:494–7.
76. Monson ST, Ryan JR. Subtalar dislocation. J Bone Joint Surg. 1981;63A:1156–8.
77. Pinzur MS, Meyer PR Jr. Complete posterior dislocation of the talus: case report and discussion. Clin Orthop. 1978;131:205–9.
78. Tucker DJ, Burian G, Boylan JP. Lateral subtalar dislocation: review of the literature and a case presentation. J Foot Ankle Surg. 1998;3:239–47.
79. Sanders DW. Fractures of the talus. In: Heckman JD, editor. Rockwood & Green's fractures in adults. 6th ed. Philadelphia: Lippincott Williams & Wilkins; 2006. p. 2249–93.
80. Krishnan KM, Sinha AK. True posterior dislocation of subtalar joint: a case report. J Foot Ankle Surg. 2003;42:363–5.
81. Bibbo C, Anderson RB, Davis WH. Injury characteristics and the clinical outcome of subtalar dislocations: a clinical and radiographic analysis of 25 cases. Foot Ankle Int. 2003;24:158–63.
82. Woodruff MJ, Brown JN, Mountney J. A mechanism for entrapment of the tibialis posterior tendon in lateral subtalar dislocation. Injury. 1996;27:193–4.
83. Simon LC, Schulz AP, Faschingbauer M, et al. "Basketball foot"-long-time prognosis after peritalar dislocation. S portverletz Sportschaden. 2008;22:31–7.
84. Wagner R, Blattert TR, Weckbach A. Talar dislocations. Injury. 2004;35(Suppl 2):SB36–45.
85. Buckingham WW Jr. Subtalar dislocation of the foot. J Trauma. 1973;13:753–65.
86. Straus DC. Subtalar dislocation of the foot. Am J Surg. 1935;30:427–34.
87. Merchan EC. Subtalar dislocations: long-term follow-up of 39 cases. Injury. 1992;23:97–100.
88. Gross RH. Medial peritalar dislocation associated foot injuries and mechanism of injury. J Trauma. 1975;15:682–8.
89. Bibbo C, Lin SS, Abidi N, et al. Missed and associated injuries after subtalar dislocation: the role of CT. Foot Ankle Int. 2001;22(4):324–8.
90. Bohay DR, Manoli A 2nd. Occult fractures following subtalar joint injuries. Foot Ankle Int. 1996;17:164–9.
91. Perugia D, Basile A, Massoni C, et al. Conservative treatment of subtalar dislocations. Int Orthop. 2002;26(1):56–60.
92. Haliburton RA, Barber JR, Fraser RL. Further experience with peritalar dislocation. Can J Surg. 1967;10:322–4.
93. Leitner B. Obstacles to reduction in subtalar dislocations. J Bone Joint Surg. 1954;36A:299–306.
94. Taylor LJ, Burke. Irreducible dislocation of the subtalar joint: a report of two cases. Injury. 1988;19:447–9.
95. Heck BE, Ebraheim NA, Jackson WT. Anatomical considerations of irreducible medial subtalar dislocation. Foot Ankle Int. 1992;17:103–6.
96. Garofalo R, Moretti B, Ortolano V, et al. Peritalar dislocations: a retrospective study of 18 cases. J Foot Ankle Surg. 2004;43:166–72.
97. Lancaster S, Horowitz M, Alonso J. Subtalar dislocations: a prognosticating classification. Orthopedics. 1985;8:1234–40.
98. Goldner JL, Poletti SC, Gates HS 3rd, et al. Severe open subtalar dislocations. Long-term results. J Bone Joint Surg Am. 1995;77A:1075–9.
99. Janssen T, Kopta J. Bilateral recurrent subtalar dislocation: case report. J Bone Joint Surg. 1985;67A:1432–3.

8 Combined Medial Pathology in Patients with Lateral Chronic Ankle Instability: Rotational Instability of the Ankle?

Hélder Pereira, Bruno Pereira, Nasef Abdelatif, and Jorge Batista

8.1 Introduction

"There is no such thing as a simple ankle sprain" [1]. This statement summarizes the current perspective from the scientific community concerning this entity, which remains one of the most frequent injuries, particularly during sports activity [1].

It affects mostly a young population, and its management depends on patient-related factors (e.g., expectations, activity-level, anatomy) and also on concomitant or subsequent pathologies which might also require treatment, either surgical or conservative [2].

Chronic ankle instability (CAI) can also be linked to loose bodies, cartilage or osteochondral defects, joint impingement (anterior and/or posterior) among others [2].

One topic gathering growing interest is the combination of lateral and medial instability which determines specific clinical and biomechanical implications and adequate treatment.

There is increasing research on the topic but only few reports so far.

Herein, the basic principles of the so-called rotational ankle instability pattern including biomechanical changes and options for management are described (Fact Box 1).

H. Pereira (✉)
Orthopedic Department of Póvoa de Varzim, Vila do Conde Hospital Centre, Póvoa de Varzim, Portugal

Ripoll y De Prado Sports Clinic: Murcia-Madrid FIFA Medical Centre of Excellence, Murcia, Spain

International Centre of Sports Traumatology of the Ave, Vila do Conde, Portugal

ICVS/3B's—PT Government Associated Laboratory, University of Minho, Braga-Guimarães, Portugal

i3B's Research Group–Biomaterials, Biodegradables and Biomimetics, University of Minho, Headquarters of the European Institute of Excellence on Tissue Engineering and Regenerative Medicine, AvePark, S. Cláudio de Barco, Taipas, Guimarães, Portugal

B. Pereira
Orthopedic Surgery Department, Hospital Santa Maria Maior, EPE—Barcelos, Barcelos, Portugal

Clínica do Dragão, Espregueira-Mendes Sports Centre—FIFA Medical Centre of Excellence, Porto, Portugal

Facultad de Medicina, University of Barcelona, Casanova 143, Barcelona, Spain

N. Abdelatif
Orthopedics and Reconstructive Foot and Ankle Surgery, Cairo, Egypt

J. Batista
Clinical Department Club Atletico Boca Juniores, CAJB—Centro Artroscopico, Buenos Aires, Argentina

H. Pereira et al. (eds.), *Lateral Ankle Instability*, https://doi.org/10.1007/978-3-662-62763-1_8

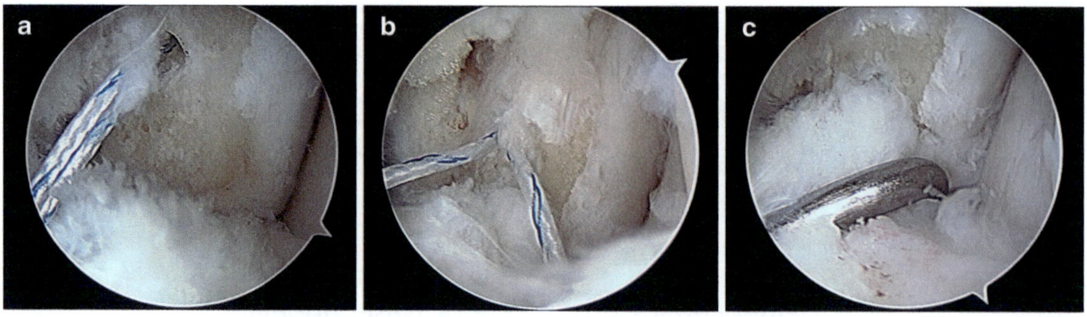

Fig. 8.1 (**a**) Arthroscopic anterior tibiofibular ligament (ATFL) repair by means of all-soft suture anchor requiring a 1.4 mm tunnel; (**b**) the suture involves the ATFL by all-inside technique. (**c**) The ATFL is brought to its native place on the distal fibula with adequate tension (hook probe)

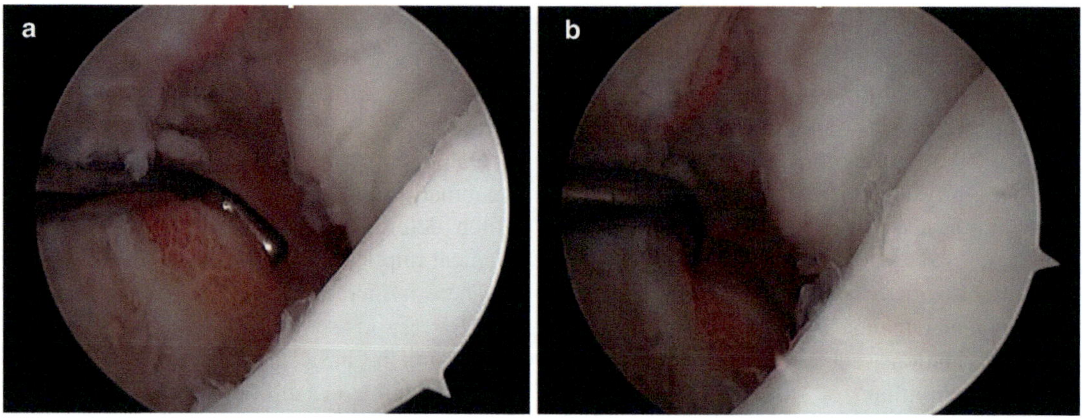

Fig. 8.2 (**a**, **b**) Arthroscopic inspection of the medial side on a patient operated for chronic ankle instability. The injury of the deltoid ligament is visible

8.2 Clinical Implications, Management, and Outcome

The clinical presentation of rotational CAI includes pain and tenderness on both sides of the ankle joint combined with feeling of giving way and repetitive sprains due to instability [3].

During weight-bearing situations, ankle joints with insufficient ATFL present a substantial increase in anterior translation, internal rotation, and superior translation of the talus [4]. This causes increased stress either in the normal or injured deltoid ligament thus aggravating acute injuries or leading to chronic medial insufficiency.

When in presence of combined insufficiency of the anterior talofibular ligament (ATFL) with lesion of anterior parts of the deltoid ligament complex (the superficial and deep part of the deltoid), the talus is prone to change its position into a "fixed anterior drawer." This anatomic disarrangement will lead to limited dorsiflexion once it will cause early osseous contact between the distal tibial edge and the talus thus diminishing the range of motion in dorsiflexion [5].

In summary, RAI patients abnormal increase of talar rotation within the tibiofibular mortise, which may cause further damage to the ankle joint.

The repair/reconstruction of medial and lateral ligament complexes will correct the talar position to the anatomic one, consequently improving the range of motion and protecting the joint from further damage [5].

Despite classically, the initial treatment approach of CAI patients is conservative treatment [6], when in presence of RAI, the authors suggest surgical repair and restoring anatomy, based in our own series and in the few studies reporting the outcome of surgical treatment [3, 5, 7].

The repair of this situation affecting both the medial and the lateral ligament complex can be performed by open, mini-open, or endoscopic-assisted (Figs. 8.1 and 8.2).

The use of suture anchors has made such repairs easier representing a significant technical advance, particularly those small ones which create minimal bone damage such as all-soft suture anchors (Fig. 8.1).

Take-Home Message

Rotational ankle instability (RAI) describes a condition that combines injuries of both lateral and medial ankle ligamen complexes.

The diagnosis of this condition is not easy either by clinical or radiological (including MRI) features.

Arthroscopic inspection and testing under anesthesia might play a role.

This situation leads to biomechanical changes which ultimately will aggravate joint damage.

There is increased talar rotation within the ankle mortise.

RAI is linked to changes in the placement of the talus and diminished range of motion.

Despite the classical approach for treatment of CAI includes conservative treatment as first approach, the authors consider that, when in presence or suspicion of RAI, surgical treatment is advised.

Fact Box 1 Rotational Ankle Instability (RAI)

- RAI is a condition that combines injuries of both lateral and medial ankle ligamen complexes.
- Difficult diagnosis by clinical or radiological (including MRI) features. Arthroscopic inspection and testing under anesthesia might play a role.
- RAI leads to biomechanical changes which ultimately will aggravate joint damage.
- The authors consider that, when in presence or suspicion of RAI, surgical treatment is advised.

References

1. van Dijk CN, Vuurberg G. There is no such thing as a simple ankle sprain: clinical commentary on the 2016 International Ankle Consortium position statement. Br J Sports Med. 2017;51(6):485–6. https://doi.org/10.1136/bjsports-2016-096733.
2. Pereira H, Vuurberg G, Spennacchio P, Batista J, D'Hooghe P, Hunt K, Van Dijk N. Surgical treatment paradigms of ankle lateral instability, osteochondral defects and impingement. Adv Exp Med Biol. 2018;1059:85–108. https://doi.org/10.1007/978-3-319-76735-2_4.
3. Alrashidi Y, Stelzenbach C, Herrera-Perez M, Wiewiorski M, Valderrabano V. Chronic rotational ankle instability—a case series study. Sports Orthop Traumatol. 2015;31:200–5.
4. Caputo AM, Lee JY, Spritzer CE, Easley ME, DeOrio JK, Nunley JA 2nd, DeFrate LE. In vivo kinematics of the tibiotalar joint after lateral ankle instability. Am J Sports Med. 2009;37(11):2241–8. https://doi.org/10.1177/0363546509337578.
5. Buchhorn T, Sabeti-Aschraf M, Dlaska CE, Wenzel F, Graf A, Ziai P. Combined medial and lateral anatomic ligament reconstruction for chronic rotational instability of the ankle. Foot Ankle Int. 2011;32(12):1122–6. https://doi.org/10.3113/FAI.2011.1122.
6. Guelfi M, Zamperetti M, Pantalone A, Usuelli FG, Salini V, Oliva XM. Open and arthroscopic lateral ligament repair for treatment of chronic ankle instability: a systematic review. Foot Ankle Surg. 2018;24(1):11–8. https://doi.org/10.1016/j.fas.2016.05.315.
7. Vega J, Allmendinger J, Malagelada F, Guelfi M, Dalmau-Pastor M. Combined arthroscopic all-inside repair of lateral and medial ankle ligaments is an effective treatment for rotational ankle instability. Knee Surg Sports Traumatol Arthrosc. 2020;28(1):132–40. https://doi.org/10.1007/s00167-017-4736-y.

Part II

Non-operative Approach

Prevention Strategies and Prehab for Lateral Ankle Instability

9

Jon Fearn, Chris Pearce, Bas Pijnenburg, and James Calder

9.1 Introduction

Ankle sprains are one of the commonest musculoskeletal injuries in sport and particularly in multidirectional sports such as football [1, 2]. Injury to the lateral ligament complex (consisting of the Anterior Talofibular, Calcaneaofibular, and Posterior Talofibular ligaments) that provide stability to the lateral aspect of the ankle, account for the majority of these.

The terms "ankle ligament laxity" and "ankle ligament instability" are often used interchangeably but they are in fact clinically distinct entities.

Ligamentous laxity is an individual characteristic of the collagen resulting in excessive joint mobility but no injury has been sustained.

Instability can be either mechanical or functional. "Mechanical instability" or laxity is a physical sign that occurs after injury and is objectively detected on examination indicating excessive movement of the joint involved. "Functional instability" is a symptom resulting from the damaged ligaments' inability to control the joint during functional movements, such as running, cutting, or turning. Patients with chronic lateral ankle instability (CLAI) may experience symptoms such as persistent ankle stiffness, swelling, pain, muscle weakness, or frequent giving way [3]. These repeated episodes of ankle sprains are known as "chronic ankle instability." [4]

In every case, a thorough examination is required in order to reach an accurate diagnosis and plan the most appropriate management program.

9.2 Epidemiology

Ankle sprains commonly affect athletes participating in sports involving frequent changes of direction. Lateral ankle sprains account for 85% of all ankle injuries in the general athletic population [5]. The most common risk factor to suffering a lateral ankle sprain is a history of at least one previous ankle sprain [6–8].

In basketball, 70% of players report a history of lateral ankle sprain with 80% of these individuals reporting recurrent sprains [8]. In football,

J. Fearn
Fortius Clinic, London, UK
e-mail: Jon.fearn@chelseafc.com

C. Pearce (✉)
National University Health System, Singapore, Singapore
e-mail: chris.pearce@doctors.net.uk

B. Pijnenburg
ACIBADEM International Medical Center, Amsterdam, The Netherlands

J. Calder
Fortius Clinic, London, UK

Chelsea Football Club Medical Department, London, UK
e-mail: James.Calder@fortiusclinic.com

H. Pereira et al. (eds.), *Lateral Ankle Instability*, https://doi.org/10.1007/978-3-662-62763-1_9

Table 9.1 Number of lateral ankle stability cases between seasons 2011 and 2017

Between 2011 and 2017	Total number of ankle injuries	Lateral complex injuries	Lead to ankle instability
Academy (U9–23)	102	78	3[a]
Professional squad	31	20	0

[a]NB: Of these three cases, two cases were in the U18 squad and one in the U23 squad

lateral ankle sprains account for approximately 20% of all injuries sustained [9, 10].

Injury audit data analyzed from Chelsea Football Club (CFC) between the 2011 and 2017 seasons (Table 9.1) showed a total of 133 ankle sprains were sustained (Academy and Professional squad) which represented 11% of the total injuries sustained at the club during that time period. Injuries to the lateral ligament complex made up 70% of total ankle ligament injuries sustained between 2011 and 2017.

Ankle instability has been suggested to affect between 10 and 20% of the athletic population [11, 12].

In the Academy system at CFC, following a period of rehabilitation, only 3% ($n = 3$) of players who sustained lateral ankle injuries had ongoing symptoms of instability. These individuals were then all treated with extended periods of nonsurgical management, with 2% receiving Platelet Rich Plasma (PRP) injections, and all returned to full football participation without further problems.

Within the professional squad, there were no players presenting with ankle instability following their initial period of rehabilitation after an acute ankle injury. Worthy of note is that all of these were treated nonsurgically using a standard treatment program (discussed later) which has an emphasis on developing the players' level of football-specific functional movement.

9.3 Prehabilitation and Prevention

Prehabilitation or "prehab" is a proactive approach to avoid future pain or injury. This is essentially the same as injury prevention where strategies are implemented to reduce the risk of a particular injury occurring. Preventing post-injury lateral ankle instability requires an effective and comprehensive rehabilitation process which begins immediately after the initial injury is sustained, and continues until the player returns to play.

Immediately following the initial injury, for example, we do not immobilize the ankle or use crutches unless it is absolutely essential to prevent the player from mobilizing on the injured ankle. We encourage the best possible gait pattern when walking, without using any immobilization or mobility aids. This is the start of the functional rehabilitation approach.

9.4 "Functional Rehabilitation" Biased Approach

The philosophy is based on the concept that the sooner the patient can start to move in a safe and pain-free manner the healing tissue will positively respond.

"Pain-free movement is therapeutic"

In this approach, local and specific ankle treatment are complimented with progressive functional loading utilizing different modalities and environments. Players are closely supervised and logically progressed in these environments which allows gradually increasing load and demands on the healing tissue in a safe manner.

These include:

- Aquatic therapy: using a varying depth of the pool and underwater treadmills such as the hydroworx.
- Anti-gravity treadmills such as Alter G.
- On-field rehabilitation (discussed later in this chapter).

Most players begin their functional movement progression in the water, where the qualities of an aquatic environment create a safe and productive way for the players to progress. One such water quality is that of buoyancy, which acts to reduce the relative weight-bearing status of an individual according to depth submerged. This effect has a linear relationship where the greater the depth of submersion the greater the degree of relative weight-bearing offload, so often players start walking in water at shoulder depth. As comfort and quality of functional pattern improve at one water level, then the water depth is reduced, which increases relative weight-bearing and progresses the individual towards full weight-bearing functional movement. As soon as the player is able to walk effectively and is symptom-free, he is then progressed onto running drills.

During this process, the functional capabilities of the ankle are continuously monitored by the medical team. Early mobilization in the water not only allows the ankle to be moving functionally in a safe, stable environment but also allows early proprioceptive stimulation to occur. The ultimate functional aim for the structure is always appreciated during this process and the movement is pain-free. This is not just important when appreciating what sport/activity an individual performs, such as football, but even the position in the sport they play, e.g., goal-keeper versus a defender, as the functional demands on the ankle may vary.

Progressing function takes many forms:

- From partial to full weight-bearing in the Aquatic environment.
- Direction of movement: Initially linear (straight line) movements in order to protect the lateral ankle ligamentous complex before progressing onto lateral or rotational movements that require more ankle joint stability.
- Develop Time/Speed/Intensity of movement: Gradually build the amount of time (volume) of functional work as well as the intensity (speed) as their ability allows.

It is important to continually monitor the ankles' response to any treatment or intervention. This may be in the form of increasing pain, swelling, reduced mobility, and then adjust future management accordingly.

This "functional rehabilitation" approach is combined with manual therapy to mobilize and stimulate tissue healing to the affected region safely without compromise to the damaged structures; electrotherapy techniques to maximize the quality of the healing; and proprioceptive neuromuscular control exercises and on occasions PRP is used.

This multidisciplinary approach involves numerous medical professionals. We are able to offer one-to-one physiotherapy to player care which ensures compliance and effective progression. A typical day involves an MDT assessment review, manual therapy, functionally based rehabilitation (e.g., in the pool or on-field with the ball) together with proprioceptive exercises and electrotherapy and can take over 4–5 h in any given day.

By following a comprehensive "functional" biased rehabilitation process for ankle injuries, we have minimized the risk of further injury and cases of instability as well as the necessity for surgical intervention. It is also essentially the same approach when implementing a post-injury "prehab" program, i.e., addressing the areas highlighted following a thorough examination.

There are many different approaches to managing musculoskeletal injuries/lateral ankle instability but this is one proposed approach.

> *"The best prevention from football injuries is to play football"*

9.5 Chelsea FC Medical Department Philosophy

- We work as a multidisciplinary team.
- We aim to have highly experienced medical staff with a varied skill mix, allowing us to deliver a wide variety of unique skills and modalities appropriate at different aspects of the rehab process.
- We feel it is essential to achieve a correct diagnosis to ensure an efficient rehabilitation process is undertaken.
- The assessment and diagnosis process must be undertaken with both a doctor, a physiotherapist and potentially other medical department staff members present.
- After the assessment (which can be led by any staff member) is complete, the player leaves the room while the staff members discuss the

presentation and come to an agreement of a single diagnosis and plan.

- The player is then invited back into the room and is given a single "team" diagnosis and a plan which the player can then also ask questions about and contribute to as they wish.
- Further investigations are undertaken as appropriate but are not always essential.
- The implementation of the injury management plan is then led by a physiotherapist.
- Regular feedback and communication with the medical team regarding progress, challenges, and management are delivered on a daily basis with group reviews being undertaken as required.

9.6 CFC Injury Management Philosophy

The goal of any rehabilitation program is to return the individual to their previous level of function as soon as it is safe and minimizing the risk of re-injury. For a footballer that is to play football. For a tennis player, that is to play tennis. Therefore, the functional movements mimicking the movements required should be initiated as soon as is safe to do so.

At CFC, there is a combined management approach facilitating the "local" ankle injury to heal in response to the football-like functional demands expected. This is achieved by carrying out functional tasks in protective environments hence the "functional based approach."

This philosophy is delivered by the medical staff throughout Chelsea Football Club in all squads and at all ages (Professional squad, Academy system U9–23, Ladies squads) and adapted accordingly.

9.7 Prevention of Lateral Ankle Instability

Following a thorough clinical examination of the ankle, it is essential to analyze the possible causes of the lateral instability in order to plan the most effective intervention program.

The aim of management is to normalize these areas as much as possible. Previous screening can help to indicate the level or ability that was previously attained.

The fundamentals of preventing ankle instability essentially fall into three categories:

9.8 "Ankle-Specific" Targeted Interventions

Following a thorough examination, areas that may need to be addressed may include:

- The level and extent of anatomical injury sustained in order to plan the direction of treatment.
- Morphotype and pathomechanics of the individual (e.g., Pes cavus, Genu Varum) which may predispose the individual to lateral ankle instability.
- Mobilizing related joints are involved to gain the optimal range of movement required.
- Strengthening of the muscles affecting the ankle, particularly muscles controlling ankle eversion and plantarflexion.
- Neuromuscular control and proprioception of the ankle. This is probably the most important aspect.
- Improving neuromuscular control can start with drills in controlled environments such as the pool. By making functional movements more dynamic, such as walking to running and changing direction, this can increase proprioceptive demand to the ankle.
- The ankle complex can be proprioceptively challenged more specifically with balance challenging exercises with a particular bias to the plantarflexion/inversion control where the ankle may feel more vulnerable. For example, during single leg balance exercises on unstable surfaces or simply by closing the individual's eyes (Fig. 9.1).
- As a part of a comprehensive rehabilitation process the inclusion of balance challenging tasks with increasing difficulty and their specificity to function is essential to minimize functional instability. This follows the constraints-

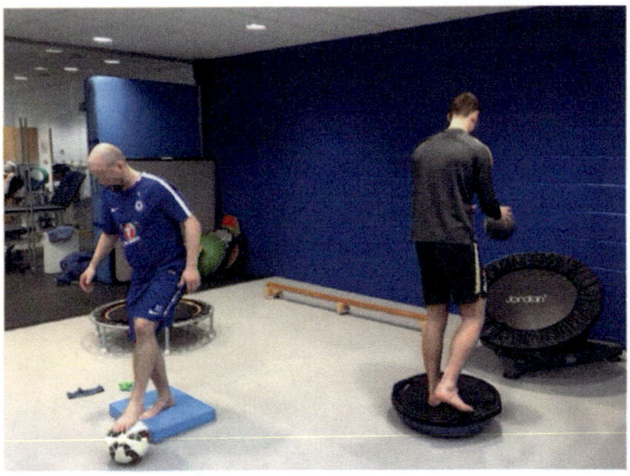

Fig. 9.1 Area dedicated to improve neuromuscular control in a gym environment. It is managed by a physiotherapist and permits innovative and football-like movements

based balance training approach discussed by Wikstrom in 2013 and has been shown to have significant improvement in self-assessed disability and postural control [13].

- We have an area designated for improving an individual's neuromuscular control within the gym environment. This is manned by a physiotherapist and allows effective, innovative, and football-like movements to be challenged and developed (Fig. 9.1).

Interventions vary according to the stage and state of the healing tissue. Different interventions are necessary at different healing stages and vary in their effectiveness, but are implemented however small the potential gain, i.e., marginal gains. These include:

- Manual Therapy (to improve joint and soft tissue mobility)
- Rest/Passive Therapy to allow the tissue to heal but enhance joint mobility.
- Electrotherapy (to optimize the healing/inflammatory response), e.g., SWD, magnetic therapy in the acute stages as well as therapeutic ultrasound during the proliferative and remodeling phase. Compex/TENS stimulation is also useful for pain control.
- Intermittent Pneumatic Compression device application to reduce excessive swelling.
- Thermal therapy to either dampen the inflammatory response in the initial stages, e.g., cold/ice, or further facilitate healing response accordingly depending on the stage of healing.
- Medication use of pain control and NSAIDs, particularly to facilitate effective function by reducing pain in the early stages.
- Injection therapy, additional benefits of PRP therapy to facilitate the healing response. Note that we never use cortisone steroid therapy in cases of lateral instability.
- Exercise therapy, together with adjuncts such as muscle stimulation, to improve neuromuscular control and strength.

9.8.1 Taping and Bracing of the Ankle

In addition to other interventions, taping (or bracing) at the ankle can be used to enhance a player's confidence to undertake functional tasks through physical and proprioceptive joint support.

- Taping and/or bracing (Fig. 9.2) can be used as part of the rehabilitation process and used to prevent further episodes of functional instability. It is clear that both taping and bracing can reduce mechanical instability but there is no guarantee this projects into reducing functional instability of the ankle.
- Taping or bracing techniques are thought to facilitate the ankles' proprioceptive response and the neuromuscular control of the ankle during functional tasks [14].
- The effectiveness of taping and bracing is very dependent on the expertise of the clinician. Not only does an experienced clinician have a greater understanding of the wide range of products, materials, and techniques at their disposal but will also be more skilled when applying a strapping or a brace aiming at controlling the ankle instability present.
- Taping by an experienced clinician is often tolerated better with function than a brace. We know however that taping is not as effective at limiting mechanical instability after approximately 20 min whereas bracing, due to its more rigid design, does limit the ankle's mobility and

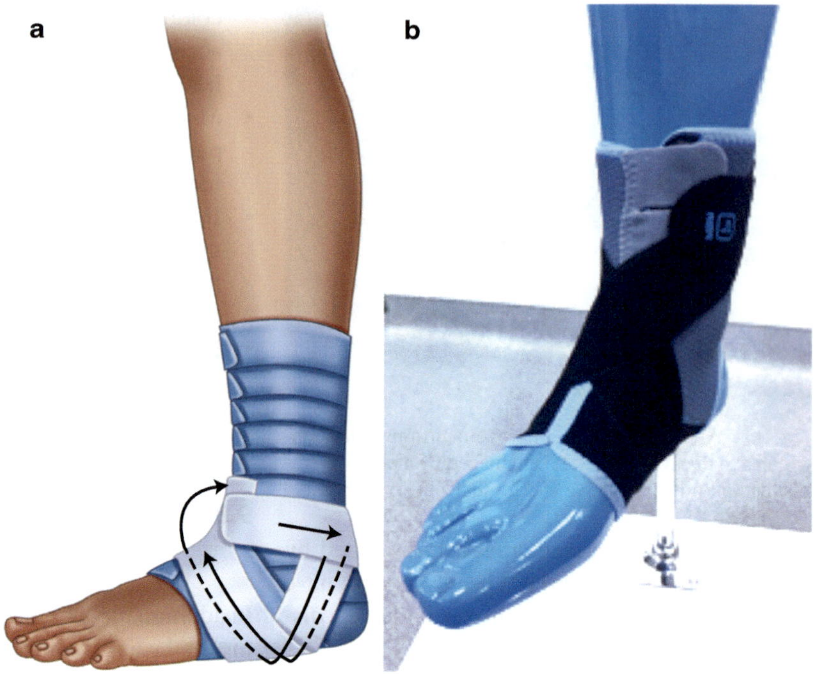

Fig. 9.2 Schematic drawing of ankle taping (**a**) and one ankle brace (**b**), indicated in lateral ankle instability management

potentially reduces mechanical instability for longer periods. Therefore, consideration of these aspects needs to be taken into consideration when choosing the most suitable option at that time in the rehabilitation process.

- It is worth noting that the nature of elite football performance requires a high level of fine motor foot control and taping or bracing can compromise this control. Therefore, a balance between the degree of control and movement freedom needs to be achieved at any time in the rehab process.
- It is important to stress that taping and bracing techniques are not a substitute for improving the neuromuscular control of the ankle complex and therefore control should be continually developed. The goal of taping should be to provide support early on, however, this need for additional control should be reduced as the player's own dynamic control and functional proprioceptive strength recover.

9.8.2 On-Field Rehabilitation

If the player is unable to train or perform their normal sporting activities it is important they optimize the "functional rehabilitation" recovery process in a more controlled environment. This may take the form of on-field rehabilitation.

As soon as the player has been able to do quality movement patterns in a reduced weight-bearing environment, such as the water, then both the clinician and the player will have confidence in making the transition to full weight-bearing function. If you have not been able to do this, then you need to introduce the activity in its most basic form and build up the complexity as they tolerate each step.

Although the functional movement approach aims to focus on function rather than the pathology, the nature and type of movement you are going to include in your first sessions on the grass will be influenced in part by the pathology you are dealing with.

Worthy of note is that, as per the functional movement philosophy, as soon as you can do something you should. If, for example, you have been doing light multidirectional movements in the water and the player has tolerated these well, then you can introduce low-intensity versions of these movements early, even in the first session.

The sessions are then progressed accordingly by increasing the intensity or speed of the exercises, the amount of time spent on field, and the increasing complexity and stress on the lateral structures of the ankle.

As previously mentioned, start with linear, straight line drills (Fig. 9.3) at a low pace which ensures the ankle complex is protected and the neuromuscular control progressed.

Figure 9.3 represents an example of an early linear drill a player may execute on the field.

The player is then progressed onto lateral cutting or rotational movements with increasing speed (Fig. 9.4). Also by introducing external cues and obstacles such as the ball are all subtle way of increasing the complexity and demand of the exercise.

Figure 9.4 demonstrates an example of a more advanced controlled on-field drill for an attacking footballer. With problem-free execution of drills such as this, the player will be close to return to modified training.

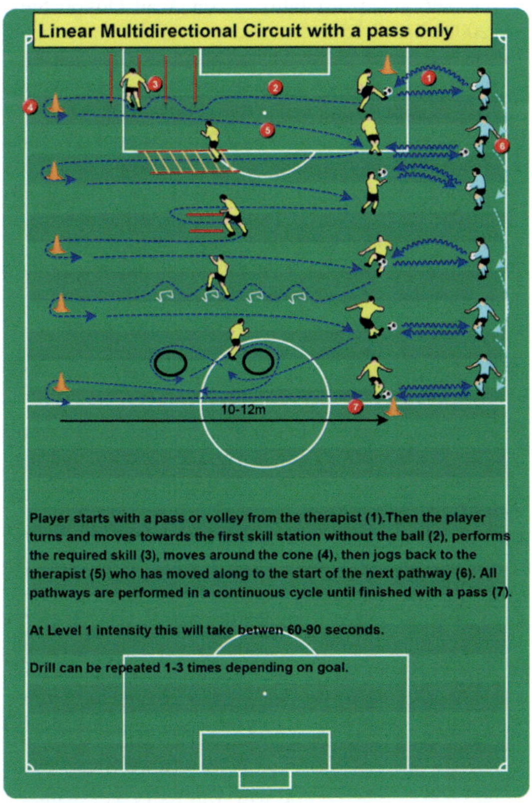

Fig. 9.3 Example of an early multidirectional drill which the player may execute on the pitch

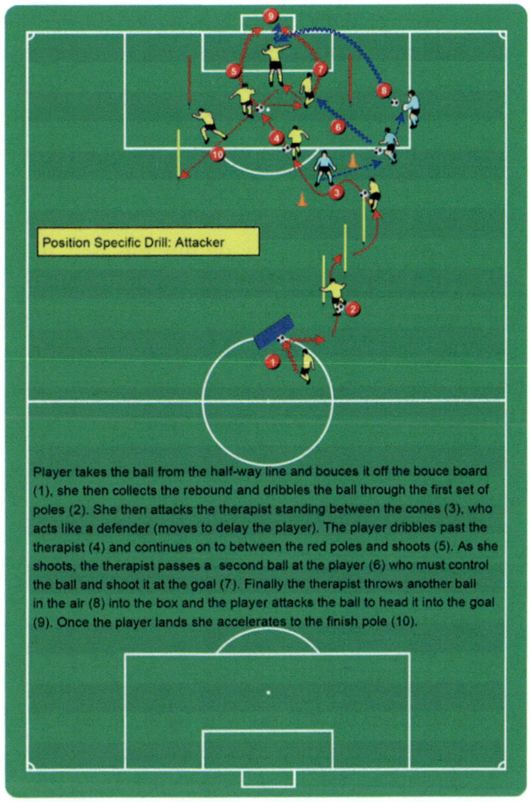

Fig. 9.4 Example of a more advanced controlled exercise for an attacking footballer with an increase in training performance

Take-Home Message: The Injury Prevention Unit at Chelsea Football Club

A "Prevention Unit" is currently under development to ensure that our injury prevention philosophy is mirrored throughout the football club.

This involves all squads of all ages, ranging from professional, academy, and ladies, as well as the foundation and developmental squads.

The unit is multidisciplinary involving doctors, physios, coaches, fitness coaches, and sports scientists representing all the squads involved.

As a club, there is a common message for all players to be educated in the importance of health essentials such as nutrition, sleep, lifestyle, mental, and physical well-being.

Similarly, it is the prevention unit's role to look at areas to improve a player's locomotor control and performance as well as lowering the injury rate.

By having a prevention unit delivering the same message, our hope is to ensure that our philosophy is followed from the first team squad down to the youngest age group of 8-year olds throughout the club and ensure our players are able to play and enjoy their football as much as possible.

It is worth noting that within the first team squad, due to players' playing commitments for both club and country with regular periods where there are only 2–3 days between competitive games, having the time to implement injury prevention strategies can be challenging.

Fact Box 1

- Ankle (or musculoskeletal) injury prevention program requires a multidisciplinary team.
- Implementing an injury prevention program might be challenging in some situations given the lack of time in highly competitive clubs. However, the benefits worth the challenge, starting even at younger ages of athletic competition or training.
- The philosophy supporting any injury prevention program should be delivered by the medical staff throughout any level of competition, all squads, genders, and at all ages.

Fact Box 2 "Ankle Specific" Assessment Topics Aiming for Injury Prevention

- Proper assessment of acute anatomical injury as well as history of previous injuries.
- Identify patient-specific risk factors which may predispose the athlete to lateral ankle instability, such as individual's morphotype and pathomechanics (e.g., Pes cavus, Genu Varum).
- Optimizing range of motion of ankle related joints in order to gain best performance and lower injury rate.
- Strengthening of the muscles controlling ankle eversion and plantarflexion.
- Choice of adequate shoe wear, insoles, bracing, taping, etc.
- Improvement of neuromuscular control and proprioception of the ankle—possibly the most important aspect.

References

1. Lassiter TE Jr, Malone TR, Garrett WE. Injury to the lateral ligaments of the ankle. Orthop Clin North Am. 1989;20:629–40.
2. McConkey JP. Ankle sprains, consequences and mimics. Med Sport Sci. 1987;18:39–55.
3. Renstrom P, Lynch SA. Ankle ligament injuries. Rev Bras Med Esporte. 1998;4:71–81.
4. Hansen H, Damholt V, Termansen NB. Clinical and social status following injury to the lateral ligaments of the ankle. Acta Othrop Scand. 1979;50:699–704.
5. Maffulli N, Ferran NA. Management of acute and chronic ankle instability. J Am Acad Orthop Surg. 2008;16:608–15.
6. Bahr R, Bahr IA. Incidence of acute volleyball injuries: a prospective study of injury mechanisms and risk factors. Scand J Med Sci Sports. 1997;7:166–72.
7. Milgrom C, Shlamkovitch N, Finestone A. Risk factors for lateral ankle sprain: a prospective study among military recruits. Foot Ankle. 1991;12:26–30.
8. Smith R, Reischl S. Treatment of ankle sprains in young athletes. Am J Sports Med. 1986;14:465–58.
9. Ekstrand J, Tropp H. The incidence of ankle sprains in soccer. Foot Ankle. 1990;11:41–4.
10. Peterson L, Junge A, Chomiak J, Graf-Baumann T, Dvorak J. Incidence of football injuries and complaints in different age groups and skill levels. AJSM. 2000;28:S51–7.
11. Lentell G, Baas B, Lopez D, et al. The contributions of proprioceptive deficits, muscle function and anatomic laxity to functional instability of the ankle. J Orthop Sports Phys Ther. 1995;21(4):206–15.
12. Michelson JD, Hutchins C. Mechanoreceptors in human ankle ligaments. J Bone Joint Surg Br. 1995;77:219–24.
13. Wikstrom EA, Hubbard-Turner T, McKeon PO. Understanding and treating lateral ankle sprains and their consequences. Sports Med. 2013;43:385–93.
14. Drez DJ, Kaveney MF. Ankle ligament injuries. Practical guidelines for examination and treatment. J Musculoskel Med. 1989;6:21–36.

10 Current Concepts in Ankle Sprain Treatment

Gwendolyn Vuurberg, P. Spennacchio, L. Laver, J. P. Pereira, P. Diniz, and G. M. M. J. Kerkhoffs

10.1 Introduction

Lateral ankle sprains (LAS) have been reported as the most common musculoskeletal injury [1, 2]. Of all traumatic ankle injuries, 40% occur during sports [3]. An incidence of seven lateral ankle sprains (LAS) per 1000 exposures has been reported for indoor sports [4]. These account for about 14% of all sports-related injuries [5]. Despite this high reported prevalence and incidence, only approximately 50% of the patients who sustained a LAS seek medical attention [6]. Adequate treatment of those who seek professional help is essential to prevent residual chronic symptoms, such as chronic ankle instability (CAI) or post-traumatic impingement syndrome [7–10]. Reported incidences for residual symptoms after lateral ankle sprain are as high as 55–72% at 6 weeks to 18 months [11, 12].

10.2 Injury Mechanism

LAS usually occur during sports involving activities such as running, cutting, jumping, diving, landing, and contact with others [1, 2, 5, 13]. Player contact in football has shown to be responsible for up to 59% of the injuries and non-contact situations accounted for 39% of all injuries [2]. The most common injury contact situations are

G. Vuurberg (✉) · G. M. M. J. Kerkhoffs
Department of Orthopedic Surgery, Amsterdam UMC location AMC, University of Amsterdam, Amsterdam Movement Sciences, Amsterdam, The Netherlands

Academic Center for Evidence Based Sports medicine (ACES), Amsterdam, The Netherlands

Amsterdam Collaboration for Health and Safety in Sports (ACHSS), Amsterdam UMC, Amsterdam, The Netherlands
e-mail: g.vuurberg@amsterdamumc.nl; g.m.kerkhoffs@amsterdamumc.nl

P. Spennacchio
Department of Trauma and Orthopaedics, University Hospitals Coventry and Warwickshire, Coventry, UK

L. Laver
Deptartment of Arthroscopy, The Royal Orthopaedic Hospital, Birmingham, UK

Clinique du Sport, Centre Hospitalier Luxembourg, Luxembourg, Luxembourg

J. P. Pereira
Ripoll y De Prado Sports Clinic: Murcia-Madrid FIFA Medical Centre of Excellence, Murcia, Spain

H.P. Orthopedics and Research Centre—International Centre of Sports Traumatology of the Ave, Vila do Conde, Portugal

P. Diniz
Department of Orthopaedic Surgery, Hospital de Sant'Ana, Parede, Portugal

Institute for Bioengineering and Biosciences, Instituto Superior Técnico, Universidade de Lisboa, Lisbon, Portugal

Fisiogaspar, Lisbon, Portugal

H. Pereira et al. (eds.), *Lateral Ankle Instability*, https://doi.org/10.1007/978-3-662-62763-1_10

defined as tackling (36%) and being tackled (18%). The most common non-contact situations are landing (36%), twisting/turning (21%), and diving (10%) [2].

The fibula extends further caudally than the medial malleolus, this creates a block to eversion and allows a greater Range of Motion (ROM) to inversion than eversion. Forced inversion lesion represents the most frequent injury pattern among LAS. An inversion sprain is a combination of internal rotation of the foot, plantar flexion of the tibiotalar joint with the subtalar joint adducting and inverting [11, 14]. This mechanism results in strain of the lateral ankle ligamentous complex. The anterior talofibular ligament (ATFL), which is a thin structure with a low ultimate load [11], is the first ligament to be damaged, followed by the calcaneofibular ligament (CFL) [11]. Isolated lesion of the ATFL occurs in 65% of all injuries, while combined rupture of the ATFL and CFL occurs in approximately 20%. Isolated ruptures of the CFL are rare. In approximately 10–15% of all inversion injuries, there is a total rupture of the lateral ankle ligaments [11].

Even though the isolated involvement of the lateral ligamentous complex (ATFL with/without CFL involvement) is by far the most frequent lesion pattern after an ankle sprains, the physician should always consider through the diagnostic process a syndesmotic and/or medial ligamentous complex injury. These lesions share a similar injury mechanism, which is a forced external rotation with the ankle in dorsiflexion, and have specific therapeutic consequences [15]. Syndesmotic and deltoid complex lesions will not be discussed in this chapter, which focuses on inversion LAS.

10.3 Diagnostics

A precise definition of the ligamentous injury severity after a LAS is crucial to establish adequate treatment, and reduce the risk of residual chronic symptoms. Kannus et al. [16] reported that the degree of damage of the most severely injured ligament has a superior clinical impact than the number of involved ligaments.

One common classification system to classify ankle lateral ligament sprain includes grade I (mild), grade II (moderate/micro lesions), and grade III (severe/full lesion) injuries (Table 10.1) [17]. From a practical point of view, the most important issue is to differentiate between "simple" grade I ligament stretch injuries and unstable grade II and III injuries, which mean partial and complete rupture of at least one ligament, respectively. Recent guidelines frequently group together grade II and III injuries, with equal therapeutic indication [18].

In the acute diagnostic setting of a LAS, the Ottawa Ankle Rules should be applied to discern whether the radiographic examination of the ankle is indicated, to rule out an ankle fracture [14].

Observations made during clinical and diagnostic examination should be considered when classifying ankle injuries. First of all severe (concomitant) injuries should be treated [14]. Harmon et al. [19] described in a five-step systematic approach that aims to avoid missing potentially serious injuries:

1. palpation of bony structures;
2. palpation of ligamentous structures;
3. assessment of range of motion (ROM) of the ankle;
4. testing of ankle muscles;
5. performance of (joint) specific tests.

Additionally, the Anterior Drawer Test (ADT) might help distinguish between a stable and unstable ankle joint [20]. Excessive swelling and pain can limit adequate physical examination up to 48h after injury [1]. Therefore, it is recommended to repeat the physical examination after 3–5 days. A delayed physical examination has been shown to have specificity and sensitivity of 84% and 96%, respectively for the detection of a lateral ankle ligament rupture [18, 21], whereas examination within 48h had a sensitivity of 71% and a specificity of 33% [22]. The high specificity of the delayed physical examination permits a reliable recognition of LAS without ankle ligament rupture [21].

Diagnostic imaging modalities may consist of ultrasonography (US) (sensitivity 92%; specificity 64%) [22, 23] or MRI (sensitivity 93–96%; specificity 100%) [24–28]. As US lacks sensitiv-

Table 10.1 Classification and related treatment focus [17, 20]

Classification	Characteristics	Treatment focus	Treatment modality
Sprain severity			
– Grade I	Mild ligament injury	Symptoms	NSAIDs[a] Exercise therapy
– Grade II	Moderate ligament injury/micro lesions	Symptoms, function	NSAIDs[a] Functional support Exercise therapy
– Grade III	Severe ligament injury/full tear	Symptoms, function, and prevention progressive joint damage	NSAIDs[a] Immobilization Surgical repair followed by exercise therapy

[a]Consider NSAIDs in case pain limits rehabilitation as it might inhibit tissue recovery

ity and specificity compared to delayed physical examination, it can only be used if available at the emergency room (ER) and reliability is dependent on the experience of the technician handling the probe. It may not be the first choice in patients who suffered from an ankle sprain [22, 23]. An MRI may be of added value if there is a suspicion of high-grade ligament injuries (both medial and lateral), osteochondral defects (OCDs), syndesmotic sprains and occult fractures [23]. Poor availability of MRI scans in the ER setting together with the high prevalence of LAS limits, however, its use in acute settings.

10.4 Treatment Modalities

Although ankle inversion sprains are very common, treatment selection remains controversial. As already mentioned, the distinction between Grade I simple stable injuries and Grade II and III partial/full ligament ruptures is the first step to an adequate treatment. The literature shows that treatment of an acute lateral ligament rupture too short in duration and/or with insufficient support of the ankle joint tends to result in more residual symptoms [29].

10.4.1 Rest Ice Compression Elevation (RICE)

RICE is a classic initial treatment modality, often applied in acute situations, to diminish swelling and pain associated with more severe LAS, and facilitate a quick rehabilitation strategy. Even though its effectiveness on LAS symptoms is not supported by strong evidence [30–36] cryotherapy in combination with exercise therapy (Fig. 10.1) has shown to reduce swelling and improve ankle function [32, 37]. There is no conclusive evidence on the effectiveness of compression therapy alone to reduce swelling during the first post-traumatic 48h [33–35].

10.4.2 Non-Steroidal Anti-Inflammatory Drugs (NSAIDs)

Non-Steroidal Anti-inflammatory Drugs (NSAIDs) are more and more commonly prescribed for patients who sustained a LAS to primarily reduce pain. Recent studies have shown that the use of oral or topical NSAIDs lightens pain without significantly increasing the risk of adverse events, compared to placebo [38–42]. Opioid analgesics have shown equal effects for pain relief but lead to significantly more side effects [43, 44]. Additionally, it should be noted that the use of NSAIDs may delay the natural healing process due to suppression of the inflammation which is a necessary component of tissue recovery [45].

10.4.3 Functional Treatment

Functional treatment is a relatively new concept including treatment modalities which aim to preserve joint function and mobility, as much as permitted by the initial diagnosis. Taping or bracing (Fig. 10.2) instead of cast immobilization, and

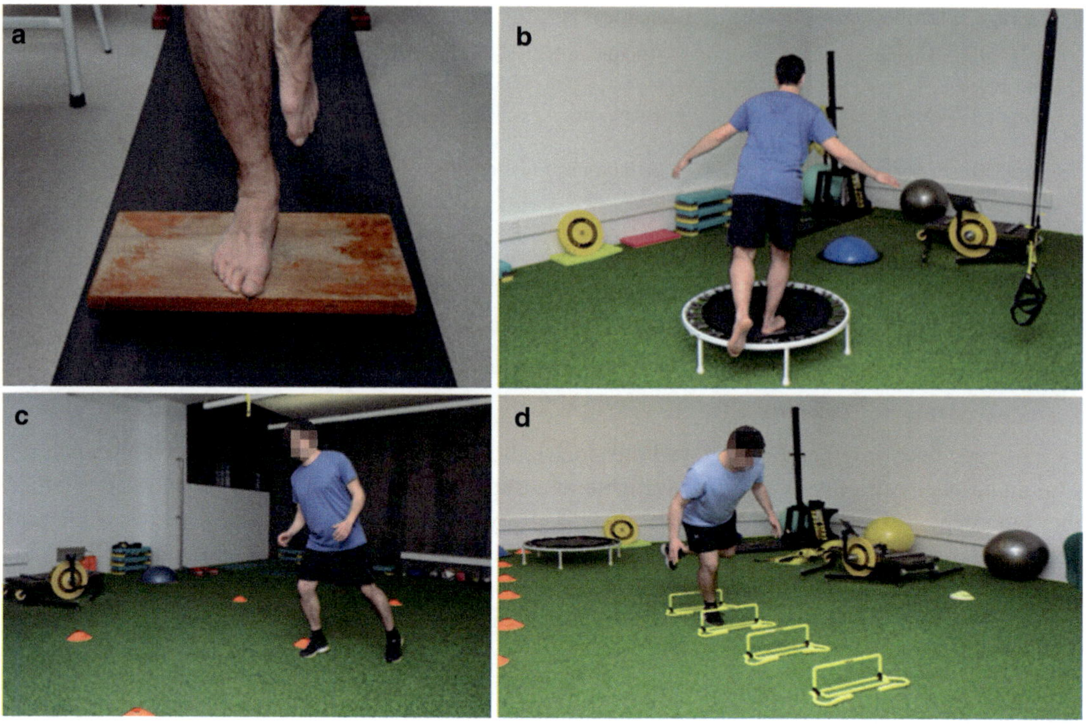

Fig. 10.1 Exercise therapy, including proprioception Freeman's protocol in unstable platforms (**a**), trampoline (**b**), lateral mobility (**c**), and jumping exercises (**d**)

early joint mobilizations are typical examples of a functional treatment strategy.

Ankle sprain without lateral ligament rupture (Grade I) can be treated with early functional rehabilitation, preserving joint mobility and weight-bearing status, as allowed by the pain. Ruptured lateral ankle ligaments (Grade II and III) require 4–6 weeks of protection with bracing or taping to limit the Range of Motion (ROM) of the ankle and allow the apposed ruptured ligament ends to heal. Treatment with functional ankle support, regardless of whether it was tape or brace, showed superior results compared to treatment with less adequate support such as a compression bandage or a tubigrip [9, 46]. Despite the conflicting results on superiority of any type of functional support over another [47–49], an ankle brace may be preferred as it shows slightly better functional outcome [47, 50, 51].

Prolonged cast immobilization is discouraged, because of potential decreased ROM and physical impairments compared to an active rehabilitation program [52, 53]. Nevertheless, recent evidence has shown that a short immobilization period of maximal 10 days, especially in Grade II and III sprains, in the acute phase can have a positive effect in terms of decreasing pain and edema [46, 54–56].

Exercise therapy is one of the main components of treatment programs for patients who sustained a LAS. The main focus of exercise programs currently are neuromuscular and proprioceptive exercises (Figs. 10.3 and 10.4). Exercise therapy may have multiple effects among which reducing the prevalence of recurrent injuries [57–59], as well as the prevalence of functional ankle instability [58, 60]. Supervised exercise therapy (Fig. 10.5) has shown superior results concerning recovery compared to home-based exercise [57, 60–67] and lead to improvement in ankle strength [67] and proprioception [67], and faster return to work [68] and sport [61].

Manual joint mobilization is a final category belonging to functional treatment. It is mainly performed with the objective to improve ankle ROM [58, 59, 69–73]. Studies have also shown

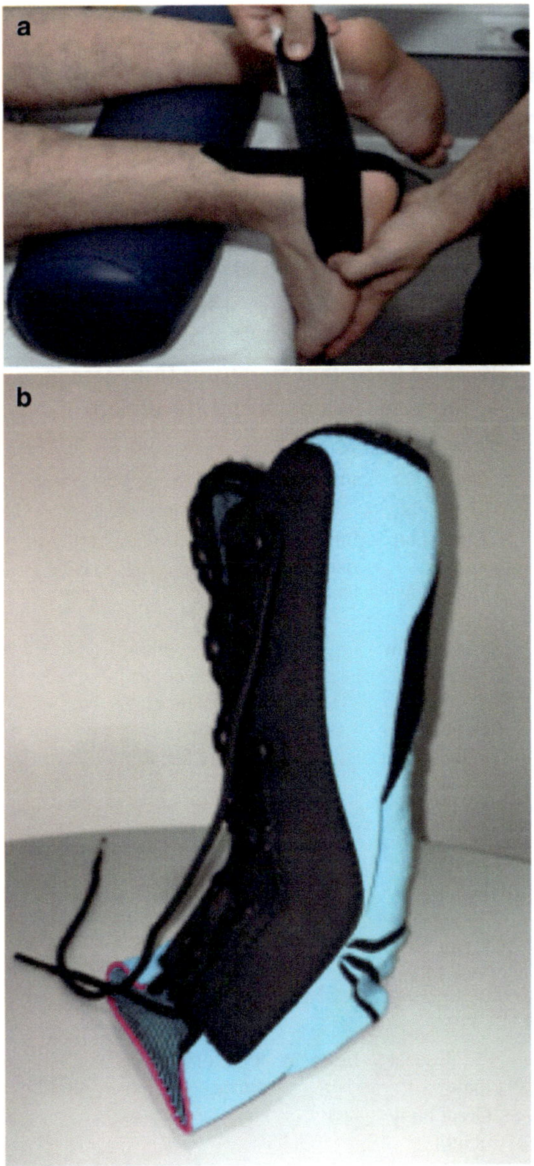

Fig. 10.2 Example of taping (**a**) and ankle brace (**b**)

that manual mobilization can be used to decrease pain [69]. The effects established by manual therapy are enhanced when combined with exercise therapy [66].

10.4.4 Other Therapies

Other treatment modalities that have been studied and are less frequently used in clinical practice

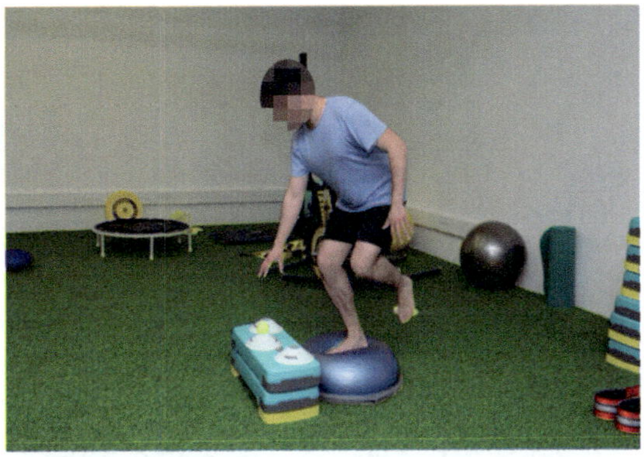

Fig. 10.3 Exercise therapy using the BOSU® device for balance, proprioception, flexibility, and muscle strengthening

include ultrasound [74, 75], electrotherapy [76–78], laser therapy [79], and shock-wave therapy [80–84] All these modalities showed no effect on pain, swelling, function, or return to play. Acupuncture has received much attention regarding treatment effect, but results remain inconclusive [85, 86]. Potential beneficial effects were found in two small studies for local vibration therapy [87] and Bioptron light therapy in combination with cryotherapy [88].

10.4.5 Modifiable Risk Factors

Modifiable risk factors may be the target of treatment to increase the chance of successful rehabilitation (Box 10.1). One of the targets of the treatment of patients who suffered from a lateral ankle sprain (LAS) is to identify and treat risk factors for further sprains or progression to instability [89]. Risk factors can be classified as modifiable and non-modifiable. The former can be further classified as intrinsic and extrinsic factors. Modifiable risk factors should be recognized and addressed during rehabilitation as part of a personalized injury prevention strategy [90, 91]; intrinsic type factors include limited range of motion (ROM) [91–93], deficits in proprioception [90, 93–96], postural control and balance [94–101], strength [90, 93–96, 102], coordination [98], and muscle latency [90, 93–96].

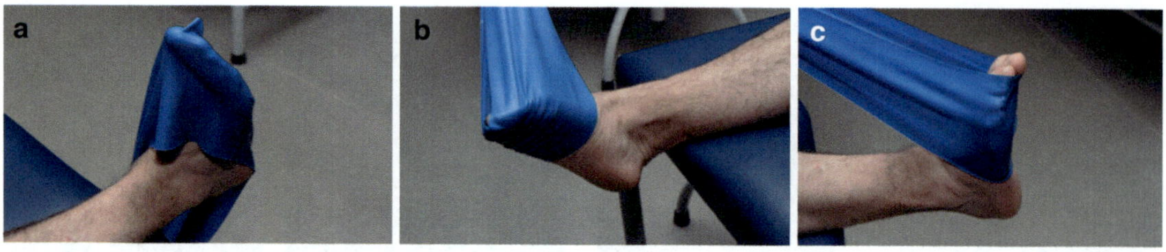

Fig. 10.4 Exercise therapy using rubber band (**a**), to work the inversion (**b**), and eversion (**c**) muscles

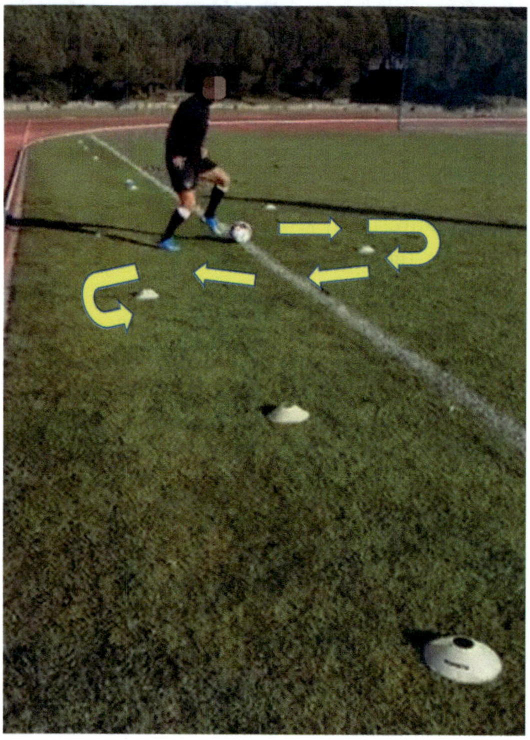

Fig. 10.5 Supervised exercise therapy, with an athlete in the pitch while training ball control while running and changing directions (yellow arrows)

Box 10.1 Important Modifiable Risk Factors as Target for Treatment and Prevention Programs

Targets for treatment		Targets for prevention	
Modifiable		Modifiable	
Altered hip joint kinematics	Intrinsic risk factor	Coordination deficits	Intrinsic risk factor
Balance impairment		Deficits in proprioception, postural control, and balance	
Deficiencies in dynamic postural control		Increased muscle latency	
Increased BMI		Limited range of motion	
Increased ligament laxity		Strength deficits	
Non-modifiable		Sports type and level of participation	Extrinsic risk factor
Adolescent male	Intrinsic risk factor	Type of playing surface	
Great body height			

Specific sports types such as basketball, indoor volleyball, handball, field sports, and climbing [103–106] have the highest risk at sustaining a LAS, and level of participation [103–105], role (defender) [107, 108], and surface type (natural grass) [109–111] have been recognized as risk factors and warrant special caution when returning to the field. As the same applies for workload guidance in return to work should not be forgotten [112].

10.4.6 Non-modifiable Risk Factors

The most common non-modifiable factors may be considered extrinsic factors as they often lie outside of the patients doing. One of these, extensively described, includes a history of an ankle sprain, showing no increased risk when assessed in a meta-analysis [93, 95, 96, 113–115].

Other intrinsic non-modifiable factors include gender, where girls have shownd an overall

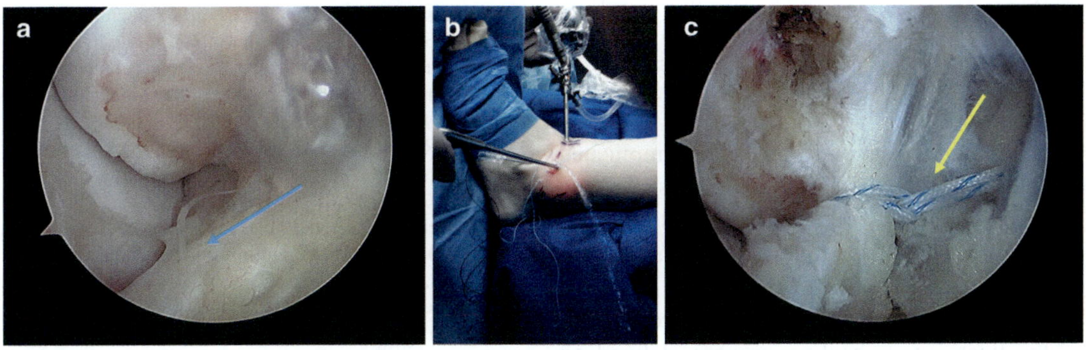

Fig. 10.6 Arthroscopic view (**a**) of an elongated anterior talofibular ligament (ATFL—blue arrow); (**b**) external view of ATFL arthroscopic repair using suture anchor; (**c**) re-tensioning of the ATFL using suture-anchor (yellow arrow)

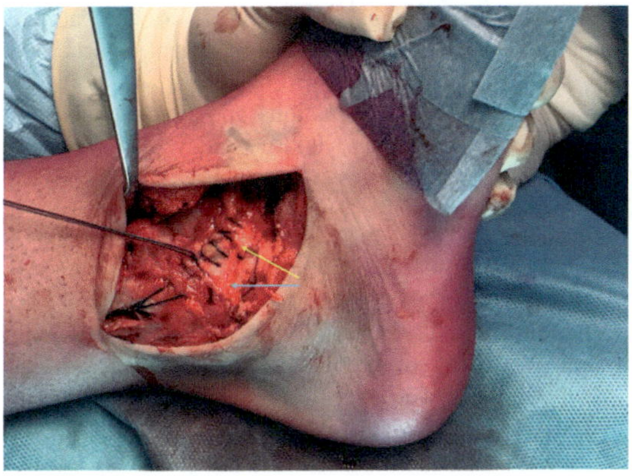

Fig. 10.7 Open approach for "Brostrom" repair of anterior talofibular ligament (ATFL—yellow arrow) and calcaneofibular ligament (CFL—blue arrow), using transosseous sutures

increased risk of a LAS while comparatively boys showed an increased risk of a LAS due to their competitive attitude [105, 116]. Other factors that have gained some attention and have been described as potential risk factors include a different ankle joint geometry and foot posture index and greater body height [101, 105, 117–120].

10.4.7 Surgical Therapy

Although surgical therapy (Figs. 10.6 and 10.7) is not the primary treatment option in patients who sustained an acute lateral ligament rupture, it may still be considered in selected cases, as high-demand athletes. Overall surgery seems superior to conservative treatment in decreasing the prevalence of recurrent LAS [121]. Moreover, in patients treated surgically, there is only limited evidence for improved recovery times, higher incidences of ankle stiffness, impaired ankle ROM, and complications compared with conservatively treated acute lateral ligament ruptures [122]. Additionally, recent studies show better outcomes in terms of recovery of ankle activity and instability compared to functionally treated patients compared to surgery [123].

One of the main advantages of surgery is that the ankle ligament laxity, which predisposes patients at sustaining recurrent sprains, is resolved by means of surgical treatment [124]. This suggests surgical therapy helps prevent recurrent ankle sprains. However, as 60–70% of patients respond well to functional treatment, and to avoid needless unnecessary invasive surgery, the decision of surgical treatment should be made on an individual basis [3].

10.5 Conclusion

In the treatment of patients who sustained a LAS, it is important to design a personalized program. Due to the great number of risk factors and prognostic factors it is essential to address these during rehabilitation to minimize the risk of recurrent ankle sprains and in time chronic ankle instability.

Take-Home Message

- Delayed physical examination is a reliable diagnostic tool to define the severity of a ligament injury;
- For the diagnosis of complete uncomplicated anterior talofibular ligament lesions, US and MRI are not needed as the sensitivity and specificity of delayed physical examination is sufficient;
- Functional treatment should take into account the ligamentous healing process, defined on the basis of the severity of the ligamentous injury;
- Acute lateral ligament rupture is not a mandatory surgical indication. Nevertheless, evidence from the literature show acute operative treatment as a viable option in selected cases;
- Up to 40% of patients who sustain a LAS develop CAI, suggesting not all factors contributing to the success or failure of rehabilitation are known.

References

1. Ivins D. Acute ankle sprain: an update. Am Fam Physician. 2006;74(10):1714–20.
2. Woods C, et al. The football association medical research Programme: an audit of injuries in professional football: an analysis of ankle sprains. Br J Sports Med. 2003;37(3):233–8.
3. Hershkovich O, et al. A large-scale study on epidemiology and risk factors for chronic ankle instability in young adults. J Foot Ankle Surg. 2015;54(2): 183–7.
4. Doherty C, et al. The incidence and prevalence of ankle sprain injury: a systematic review and meta-analysis of prospective epidemiological studies. Sports Med. 2014;44(1):123–40.
5. Fong DT, et al. Understanding acute ankle ligamentous sprain injury in sports. Sports Med Arthrosc Rehabil Ther Technol. 2009;1:14.
6. Verhagen EA, van Mechelen W, de Vente W. The effect of preventive measures on the incidence of ankle sprains. Clin J Sport Med. 2000;10(4):291–6.
7. Gribble PA, et al. Evidence review for the 2016 International Ankle Consortium consensus statement on the prevalence, impact and long-term consequences of lateral ankle sprains. Br J Sports Med. 2016;50:1496–505.
8. Gribble PA, et al. 2016 Consensus statement of the International Ankle Consortium: prevalence, impact and long-term consequences of lateral ankle sprains. Br J Sports Med. 2016;50:1493–5.
9. Pijnenburg AC, et al. Treatment of ruptures of the lateral ankle ligaments: a meta-analysis. J Bone Joint Surg Am. 2000;82(6):761–73.
10. van Rijn RM, et al. What is the clinical course of acute ankle sprains? A systematic literature review. Am J Med. 2008;121(4):324–31. e6
11. Hertel J. Functional anatomy, pathomechanics, and pathophysiology of lateral ankle instability. J Athl Train. 2002;37(4):364–75.
12. Gerber JP, et al. Persistent disability associated with ankle sprains: a prospective examination of an athletic population. Foot Ankle Int. 1998;19(10):653–60.
13. Dubin JC, et al. Lateral and syndesmotic ankle sprain injuries: a narrative literature review. J Chiropr Med. 2011;10(3):204–19.
14. Lynch SA, Renstrom PA. Treatment of acute lateral ankle ligament rupture in the athlete. Conservative versus surgical treatment. Sports Med. 1999;27(1):61–71.
15. Mulligan EP. Evaluation and management of ankle syndesmosis injuries. Phys Ther Sport. 2011;12(2):57–69.
16. Kannus P, Renstrom P. Treatment for acute tears of the lateral ligaments of the ankle. Operation, cast, or early controlled mobilization. J Bone Joint Surg Am. 1991;73(2):305–12.
17. Konradsen L, Holmer P, Sondergaard L. Early mobilizing treatment for grade III ankle ligament injuries. Foot Ankle. 1991;12(2):69–73.
18. van Dijk CN. Management of the sprained ankle. Br J Sports Med. 2002;36(2):83–4.
19. Harmon KG. The ankle examination. Prim Care. 2004;31(4):1025–37. x
20. de Vries JS, et al. Clinical evaluation of a dynamic test for lateral ankle ligament laxity. Knee Surg Sports Traumatol Arthrosc. 2010;18(5):628–33.
21. van Dijk CN, et al. Physical examination is sufficient for the diagnosis of sprained ankles. J Bone Joint Surg Br. 1996;78(6):958–62.
22. van Dijk CN, et al. Diagnosis of ligament rupture of the ankle joint. Physical examination, arthrography, stress radiography and sonography compared in 160 patients after inversion trauma. Acta Orthop Scand. 1996;67(6):566–70.
23. Polzer H, et al. Diagnosis and treatment of acute ankle injuries: development of an evidence-based algorithm. Orthop Rev (Pavia). 2012;4(1):e5.
24. Yammine K, Fathi Y. Ankle "sprains" during sport activities with normal radiographs: incidence of associated bone and tendon injuries on MRI findings and its clinical impact. Foot (Edinb). 2011;21(4):176–8.
25. van Putte-Katier N, et al. Magnetic resonance imaging abnormalities after lateral ankle trauma in injured and contralateral ankles. Eur J Radiol. 2015;84(12):2586–92.
26. Roemer FW, et al. Ligamentous injuries and the risk of associated tissue damage in acute ankle sprains in

athletes: a cross-sectional MRI study. Am J Sports Med. 2014;42(7):1549–57.
27. Margetic P, Pavic R. Comparative assessment of the acute ankle injury by ultrasound and magnetic resonance. Coll Antropol. 2012;36(2):605–10.
28. Margetic P, Salaj M, Lubina IZ. The value of ultrasound in acute ankle injury: comparison with MR. Eur J Trauma Emerg Surg. 2009;35(2):141–6.
29. Struijs PA, Kerkhoffs GM. Ankle sprain. BMJ Clin Evid. 2010;2010:1115.
30. Bleakley C, McDonough S, MacAuley D. The use of ice in the treatment of acute soft-tissue injury: a systematic review of randomized controlled trials. Am J Sports Med. 2004;32(1):251–61.
31. van den Bekerom MP, et al. What is the evidence for rest, ice, compression, and elevation therapy in the treatment of ankle sprains in adults? J Athl Train. 2012;47(4):435–43.
32. Cote DJ, et al. Comparison of 3 treatment procedures for minimizing ankle sprain swelling. Phys Ther. 1988;68(7):1072–6.
33. Airaksinen O, Kolari PJ, Miettinen H. Elastic bandages and intermittent pneumatic compression for treatment of acute ankle sprains. Arch Phys Med Rehabil. 1990;71(6):380–3.
34. Rucinkski TJ, et al. The effects of intermittent compression on edema in postacute ankle sprains. J Orthop Sports Phys Ther. 1991;14(2):65–9.
35. Tsang KK, Hertel J, Denegar CR. Volume decreases after elevation and intermittent compression of postacute ankle sprains are negated by gravity-dependent positioning. J Athl Train. 2003;38(4):320–4.
36. Bleakley CM, McDonough SM, MacAuley DC. Cryotherapy for acute ankle sprains: a randomised controlled study of two different icing protocols. Br J Sports Med. 2006;40(8):700–5.
37. Bleakley CM, et al. Effect of accelerated rehabilitation on function after ankle sprain: randomised controlled trial. Br Med J. 2010;340:c1964.
38. van den Bekerom MP, et al. Non-steroidal anti-inflammatory drugs (NSAIDs) for treating acute ankle sprains in adults: benefits outweigh adverse events. Knee Surg Sports Traumatol Arthrosc. 2015;23(8):2390–9.
39. Campbell J, Dunn T. Evaluation of topical ibuprofen cream in the treatment of acute ankle sprains. J Accid Emerg Med. 1994;11(3):178–82.
40. Predel HG, et al. Efficacy and safety of diclofenac diethylamine 2.32% gel in acute ankle sprain. Med Sci Sports Exerc. 2012;44(9):1629–36.
41. Predel HG, et al. A randomized, double-blind, placebo-controlled multicentre study to evaluate the efficacy and safety of diclofenac 4% spray gel in the treatment of acute uncomplicated ankle sprain. J Int Med Res. 2013;41(4):1187–202.
42. Serinken M, Eken C, Elicabuk H. Topical ketoprofen versus placebo in treatment of acute ankle sprain in the emergency department. Foot Ankle Int. 2016;37(9):989–93.
43. Ekman EF, et al. The COX-2 specific inhibitor Valdecoxib versus tramadol in acute ankle sprain: a multicenter randomized, controlled trial. Am J Sports Med. 2006;34(6):945–55.
44. Aghababian RV. Comparison of diflunisal and acetaminophen with codeine in the management of grade 2 ankle sprain. Clin Ther. 1986;8(5):520–6.
45. Stovitz SD, Johnson RJ. NSAIDs and musculoskeletal treatment: what is the clinical evidence? Phys Sportsmed. 2003;31(1):35–52.
46. Prado MP, et al. A comparative, prospective, and randomized study of two conservative treatment protocols for first-episode lateral ankle ligament injuries. Foot Ankle Int. 2014;35(3):201–6.
47. Kerkhoffs GM, et al. Different functional treatment strategies for acute lateral ankle ligament injuries in adults. Cochrane Database Syst Rev. 2002;3:CD002938.
48. van den Bekerom MP, et al. Randomized comparison of tape versus semi-rigid and versus lace-up ankle support in the treatment of acute lateral ankle ligament injury. Knee Surg Sports Traumatol Arthrosc. 2016;24(4):978–84.
49. Kemler E, et al. Effects of soft bracing or taping on a lateral ankle sprain: a non-randomised controlled trial evaluating recurrence rates and residual symptoms at one year. J Foot Ankle Res. 2015;8:13.
50. Kemler E, et al. A systematic review on the treatment of acute ankle sprain: brace versus other functional treatment types. Sports Med. 2011;41(3):185–97.
51. Raymond J, et al. The effect of ankle taping or bracing on proprioception in functional ankle instability: a systematic review and meta-analysis. J Sci Med Sport. 2012;15(5):386–92.
52. Kerkhoffs GM, et al. Immobilisation and functional treatment for acute lateral ankle ligament injuries in adults. Cochrane Database Syst Rev. 2002;3:CD003762.
53. Naeem M, et al. Assessment of functional treatment versus plaster of Paris in the treatment of grade 1 and 2 lateral ankle sprains. J Orthop Traumatol. 2015;16(1):41–6.
54. Uslu M, et al. Cohesive taping and short-leg casting in acute low-type ankle sprains in physically active patients. J Am Podiatr Med Assoc. 2015;105(4):307–12.
55. Lamb SE, et al. Mechanical supports for acute, severe ankle sprain: a pragmatic, multicentre, randomised controlled trial. Lancet. 2009;373(9663):575–81.
56. Bilgic S, et al. Comparison of two main treatment modalities for acute ankle sprain. Pak J Med Sci. 2015;31(6):1496–9.
57. Zech A, et al. Neuromuscular training for rehabilitation of sports injuries: a systematic review. Med Sci Sports Exerc. 2009;41(10):1831–41.
58. van der Wees PJ, et al. Effectiveness of exercise therapy and manual mobilisation in ankle sprain and functional instability: a systematic review. Aust J Physiother. 2006;52(1):27–37.

59. Bleakley CM, McDonough SM, MacAuley DC. Some conservative strategies are effective when added to controlled mobilisation with external support after acute ankle sprain: a systematic review. Aust J Physiother. 2008;54(1):7–20.
60. Postle K, Pak D, Smith TO. Effectiveness of proprioceptive exercises for ankle ligament injury in adults: a systematic literature and meta-analysis. Man Ther. 2012;17(4):285–91.
61. van Rijn RM, et al. Effectiveness of additional supervised exercises compared with conventional treatment alone in patients with acute lateral ankle sprains: systematic review. BMJ. 2010;341:c5688.
62. Bleakley CM, et al. Effect of accelerated rehabilitation on function after ankle sprain: randomised controlled trial. BMJ. 2010;340:c1964.
63. Hultman K, Fältström A, Öberg U. The effect of early physiotherapy after an acute ankle sprain. Adv Physiother. 2010;12(2):65–73.
64. Ismail MM, et al. Plyometric training versus resistive exercises after acute lateral ankle sprain. Foot Ankle Int. 2010;31(6):523–30.
65. van Rijn RM, et al. Some benefit from physiotherapy intervention in the subgroup of patients with severe ankle sprain as determined by the ankle function score: a randomised trial. Aust J Physiother. 2009;55(2):107–13.
66. Cleland JA, et al. Manual physical therapy and exercise versus supervised home exercise in the management of patients with inversion ankle sprain: a multicenter randomized clinical trial. J Orthop Sports Phys Ther. 2013;43(7):443–55.
67. Feger MA, et al. Supervised rehabilitation versus home exercise in the treatment of acute ankle sprains: a systematic review. Clin Sports Med. 2015;34(2):329–46.
68. van Os AG, et al. Comparison of conventional treatment and supervised rehabilitation for treatment of acute lateral ankle sprains: a systematic review of the literature. J Orthop Sports Phys Ther. 2005;35(2):95–105.
69. Loudon JK, Reiman MP, Sylvain J. The efficacy of manual joint mobilisation/manipulation in treatment of lateral ankle sprains: a systematic review. Br J Sports Med. 2014;48(5):365–70.
70. Brantingham JW, et al. Manipulative therapy for lower extremity conditions: expansion of literature review. J Manip Physiol Ther. 2009;32(1):53–71.
71. Mobarakeh M, Hafidz HJOA. Effect of friction technique on ankle sprain grade II treatment. Biomed Pharmacol J. 2015;8:523–8.
72. Truyols-Domi Nguez S, et al. Efficacy of thrust and nonthrust manipulation and exercise with or without the addition of myofascial therapy for the management of acute inversion ankle sprain: a randomized clinical trial. J Orthop Sports Phys Ther. 2013;43(5):300–9.
73. Cosby NL, et al. Immediate effects of anterior to posterior talocrural joint mobilizations following acute lateral ankle sprain. J Man Manip Ther. 2011;19(2):76–83.
74. Van Der Windt DA, et al. Ultrasound therapy for acute ankle sprains. Cochrane Database Syst Rev. 2002;1:CD001250.
75. van den Bekerom MP, et al. Therapeutic ultrasound for acute ankle sprains. Eur J Phys Rehabil Med. 2012;48(2):325–34.
76. Mendel FC, et al. Effect of high-voltage pulsed current on recovery after grades I and II lateral ankle sprains. J Sport Rehabil. 2010;19(4):399–410.
77. Feger MA, et al. Electrical stimulation as a treatment intervention to improve function, edema or pain following acute lateral ankle sprains: a systematic review. Phys Ther Sport. 2015;16(4):361–9.
78. Sandoval MC, et al. Effect of high-voltage pulsed current plus conventional treatment on acute ankle sprain. Rev Bras Fisioter. 2010;14(3):193–9.
79. de Bie RA, et al. Low-level laser therapy in ankle sprains: a randomized clinical trial. Arch Phys Med Rehabil. 1998;79(11):1415–20.
80. Barker AT, Barlow PS, Porter J. A double-blind clinical trial of lower power pulsed shortwave therapy in the treatment of a soft tissue injury. Phys Ther. 1985;71:500–4.
81. Michlovitz SL, Smith W, Watkins M. Ice and high voltage pulsed stimulation in treatment of acute lateral ankle sprains*. J Orthop Sports Phys Ther. 1988;9(9):301–4.
82. Pasila M, Visuri T, Sundholm A. Pulsating shortwave diathermy: value in treatment of recent ankle and foot sprains. Arch Phys Med Rehabil. 1978;59(8):383–6.
83. Pennington GM, et al. Pulsed, non-thermal, high-frequency electromagnetic energy (DIAPULSE) in the treatment of grade I and grade II ankle sprains. Mil Med. 1993;158(2):101–4.
84. Wilson DH. Treatment of soft-tissue injuries by pulsed electrical energy. Br Med J. 1972;2(5808):269–70.
85. Park J, et al. Acupuncture for ankle sprain: systematic review and meta-analysis. BMC Complement Altern Med. 2013;13:55.
86. Kim TH, et al. Acupuncture for treating acute ankle sprains in adults. Cochrane Database Syst Rev. 2014;6:CD009065.
87. Peer KS, Barkley JE, Knapp DM. The acute effects of local vibration therapy on ankle sprain and hamstring strain injuries. Phys Sportsmed. 2009;37(4):31–8.
88. Stasinopoulos D, et al. The use of Bioptron light (polarized, polychromatic, non-coherent) therapy for the treatment of acute ankle sprains. Disabil Rehabil. 2017;39(5):450–7.
89. Kerkhoffs GM, et al. Diagnosis, treatment and prevention of ankle sprains: an evidence-based clinical guideline. Br J Sports Med. 2012;46(12):854–60.
90. Kobayashi T, Tanaka M, Shida M. Intrinsic risk factors of lateral ankle sprain: a systematic review and meta-analysis. Sports Health. 2016;8(2):190–3.

91. Kobayashi T, et al. Intrinsic predictive factors of noncontact lateral ankle sprain in collegiate athletes: a case-control study. Orthop J Sports Med. 2013;1(7):2325967113518163.
92. Pope R, Herbert R, Kirwan J. Effects of ankle dorsiflexion range and pre-exercise calf muscle stretching on injury risk in Army recruits. Aust J Physiother. 1998;44(3):165–72.
93. de Noronha M, et al. Do voluntary strength, proprioception, range of motion, or postural sway predict occurrence of lateral ankle sprain? Br J Sports Med. 2006;40(10):824–8; discussion 828.
94. Tropp H, Ekstrand J, Gillquist J. Stabilometry in functional instability of the ankle and its value in predicting injury. Med Sci Sports Exerc. 1984;16(1):64–6.
95. McGuine TA, Keene JS. The effect of a balance training program on the risk of ankle sprains in high school athletes. Am J Sports Med. 2006;34(7):1103–11.
96. de Noronha M, et al. Intrinsic predictive factors for ankle sprain in active university students: a prospective study. Scand J Med Sci Sports. 2013;23(5):541–7.
97. Trojian TH, McKeag DB. Single leg balance test to identify risk of ankle sprains. Br J Sports Med. 2006;40(7):610–3; discussion 613.
98. Willems TM, et al. Intrinsic risk factors for inversion ankle sprains in male subjects: a prospective study. Am J Sports Med. 2005;33(3):415–23.
99. Hrysomallis C, McLaughlin P, Goodman C. Balance and injury in elite Australian footballers. Int J Sports Med. 2007;28(10):844–7.
100. Wang HK, et al. Risk-factor analysis of high school basketball-player ankle injuries: a prospective controlled cohort study evaluating postural sway, ankle strength, and flexibility. Arch Phys Med Rehabil. 2006;87(6):821–5.
101. Watson AW. Ankle sprains in players of the field-games Gaelic football and hurling. J Sports Med Phys Fitness. 1999;39(1):66–70.
102. Hagen M, et al. The angle-torque-relationship of the subtalar pronators and supinators in male athletes: a comparative study of soccer and handball players. Technol Health Care. 2016;24(3):391–9.
103. Fong DT, et al. A systematic review on ankle injury and ankle sprain in sports. Sports Med. 2007;37(1):73–94.
104. Verhagen EA, et al. A one season prospective cohort study of volleyball injuries. Br J Sports Med. 2004;38(4):477–81.
105. Waterman BR, et al. Epidemiology of ankle sprain at the United States military academy. Am J Sports Med. 2010;38(4):797–803.
106. Laver L, Myklebust G. Handball injuries: epidemiology and injury characterization. Sports Injuries. 2014:1–17.
107. Kofotolis N, Kellis E. Ankle sprain injuries: a 2-year prospective cohort study in female Greek professional basketball players. J Athl Train. 2007;42(3):388–94.
108. Kofotolis ND, Kellis E, Vlachopoulos SP. Ankle sprain injuries and risk factors in amateur soccer players during a 2-year period. Am J Sports Med. 2007;35(3):458–66.
109. Ekstrand J, Timpka T, Hagglund M. Risk of injury in elite football played on artificial turf versus natural grass: a prospective two-cohort study. Br J Sports Med. 2006;40(12):975–80.
110. Orchard JW, Powell JW. Risk of knee and ankle sprains under various weather conditions in American football. Med Sci Sports Exerc. 2003;35(7):1118–23.
111. Hershman EB, et al. An analysis of specific lower extremity injury rates on grass and FieldTurf playing surfaces in National Football League Games: 2000-2009 seasons. Am J Sports Med. 2012;40(10):2200–5.
112. van Middelkoop M, et al. Re-sprains during the first 3 months after initial ankle sprain are related to incomplete recovery: an observational study. J Physiother. 2012;58(3):181–8.
113. McHugh MP, et al. Risk factors for noncontact ankle sprains in high school athletes: the role of hip strength and balance ability. Am J Sports Med. 2006;34(3):464–70.
114. Verhagen E, et al. The effect of a proprioceptive balance board training program for the prevention of ankle sprains: a prospective controlled trial. Am J Sports Med. 2004;32(6):1385–93.
115. Engebretsen AH, et al. Intrinsic risk factors for acute ankle injuries among male soccer players: a prospective cohort study. Scand J Med Sci Sports. 2010;20(3):403–10.
116. Swenson DM, et al. Epidemiology of U.S. high school sports-related ligamentous ankle injuries, 2005/06-2010/11. Clin J Sport Med. 2013;23(3):190–6.
117. Rice H, et al. High medial plantar pressures during barefoot running are associated with increased risk of ankle inversion injury in Royal Marine recruits. Gait Posture. 2013;38(4):614–8.
118. Onate JA, et al. Physical exam risk factors for lower extremity injury in high school athletes: a systematic review. Clin J Sport Med. 2016;26(6):435–44.
119. Frigg A, et al. The effect of osseous ankle configuration on chronic ankle instability. Br J Sports Med. 2007;41(7):420–4.
120. Magerkurth O, et al. Frontal and lateral characteristics of the osseous configuration in chronic ankle instability. Br J Sports Med. 2010;44(8):568–72.
121. Pihlajamaki H, et al. Surgical versus functional treatment for acute ruptures of the lateral ligament complex of the ankle in young men: a randomized controlled trial. J Bone Joint Surg Am. 2010;92(14):2367–74.
122. Kerkhoffs GM, et al. Surgical versus conservative treatment for acute injuries of the lateral ligament complex of the ankle in adults. Cochrane Database Syst Rev. 2007;(2):Cd000380. https://doi.org/10.1002/14651858.CD000380.

123. Han LH, et al. A meta-analysis of treatment methods for acute ankle sprain. Pakistan J Med Sci. 2012;28(5):895–9.
124. Rowden A, et al. Double-blind, randomized, placebo-controlled study evaluating the use of platelet-rich plasma therapy (PRP) for acute ankle sprains in the emergency department. J Emerg Med. 2015;49(4):546–51.

Level of Evidence for Nonoperative Treatment on Chronic Ankle Instability

11

Francisco Guerra-Pinto, Chris DiGiovanni, Hélder Pereira, and Nuno Côrte-Real

Fact Box 1 Chronic Ankle Instability Models

- Inconsistencies in CAI research may be explained, in part, by the common assumption that CAI is a homogeneous condition.
- Freeman, in 1965, reported that "mechanical instability of the ankle can only rarely be the initial cause of the symptom of functional instability of the foot."
- Although the definition of mechanical instability is universally accepted as pathologic ligamentous laxity about the ankle-joint complex, there is currently no gold standard for diagnosing CAI.
- Hertel proposed a model involving mechanical and functional insufficiencies that is widely accepted. In this model, mechanical and functional insufficiencies are not mutually exclusive but part of a continuum, and recurrent sprain occurs when both conditions are present
- Hiller proposed an evolution of the Hertel model, with three different types of CAI patients: "mechanical instability," "perceived instability," and "recurrent sprains." The combinations of these three types fulfill seven subgroups of CAI.

F. Guerra-Pinto (✉)
Department of Orthopaedics, Hospital Ortopédico de Sant'Ana, Parede, Portugal

Department of Orthopaedics, Hospital da Cruz Vermelha Portuguesa, Lisboa, Portugal

NOVA Medical School, Lisbon NOVA University, Lisbon, Portugal

C. DiGiovanni
Division of Foot & Ankle Surgery, Department of Orthopaedic Surgery, Massachusetts General Hospital/Newton-Wellesley Hospital, Harvard Medical School, Boston, MA, USA
e-mail: cwdigiovanni@partners.org

H. Pereira
Orthopedic Department of Póvoa de Varzim, Vila do Conde Hospital Centre, Póvoa de Varzim, Portugal

Ripoll y De Prado Sports Clinic: Murcia-Madrid FIFA Medical Centre of Excellence, Murcia, Spain

International Centre of Sports Traumatology of the Ave, Vila do Conde, Portugal

ICVS/3B's—PT Government Associated Laboratory, University of Minho, Braga-Guimarães, Portugal

N. Côrte-Real
Cascais Hospital, Lisbon, Portugal

H. Pereira et al. (eds.), *Lateral Ankle Instability*, https://doi.org/10.1007/978-3-662-62763-1_11

Fact Box 2 Ankle Mechanoreceptors

- In addition to altering ankle mechanics, injury to the lateral ankle ligaments is thought to damage the mechanoreceptors in the ligamentous and capsular tissues supporting the ankle.
- Mechanoreceptors have been identified in both human and animal joints. The classification of sensory receptors is based on the description proposed by Freeman and Wyke which classified mechanoreceptors into four types according to the morphology and function
- There might be a continuation of pathology between functional instability, microinstability, and mechanical instability.
- The conservative treatment should be the first-line treatment for the vast majority of our patients. ESSKA consensus recommends 3–6 weeks of conservative treatment before considering surgery.

Fact Box 3 External Support in CAI

- There is limited evidence on the impact of the plantar orthosis on the postural control and balance during functional in CAI patients. The onset times of peroneus longus is significantly earlier with shoes and shoes with customized foot orthosis compared to barefoot.
- Despite the evolution in shoe industry, the reviews outline that the evidence for modified footwear is inconclusive in the prevention of ankle sprain or its recurrence.
- Adhesive contentions are divided into taping (nonelastic), strapping (elastic), and kinesio. The use of taping proved to give the greatest decrease of the talar tilt angle in mechanical CAI
- Commercial ankle orthosis might be described according to its mobility: constrictive, hinged, or simple (non-constrictive). Bracing provides supplemental external **joint** stiffness and/or improved proprioceptive acuity.
- Systematic reviews on this topic report that bracing is effective at preventing a recurrence of ankle sprain.

Fact Box 4 Rehabilitation in CAI

- The rehabilitation modalities are divided into three big groups:
  - Manipulation and massage (STAR)
  - Strength training
  - Proprioceptive training.
- Sensory-targeted ankle rehabilitation strategies (STARS) for CAI have several components: joint mobilization, plantar massage, triceps surae stretching, or control.
- STARS improved patient-oriented outcomes but had no clinically relevant impact on laboratory-oriented measures
- There is evidence on changes in peroneal reaction time and eversion strength deficits in CAI. Strength training protocols might be applied as resistance tubing or through manual resistance.
- Proprioceptive training has many modalities. It uses some type of unstable or irregular surface where the patient trains his balance and postural control, in a closed-chain exercise
- Stabilization exercises for 6 weeks showed improved self-reported function and neuromuscular control: preparatory muscle activation, reactive muscle activation, and muscle onset time.

11.1 Chronic Ankle Instability Models

Chronic ankle instability (CAI) has been defined as "repetitive bouts of lateral ankle instability resulting in numerous ankle sprains" [1]. The most commonly cited characteristics of CAI include giving way of the ankle, mechanical instability, pain and swelling, loss of strength, recurrent sprain, and functional instability.

The clinical picture might be grouped in the following presentations:

- A first acute sprain followed by pain
- Repetitive sprains with symptom-free intervals
- Repetitive sprains with pain between them

It is not uncommon for patients to report progressive pain between the sprains, which tells the clinician that the prognosis is deteriorating.

Terada defined individuals with CAI according to the presence of (a) a previous history of an acute lateral ankle sprain which caused swelling, pain, and temporary loss of function at least 1 day; (b) repeated episodes of "giving way" for 6 months; (c) recurrent ankle sprains; and/or (d) perceived ankle instability assessed by the Ankle Instability Instrument (AII) and Identification of Functional Ankle Instability (IdFAI) [2].

Inconsistencies in CAI research may be explained, in part, by the common assumption that CAI is a homogeneous condition. Not only the pain has variable locations, and might suggest other underlying injured structures (cartilage, peroneal tendons, impingement) besides the ligament rupture, but also several terms have historically been used interchangeably to describe the phenomenon of ankle instability: chronic ankle instability, chronic lateral ankle instability, ankle instability, residual ankle instability, chronic instability, recurrent instability, recurrent lateral ankle instability, and chronic ankle sprain [1].

Although the idea of CAI as a homogeneous condition is still present, the literature regarding different subgroups of patients with CAI starts in the 1950s. Wiles reported on a group of patients that, following a sprain, developed a foot which tends to "give way," but in which no abnormality is detectable on examination." Freeman, in 1965, labels all patients with chronic disability after a lateral sprain as "functional instability." Although many authors quote the contribution of Freeman in recalling that some patients did not have "mechanical instability" in stress x-rays (while other had it), his exact words were "this study suggests that mechanical instability of the ankle can only rarely be the initial cause of the symptom of functional instability of the foot" [3].

Although the definition of mechanical instability is universally accepted as pathologic ligamentous laxity about the ankle-joint complex, there is currently no gold standard for diagnosing CAI. Expert recommendations for clinicians and researchers rely on self-report function questionnaires and injury history instead of objective clinical or laboratory tests [4].

Post-traumatic laxity, defined as excessive joint range of motion beyond the normal physiologic range of motion, has been demonstrated in an acute sprain population and up to 8 weeks post-trauma [5].

While established in an acute post-injury population, there is limited consensus on the role mechanical ligamentous laxity plays in those with CAI. A systematic review indicated that those with CAI tended to have more laxity than those not suffering from CAI; however, a consensus is still lacking regarding the role mechanical laxity plays in those with CAI. Laxity may only be affecting a portion of those with perceived instability (Hiller et al., 2011), and methods and instruments to measure laxity may lack validity and reliability [1, 6]

Hertel proposed a model involving mechanical and functional insufficiencies that is widely accepted (Fig. 11.1). In this model, mechanical and functional insufficiencies are not mutually exclusive but part of a continuum, and recurrent sprain occurs when both conditions are present. Functional instability is proposed to result from functional insufficiencies such as strength defi-

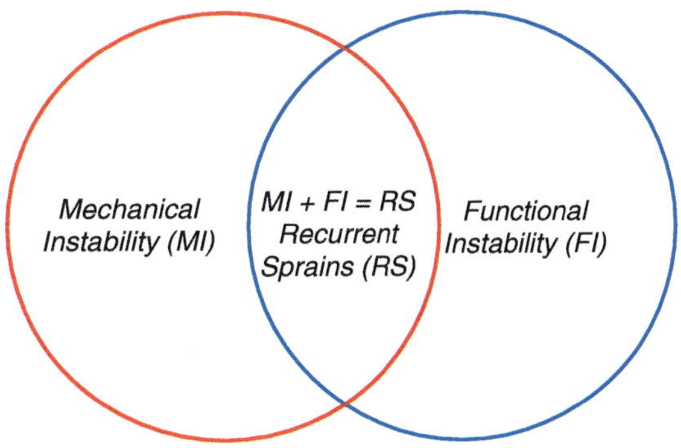

Fig. 11.1 Hertel's chronic ankle instability model

cits, impaired proprioception, and impaired neuromuscular or postural control [7].

At this point, a patient is considered to have mechanical instability when there is documented increased laxity on the symptomatic ankle (when compared with the other side) either on the clinical examination, stress X-rays, or stress sonography. The patients in whom this laxity cannot be documented (40% in Freeman series, 37% in Lohrer studies) are considered to have functional instability [3, 8].

This is the most known and accepted model, despite the fact that some patients do not fit this model. Hiller proposed an evolution of the Hertel model (Fig. 11.2), with three different types of CAI patients: "mechanical instability," "perceived instability," and "recurrent sprains." The combinations of these three types fulfill seven subgroups of CAI. The authors state that, for example, it is possible to have mechanical instability and perceived instability without recurrent sprains. They even consider another factor—hypomobility—that "may constitute the basis for an additional subgroup and should be further investigated," because "hypomobility, rather than mechanical instability, can also be associated with ankle sprain" and "the presence of participants with hypomobility in CAI studies may, therefore, "washout" significant findings and provide one explanation for inconsistent results" [1].

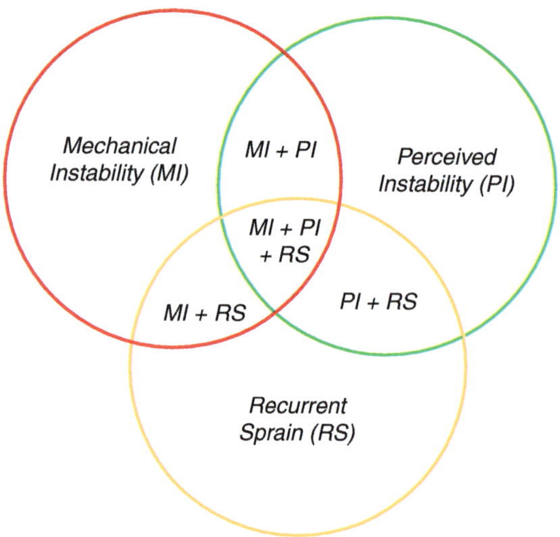

Fig. 11.2 Hiller's chronic ankle instability model

Another useful concept is that some patients do not develop chronic complaints, and these are named "copers" [9]. These patients experienced severe lateral ankle sprain and ultimately do not develop CAI or have no perceived instability. Rosen distinguished these from healthy ankles describing copers as those patients with one or two lateral ankle sprains on one limb and a Cumberland Ankle Instability Tool (CAIT) score equal or bigger than 28, indicating good ankle function. His Healthy controls ($n = 32$) had no history of lateral ankle sprain, and had CAIT scores of 29 or 30, indicating no loss of function. Croy defined copers as those who had one ankle sprain for more than 1 year and without instability symptoms.

An interesting point while mentioning the copers is its conventional definition: a patient who had two sprains might be considered a coper in absence of other complaints, but a patient who suffered three sprains is considered to have CAI. This brings up another group of patients to be identified, besides already proposed Hiller, adding up nine groups of patients to be recognized after a severe lateral ankle sprain.

- Mechanical Instability (MI)
- Perceived Instability (PI)
- Recurrent Sprain (RS)
- MI + PI
- MI + RS
- PI + RS
- MI + PI + RS
- Any of the above with hypomobility (which might double the previous categories)
- Copers (if only two sprains; changes to CAI if third episode occurs)

Interestingly enough, these classifications merely increase the awareness of CAI diagnosis. They do not assist the clinician in deciding if, and when, a patient should have surgical treatment.

They do, on the other hand, lead us into wondering why mechanically stable ankles make up more than half of all CAI patients.

11.2 Ankle Mechanoreceptors

Ankle ligaments have two functions: biomechanical and proprioceptive.

In addition to altering ankle mechanics, injury to the lateral ankle ligaments is thought to damage the mechanoreceptors in the ligamentous and capsular tissues supporting the ankle. Disruption to these mechanoreceptors may impair the ankle's joint position sense [10].

Changes in the conscious perception of afferent somatosensory information, reflex responses, and efferent motor control deficits are present with ankle instability [11].

The theory of articular deafferentation secondary to direct injury of ligamentous proprioceptors and arthrogenic muscle inhibition is central to current rehabilitation principles following ankle sprain [12].

The proprioceptive loss and restoration in lateral ankle sprain and chronic ankle instability are becoming a hot spot in sports medicine and orthopedics research.

The motor and sensory supplies to the ankle complex stem from the lumbar and sacral plexus. The motor supply to the muscles comes from the tibial, deep peroneal, and superficial peroneal nerves. The sensory supply comes from these three mixed nerves and two sensory nerves: the sural and saphenous nerves. The lateral ligaments and joint capsules of the talocrural and subtalar joints have been shown to be extensively innervated by mechanoreceptors that contribute to proprioception.

Mechanoreceptors have been identified in both human and animal joints. In the cat knee, the mechanoreceptors were identified in joint capsule as well as in ligament parenchyma. The classification of sensory receptors is based on the description proposed by Freeman and Wyke which classified mechanoreceptors into four types according to the morphology and function [13].

It is likely that ligaments healed with elongation have worse function of the mechanoreceptors. Hinterman described the arthroscopic examination of 148 patients with symptomatic chronic ankle instability, reporting rupture or elongation of the anterior talofibular ligament in 86% of ankles, of the calcaneofibular ligament in 64%, and of the deltoid ligament in 40% [14].

The clinical impact of this laxity on mechanoreceptors is easily understood if we quote the words of Van Dijk:

> "The ATFL plays a key role in transmitting rotational forces from fibula to talus. (…) The type III nerve endings, which are confined to the extremities of the joint ligaments, are only excited when stress is applied to the ligament. In the case of laxity, they only start providing information when a subluxation of the talus is already present. (…) Freeman 1965 regards this as the explanation of the giving way sensation felt in proven stable ankles. In every ankle ligament rupture, there is at the same time a capsule rupture that disrupts parts of the type I and II nerve-ending system. In situations where disruption is slight or where proprioception training can compensate for loss of sensation then there is still a problem when considering the elongated ligament. (…) … Whenever a forced endorotation of the foot occurs, specially with the foot in plantar flexion, information relayed by type III fibers will only result in reaction when the joint has subluxated." [15]

This explanation suggests that there is always a pathological laxity of the ligaments when the patient is symptomatic. There might be a continuation of pathology between functional instability, microinstability, and mechanical instability. Cases in which this can be perceived and/or documented by the clinician are classified as mechanical CAI. Patients in whom this mechanical laxity cannot be accessed—possibly due to diagnostic limitations of the clinical examination or arthrometric measurement—are labeled as functional CAI. Microinstability is perhaps something in between, although difficult to precise because the amount of pathologic laxity is yet to be determined. This rationale might also be the reason for the success of the Brostrom technique, which is not a true reconstruction but a re-tensioning technique. The same re-tensioning principle could not be applied in lateral knee instability, in which a true reconstruction is needed. The precise proprioceptive role of all body ligaments is yet to be defined.

It might be difficult to distinguish microinstability from functional instability. Maybe they behave similarly when we take into consideration that ligament elongation might cause a "shutdown" in mechanoreceptors with proprioception impairment. For these reasons, conservative treatment should be the first-line treatment for the vast majority of our patients. ESSKA consensus recommends 3–6 weeks of conservative treatment before considering surgery [16].

11.3 What Are the Options for Nonoperative Treatment

Vigilance
External Support

- plantar orthosis
- custom-made shoes
- taping and other adhesive contentions
- ankle orthosis

Rehabilitation

- STARS
- Strength Training
- Proprioceptive Training

11.3.1 Vigilance/Natural History

In a strict sense, all the options for nonoperative treatment include lack of treatment, which means the natural history. The natural history of CAI is, by definition, chronic. This means that patients do not get better with time, they keep the same complaints or, possibly, they get worse. The lack of lateral ankle ligaments will allow recurrent tibiotalar joint subluxations and pathological movements that will cause an accelerated cartilage wear and degeneration, resulting in ankle arthritis [17]. The typical pathological joint wear is asymmetrical and affects the medial talus [18].

11.3.2 External Support: Braces/Orthosis/Taping

A literature review of external support devices for CAI should consider the evidence related to acute ankle instability. In other words, it is likely that some kind of protection might increase the chances of normal ligament healing in the acute severe sprain. Once the ligament failed to heal, or is healed with elongation, an external support will benefit the patient's symptoms but might not interfere in the long-term prognosis.

There are four kinds of external stabilizers of the ankle

- Plantar orthosis/insoles
- Custom-made shoes
- Taping and other adhesive contentions
- Ankle orthosis

11.3.2.1 Plantar Orthosis

The goal of plantar orthosis is to change the stance phase ankle alignment. This might be a logical choice when there is some ankle or hindfoot condition driving the ankle into a varus position that might predispose to lateral sprain, as long as the undesired deformity is flexible. The typical case is a patient with a flexible cavus foot. There is limited evidence on the impact of the plantar orthosis on the postural control and balance during functional in CAI patients.

In a recent systematic review, Molsan reported on the slight angular adjustments in CAI compared to the control groups. No difference was reported for the hip and knee kinematics [19].

Baur reported higher peroneal preactivity but no effect on the timing of peroneus longus activation after an 8-week foot-orthoses intervention in participants with running-related overuse injuries [20].

Dingenen compared latencies of muscle activation onset for peroneus longus activity with different shoes and foot orthosis, in CAI, during the transition from double-leg stance to single-leg stance. The onset times of peroneus longus were significantly earlier with shoes ($P = 0.029$) and shoes with customized foot orthosis ($P = 0.001$) compared to barefoot [21].

An earlier onset of muscle activity was also reported in the other study that analyzed nine lower extremity muscles using surface electromyography. Earlier muscle activation onset times were observed in the shoes with customized foot orthosis than in the barefoot condition for the *peroneus longus* ($P < 0.001$), tibialis anterior ($P = 0.003$), *vastus medialis obliquus* ($P = 0.04$), and *vastus lateralis* ($P = 0.005$). Furthermore, the *peroneus longus* was activated earlier in the shoes-only ($P = 0.02$) and shoes-with-standard-foot-orthoses ($P = 0.03$) conditions than in the barefoot condition [22].

Custom-made foot orthosis has, therefore, some effect on the peroneal activation time and might be considered as a potential tool.

11.3.2.2 Orthopedic Shoes/Custom-Made Shoes

It is difficult to find the clinical difference between custom-made insoles and custom-made shoes, also known as orthopedic shoes. Custom-made shoes might include any item of the External Support menu, like insoles and tight ankle contentions. Customized high shoes might even include semi-rigid lateral supports when ordered.

Herb described that Patients with CAI presented with differences in their landing strategies. In his cohort ($n = 24$) patients with CAI had greater inversion from 107 to 200 ms post-contact (difference = 4.01°±2.55°). Kinematic and kinetic changes after ground contact may be related to a faulty landing strategy. This author suggests that drop-vertical-jump task should be considered for rehabilitation protocol [23]. This might sustain the current option of wearing high top shoes in basketball players, despite the fact that its role in preventing ankle sprains has not been shown [24].

Shod CAI subjects may adjust their gait in order to successfully accomplish the given task in jogging conditions [25].

Ramanathan studied 35 healthy subjects on the protective function of the peroneus longus muscle during unanticipated foot inversion. He compared barefoot, standard training shoe, shoe with a sole flare, and an above the **ankle** laced boot. The muscle was responding earlier in the shod conditions compared to the barefoot. The standard shoe and the flared sole design showed greater statistically significant differences from the unshod condition than the boot [26].

Despite the continuous efforts in shoe industry, the reviews outline that the evidence for modified footwear is inconclusive in the prevention of ankle sprain or its recurrence [27].

11.3.2.3 Taping and Other Adhesive Contentions

Taping is one of the most popular methods of external contention (Fig. 11.3). It is cheap and easily accessible. The stabilizing effects on the ankle have been related to three main mechanisms:

- mechanical stability of the ankle
- improved neuromuscular function
- positive psychological impact

Among the many taping techniques the three main types are nonelastic, elastic, and kinesio [28].

The nonelastic (usually referred as taping) is frequently applied on the lateral ankle surface or in a figure of 8 around the ankle. Its tightness might lead to skin complications, including necrosis. Elastic adhesive bandage, sometimes called strapping, allows improved motion, at the obvious expense of stability. When comparing in healthy volunteers nonelastic adhesive taping was slightly superior to elastic taping. While total inversion did not differ between tape conditions, the rate of inversion in the nonelastic condition was lower than the elastic adhesive condition [29, 30].

Vaes compared strapping and taping in 51 patients with *mechanical* CAI (documented in stress X-rays). A comparative radiological study was carried out to test the stabilizing value of ankle strapping and taping on unstable tibiotalar joints. Unstable ankle joints of 51 sportsmen were examined without bandages, with strapping, and with taping before and after an activity program. The use of **taping** proved to give the

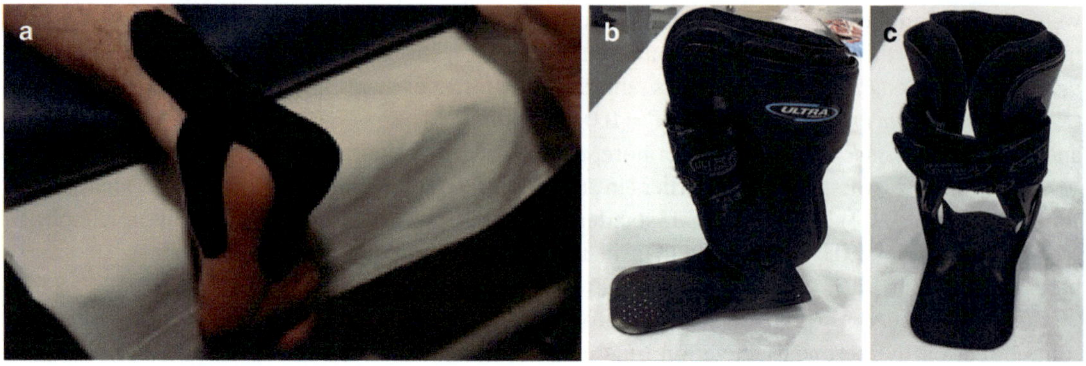

Fig. 11.3 Ankle taping for instability (**a**). Hinged orthosis permits sagittal plane controlled mobility while aiming for coronal and axial stability (**b** and **c**)

greatest decrease of the talar tilt angle. This improvement was still greater, even after activity, than the stabilization obtained by **strapping**, before any activity [31].

This author also analyzed the impact of taping in 220 *functionally* unstable ankles. A standard surface EMG controlled stress Roentgen test protocol was used, measuring talar tilt (TT) without support and with tape bandage or brace. Tape bandage and two braces had a highly significant influence on the talar tilt [32].

The kinesio taping is gaining popularity in the sports population. It uses an elastic adhesive band, which allows 140% of stretching, therefore, with small constraining of the movements. The goal is not to limit the motion but to stimulate the proprioception.

In a systematic review that included 10 papers, Wang reported The Star Excursion Balance Test results indicated that Kinesio taping was superior to other taping methods in the studies in which vertical jump height was measured. His population was healthy individuals and patients with ankle sprain (no CAI patients). This suggests a smaller constraining of the ankle during that task [33].

Bicici measured the effect of athletic taping and kinesio taping on measurements of functional performance in basketball players with chronic inversion ankle sprains. Faster performance times were measured with kinesio taping and athletic tape in single-limb hurdle test when compared to placebo and non-taped conditions (athletic **taping** versus placebo **taping**: $p = 0.03$; athletic **taping** versus non tape $p = 0.016$; kinesio taping versus placebo **taping** $p = 0.042$; kinesio taping versus non tape $p = 0.016$) [34].

De la Torre performed a randomized trial (15 vs. 15) with kinesiology tape versus placebo using the Sensory Organization Test (SOT). Post hoc analysis showed that both groups obtained improvements in composite Sensory Organization Test scores immediately after tape application and 7 days of use, with no significant difference. The authors report these results to a subjective increase in confidence after the tape application [35].

11.3.2.4 Orthosis

One way of reducing the possibility of ankle joint injury is using external ankle supports, e.g., ankle orthoses (Fig. 11.3) [36]. Evidence shows that the use of ankle orthoses in individuals with CAI can reduce ankle sprains in high-risk sports such as basketball [37].

If we exclude the previously described orthosis (insoles, custom-made shoes, and taping) the ankle orthosis might include orthosis that includes two or more joints, like the ankle-foot-orthosis and the knee-ankle-foot orthosis, or merely the ankle joint.

An orthosis prescription should mention:

- the affected joint/segment to be considered
- the diagnosis

- the degree of mobility desired
- if the deformity/condition is flexible
- the purpose of the orthosis: correction, accommodation, stability
- the material desired (although this is mostly defined by the orthosis technician

These indications are interrelated. Generally speaking, the corrective orthosis are semi-rigid and the accommodative are flexible. If we consider the previous example of a CAI patient with flexible cavus feet an appropriate in-sole prescription would order for a plantar orthosis for chronic ankle instability associated with a flexible cavus foot. The orthosis goal is correction of the cavus; therefore, it needs to be semi-rigid/rigid. A lateral heel wedge with first metatarsal recess is a good option.

Commercial ankle orthosis might be described according to its mobility: constrictive, hinged, or simple (non-constrictive). Constrictive (or solid) ankle orthosis place the ankle in a fixed position. These are shaped to accommodate the foot and may come with padding to relieve pressure at key pressure points. Its simpler design consists of one solid piece of plastic shaped to fit around the heel. They offer maximal stability by placing the ankle in a fixed position. Its role in CAI patients is limited. These AFOS are most commonly used to treat foot drop associated with cerebral vascular accidents or cerebral palsy. Some clinicians might find it useful for short-time pain management after an acute sprain or relapse.

Hinged orthosis allows sagittal plane controlled mobility with coronal and axial stability (Fig. 11.3).

Simple orthosis are usually called braces. Nomenclature is misleading in the sense that it is not simple to understand the type of device used in many papers. There are soft braces, with non-rigid components like stirrups, and semi-rigid braces with some kind of plastic medial and lateral pieces for coronal plane movement control. Kerkhoffs calls them lace-up **ankle** support and semi-rigid **ankle** support [38].

A recent review on the effect of braces on acute ankle sprains described that few individual studies reported positive outcomes after treatment with an ankle brace compared with other functional methods. The two high-quality studies that measured ankle instability as an outcome variable reported no difference with the application of a brace. The author concludes that braces are a cost-effective method, so its use after acute ankle sprains should be considered. If we apply this rationale in CAI patients it might be of clinical use after a relapse, although it has no influence on the prognostic or ligament healing [39].

Bracing provides supplemental external **joint** stiffness and/or improved proprioceptive acuity.

Webster assessed the effects of two ankle braces on joint position sense and ankle stiffness, and determined whether bracing effects are reduced with localized muscle fatigue. Fatigue increased absolute joint position sense errors by 0.3° (6–12%) across all conditions.

Stiffness was unaffected by fatigue among females.

Among males, fatigue increased stiffness by 0.75 Nm/rad (3.3%) with the semi-rigid brace and decreased stiffness by 0.32 Nm/rad (1.5%) with no brace. The conclusions were that the semi-rigid plastic brace provides more effective ankle support compared to no brace or neoprene ankle wrap brace conditions. The semi-rigid brace improved joint position sense after initial application (pre-fatigue), and it helped to maintain ankle effective stiffness after fatigue. The neoprene ankle wrap brace may provide an increase in effective stiffness when initially applied, but as an adult with CAI fatigues, it may not compensate for losses in physiological stiffness [40].

Doherty reported on nine systematic reviews on this topic. His review analyzed 39 papers (15 RCTs, 24 non-RCTs; $N = 8734$; 90% male, 10% female) that evaluated some kind of external support for the treatment of CAI. Although it remains unclear whether bracing or taping are effective interventions for the primary prevention of an ankle sprain, there was unanimous consensus among the reviews that bracing is effective at preventing a recurrence of an ankle sprain [27].

11.3.3 Physiotherapy

The rehabilitation modalities are divided into three big groups:

- Manipulation and massage (Sensory-targeted ankle rehabilitation strategies: STARS)
- Strength training
- Proprioceptive training.

These three rehabilitation groups are frequently called "physiotherapy." In a strict sense, if a patient reports that his CAI symptoms get better by walking on the beach (or any home-based training) he is doing his own "physiotherapy" (healing through movement or exercise) [41].

Again, it is useful to mention that this option is of paramount effect in CAI patients. In the acute setting (first episode), the rate of reinjury was considered similar in 204 young athletes in a prospective study from the Savoie University, whether that had, or not, supervised rehabilitation: 54% of patients without guided rehabilitation had a relapse, as well as 57% of those patients who had the same treatment [42].

11.3.3.1 Manipulation and Massage (STARS)

The rationale behind these treatments is that deficient sensory input from damaged ankle ligament receptors is thought to contribute to sensorimotor deficits in those with CAI. Targeting other viable sensory receptors may then enhance sensorimotor control in these patients. Sensory-targeted ankle rehabilitation strategies (STARS) for CAI have several components: joint mobilization, plantar massage, triceps surae stretching, or control.

These have been compared in a randomized study (n = 80 patients) where all STARS groups improved patient-oriented outcomes. Joint mobilization had the most meaningful effect immediately after the intervention and plantar massage at the 1-month follow-up [43].

That said, the same authors that published on the impact of STARS on patient-oriented outcomes reported that these strategies had no clinically relevant impact on laboratory-oriented measures of single-leg balance in those with chronic ankle instability [44].

STARS substantially improve single-leg postural control after one treatment, but these changes are short-lived. No substantial benefit of any of the interventions was found after 2 weeks of treatment, regardless of the treatment group [45].

11.3.3.2 Strength Training

There is evidence on peroneal strength deficits in patients with CAI. Willems, Terrier, Sakai, and others reported on the diminished eversion muscle strength [46, 47]. This deficit has been identified in strength tests, personal reaction time [48], and electromyography. This deficit has been reported in both plantarflexion and neutral ankle positions. The force measures correlated with sEMG amplitudes in the healthy group but not in the group with CAI [49].

David considers that the rehabilitation programs for unstable ankle patients must be focused on the motor control of eccentric contractions of the ankle evertors and invertors [50].

Apparently, copers do not suffer from this weakness, which has been related to an increase in muscle adipose tissue in peroneus longus muscle, although the cross-sectional area remained unchanged on the CAI side [51].

This finding was reported in research on the effect of peroneal Muscle Strength after the Modified Broström Procedure in CAI. The deficit ratio of peak torque for eversion significantly improved from a mean 38.6–17.4%. This meant a restoration of peroneal strength postoperatively of about 82.6% of the unaffected ankle [52].

This problem seems to be multi-planar. Abdel-Aziem compared the eccentric evertor/invertor and dorsiflexor/plantarflexor ratios in subjects with CAI. The eccentric contraction dorsiflexion/plantarflexion (Fig. 11.4) ratio of CAI group was significantly higher than the normal group, as well as a deficit in inversion and eversion eccentric torques [53].

In Thompson's meta-analysis of systematic reviews there is a strong evidence to support the

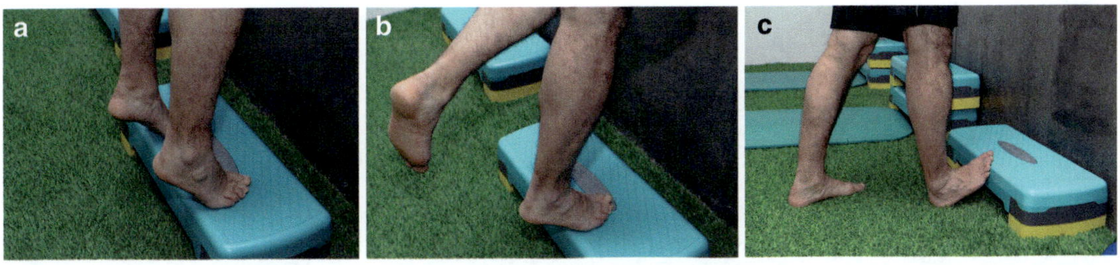

Fig. 11.4 Exercise therapy with elongation, strengthening, and eccentric training (**a**–**c**). This should include working the evertors/invertors as well as dorsiflexion and plantarflexion

contribution of dynamic balance, peroneal reaction time, and eversion strength deficits and moderate evidence for proprioception and static balance deficits to nonspecific ankle instability [54].

Strength training protocols might be applied as resistance tubing or through manual resistance. Active postural exercises, as wobble-board balance training, are considered proprioceptive training, despite the fact that they, too, imply strength training. A good way to differentiate might be considering that all open-chain training are merely strength training. Closed-chain exercises are part of postural/proprioceptive training, despite the evidence that they improved muscle strength [55, 56].

The strength training usually refers to ankle evertors. Kim analyzed isokinetic ankle-evertor strength (peak torque, total work) at 30°/s, 60°/s, 90°/s, and 120°/s, mediolateral stability index, and dynamic stability test. Data were recorded at baseline, 6 week and 24 week. The CAI group exhibited significant increases in concentric/eccentric evertor peak torque and total work at 120°/s in comparison with the control group [57].

11.3.3.3 Proprioceptive Training

This is the single best option in CAI treatment. Proprioceptive deficits lead to a delay in peroneal reaction time, which appears to be a peripheral reflex. Balance and postural control of the ankle are diminished after a lateral ankle sprain and can be restored through training that is mediated through central nervous mechanisms (Fig. 11.5). Basically, every author mentioned the importance of the neuromuscular training for joint protection [58].

Ankle inversion is a physiological movement. It becomes pathological due to the (micro or macro) joint incongruence (or instability) in the absence of the lateral ligaments or active eversion movement. In Konradsen words, “if the ankle has become subject to an inversion torque, injury can still be prevented if the reaction to counteract the inversion torque is sufficiently fast and powerful” [59].

Ko reported that there seems to be no strong association between deficits in postural stability and weakness in ankle strength [60].

The timing in which the active stabilizers work is as important as its power [61].

Copers showed greater activation of the tibialis anterior and peroneus longus muscles, during the posteromedial reach of the Star Excursion Balance Test. This greater activation was significantly bigger than the one observed in healthy ankles, and bigger (without significance) [62].

CAI is frequently felt like recurrent bouts of ankle sprain. The absence of an objective mechanical instability, like previously described, does not change the clinical diagnosis of chronicity. It might, nonetheless, guide the doctor into a bigger investment in proprioceptive and neuromuscular training. Some patients with mechanical CAI might also solve their symptoms with rehabilitation. Every patient has his own needs. A low demand patient might feel little limitation in his activities and a high-level athlete might report an inferior performance even in the presence of a slight functional instability.

Like every conservative option mentioned this far, proprioceptive training has many varieties [63]. Basically, they imply some type of unstable or irregular surface where the patient trains his

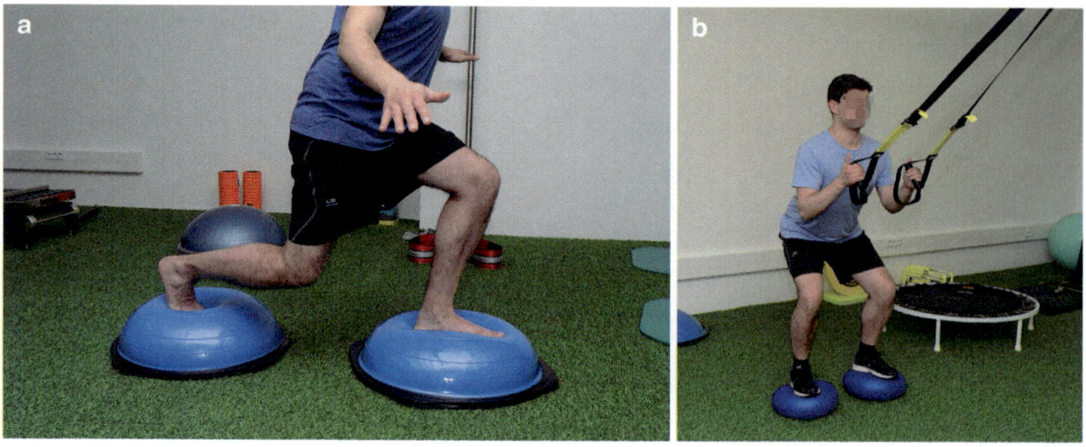

Fig. 11.5 Training neuromuscular and proprioceptive control using instability exercises (**a**, **b**); combined exercises with strength training combined with proprioception and neuromuscular balance improvement

balance and postural control, in a closed-chain exercise [64].

Forestier showed that using an ankle destabilization device (in the sole of a shoe) caused a pre-activation of the peroneus longus and brevis between 10 and 20 ms before the heel strike in stance phase, in contrast to its regular activation, which occurs 20 ms after heel strike [65].

Burcal compared Balance Training Versus Balance Training With STARS (sensory-targeted Ankle Rehabilitation Strategies) in Patients With Chronic Ankle Instability in a 4-week program. Both groups demonstrated improvements in all outcome categories after the interventions ($P < 0.10$) [66].

Hop stabilization exercises for 6 weeks showed improving neuromuscular control (preparatory muscle activation, reactive muscle activation, and muscle onset time) and self-reported function in collegiate basketball players with CAI [67].

A 6-week neuromuscular training program was also effective in women's field hockey players. Following the 6-week training, the CAI participants demonstrated a less everted ankle at heel strike during walking and running (−1.77° and −1.76°) compared to the previous positions. They also showed less ankle eversion at mid-stance (−5.14° and −4.19°).

Ankle orientation at toe-off changed significantly to an inverted ankle position (from −0.26° to 4.11°). The ankle kinematics was restored back to the previous positions at 24 weeks except for landing but not during walking and running [68].

Basically, this shows that personal pre-activation needs a neuromuscular training, which should be based on dynamic exercises. Irregular surfaces, BOSU, foam, wobble boards are just a few more options to this rehabilitation modality [69].

At last, besides the unstable surface or destabilization devices, there might be a place for vibration platform. Sierra-Guzman studied the effects of a 6-week WBV training program on a soft, unstable surface, on peak torque, reaction time, and the electrical activity of ankle muscles in 50 recreational athletes with chronic ankle instability [70].

11.4 Conclusion and Take-Home Message

The vast majority of CAI patients should have conservative treatment before considering surgery. External support measures, like taping or bracing, help the patient in everyday and sports activities.

Proprioceptive deficits lead to a delay in peroneal reaction time, as well as balance and postural control impairment. These can be improved through training that is mediated by central nervous mechanisms. Proprioceptive training should be included in the rehabilitation of all CAI patients.

References

1. Hiller CE, Kilbreath SL, Refshauge KM. Chronic ankle instability: evolution of the model. J Athl Train. 2011;46:133–41. https://doi.org/10.4085/1062-6050-46.2.133.
2. Terada M, Bowker S, Hiller CE, Thomas AC, Pietrosimone B, Gribble PA. Quantifying levels of function between different subgroups of chronic ankle instability. Scand J Med Sci Sports. 2017;27:650–60. https://doi.org/10.1111/sms.12712.
3. Freeman MA. Instability of the foot after injuries to the lateral ligament of the ankle. J Bone Joint Surg Br. 1965;47:669–77.
4. Gribble PA, Delahunt E, Bleakley CM, Caulfield B, Docherty CL, Fong DT-P, Fourchet F, Hertel J, Hiller CE, Kaminski TW, McKeon PO, Refshauge KM, van der Wees P, Vicenzino W, Wikstrom EA. Selection criteria for patients with chronic ankle instability in controlled research: a position statement of the International Ankle Consortium. J Athl Train. 2014;49:121–7. https://doi.org/10.4085/1062-6050-49.1.14.
5. Hubbard TJ, Cordova M. Mechanical instability after an acute lateral ankle sprain. Arch Phys Med Rehabil. 2009;90:1142–6. https://doi.org/10.1016/j.apmr.2009.01.020.
6. Cordova ML, Sefton JM, Hubbard TJ. Mechanical joint laxity associated with chronic ankle instability: a systematic review. Sports Health. 2010;2:452–9. https://doi.org/10.1177/1941738110382392.
7. Hertel J. Functional anatomy, pathomechanics, and pathophysiology of lateral ankle instability. J Athl Train. 2002;37:364–75.
8. Lohrer H, Nauck T, Gehring D, Wissler S. Differences between mechanically stable and unstable chronic ankle instability subgroups when examined by arthrometer and FAAM-G. J Orthop. 2015;10:32.
9. Rosen AB, Ko J, Brown CN. Diagnostic accuracy of instrumented and manual talar tilt tests in chronic ankle instability populations. Scand J Med Sci Sports. 2015;25:e214–21. https://doi.org/10.1111/sms.12288.
10. Kirby JL, Houston MN, Gabriner ML, Hoch MC. Relationships between mechanical joint stability and somatosensory function in individuals with chronic ankle instability. Foot (Edinb). 2016;28:1–6. https://doi.org/10.1016/j.foot.2016.04.001.
11. Hertel J. Sensorimotor deficits with ankle sprains and chronic ankle instability. Clin Sports Med. 2008;27:353–70. https://doi.org/10.1016/j.csm.2008.03.006.
12. Bosman HA, Robinson AHN. Treatment of ankle instability with an associated cavus deformity. Foot Ankle Clin. 2013;18:643–57. https://doi.org/10.1016/j.fcl.2013.08.005.
13. Wu X, Song W, Zheng C, Zhou S, Bai S. Morphological study of mechanoreceptors in collateral ligaments of the ankle joint. J Orthop Surg Res. 2015;10(92) https://doi.org/10.1186/s13018-015-0215-7.
14. Hintermann B, Boss A, Schäfer D. Arthroscopic findings in patients with chronic ankle instability. Am J Sports Med. 2002;30:402–9.
15. van Dijk CN. On diagnostic strategies in severe ankle sprain. Amsterdam: Rodopi; 1994.
16. Michels F, Pereira H, Calder J, Matricali G, Glazebrook M, Guillo S, Karlsson J, ESSKA AFAS Ankle Instability Group, Acevedo J, Batista J, Bauer T, Calder J, Carreira D, Choi W, Corte-Real N, Glazebrook M, Ghorbani A, Giza E, Guillo S, Hunt K, Karlsson J, Kong SW, Lee JW, Michels F, Molloy A, Mangone P, Matsui K, Nery C, Ozeki S, Pearce C, Pereira H, Perera A, Pijnenburg B, Raduan F, Stone J, Takao M, Tourne Y, Vega J. Searching for consensus in the approach to patients with chronic lateral ankle instability: ask the expert. Knee Surg Sports Traumatol Arthrosc. 2017. doi: https://doi.org/10.1007/s00167-017-4556-0
17. Harrington KD. Degenerative arthritis of the ankle secondary to long-standing lateral ligament instability. J Bone Joint Surg. 1979;61:354–61.
18. Caputo AM, Lee JY, Spritzer CE, Easley ME, DeOrio JK, Nunley JA, DeFrate LE. In vivo kinematics of the tibiotalar joint after lateral ankle instability. Am J Sports Med. 2009;37:2241–8. https://doi.org/10.1177/0363546509337578.
19. Moisan G, Descarreaux M, Cantin V. Effects of chronic ankle instability on kinetics, kinematics and muscle activity during walking and running: a systematic review. Gait Posture. 2017;52:381–99. https://doi.org/10.1016/j.gaitpost.2016.11.037.
20. Baur H, Hirschmüller A, Müller S, Mayer F. Neuromuscular activity of the peroneal muscle after foot orthoses therapy in runners. Med Sci Sports Exerc. 2011;43:1500–6. https://doi.org/10.1249/MSS.0b013e31820c64ae.
21. Dingenen B, Peeraer L, Deschamps K, Fieuws S, Janssens L, Staes F. Influence of shoes and foot orthoses on lower extremity muscle activation onset times in healthy subjects during the transition from double-leg stance to single-leg stance. J Sports Med Phys Fitness. 2015;55:16–24.
22. Dingenen B, Peeraer L, Deschamps K, Fieuws S, Janssens L, Staes F. Muscle-activation onset times with shoes and foot orthoses in participants with chronic ankle instability. J Athl Train. 2015;50:688–96. https://doi.org/10.4085/1062-6050-50.2.02.
23. Herb CC, Grossman K, Feger MA, Donovan L, Hertel J. Lower extremity biomechanics during a drop-vertical jump in participants with or without chronic

ankle instability. J Athl Train. 2018;53:364–71. https://doi.org/10.4085/1062-6050-481-15.
24. Barrett JR, Tanji JL, Drake C, Fuller D, Kawasaki RI, Fenton RM. High- versus low-top shoes for the prevention of ankle sprains in basketball players. A prospective randomized study. Am J Sports Med. 1993;21:582–5. https://doi.org/10.1177/036354659302100416.
25. Chinn L, Dicharry J, Hertel J. Ankle kinematics of individuals with chronic ankle instability while walking and jogging on a treadmill in shoes. Phys Ther Sport. 2013;14:232–9. https://doi.org/10.1016/j.ptsp.2012.10.001.
26. Ramanathan AK, Wallace DT, Arnold GP, Drew TS, Wang W, Abboud RJ. The effect of varying footwear configurations on the peroneus longus muscle function following inversion. Foot (Edinb). 2011;21:31–6. https://doi.org/10.1016/j.foot.2010.11.001.
27. Doherty C, Bleakley C, Delahunt E, Holden S. Treatment and prevention of acute and recurrent ankle sprain: an overview of systematic reviews with meta-analysis. Br J Sports Med. 2017;51:113–25. https://doi.org/10.1136/bjsports-2016-096178.
28. Tourne Y, Mabit C. La Cheville Instable; 2015.
29. Trégouët P, Merland F, Horodyski MB. A comparison of the effects of ankle taping styles on biomechanics during ankle inversion. Ann Phys Rehabil Med. 2013;56:113–22. https://doi.org/10.1016/j.rehab.2012.12.001.
30. Kuni B, Mussler J, Kalkum E, Schmitt H, Wolf SI. Effect of kinesiotaping, non-elastic taping and bracing on segmental foot kinematics during drop landing in healthy subjects and subjects with chronic ankle instability. Physiotherapy. 2016;102:287–93. https://doi.org/10.1016/j.physio.2015.07.004.
31. Vaes P, De Boeck H, Handelberg F, Opdecam P. Comparative radiological study of the influence of ankle joint strapping and - - taping on ankle stability*. J Orthop Sports Phys Ther. 1985;7:110–4.
32. Vaes P, Duquet W, Handelberg F, Casteleyn PP, Van Tiggelen R, Opdecam P. Objective roentgenologic measurements of the influence of ankle braces on pathologic joint mobility. A comparison of 9 braces. Acta Orthop Belg. 1998;64:201–9.
33. Wang Y, Gu Y, Chen J, Luo W, He W, Han Z, Tian J. Kinesio taping is superior to other taping methods in ankle functional performance improvement: a systematic review and meta-analysis. Clin Rehabil. 2018;32:1472–81. https://doi.org/10.1177/0269215518780443.
34. Bicici S, Karatas N, Baltaci G. Effect of athletic taping and kinesiotaping® on measurements of functional performance in basketball players with chronic inversion ankle sprains. Int J Sports Phys Ther. 2012;7:154–66.
35. de-la Torre-Domingo C, Alguacil-Diego IM, Molina-Rueda F, López-Román A, Fernández-Carnero J. Effect of kinesiology tape on measurements of balance in subjects with chronic ankle instability: a randomized controlled trial. Arch Phys Med Rehabil. 2015;96:2169–75. https://doi.org/10.1016/j.apmr.2015.06.022.
36. Faraji E, Daneshmandi H, Atri AE, Onvani V, Namjoo FR. Effects of prefabricated ankle orthoses on postural stability in basketball players with chronic ankle instability. Asian J Sports Med. 2012;3:274–8.
37. Quinn K, Parker P, de Bie R, Rowe B, Handoll H. Interventions for preventing ankle ligament injuries. Cochrane Database Syst Rev. 2000:CD000018. https://doi.org/10.1002/14651858.CD000018.
38. Kerkhoffs GMMJ, Struijs PAA, Marti RK, Blankevoort L, Assendelft WJJ, van Dijk CN. Functional treatments for acute ruptures of the lateral ankle ligament: a systematic review. Acta Orthop Scand. 2003;74:69–77. https://doi.org/10.1080/00016470310013699.
39. Kemler E, van de Port I, Backx F, van Dijk CN. A systematic review on the treatment of acute ankle sprain: brace versus other functional treatment types. Sports Med. 2011;41:185–97. https://doi.org/10.2165/11584370-000000000-00000.
40. Webster CA, Nussbaum MA, Madigan ML. Stiffness and proprioceptive contributions of ankle braces and the influence of localized muscle fatigue. J Electromyogr Kinesiol. 2017;34:37–43. https://doi.org/10.1016/j.jelekin.2017.02.009.
41. De Ridder R, Willems TM, Vanrenterghem J, Roosen P. Effect of a home-based balance training protocol on dynamic postural control in subjects with chronic ankle instability. Int J Sports Med. 2015;36:596–602. https://doi.org/10.1055/s-0034-1396823.
42. Tourne Y, Mabit C (2015) La cheville instable. Elsevier Masson
43. McKeon PO, Wikstrom EA. Sensory-targeted ankle rehabilitation strategies for chronic ankle instability. Med Sci Sports Exerc. 2016;48:776–84. https://doi.org/10.1249/MSS.0000000000000859.
44. Wikstrom EA, McKeon PO. Predicting manual therapy treatment success in patients with chronic ankle instability: improving self-reported function. J Athl Train. 2017;52:325–31. https://doi.org/10.4085/1062-6050-52.2.07.
45. McKeon PO, Wikstrom EA. The effect of sensory-targeted ankle rehabilitation strategies on single-leg center of pressure elements in those with chronic ankle instability: a randomized clinical trial. J Sci Med Sport. 2018; https://doi.org/10.1016/j.jsams.2018.08.017.
46. Willems T, Witvrouw E, Verstuyft J, Vaes P, De Clercq D. Proprioception and muscle strength in subjects with a history of ankle sprains and chronic instability. J Athl Train. 2002;37:487–93.
47. Terrier R, Degache F, Fourchet F, Gojanovic B, Forestier N. Assessment of evertor weakness in patients with chronic ankle instability: Functional versus isokinetic testing. Clin Biomech (Bristol, Avon). 2017;41:54–9. https://doi.org/10.1016/j.clinbiomech.2016.12.002.
48. Schmidt R, Becker HP, Rauhut F, Tannheimer M. Neuromuscular deficits in chronic ankle instability. Frequency and significance—multicenter

study. Unfallchirurg. 2014;117:710–5. https://doi.org/10.1007/s00113-013-2392-3.
49. Donnelly L, Donovan L, Hart JM, Hertel J. Eversion strength and surface electromyography measures with and without chronic ankle instability measured in 2 positions. Foot Ankle Int. 2017;38:769–78. https://doi.org/10.1177/1071100717701231.
50. David P, Halimi M, Mora I, Doutrellot P-L, Petitjean M. Isokinetic testing of evertor and invertor muscles in patients with chronic ankle instability. J Appl Biomech. 2013;29:696–704.
51. Sakai S, Urabe Y, Morikawa M, Fujishita H, Komiya M, Sasadai J, Fujishita H, Maeda N. Quantity and quality of the peroneus longus assessed using ultrasonography in leg with chronic ankle instability. J Phys Ther Sci. 2018;30:1396–400. https://doi.org/10.1589/jpts.30.1396.
52. Cho B-K, Park J-K, Choi S-M, Kang S-W, SooHoo NF. The peroneal strength deficits in patients with chronic ankle instability compared to ankle sprain copers and normal individuals. Foot Ankle Surg. 2017; https://doi.org/10.1016/j.fas.2017.10.017.
53. Abdel-aziem AA, Draz AH. Chronic ankle instability alters eccentric eversion/inversion and dorsiflexion/plantarflexion ratio. J Back Musculoskelet Rehabil. 2014;27:47–53. https://doi.org/10.3233/BMR-130418.
54. Thompson C, Schabrun S, Romero R, Bialocerkowski A, van Dieen J, Marshall P. Factors contributing to chronic ankle instability: a systematic review and meta-analysis of systematic reviews. Sports Med. 2018;48:189–205. https://doi.org/10.1007/s40279-017-0781-4.
55. Wright CJ, Linens SW, Cain MS. A randomized controlled trial comparing rehabilitation efficacy in chronic ankle instability. J Sport Rehabil. 2017;26:238–49. https://doi.org/10.1123/jsr.2015-0189.
56. Blackburn JR, Morrissey MC. The relationship between open and closed kinetic chain strength of the lower limb and jumping performance. J Orthop Sports Phys Ther. 1998;27:430–5. https://doi.org/10.2519/jospt.1998.27.6.430.
57. Kim T, Kim E, Choi H. Effects of a 6-week neuromuscular rehabilitation program on ankle-evertor strength and postural stability in elite women field hockey players with chronic ankle instability. J Sport Rehabil. 2017;26:269–80. https://doi.org/10.1123/jsr.2016-0031.
58. Richie DH. Functional instability of the ankle and the role of neuromuscular control: a comprehensive review. J Foot Ankle Surg. 2001;40:240–51.
59. Konradsen L. Sensori-motor control of the uninjured and injured human ankle. J Electromyogr Kinesiol. 2002;12:199–203.
60. Ko KR, Lee H, Lee W-Y, Sung K-S. Ankle strength is not strongly associated with postural stability in patients awaiting surgery for chronic lateral ankle instability. Knee Surg Sports Traumatol Arthrosc. 2018; https://doi.org/10.1007/s00167-018-4960-0.
61. Sousa ASP, Valente I, Pinto A, Soutelo T, Silva M. Short and medium latency responses in participants with chronic ankle instability. J Athl Train. 2018;53:679–86. https://doi.org/10.4085/1062-6050-120-17.
62. Pozzi F, Moffat M, Gutierrez G. Neuromuscular control during performance of a dynamic balance task in subjects with and without ankle instability. Int J Sports Phys Ther. 2015;10:520–9.
63. Eils E, Rosenbaum D. A multi-station proprioceptive exercise program in patients with ankle instability. Med Sci Sports Exerc. 2001;33:1991–8.
64. Faizullin I, Faizullina E. Effects of balance training on post-sprained ankle joint instability. Int J Risk Saf Med. 2015;27(Suppl 1):S99–S101. https://doi.org/10.3233/JRS-150707.
65. Forestier N, Toschi P. The effects of an ankle destabilization device on muscular activity while walking. Int J Sports Med. 2005;26:464–70. https://doi.org/10.1055/s-2004-830336.
66. Burcal CJ, Trier AY, Wikstrom EA. Balance training versus balance training with STARS in patients with chronic ankle instability: a randomized controlled trial. J Sport Rehabil. 2017;26:347–57. https://doi.org/10.1123/jsr.2016-0018.
67. Minoonejad H, Karimizadeh Ardakani M, Rajabi R, Wikstrom EA, Sharifnezhad A. Hop stabilization training improves neuromuscular control in collegiate basketball players with chronic ankle instability: a randomized controlled trial. J Sport Rehabil. 2018:1–25. https://doi.org/10.1123/jsr.2018-0103.
68. Kim E, Choi H, Cha J-H, Park J-C, Kim T. Effects of neuromuscular training on the rear-foot angle kinematics in elite women field hockey players with chronic ankle instability. J Sports Sci Med. 2017;16:137–46.
69. Hupperets MDW, Verhagen EALM, van Mechelen W. The 2BFit study: is an unsupervised proprioceptive balance board training programme, given in addition to usual care, effective in preventing ankle sprain recurrences? Design of a randomized controlled trial. BMC Musculoskelet Disord. 2008;9:71. https://doi.org/10.1186/1471-2474-9-71.
70. Sierra-Guzmán R, Jiménez JF, Ramírez C, Esteban P, Abián-Vicén J. Effects of synchronous whole body vibration training on a soft, unstable surface in athletes with chronic ankle instability. Int J Sports Med. 2017;38:447–55. https://doi.org/10.1055/s-0043-102571.

Part III

Surgical Treatment

12 Surgical Treatment for Acute Ankle Sprain: "State of the Art"

Arul Ramasamy, Anthony Perera, and James Calder

12.1 Introduction

The management of severe acute ankle sprain has evolved over the past 30 years. With the advent of anatomic ligament repair advocated by Broström in 1966 which provided a reproducible, effective reconstruction without the complications and side effects of previous nonanatomic repairs, this soon became the gold standard surgical repair in the young active population [1, 2].

However, the pendulum began to swing towards functional non-operative rehabilitation following the publication of a number of studies in the 1990s demonstrating equivalent and even superior results to surgery [3, 4]. The evolution of rehabilitation protocols promoting early mobilization and functional rehabilitation again led to improved outcomes compared to the previous management of cast immobilization [5]. Thus, it is now accepted that Grade I and II lateral ligament injuries can be treated non-operatively and that even in Grade III injuries, non-operative treatment remains an appropriate treatment modality for the vast majority of patients. Consequently, surgical repair was often reserved for patients with chronic, symptomatic lateral ligament laxity [6].

The role of surgery in the acute ankle sprain has become questioned. A Cochrane review undertaken by Kerkhoffs et al. in 2007 could not demonstrate a significant difference between non-operative treatment and surgery in the management of Grade III lateral ligament injuries [7, 8]. Although there was no significant difference in the primary outcome measures of pain, recurrence of instability, return to activity, or subjective instability, there was evidence that objective instability (e.g., anterior drawer test, talar tilt) were significantly reduced in the surgical group.

Optimal treatment for these injuries in high-demand athletes has been controversial for many years. Most of the literature related to the management of ankle sprains is based on recreational athletes and non-athletic populations and therefore those findings cannot be completely extrapolated to the high-level professional athlete [9]. Proponents of surgical reconstruction suggest

A. Ramasamy (✉)
Fortius Clinic London, London, UK

Academic Department of Military Surgery and Trauma, Royal Centre for Defence Medicine, Birmingham, UK

Department of Bioengineering, Imperial College London, London, UK
e-mail: a.ramasamy09@imperial.ac.uk

A. Perera
University Hospital of Wales, Cardiff, UK

J. Calder
Fortius Clinic London, London, UK

Department of Bioengineering, Imperial College London, London, UK
e-mail: james.calder@fortiusclinic.com

H. Pereira et al. (eds.), *Lateral Ankle Instability*, https://doi.org/10.1007/978-3-662-62763-1_12

that the reduction of objective instability is a compelling reason to consider surgery. Objective instability is a known predictor for future ankle sprains which in turn can result in prolonged delays in returning to competitive sport as well as affecting the athletes' confidence in the stability of his/her ankle. In addition, current consensus suggests that short-term outcomes following surgery are likely to better in the hands of an experienced foot and ankle surgeon which may further sway the decision towards earlier surgical intervention in this selected patient population [10]. Hence, there is now a growing consensus that surgery may be indicated in the high-level professional athlete [11].

12.2 Assessment of the Ankle Sprain in the Elite Athlete

The assessment of the acute ankle sprain in the elite athlete can frequently be challenging. The mode and force of injury, as well as the patient's inability to keep on playing or even weight-bearing is often a useful indicator of a more severe injury. Many athletes will often have a plain radiograph performed to exclude a fracture even when they may be outside the Ottawa guidelines for radiography and frequently there is a low threshold to perform an MRI scan.

Tenderness alone is ineffective in determining ligamentous injury. In contrast, tenderness combined with significant discoloration or hematoma formation has a sensitivity of 90% in determining ligamentous disruption. Isolated anterior drawer has a sensitivity of 73% and a specificity of 97%. When all three findings are present, then there is a sensitivity of 100% and a specificity of 73% [12].

The timing of clinical examination also has a significant bearing on the accuracy of clinical diagnosis. Van Dijk et al. demonstrated that the specificity and sensitivity of clinical examination within 48 h post-injury was 71% and 33% respectively, but at 5 days after injury increased significantly to 96% and 84% [13].

In terms of preoperative imaging, MRI remains a useful adjunct in identifying additional pathologies like osteochondral lesions, which will need to be addressed at surgery. However, imaging alone cannot substitute clinical examination. Although demonstrating good specificity (100% for ATFL and 83% for CFL), it has a relatively low sensitivity (56% for ATFL and 50% for CFL) [14–16]. Ultrasound may also be a useful imaging modality although it remains highly operator-dependent.

The decision to consider acute reconstruction in the high-level athlete must be individually tailored to the athlete's needs. Several factors such as the time of the season, athletes' expectation, sports-specific ankle demands, stage of career, and collateral ankle joint pathology are all features that need to be considered when contemplating surgery. The competing interests of returning to sport quickly and the possible increased time loss after surgical repair is a significant factor in some athletes avoiding surgery. However, with current postsurgical rehabilitation programs, the time to recover from surgery has been significantly reduced compared to previously when plaster immobilization for several weeks after surgery was the norm.

Another important factor to consider is the potential increased risk of re-injury after non-operative management, which in itself can also lead to significant time away from competitive sport [11]. Surgery should therefore be offered on an individual basis.

12.3 Surgical Management

Surgical treatment of lateral ligament instability can be broadly categorized into either anatomic reconstruction involving direct repair of the lateral ligament complex or nonanatomic reconstruction where tendons (usually the peroneal tendons) are rerouted to recreate the complex. In 1966, Broström described direct ligament repair of the ATFL and CFL. Later the Gould modification incorporated the inferior extensor retinaculum, which has been demonstrated to improve biomechanical strength by 60% [17, 18]. Since that time, the Broström-Gould procedure has become the gold standard of surgical treatment of ankle instability. Within the context of the acute ankle sprain, direct anatomic repair should be considered the primary procedure of choice.

While open lateral ligament repair is the most widely performed procedure, the development of arthroscopic techniques has become more widespread. Proponents suggest that the potential advantages of an arthroscopic ligament repair include quicker recovery, decreased morbidity as well as the ability to address intra-articular pathology with a single minimally invasive approach [19]. Biomechanical studies have also demonstrated that there is no difference in the strength or stiffness of a traditional open repair compared with an arthroscopic anatomic repair [20].

In a systematic review comparing open versus arthroscopic lateral ligament anatomic repair, both demonstrated excellent AOFAS scores (open 90.1 vs arthroscopic 92.4) [21]. However, surgery-related complications occurred in 7.9% (40/505 ankles) of open procedures compared to 15.2% (30/216) of arthroscopic procedures. Residual instability was reported as 0.99% in the open group compared to 2.3% in the arthroscopic group. Despite the increased complication rate, both procedures resulted in extremely high patient satisfaction rates of 91.7% (open) and 96.4% (arthroscopic).

Although the Broström-Gould procedure has been shown to result in excellent clinical results with extremely low recurrence rates, cadaveric studies have reported that ATFL direct suture repair or the use of bone suture anchors still resulted in a repair that has inferior strength to a native ATFL [22]. This has led some authors to suggest that the ATFL repair will need to be protected in the short-term to prevent failure or lengthening of the ligament. As a result, the concept of a high-strength nonabsorbable suture tape has been proposed as a potential augmentation to the repair and thereby enable faster rehabilitation. Biomechanical studies have reported statistically superior performance of direct ligament repair augmented with suture tape compared to the standard Broström-Gould repair [23]. Clinically, Yoo et al. showed that the AOFAS scores in the suture tape augmentation group were better than the standard repair group at the 6 and 12-week stage but the results were the same at 6 months following surgery [24]. These early differences may be attributed to the different rehabilitation protocols used, where the tape augmentation group was allowed to weight bear straight after surgery and were not immobilized in a cast whereas the standard group was immobilized in a cast for 4 weeks. Despite the lack of protection in the suture tape augmentation group, no recurrent instability was noted in either group.

12.4 Surgical Procedure

Following administration of the general anesthetic, an examination under anesthesia is performed to confirm genuine anterior drawer and talar tilt tests. Intravenous antibiotics, cephalosporin, is infused prior to inflation of a thigh tourniquet. Anterior ankle arthroscopy is performed in all cases, washing out any hematoma and enabling direct visual assessment of the ligamentous structures and the articular surface. Care must be taken to ensure that the soft tissue envelope is not over-distended and it is recommended that intra-articular fluid pressures are maintained at or below 30 mm Hg utilizing a fluid management system. At this stage, any intra-articular pathology is addressed, with osteochondral lesions treated with debridement, curettage, and microfracture. In addition, complete deltoid ligament ruptures (grade III injuries) should also be repaired using either bone tunnel sutures or bone anchors.

The lateral ligament reconstruction is performed using a modified Broström-Gould procedure [17]. A 6 cm curved skin incision is made along the anterior-distal border of the fibula, taking care to avoid damage to the sural nerve and cutaneous branch of the superficial peroneal nerve and a superficial dissection on to the distal fibula is performed. The peroneal tendons are identified and retracted to visualize the CFL located beneath. The ATFL is then identified. Using sharp dissection, the ATFL and CFL are resected from the distal fibula. A periosteal elevator or scalpel is then used to lift a periosteal flap proximally/posteriorly away from the anterior-distal border of the fibula. The distal fibula is prepared by using a rongeur to roughen up the bone. Once the fibula is prepared, two suture anchors are inserted into the bone and two sutures are placed each in the ATFL and the CFL footprint, 7–8 mm from the leading edge in order to advance and tighten the ligament reconstruction. When tying the sutures, it is important to dorsiflex and evert the ankle to ensure that the ATFL and CFL repair is snug against the bone. To reinforce the repair, the extensor retinaculum is dissected as a separate layer, ensuring that the superficial peroneal nerve is not injured. Occasionally it is observed that the ATFL is avulsed from its talar attachment and the bone anchor may therefore be placed in the ATFL footprint of the talus enabling anatomical reconstruction. The retinaculum is then sutured up onto the repaired ATFL. The previously elevated periosteal flap is then brought down over the repair to further reinforce it as well as covering the surgical knots to prevent superficial irritation. The wound is then closed and protected by dressings and a below-knee Plaster of Paris is applied. On discharge, the patient is advised to non weight bear for the first 2 weeks and to keep the limb elevated until the wound is inspected and sutures removed.

12.5 Rehabilitation

Optimal outcome following acute ankle ligament reconstruction is reliant upon the implementation and strict adherence to a postoperative regimen that aims to avoid complications and re-injury. Within the modern professional sporting environment, there exists an imperative for accelerated rehabilitation programs to return to play as quickly as possible. With increasing awareness of issues of thromboembolic disease, neuromuscular deconditioning, and chronic regional pain syndrome associated with prolonged immobilization, the pendulum has swung towards earlier mobilization and weight-bearing. Protection of the ankle in a boot or brace is usually recommended for 4 weeks following removal of the plaster cast and sutures with a functional rehabilitation program starting immediately. Partial weight-bearing may commence at this 2-week stage, building up to full weight-bearing by 4 weeks postoperatively. In a case series of 49 patients with chronic ankle instability undergoing a modified Broström repair followed by immediate weight-bearing, Petrera et al. reported a return to sport rate of 94% at 42 months follow-up [25]. However, there remain concerns regarding rehabilitating patients too quickly. In an epidemiological review of professional rugby union players, Pearce et al. noted that re-injuries kept players out of the game on average 3.5 times longer than the original injury, highlighting the dangers of not allowing for a complete recovery [26].

When designing a rehabilitation protocol following acute ankle ligament reconstruction surgery, several factors need to be considered:

- Strength of the initial repair in relation to the loads applied to it during weight-bearing and ankle movements.
- The mechanism by which the ligament repair/reconstruction heals to bone.
- Prevention of re-injury by safely returning the patient to sport-specific activities based on an objective assessment of strength and neuromuscular control.

12.5.1 Tissue Healing

One of the critical aspects of tissue healing, especially following the implantation of foreign material is the wound. Delayed wound healing in the oedematous limb and subsequent increase in prolonged wound exudate is likely to contribute to increased wound infection rates which in turn may result in prolonged rehabilitation and delayed return to sport. Although small studies have demonstrated that immediate weight-bearing following ankle reconstruction was not associated with increased wound complication rates, most surgeons questioned in a survey of the Ankle Instability Group section of the European

Society for Sports Traumatology, Knee Surgery and Arthroscopy (ESSKA-AFAS) advocated a short (10–14) day period of immobilization and elevation of the limb until the wound has healed [25, 27, 28].

12.5.2 Reconstitution of Bone Ligament Repair Interface

From an engineering perspective, ligaments can be analogous to machines with multiple moving parts (fibrils, fibers, and fascicles) whose basic function is of force transfer to and from the skeleton. Their complex response to loading allows for multi-axis bending which adds to the stress concentration to the region where they attach to bone (enthesis) [29]. Within the attachment of the ATFL and CFL to the fibula, a fibrocartilaginous enthesis occurs consisting of four zones of tissue: (i) pure dense fibrous connective tissue, uncalcified fibrocartilage, calcified fibrocartilage, and bone. The differing mechanical properties of these tissue zones enable a smooth stress distribution, eliminate singularities in stress, reduce stress concentration, improve the strength of the bonding, and decrease the risk of failure [30]. Therefore, the success of an acute ligament reconstruction relies on the ability to reconstitute the mechanical properties of the enthesis to prevent failure.

It is well known that mechanical loading of both bone and ligaments are crucial for homeostasis, and a lack of this loading leads to a decrease in the mechanical properties of both. Without the appropriate biological and mechanical environment, the four-zone enthesis complex is not produced and fibrous scar tissue forms in its stead [31]. Further animal models suggest that controlled mechanical loads after a delay to allow resolution of acute postoperative inflammation may be most favorable to the healing enthesis [32]. These studies would suggest that early controlled weight-bearing rehabilitation protocols would provide optimal conditions following acute ankle ligament reconstruction.

12.5.3 Neuromuscular Rehabilitation

It is well recognized that ankle instability is generally associated with motor deficits such as peroneal weakness, lower evertor activation, deficits of central organization of movement, and corticomotor excitability of peroneal muscles [33].

A number of studies have demonstrated that even short periods of immobilization (greater than 48 h) can result in functional deconditioning with cortical reorganization [34, 35]. Hence, early supervised joint movements (such as plantar/dorsiflexion) that will not interfere with tissue healing are likely to be advantageous in terms of neuromuscular rehabilitation.

The aim of this phase of rehabilitation is to:

- Strengthen the active stabilizers of the ankle.
- Restoration of the proprioceptive acuity.

The role of the ankle evertors is to control potentially traumatic ankle inversion movements and weakness of these muscles is known to be one of the main factors leading to chronic instability. Hence, any rehabilitation program should include both functional and targeted strengthening of the evertors including eccentric muscle recruitment.

Restoration of proprioceptive acuity is required to reduce functional deficits, improve symptoms of giving way, improve postural control, and thereby diminish the risk of re-injury. Traditionally proprioceptive training following ankle injury has involved performing balance exercises on unstable platforms such as plates, foam blocks, etc. However more recent research has determined that these types of exercises do not specifically target proprioception. Forestier et al. performed a study examining the effects on ankle muscular proprioceptive signals on healthy volunteers placed on three surfaces (stable, unstable unspecific—foam block, and unstable specific—unstable hindfoot and anchored forefoot). They found that the unstable specific surface was associated with the greatest peroneal muscle activation and greater postural agitation.

The authors concluded that specific exercises that focus purely on the hindfoot may be more effective in restoring proprioceptive function [33]. Although it is uncertain whether this focused treatment could accelerate the rehabilitation process, it would appear to be an area worthy of future research.

12.5.4 Return to Sport

The return to sport phase falls between 8 weeks and 4 months postsurgery. Progression in this phase relies on the patient's ability to demonstrate >90% function compared to the unaffected side with jogging progressing to running with directional changes. Agility drills are also included in this phase of rehabilitation. Once a patient can participate in practice without increased symptoms, return to competitive play should be considered. A prophylactic brace or taping is recommended during the initial return to the competition to help reduce the risk of re-injury. It is important to remember that continued assessment of stability and reinforcement of strength and proprioceptive exercises will be required to prevent further re-injury. Within this institution, White et al. reported on 42 professional athletes undergoing early reconstruction of severe (Grade III) acute lateral ligament injuries. The median return to training was 63 days and return to competitive sports was 77 days with no recurrent instability noted at 2 years follow-up [36]. They also noted that in the presence of concomitant injuries (OCD or deltoid injury) the return to training and return to play was significantly longer (86 days and 105 days, respectively).

12.6 Conclusion

Despite the good functional results obtained with non-operative treatment for the clear majority of patients with an acute lateral ankle ligament injury, there exists a role for acute surgical repair in high functioning athletes with a severe Grade III injury. In these patients, lateral ligament reconstruction can be a safe and effective treatment that can lead to an early return to competitive sport. Prompt diagnosis, early surgery, and a controlled accelerated rehabilitation program remain key to obtaining optimal results.

References

1. Staples OS. Ruptures of the fibular collateral ligaments of the ankle. Result study of immediate surgical treatment. J Bone Joint Surg Am. 1975;57:101–7.
2. Haapasalo H, Kannus P, Laine H-J, et al. Scientific evidence and reduced surgical treatment in acute ligament ruptures of the ankle. Scand J Med Sci Sports. 2015;25:299–300. https://doi.org/10.1111/sms.12179.
3. Kannus P, Renström P. Treatment for acute tears of the lateral ligaments of the ankle. Operation, cast, or early controlled mobilization. JBJS(Am). 1991;73:305–12.
4. Kaikkonen A, Kannus P, Jarvinen M. Surgery versus functional treatment in ankle ligament tears. A prospective study. Clin Orthop Relat Res. 1996;326:194–202.
5. Seah R, Mani-Babu S. Managing ankle sprains in primary care: what is best practice? A systematic review of the last 10 years of evidence. Br Med Bull. 2011;97:105–35. https://doi.org/10.1093/bmb/ldq028.
6. Doherty C, Bleakley C, Delahunt E, Holden S. Treatment and prevention of acute and recurrent ankle sprain: an overview of systematic reviews with meta-analysis. Br J Sport Med. 2017;51:113–25. https://doi.org/10.1136/bjsports-2016-096178.
7. Kerkhoffs GM, Handoll HH, de Bie R, et al (2007) Surgical versus conservative treatment for acute injuries of the lateral ligament complex of the ankle in adults. Cochrane Database Syst Rev doi: https://doi.org/10.1002/14651858.CD000380.pub2.
8. Chaudhry H, Simunovic N, Petrisor B. Cochrane in CORR ®: surgical versus conservative treatment for acute injuries of the lateral ligament complex of the ankle in adults (review). Clin Orthop Relat Res. 2015;473:17–22. https://doi.org/10.1007/s11999-014-4018-7.
9. Kerkhoffs GMMJ, Van Dijk CN. Acute lateral ankle ligament ruptures in the athlete: the role of surgery. Foot Ankle Clin. 2013;18:215–8. https://doi.org/10.1016/j.fcl.2013.02.003.
10. van Dijk CN. The athletes' ankle: lateral ligament injury. Consens. Meet. ESSKA-AFAS; 2011.
11. Kerkhoffs GM, Tol JL. A twist on the athlete's ankle twist: some ankles are more equal than others. Br J Sports Med. 2012;46:835–6. https://doi.org/10.1136/bjsports-2012-091493.
12. van Dijk CN. Diagnosis of ankle sprain: history and physical examination. In: Chan K-M, Karlsson J, edi-

tors. World Consens. Conf. Ankle Instab. Stockholm: ISAKOS–FIMS; 2005. p. 21–2.
13. van Dijk CN, Lim LS, Bossuyt PM, Marti RK. Physical examination is sufficient for the diagnosis of sprained ankles. J Bone Joint Surg Br. 1996;78:958–62.
14. Verhaven EFC, Shahabpour M, Handelberg FWJ, et al. The accuracy of three-dimensional magnetic resonance imaging in the diagnosis of ruptures of the lateral ligaments of the ankle. Am J Sports Med. 1991;19:583–7. https://doi.org/10.1177/036354659101900605.
15. Kreitner K-F, Ferber A, Grebe P, et al. Injuries of the lateral collateral ligaments of the ankle: assessment with MR imaging. Eur Radiol. 1999;9:519–24. https://doi.org/10.1007/s003300050703.
16. Gaebler C, Kukla C, Breitenseher MJ, et al. Diagnosis of lateral ankle ligament injuries. Comparison between talar tilt, MRI and operative findings in 112 athletes. Acta Orthop Scand. 1997;68:286–90. https://doi.org/10.3109/17453679708996703.
17. Gould N, Seligson D, Gassman J. Early and late repair of lateral ligament of the ankle. Foot Ankle. 1980;1:84–9. https://doi.org/10.1177/107110078000100206.
18. Aydogan U, Glisson RR, Nunley JA. Extensor retinaculum augmentation reinforces anterior talofibular ligament repair. Clin Orthop Relat Res. 2006;442:210–5.
19. Shakked RJ, Karnovsky S, Drakos MC. Operative treatment of lateral ligament instability. Curr Rev Musculoskelet Med. 2017;10:113–21. https://doi.org/10.1007/s12178-017-9391-x.
20. Giza E, Shin EC, Wong SE, et al. Arthroscopic suture anchor repair of the lateral ligament ankle complex: a cadaveric study. Am J Sports Med. 2013;41:2567–72. https://doi.org/10.1177/0363546513500639.
21. Guelfi M, Zamperetti M, Pantalone A, et al. Open and arthroscopic lateral ligament repair for treatment of chronic ankle instability: a systematic review. Foot Ankle Surg. 2016;24:11. https://doi.org/10.1016/j.fas.2016.05.315.
22. Waldrop NE, Wijdicks CA, Jansson KS, et al. Anatomic suture anchor versus the Broström technique for anterior talofibular ligament repair. Am J Sports Med. 2012;40:2590–6. https://doi.org/10.1177/0363546512458420.
23. Schuh R, Benca E, Willegger M, et al. Comparison of Broström technique, suture anchor repair, and tape augmentation for reconstruction of the anterior talofibular ligament. Knee Surg Sports Traumatol Arthrosc. 2016;24:1101–7. https://doi.org/10.1007/s00167-015-3631-7.
24. Yoo JS, Yang EA. Clinical results of an arthroscopic modified Brostrom operation with and without an internal brace. J Orthop Traumatol. 2016;17:353–60. https://doi.org/10.1007/s10195-016-0406-y.
25. Petrera M, Dwyer T, Theodoropoulos JS, Ogilvie-Harris DJ. Short- to medium-term outcomes after a modified Broström repair for lateral ankle instability with immediate postoperative weightbearing. Am J Sports Med. 2014;42:1542–8. https://doi.org/10.1177/0363546514530668.
26. Pearce CJ, Brooks JH, Kemp SPT, Calder JD. The epidemiology of foot injuries in professional rugby union players. Foot Ankle Surg. 2011;17:113–8. https://doi.org/10.1016/j.fas.2010.02.004.
27. Pearce CJ, TournéY, Zellers J, et al. Rehabilitation after anatomical ankle ligament repair or reconstruction. Knee Surg Sport Traumatol Arthrosc. 2016;24:1130–9. https://doi.org/10.1007/s00167-016-4051-z.
28. Miyamoto W, Takao M, Yamada K, Matsushita T. Accelerated versus traditional rehabilitation after anterior talofibular ligament reconstruction for chronic lateral instability of the ankle in athletes. Am J Sports Med. 2014;42:1441–7. https://doi.org/10.1177/0363546514527418.
29. Benjamin M, Toumi H, Ralphs JR, et al. Where tendons and ligaments meet bone: attachment sites ('entheses') in relation to exercise and/or mechanical load. J Anat. 2006;208:471–90.
30. Suresh S. Graded materials for resistance to contact deformation and damage. Science. 2001;292:2447–51. https://doi.org/10.1126/science.1059716.
31. Galatz LM, Sandell LJ, Rothermich SY, et al. Characteristics of the rat supraspinatus tendon during tendon-to-bone healing after acute injury. J Orthop Res. 2006;24:541–50. https://doi.org/10.1002/jor.20067.
32. Bedi A, Kovacevic D, Fox AJS, et al. Effect of early and delayed mechanical loading on tendon-to-bone healing after anterior cruciate ligament reconstruction. J Bone Joint Surg. 2010;92:2387–401. https://doi.org/10.2106/JBJS.I.01270.
33. Forestier N, Terrier R, Teasdale N. Ankle muscular proprioceptive signals' relevance for balance control on various support surfaces. Am J Phys Med Rehabil. 2015;94:20–7. https://doi.org/10.1097/PHM.0000000000000137.
34. Langer N, Hänggi J, Müller NA, et al. Effects of limb immobilization on brain plasticity. Neurology. 2012;78:182–8. https://doi.org/10.1212/WNL.0b013e31823fcd9c.
35. Fortuna M, Teixeira S, Machado S, et al. Cortical reorganization after hand immobilization: the beta qEEG spectral coherence evidences. PLoS One. 2013;8 https://doi.org/10.1371/journal.pone.0079912.
36. White WJ, McCollum GA, Calder JDF. Return to sport following acute lateral ligament repair of the ankle in professional athletes. Knee Surg Sport Traumatol Arthrosc. 2016;24:1124–9. https://doi.org/10.1007/s00167-015-3815-1.

13 Current Published Evidence to Support Open Surgical Treatment of Chronic Ankle Instability

D. Haverkamp, Chad Purcell, Kentaro Matsui, and Mark Glazebrook

13.1 Introduction

Ankle sprains are one of the most common injuries of the musculoskeletal system. They are a feature of daily practice in both emergency departments and family physician offices and account for as many as 40% of all athletic injuries [1].

Ankle sprains are often considered benign, self-limiting injuries; and fortunately, most heal without intervention. However, some sprains may progress to chronic ankle instability. And published studies suggest that this varies from 10 to 30% of patients who will require further treatment [2–4]. Most of these patients are initially treated with conservative methods including early mobilization and a rehabilitation program, which is the primary treatment for chronic instability [5]. Surgical intervention is indicated for patients who are refractory to nonoperative treatment [1, 2]. Many open surgical procedures for anatomic repair or reconstruction of ATFL and/or CFL have been described in the literature over the years, and recently newer minimally invasive and arthroscopic techniques have recently been reviewed [4, 6–8]. With over 50 possible procedures to select from, surgeons must consider the available range of procedures with their experience, and the patients' physical demands and lifestyle [9, 10].

13.2 Reconstruction Versus Repair

An important distinction in operative treatments for chronic ankle instability can be made between repair or reconstruction. Procedures within the reconstruction group can be further distinguished by the degree to which the correction is made anatomically to the original ligament insertion points. Reconstructive techniques were defined as the use of grafts as new ligaments to recreate connections between bones. Conversely, repair techniques were defined as reattachment or strengthening of torn or damaged ligaments.

D. Haverkamp (✉)
Xpert Orthopedie Amsterdam,
Amsterdam, The Netherlands
e-mail: D.Haverkamp@xpertorthopedie.nl

C. Purcell
Dalhousie University | Medicine Class of 2019,
Halifax, NS, Canada
e-mail: chad.purcell@dal.ca

K. Matsui
Department of Orthopaedic Surgery, Orthopaedic Trauma Center, Foot and Ankle Unit, Teikyo University School of Medicine, Tokyo, Japan
e-mail: kenor@nifty.com

M. Glazebrook
Dalhousie University | Medicine Class of 2019,
Halifax, NS, Canada

Reconstructive Foot & Ankle Surgery and Orthopaedic Sports Medicine, Queen Elizabeth II Health Sciences Center, Halifax, NS, Canada

H. Pereira et al. (eds.), *Lateral Ankle Instability*, https://doi.org/10.1007/978-3-662-62763-1_13

Nonanatomic reconstructive techniques have been described since the 1930s with the original Elmslie procedure. The Chrisman-Snook reconstruction is a modification of the original Elmslie procedure remains a commonly used reconstructive procedure [11, 12]. Other notable procedures that lead way to modifications over the past half-century include the Evans and Watson-Jones procedures [13]. Nonanatomic tenodeses are an effective method for treating CAI that show above 80% good-to-excellent results [6]. However, permanent impairment of subtalar motion is common. Tenodesis can be improved by increasing the anatomicity of the reconstruction; hence, anatomic reconstructions are becoming popularized, and many are described in the literature [6, 13].

The purpose of this chapter is to provide a comprehensive review of current published literature available to support the open treatment of Chronic Ankle instability. We classified open CAI surgical procedures into the following three main categories of the open surgical treatment and reviewed them based on their surgical procedure: Repair, Anatomic reconstruction, Nonanatomic reconstruction.

13.3 Definition of Evidence

We used the well-known classification of Wright et al. where published papers are first classified, according to the research method quality, into Level I to V by use of the Level of Evidence criteria [14]. All publications with an assigned level of evidence on a designated topic were combined to provide a grade of recommendation for each category of open surgical procedure using four levels (A, B, C, or I). In which A stands for Good evidence (Level I studies with consistent findings) for or against recommending intervention. Level B stands for Fair evidence (Level II or III studies with consistent findings) for or against recommending intervention. Level C stands for Conflicting or poor-quality evidence (Level IV or V studies) not allowing a recommendation for or against intervention. Level I stands for there is insufficient evidence to make a recommendation [15].

13.4 Evidence for Open Repair Techniques

Twenty-five articles were identified in which the open (anatomic) repair techniques were described [16–36]. No Level I studies were found for this topic. A total of six level II articles [16–21], including two RCTs [16, 21], one cohort study [17], and three prospective comparative studies [18–20] were identified.

The two RCTs of anatomic repair are the most important for defining the grade of recommendation since they are the highest quality papers published on this topic. These were both classified as level II evidence. Cho et al. [16] sought differences in modified Broström techniques, comparing a transosseous suture technique with a suture anchor technique. This was a small RCT, in which each group consisted of only 20 participants. This RCT was considered level II evidence because it is a small study that found improvement in Karlsson scores in both groups, but no significant differences between transosseous and suture anchor techniques.

Rosenbaum et al. [21] compared a modified Evans procedure with a periosteal flap anatomic repair in 20 patients randomly assigned to either group. All 10 patients in the Evans group, and none of the 10 patients in the periosteal flap group, reported subjectively improved ankle stability. This article was classified as level II evidence because it is a small study with just 10 participants per group.

The other studies are all level III–V including four level III retrospective cohort studies [22–24, 34], seven level IV case series [25–30, 35], and four level V articles [31–33, 36] describing a technique for CAI correction. In a retrospective comparative study, Pace et al. [34] found greater satisfaction among patients treated with conservative measures (immediate backslab. Elevation, ice, anti-inflammatories and diuretics, plaster casting followed by elastic dressing and rehabilitation therapy) than surgical repair (capsulosyndesmorrhaphy). This was the only article on anatomic repair that did not favor surgical intervention for CAI. Ten of the remaining 14 articles involved either a Brostrom-Gould or modified technique and the remaining 4 articles used a novel or unspecified technique.

13.4.1 Grade of Recommendation

The literature consistently reports good outcomes for treating CAI with anatomic repair. Our searches identified two poor-quality (level II) RCTs, among other level II studies and weaker evidence, supporting anatomic repair for CAI. Hence, the anatomic repair was given a grade B recommendation for surgical treatment of CAI.

13.5 Evidence for Open Anatomic Reconstruction Techniques

For anatomic open reconstruction, we could identify 18 studies investigating anatomic reconstruction [35, 37–54]. Among these articles, there is one level I article, three level III, ten level IV articles, and three level V articles.

The level I RCT identified is a prospective and randomized study assigning patients to static reconstruction (modified Windfeld) or dynamic reconstruction (Gianella and Huggler) [37]. Fifty-six patients (30 men and 26 women) were treated by static reconstruction (Group S), and 26 patients (16 men and 10 women) by dynamic reconstruction (Group D). At 25 month follow-up, “excellent” or “good” results were achieved in 54/56 (96.4%) static treated patients, and 16/26 (69.2%) dynamic treated patients ($p = 0.0017$, chi-square test). Among the nine athletes included, three were unable to return to sports. One woman from static treated, due to unrelated back pain and two from dynamic treated, due to giving way of the operated ankle. Overall, more complications were reported among those in static treated, compared with dynamic treated. The static reconstruction uses less of the peroneus brevis tendon, theoretically reducing the risk of sural nerve damage. The authors write in support of the static (Windfeld) reconstructive technique, stating advantages include the anatomic positioning of the malleolar in accordance with the original ligaments, hiding the tendon graft in bone, and the customizability of tendon graft positioning depending on the type of instability.

Other studies included one level III case control trial [38], two level III prospective cohorts [39, 40], nine level IV case series [35, 41–46, 48, 49], one case report [47], and two level V technique articles [52, 53].

Becker et al. [38] compared modified Evan’s (nonanatomic reconstruction) with carbon fiber anatomic reconstruction and was classified as level III evidence for both nonanatomic and anatomic reconstruction.

Three level III articles compared modified Evans (n = 30) vs. carbon fiber anatomic reconstruction (n = 23) [38], modified Broström-Evans (n = 20) vs. contralateral uninjured ankle [39], and a novel anatomic reconstruction (n = 15) vs. anatomic repair (n = 17) [40]. All three articles reported satisfactory results among treated patients and concluded in support of nonanatomic reconstruction.

Level IV–V articles include a variety of techniques, including novel reconstructions [34, 43, 50, 52, 55, 56], Weber [42], Colville [44], Evans [45], Modified Evans [46], Modified Chrisman-Snook [50], Modified Mukherjee and Gangopadhyay [49], Modified Elmslie [52], and Dockery [51]. Each of these articles support use of anatomic reconstructive techniques for treatment of CAI.

13.5.1 Grade of Recommendation

We identified strong (Level I) evidence with corroborating weaker evidence in support of anatomic reconstruction for CAI. This warrants a grade A recommendation for use of anatomic reconstructive procedures in practice.

13.6 Evidence for Open Nonanatomic Reconstruction Techniques

For the open nonanatomic reconstruction procedures we could identify 29 articles for the treatment of CAI [21, 26, 38, 50, 51, 55–81]. These include one level II, four level III, 23 level IV, and one level V studies. No level I studies were identified.

We identified one level II study using nonanatomic reconstruction as a treatment for CAI

[21]. This article is a poor-quality RCT ($n = 20$), in which individuals were randomized to a nonanatomic reconstructive procedure (modified Evan's) or fibular periosteal flap anatomical repair. All patients in the Evans group and 9/10 in the anatomical repair group subjectively reported improved ankle stability. As mentioned in the anatomic repair section, the article by Rosenbaum et al. [21] has been classified as both level II nonanatomic reconstruction and anatomic repair.

Four level III studies were found [38, 57–59]. Articles compared Evans vs. anatomic reconstruction, Evans vs. Chrisman-Snook, modified Watson-Jones vs. contralateral ankle, Chrisman-Snook vs. Watson-Jones, and all studies supported these treatments for CAI. As mentioned in the anatomic reconstruction section, one level III article [38] has been classified as both nonanatomic and anatomic reconstruction.

Our searches identified 23 articles level IV quality. Among these, there were 21 case series [56, 60–65, 67–78, 81, 82], One retrospective comparative study [66] and one case report [55].

Among the 21 case series articles, all but two were in favor of the nonanatomic reconstructive procedure used. The two articles that did not support the intervention had both studied the modified Evans procedure [63, 65]). These studies reviewed 48 and 75 cases, respectively. Only 15 of the 48 patients reported their postoperative function as excellent, where they recovered to the pre-injury level, and 10 as "good" where the ankle was not as good as the contralateral healthy ankle, but much better than before surgery [65]. Similarly, of the 75 patients treated with the modified Evan's procedure, only 82.6% reported excellent or good results [63].

The retrospective comparative study found patient satisfaction in 17/18 people with the Evans procedure and 12/13 with the Watson-Jones procedure, with no significant differences in long-term results between procedures [66]. The case report found positive results with the Chrisman-Snook procedure with no instability, tendon subluxation, or limited function [55].

We identified one level V article describing techniques of nonanatomic reconstructive procedures for CAI [79]. The authors wrote in support of a modified Francillon technique.

13.6.1 Grade of Recommendation

Treatment of CAI with nonanatomic reconstructive procedures warrants a grade B recommendation with consistent support from level II and III evidence.

13.7 Conclusion

A comprehensive review of the literature currently available for open surgical correction of chronic ankle instability has identified predominantly Level III and IV studies. Sufficient evidence was found to assign a grade A recommendation to anatomic reconstruction procedures. There was ample level II and III evidence to support a grade B recommendation for both anatomic repair and nonanatomic reconstruction procedures. It can be concluded that good quality evidence exists to support open surgical treatment of CAI and as such, it is important to conduct high-quality studies on the new minimally invasive and arthroscopic surgical techniques for CAI to assure equal efficacy and safety to open techniques summarized here.

References

1. Colville MR. Surgical treatment of the unstable ankle. J Am Acad Orthop Surg. 1998;6(6):368–77.
2. De Vries JS, Krips R, Sierevelt IN, Blankevoort L. Interventions for treating chronic ankle instability. Cochrane Database Syst Rev. 2006;4 https://doi.org/10.1002/14651858.CD004124.pub2.
3. Del Buono A, Aweid O, Coco M, Maffulli N. Ankle instability: what do we know and what is the future? Fuss und Sprunggelenk. 2013;11(1):3–8.
4. Guillo S, Bauer T, Lee JW, Takao M, Kong SW, Stone JW, et al. Consensus in chronic ankle instability: aetiology, assessment, surgical indications and place for arthroscopy. Orthop Traumatol Surg Res. 2013;99(8 Suppl):S411–9.
5. Karlsson J, Faxen E, Eriksson BI. Ankle joint ligament injuries: prevention, evaluation and treatment. Crit Rev Phys Rehabil Med. 1996;8(3):183–200.

6. Matsui K, Burgesson B, Takao M, Stone J, Guillo S, Glazebrook M, et al. Minimally invasive surgical treatment for chronic ankle instability: a systematic review. Knee Surg Sports Traumatol Arthrosc. 2016;24:1040–8.
7. Dierckman BD, Ferkel RD. Anatomic reconstruction with a semitendinosus allograft for chronic lateral ankle instability. Am J Sports Med. 2015;43(8):1941–50.
8. Takao M, Miyamoto W, Matsui K, Sasahara J, Matsushita T. Functional treatment after surgical repair for acute lateral ligament disruption of the ankle in athletes. Am J Sports Med. 2012;40(2):447–51.
9. Karlsson J, Lansinger O. Lateral instability of the ankle joint. Clin Orthop. 1992;276:253–61.
10. Espinosa N, Smerek J, Kadakia AR, Myerson MS. Operative management of ankle instability: reconstruction with open and percutaneous methods. Foot Ankle Clin. 2006;11(3):547–65.
11. Elmslie RC. Recurrent subluxation of the ankle-joint. Ann Surg. 1934;100(2):364–7.
12. Snook GA, Chrisman OD, Wilson TC. Long-term results of the Chrisman-Snook operation for reconstruction of the lateral ligaments of the ankle. J Bone Joint Surg Am. 1985;67(1):1–7.
13. Chan KW, Ding BC, Mroczek KJ. Acute and chronic lateral ankle instability in the athlete. Bull NYU Hosp Jt Dis. 2011;69(1):17–26.
14. Wright JG, Swiontkowski MF, Heckman JD. Introducing levels of evidence to the journal. J Bone Joint Surg Am. 2003;85-A(1):1–3.
15. Wright JG, Einhorn TA, Heckman JD. Grades of recommendation. J Bone Joint Surg Am. 2005;87(9):1909–10.
16. Cho B, Kim Y, Kim D, Choi E, Shon H, Park K. Comparison between suture anchor and transosseous suture for the modified-Brostrom procedure. Foot Ankle Int. 2012;33(6):462–8.
17. Hu CY, Lee KB, Song EK, Kim MS, Park KS. Comparison of bone tunnel and suture anchor techniques in the modified Brostrom procedure for chronic lateral ankle instability. Am J Sports Med. 2013;41(8):1877–84.
18. Cho B, Kim Y, Park K, Park J, Kim D. A prospective outcome and cost-effectiveness comparison between two ligament reattachment techniques using suture anchors for chronic ankle instability. Foot Ankle Int. 2015;36(2):172–9.
19. Halasi T, Kynsburg Ã, Tallay A, Berkes I. Changes in joint position sense after surgically treated chronic lateral ankle instability. Br J Sports Med. 2005;39(11):818–24.
20. Lofvenberg R, Karrholm J, Ahlgren O. Ligament reconstruction for ankle instability: A 5-year prospective RSA follow-up of 30 cases. Acta Orthop Scand. 1994;65(4):401–7.
21. Rosenbaum D, Engelhardt M, Becker HP, Claes L, Gerngross H. Clinical and functional outcome after anatomic and nonanatomic ankle ligament reconstruction: evans tenodesis versus periosteal flap. Foot Ankle Int. 1999;20(10):636–9.
22. Fujimaki Y, Miyawaki M, Thorhauer E, Prisk V, Tashman S. In vivo kinematics of the ankle during gait following reconstruction for chronic ankle instability. Arthroscopy. 2013;29(10):e65–6.
23. Xu H, Choi M, Kim M, Park K, Lee K. Gender differences in outcome after modified Brostrom procedure for chronic lateral ankle instability. Foot Ankle Int. 2016;37(1):64–9.
24. White WJ, McCollum GA, Calder JD. Return to sport following acute lateral ligament repair of the ankle in professional athletes. Knee Surg Sports Traumatol Arthrosc. 2016;24(4):1124–9.
25. Cannon LB, Hackney RG. Anterior tibiotalar impingement associated with chronic ankle instability. J Foot Ankle Surg. 2000;39(6):383–6.
26. Cho B, Kim Y, Shon H, Park K, Cha J, Ha Y. A ligament reattachment technique for high-demand athletes with chronic ankle instability. J Foot Ankle Surg. 2015;54(1):7–12.
27. Conlin FD, Johnson PG, Sinning JE Jr. The etiology and repair of rotary ankle instability. Foot Ankle. 1989;10(3):152–5.
28. Curry EE. Brostrom-Gould lateral ankle ligament reconstruction with suture bridge modification. Tech Foot Ankle Surg. 2011;10(3):105–10.
29. Liu SH, Jacobson KE. A new operation for chronic lateral ankle instability. J Bone Joint Surg Ser B. 1995;77(1):55–9.
30. TrÄ T, Handl M, Havlas V. The anterior talofibular ligament reconstruction in surgical treatment of chronic lateral ankle instability. Int Orthop. 2010;34(7):991–6.
31. Bynum JA, Crates JM, Aziz-Jacobo J, Barber FA. Modified Brostrom technique using knotless suture anchors. Tech Foot Ankle Surg. 2010;9(1):29–31.
32. DaSilva MF, Fadale PD, Hulstyn MJ. Repair of the lateral ankle ligaments using the Mitek suture anchor system. J Orthop Tech. 1995;3(1):41–4.
33. Groth AT, Guyton GP, Schon LC. Lateral ankle ligament injuries in athletes: diagnosis and treatment. Oper Tech Sports Med. 2010;18(1):18–26.
34. Pace N, Iacono EL, Chiusaroli M, Serafini P, Basconi G, Zanoli S. A comparison between conservative treatment and operative treatment (capsulosyndesmorrhaphy) in severe acute capsuloligamentous lateral lesions of the ankle joint. Ital J Orthop Traumatol. 1990;16(1):19–24.
35. Alrashidi Y, Stelzenbach C, Herrera-Perez M, Wiewiorski M, Valderrabano V. Chronic rotational ankle instability—a case series study. Sports Orthop Traumatol. 2015;31(3):200–5.
36. Trc T, Handl M, Havlas V. The anterior talo-fibular ligament reconstruction in surgical treatment of chronic lateral ankle instability. Int Orthop. 2010;34(7):991–6.
37. Larsen E. Static or dynamic repair of chronic lateral ankle instability. A prospective randomized study. Clin Orthop. 1990;257:184–92.

38. Becker HP, Rosenbaum D, Zeithammel G, Gnann R, Bauer G, Gerngross H, et al. Tenodesis versus carbon fiber repair of ankle ligaments: A clinical comparison. Clin Orthop. 1996;325:194–202.
39. Girard P, Anderson RB, Davis WH, Isear JA Jr, Kiebzak GM. Clinical evaluation of the modified Brostrom-Evans procedure to restore ankle stability. Foot Ankle Int. 1999;20(4):246–52.
40. Jarvela T, Weitz H, Jarvela K, Alavaikko A. A novel reconstruction technique for chronic lateral ankle instability: comparison to primary repair. Int Orthop. 2002;26(5):314–7.
41. Jung HG, Shin MH, Park JT, Eom JS, Lee DO, Lee SH. Anatomical reconstruction of lateral ankle ligaments using free tendon allografts and biotenodesis screws. Foot Ankle Int. 2015;36(9):1064–71.
42. De Vries JS, Struijs PAA, Raaymakers ELFB, Marti RK. Long-term results of the weber operation for chronic ankle instability: 37 patients followed for 20-30 years. Acta Orthop. 2005;76(6):891–8.
43. Et-Titi A, Ismaiel A. A new method of lateral ankle joint reconstruction for chronic instabillity: preliminary report. Foot. 1995;5(1):24–6.
44. Keklikai K, Åžahin O, Yildirim C, Solakoglu C, Kiral A, Pehlivan O, et al. Treatment of chronic lateral instability of the ankle with the Colville technique: a prospective analysis with minimum five years of follow-up. Eklem Hastaliklari ve Cerrahisi. 2012;23(1):35–9.
45. Kristiansen B. Surgical treatment of ankle instability in athletes. Br J Sports Med. 1982;16(1):40–5.
46. Levy M. Newly modified Evans operation enables immediate mobilization. Reinforcement band stabilizes ankle, no cast is used. Orthop Rev. 1986;15(9):600–4.
47. Leyshon RL. Chronic lateral ligament instability of the ankle—bilateral repair using flexible carbon fibre in an international sportsman. Br J Sports Med. 1982;16(3):172–3.
48. Morelli F, Guidi M, Ferretti A. Anatomical tenodesis for the treatment of chronic lateral ankle instability: a new surgical technique. J Orthop Traumatol. 2013;14(1):S31.
49. Westlin NE, Vogler HW, Albertsson MP, Arvidsson T, Montgomery F. Treatment of lateral ankle instability with transfer of the extensor digitorum brevis muscle. J Foot Ankle Surg. 2003;42(4):183–92.
50. Dockery GL, Gusman DN, Vickers MB. An autogenous free graft technique for lateral ankle stabilization. J Foot Surg. 1989;28(4):319–24.
51. Evans RD, Feller SR, Heath NS. Review of the Dockery procedure for lateral ankle instability. A seven-year retrospective analysis. J Am Podiatr Med Assoc. 1998;88(6):279–84.
52. Coughlin MJ, RCJ S. Technique tip: lateral ankle reconstruction. Foot Ankle Int. 2001;22(3):256–8.
53. Jeys LM, Harris NJ. Ankle stabilization with hamstring autograft: a new technique using interference screws. Foot Ankle Int. 2003;24(9):677–9.
54. Karlsson J, Bergsten T, Peterson L, Lansinger O. Anatomic reconstruction of the lateral ligaments of the ankle joint—a new procedure. Acta Orthop Scand. 1987;58(3):318.
55. Sobel M, Warren RF, Brourman S. Lateral ankle instability associated with dislocation of the peroneal tendons treated by the Chrisman-Snook procedure: a case report and literature review. Am J Sports Med. 1990;18(5):539–43.
56. Van Rappard JHA, Reinders JFM, Mahabier C, Munting JDK. Operative treatment of persistent lateral instability of the ankle—is it worse to sprain the ankle than to break it? Neth J Surg. 1987;39(2):65–7.
57. Bernhard JA, Burckhardt A. Long-term results after surgical treatment of chronic lateral instability of the ankle joint (comparison of Watson-Jones and Chrisman-Snook (modified) techniques). Swiss Surg. 1996;2(6):274–9.
58. Morelli F, Perugia D, VadalÃ A, Serlorenzi P, Ferretti A. Modified Watson-Jones technique for chronic lateral ankle instability in athletes: clinical and radiological mid- to long-term follow-up. Foot Ankle Surg. 2011;17(4):247–51.
59. Thermann H, Zwipp H, Tscherne H. Treatment algorithm of chronic ankle and subtalar instability. Foot Ankle Int. 1997;18(3):163–9.
60. Andersen E, Hvass I. Treatment of lateral instability of the ankle. A new modification of the Evans repair. Arch Orthop Trauma Surg. 1986;106(1):15–7.
61. Ateşalp S, Demiralp B, Ozkal UB, Uğurlu M, Bozkurt M, Başbozkurt M. Modified evans technique improves plantar pressure distribution in lateral ankle instability. Eklem Hastaliklari ve Cerrahisi. 2009;20(1):41–6.
62. Barbari SG, Brevig K, Egge T. Reconstruction of the lateral ligamentous structures of the ankle with a modified Watson-Jones procedure. Foot Ankle. 1987;7(6):362–8.
63. Becker HP, Zeithammel G, Danz B, Rosenbaum D, Gerngross H. Clinical and radiological results 5 years after modified Evans repair for chronic lateral instability of the ankle. Unfallchirurg. 1995;98(6):333–7.
64. Canadell JM, Valenti JR, Martinez A. Chronic lateral instability of the ankle. Arch Orthop Trauma Surg. 1982;99(3):189–93.
65. Kaikkonen A, Lehtonen H, Kannus P, Järvinen M. Long-term functional outcome after surgery of chronic ankle instability. A 5-year follow-up study of the modified Evans procedure. Scand J Med Sci Sports. 1999;9(4):239–44.
66. Kitaoka HB, Lee MD, Morrey BF, Cass JR. Acute repair and delayed reconstruction for lateral ankle instability: twenty-year follow-up study. J Orthop Trauma. 1997;11(7):530–5.
67. Langstaff RJ, Handley CH. Functional ankle instability in members of the armed forces, the results of the extensor digitorum brevis transfer operation. Injury. 1991;22(2):105–7.
68. Orava S, Jaroma H, Weitz H. Radiographic instability of the ankle joint after Evans' repair. Acta Orthop Scand. 1983;54(5):734–8.

69. Pieron AP. Lateral ankle instability correction by translocation of the intact peroneus brevis tendon: a prospective study of 45 cases. J South Orthop Assoc. 1998;7(3):187–91.
70. Pieron AP. Dynamic peroneus tendon transfer for repair of the unstable ankle. Can J Surg. 1982;25(6):672–5.
71. Reinherz RP, Sharon SM, Knudsen HA. Surgical repair of lateral ankle instability by modification of traditional approaches. J Foot Surg. 1978;17(1):12–5.
72. Sammarco GJ, DiRaimondo CV. Surgical treatment of lateral ankle instability syndrome. Am J Sports Med. 1988;16(5):501–11.
73. Shibuya N, Bazán DI, Evans AM, Agarwal MR, Jupiter DC. Efficacy and safety of split peroneal tendon lateral ankle stabilization. J Foot Ankle Surg. 2015;55:812–6.
74. Sugimoto K, Takakura Y, Akiyama K, Kamei S, Kitada C, Kumai T. Long-term results of Watson-Jones tenodesis of the ankle: clinical and radiographic findings after ten to eighteen years of follow-up. J Bone Joint Surg Ser A. 1998;80(11):1587–96.
75. Usami N, Inokuchi S, Hiraishi E, Miyanaga M, Waseda A. Clinical application of artificial ligament for ankle instability—long-term follow-up. J Long Term Eff Med. 2000;10(4):239–50.
76. Zenni EJ, Grefer M, Krieg JK. Lateral ligamentous instability of the ankle: a method of surgical reconstruction by a modified Watson Jones technique. Am J Sports Med. 1977;5(2):78–83.
77. Benard MA, Morgan J, Dikes N, Hambrecht S, Meis CM, Smith S. The use of tensor fascia lata allograft material in the foot and ankle. Lower Extremity. 1995;2(4):237–42.
78. Hsu AR, Ardoin GT, Davis WH, Anderson RB. Intermediate and long-term outcomes of the modified Brostrom-Evans procedure for lateral ankle ligament reconstruction. Foot Ankle Spec. 2016;9(2):131–9.
79. Pace N, Giacchetta AM. External ligamentoplastic of the ankle joint. Personal technique. Chirurgia del Piede. 1987;11(5):299–302.
80. Sobel M, Geppert MJ. Technique tips: repair of concomitant lateral ankle ligament instability and peroneus brevis splits through a posteriorly modified Brostrom Gould. Foot Ankle. 1992;13(4):224–5.
81. Ahlgren O, Larsson S. Reconstruction for lateral ligament injuries of the ankle. J Bone Joint Surg Ser B. 1989;71(2):300–3.
82. Cheng YM, Chang JK, Wang IM, Lin SY. Surgical reconstruction for chronic lateral instability of the ankle. Kao Hsiung I Hsueh Ko Hsueh Tsa Chih. 1994;10(3):138–44.

14 Anatomic Open Repair Procedures: Description of the Broström-Gould Technique

Michael Grant, Lyndon Mason, Hélder Pereira, Jorge Acevedo, and Andy Molloy

Surgical management of lateral ankle instability can be divided into anatomical or nonanatomical reconstructions, with most surgeons preferring anatomical reconstruction when possible [1]. Nonanatomical techniques were first described in 1932 based upon existing work in paralytic club-foot from 1913 by Gallie [2]. Gallie described a nonanatomic peroneus longus and brevis transfer to correct a chronic equinovarus deformity in a child [2]. Multiple described techniques of non-anatomical tendon-sacrificing procedures have followed, including the Watson-Jones [3], Evans [4] and Chrisman-Snook procedures [5]. These techniques involve sacrificing the peroneus brevis tendon to reconstruct the lateral ankle ligament complex, and long-term outcomes were unfavourable, with reports of pain, recurrent instability, stiffness or subtalar arthritis [2]. Likewise, multiple techniques of anatomical repair or reconstruction of the lateral ligament complex for ankle instability have been described. Anatomical open repair procedures can be divided into Isolated anatomic ligament repair or reinforced ligament repair [6] (Fig. 14.1).

M. Grant
Tr&Orth (Eng) Speciality Trainee Year 7, Health Education North West (Mersey), Liverpool, UK
e-mail: michaelgrant@doctors.org.uk

L. Mason
Trauma and Orthopaedic, Liverpool University Hospitals NHS Foundation Trust, Liverpool, UK

School of Medicine, University of Liverpool, Liverpool, UK

H. Pereira
Knee and Ankle Orthopaedic Department, Centro Hospitalar Póvoa de Varzim, Vila do Conde, Portugal

Ripoll y De Prado Sports Clinic: FIFA Medical Centre of Excellence, Murcia-Madrid, Spain

ICVS/3B's—PT Government Associate Laboratory, University of Minho, Braga/Guimarães, Portugal

J. Acevedo
Department of Orthopedics, Southeast Orthopedic Specialists, Jacksonville, FL, USA

A. Molloy (✉)
Liverpool University Hospital Foundation Trust, Spire Liverpool Hospital, University of Liverpool, Liverpool, UK

14.1 Isolated Anatomic Ligament Repair

First described by Lennart Broström in 1966 [7], this consists of re-tensioning the damaged lateral ligament and joint capsule complex, aiming to restore original anatomy where possible. Broström described a method of repair whereby the lateral ankle ligaments that had been stretched were tightened, without the use of 'weaving' procedures or supplemental tissues [8]. The technique describes how the shortened anterior talofibular ligament (ATFL) and calcaneofibular ligament (CFL) were re-fashioned to their origi-

H. Pereira et al. (eds.), *Lateral Ankle Instability*, https://doi.org/10.1007/978-3-662-62763-1_14

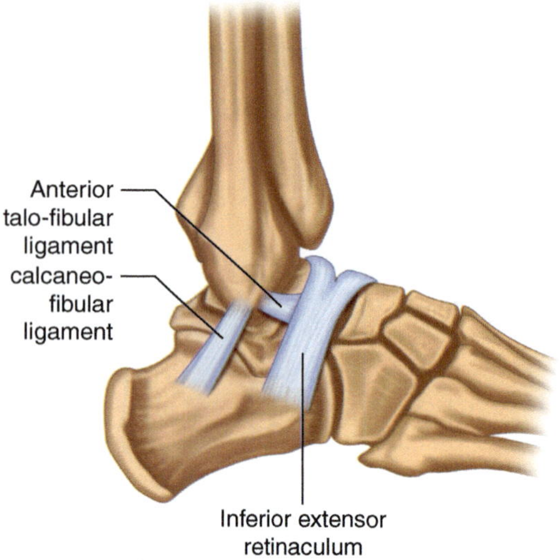

Fig. 14.1 Diagram illustrating the normal anatomy of the lateral ligamentous structures of the ankle (*ATFL* Anterior talofibular ligament, *CFL* Calcaneofibular ligament)

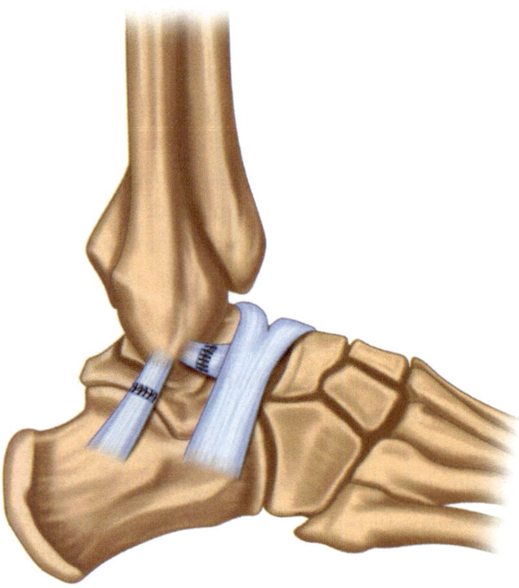

Fig. 14.2 Broström anatomical repair of the ATFL and CFL ligaments

nal lengths and sutured back to their original anatomical location thus preserving the peroneal tendons [7] (Fig. 14.2).

Broström described using this method on 60 cases of chronic ankle instability with a mean follow-up of 2.9 years. All patients returned a written questionnaire and 56 of the 60 patients underwent a physical examination; 43 out of the 60 patients were said to have complete resolution of symptoms, and only 1 patient reported no improvement. Other series of patients undergoing a Broström repair for ankle instability have also reported good outcomes, including Javors and Violet [9] who reported on a series of 15 patients who had undergone Broström repair for chronic lateral ligament instability. Out of their 15 cases, 13 were said to have achieved good or excellent results, with improvement of stability as their primary aim. Bell and colleagues [10] reported on 31 patients (32 ankles) that had undergone the original Broström procedure for ankle instability between 1975 and 1979 at their institution. Their follow-up was 26 years and the outcome measures used were questionnaires based on functional outcome [11] and a functional scale [12]. Twenty two of the thirty one original patients were included in the results, with 91% describing their ankle function as good or excellent. Though this indicates long-term results of the Broström procedure are good, limitations of this work include no radiographic or clinical follow-up, and 9 out of 31 patients were either excluded or lost to follow-up.

Fact Box 1

- Lennart Broström was the first to publish on operative treatment of ankle instability in 1966.
- His technique was advocated for both acute ruptures and chronic instability.
- He advocated a direct anatomical repair of the ATFL and also advocated repair of the CFL if indicated.
- Outcomes from this procedure are largely reported as good in the literature, though multiple modifications have since been described.

Maffuli and colleagues [13] reported on their outcomes using the anatomic Broström technique without using bone-anchors or transosseous sutures. Their post-operative protocol included a lightweight cast in neutral, weight-bearing as tolerated for the first 2 weeks, with progressive weight-bearing from 2 weeks onwards. At 4 weeks the cast was removed and physiotherapy and proprioceptive training was commenced, high-level sports were only reintroduced at 6 months. Their outcome measures included the AOFAS score, the Kaikkonen score, clinical assessment and weight-bearing radiographs. The AOFAS and Kaikkonen scores improved significantly from 51 to 90 and 45 to 90, respectively.

Karlsson and colleagues [14] described a modification of the Broström technique, a further example of an isolated anatomic ligament repair, as they found, contrary to Broström, that the ligaments were often elongated and unable to simply be sutured back in place without compromising stability. Their technique, described in 60 patients with chronic lateral ankle instability, consists of an incision posterior to the lateral malleolus, opening the peroneus tendon sheath and identifying the ATFL and CFL. The ligaments and joint capsule are then divided 1–2 mm from the anterior-inferior border of the fibula. A small bone block is taken from the anterior-inferior border of the fibula measuring 4x4mm. Five to six drill-holes are made in the fibula with a 2.0 mm drill bit, and the ligaments are tightened using mattress sutures with the foot pronated and dorsiflexed, and then a duplication procedure is performed with the periosteal flap and proximal end of the ligaments. Their post-operative regime included immobilisation in a short-walking cast for 6 weeks, followed by a 6–12-week training programme of peroneal strengthening and coordination exercises. Return to sport was once the ankle was felt to be functionally stable. Their reported results were based on return to activity, episodes of instability and pain. Eighty-eight percent of their cohort had good or excellent outcomes, with a poor result in four patients (7%).

In 1980, Duqeunnoy had described his version of isolated anatomic ligament repair, using transosseous tensioning of the ATFL and anterior capsule, reporting on 22 patients who had the procedure. Eighteen patients were followed up and 15 of those had a good result, with 1 having a poor result [15].

A further description of isolated anatomic ligament repair was presented in 1989 [16]. Ahlgren described a subperiosteal release at the tip of the lateral malleolus, creating a flap containing the ATFL and CFL and inferior retinaculum, and reattaching the flap to the fibula more proximally using transosseous sutures. This was performed on 82 ankles, with a mean follow-up of 24 months, and 95% had a good or excellent result, with only 1 episode of recurrence of instability following a further injury to the ankle [16].

14.2 Reinforced Anatomic Ligament Repair

Reinforcement of the anatomic ligament repair described by Broström was first recommended by Gould and colleagues in 1980 using the extensor retinaculum [17]. Gould and colleagues described a modification of the Broström technique by incorporating the nearby lateral talocalcaneal ligament and inferior extensor retinaculum into the repair. In their series of 50 athletes, all patients were said to have returned to the sports of their choice with no restriction in activity [17]. There are reports of improved biomechanical strength using the Broström-Gould technique of up to 60% [18]. Behrens and colleagues [19] reported on a cadaveric study assessing the biomechanical strength of the Broström and the Broström-Gould repairs and found they both had a significant improvement in stability, but there was no significant difference between the two techniques. However, given this was a cadaveric study on 10 specimens, these results may not correlate with clinical outcomes in athletes who have undergone the procedures. Hamilton [8] described using the Broström-Gould technique to treat 20 high-level professional ballet dancers who were all said to have excellent results and returned to their career. In his article, he describes a curvilinear incision along the anterior border of the distal fibula, stopping at the peroneal tendons, taking care not to encounter the sural nerve, though ligating the short saphenous vein as it

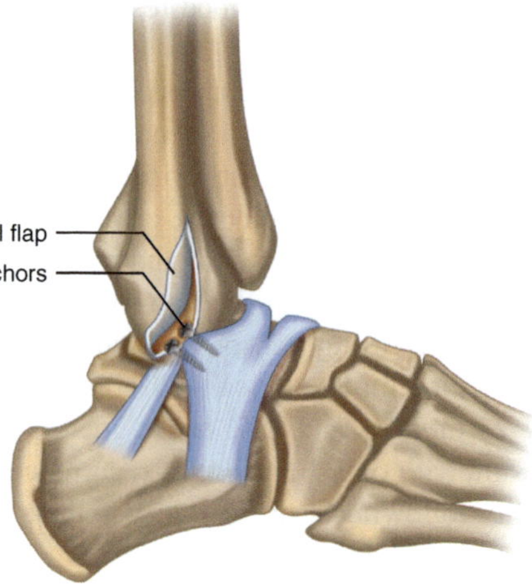

Fig. 14.3 Goulds modification of the Broström anatomical repair, with anatomical repair of the ATFL and CFL ligaments, supported by the inferior extensor retinaculum

often crosses the distal fibula at this level. The dissection continues down to the joint capsule along the anterior border of the fibula, here the lateral portion of the extensor retinaculum is identified and dissected off the capsule. This allows the extensor retinaculum to be mobilised and pulled over the repair. The joint capsule is then divided along the anterior border of the fibula, leaving a small 2–3 mm cuff, the ATFL lies within the capsule and can be identified as a thickening of the capsule. The CFL lies deep to the peroneal tendons, running obliquely and inferiorly to the calcaneum. It is often stretched or attenuated or can be found avulsed from the calcaneal origin. The ligaments are then shortened and repaired, with the ankle in neutral dorsiflexion and slight eversion, the stumps of the ligaments are pulled up, and any excess length is resected. The ligaments should then be sutured back into their anatomical locations using non-absorbable sutures, using end-to-end repair or into drill-holes. The lateral extensor retinaculum is then pulled over the repair and sutured to the tip of the fibula, this is said to reinforce the repair. The postsurgical care described by Hamilton et al. [8] included a short-leg walking cast for 3–4 weeks, which was then replaced with an air splint and commencement of range of motion and isometric peroneal exercises. A return to sport and unrestricted activities were allowed between 10 and 20 weeks postoperatively providing that full peroneal strength was present (Fig. 14.3).

In 1996, Keller and colleagues [20] described their outcomes using the Broström-Gould procedure. They discuss the variety of anchoring options that were available for reattaching the CFL, using drill-holes and various suture materials. Post-operatively their patients were immobilised non-weight-bearing for 4 weeks, followed by partial-to-full weight-bearing for the next 2 weeks. Physiotherapy was then instigated, and 'guarded' activity continued for 10–12 weeks after full weight-bearing status. Forty-four patients were included, and 39 patients were reported on, with a mean follow-up of 2.6 years. They achieved 97.5% good-to-excellent outcomes, with only 1 patient having a poor outcome.

Fact Box 2

- Nathaniel Gould was an American Orthopaedic surgeon whose modification of the Broström repair in 1980 became one of the most popularly used techniques in lateral ankle instability.
- His modification incorporates the inferior extensor retinaculum and lateral talocalcaneal ligament into the repair for added stability.
- The literature reports favourably on this repair and suggests the majority of Athletes will return to their pre-injury level of competition.
- A systematic review of 11 articles with 669 patients who underwent a Brostrom-Gould repair found the revision surgery rate to be just 1.2%.

Karlsson who had previously described a slight modification to the Broström technique compared his and Gould's modification in the form of a randomised trial [21]. Thirty patients were randomised to the Karlsson modification (Group 1) and 30 patients to the Gould modification (Group 2). Outcome measures included functional outcomes and stress radiographs, with a minimum follow-up of 2 years. Results were comparable in both groups, with satisfactory outcomes in 90% (Group 1) and 83% (Group 2). Despite good reported outcomes in both groups, there are limitations to the study, namely author bias.

Further developments to open, anatomical repair of the lateral ankle ligaments were made in the 1990s, with the development of suture anchors. Messer and colleagues [22] published their outcomes of using the modified Broström procedure utilising suture anchors. Their surgical technique comprised of the same approach as the Broström-Gould procedure, though after division of the capsule and ligaments, a subperiosteal sleeve was elevated off the distal aspect of the fibula. This is then prepared by removing further soft tissue and creating a trough with a rasp and small curette, effectively creating a 'bed' for the anchors. Suture anchors are then inserted into the normal anatomic origins of the ATFL anteriorly and the CFL posterolaterally. Tension is applied to the previously tagged ligaments with the ankle in neutral dorsiflexion and slight eversion, and the sutures are passed into the ATFL and CFL. The ligaments and capsule were then secured to the distal fibula, the periosteal sleeve sutured over the newly anchored ATFL and CFL, and as per the Gould modification, the inferior extensor retinaculum was mobilised and sutured into the lateral ankle joint capsule and periosteum of the lateral malleolus. The number of cases in this series was 24, though 22 returned the questionnaire after a mean follow-up of 34.5 months. Out of the 22 patients who returned the questionnaire, none had a poor result, with 20 having a good or excellent result.

14.3 Modern Adaptations

A further modification to the Broström procedure was proposed by Angirasa and Barrett [23] where they describe placing suture anchors into the lateral shoulder of the anterior talus, as opposed to the anatomical location of the ATFL and CFL into the distal fibula. They describe good results in 32 patients who underwent this procedure, though there is no description of outcome measures other than a negative anterior-drawer test in all patients post-operatively.

Li and colleagues [24] added an extra suture anchor to their modification of the Broström repair, using three suture anchors. Their technique follows the Broström-Gould procedure and uses suture anchors at the anatomical footprint of the ATFL and CFL, and a further suture anchor is then inserted 1 cm above the ATFL insertion. The remnants of the ATFL, CFL and a capsular-periosteal flap are then tied down to the three suture anchors with the foot in neutral dorsiflexion and slight eversion. As per Gould's modification, the extensor retinaculum that was previously mobilised is then used to reinforce the repair as it is repaired to the periosteum of the distal fibula. The post-operative protocol placed patients in a posterior and sugar-tong splint in neutral and slight eversion, and kept non-weight-bearing for the first 2 weeks, a short-leg walking cast was then applied and protected weight-bearing commenced for the next 2 weeks. At weeks 4–6, an ankle support orthosis (ASO) replaced the short cast and active-assisted range of motion exercises used. Proprioception and strength training was implemented at 6–8 weeks, and plyometric training at 8–12 weeks. Full return to sport was after 16 weeks. All the 62 patients included in their study were reported to be high-level athletes, and outcome measures included the Tegner score [25] and the Karlsson score [26]. Ten of the original sixty-two patients were lost to follow-up, and of the remaining, 94% returned to their pre-injury Tegner score at 2 years, with no unacceptable ratings in the Karlsson scores. At 2 years, 94% of patients had an equal range of motion compared to their uninjured side. Complications described included three re-ruptures following an acute injury more than a year following their original procedure.

In 2014, Molloy and colleagues [1] described a new modification of the Broström-Gould procedure. Sixteen patients were included, and outcomes included AOFAS hindfoot scoring system, along with clinical assessment and assessment of physical and sporting ability, with a mean follow-up of 25 months. An ankle arthroscopy was performed, followed by the new modification of the Broström repair using 2.9 mm suture anchors and triple breasting of the ATFL and CFL complex. Following the dissection of the subcutaneous tissues off the lateral ligament complex, a U-shaped subfibular incision is made from the anterior border of the fibula stopping short of the peroneal tendons, approximately 1 cm from the edge of the fibula border. If the CFL remnant is not visible, the dissection is continued posteriorly beneath the peroneal tendons. A subperiosteal sleeve is then elevated 2 cm off the fibula and retracted as rongeurs are used to remove the cortex from the lateral distal fibula. The suture anchors are then placed at the anatomical origin of the ATFL and CFL. All four suture strands are then passed through the distal flap which includes the lateral ligament complex and lateral joint capsule, approximately 1 cm from its edge. The foot is held in dorsiflexion and eversion for the remainder of the operation, and knots are tied sequentially from anterior to posterior, shortening the lateral ligament complex and attaching the flap to bone at the anatomical origin of the ATFL and CFL. Each strand of suture anchor is then passed through the base of the periosteal flap on the fibula, tied and then cut. It is this step that is the variation on the modified Broström-Gould procedure, and Molloy explains that this step provides a more robust anatomical repair, though the main desired effect is the prevention of tearing of the subperiosteal flap as it is drawn down during the final step of imbrication. Final imbrication is performed with horizontal mattress sutures from the distal edge of the fibula subperiosteal flap to 1 cm distal to the row of sutures from the prior placed suture anchors. Post-operative protocol includes non-weight-bearing for 2 weeks in a temporary cast, followed by 2 weeks in a weight-bearing neutral cast, and physiotherapy was commenced 4 weeks post-operatively, weight-bearing as tolerated in an unlocked range of motion walker boot. From 6 weeks post-operatively, patients were weaned out of their ROM walker boot under the supervision of the physiotherapists. From the 16 patients included in the follow-up, the mean AOFAS score improved from 53 (19–70) pre-operatively to 89 (76–100) at final follow-up. All ankles felt clinically stable with negative anterior-drawer tests and half the patients returned to pre-injury sporting level, with 8 patients reporting some reduction in the level of activity (Figs. 14.4, 14.5, 14.6, 14.7).

Recent developments have led some surgeons to augment their repair with an internal brace (IB), which acts as a secondary stabiliser to reinforce the repaired ligament, which may reduce the return to sports and reduce the recurrence of instability symptoms [27]. Schuh and colleagues in 2016 performed biomechanical cadaveric studies comparing the Broström technique with suture anchor repair and IB augmentation, demonstrating improved stability of the repair using the IB [28], but as previously this does not necessarily correlate clinically as no healing has occurred. Yoo and Yang in 2016 have compared modified arthroscopic Broström repair with augmentation using an IB, in 85 patients, 22 in the IB group with a mean follow-up of 7.4 months. In their cohort, they found no difference in AOFAS scores at final follow-up, though there were significant differences in favour of the IB group at 6 and 12 weeks post-operatively. Interestingly, there was a significant improvement in the incidence of return to sport at 12 weeks, indicating that the IB augmentation may be favourable in achieving a quicker return to sport in athletes [29].

14.4 Evidence for the Techniques

Mabit and colleagues [30] performed a systematic review and summarised the evidence. Simple anatomical ligament repair (Broström and Duquennoy techniques) documented good or excellent results between 81–96% of cases. The evidence for the anatomic repair with reinforcement (Broström-Gould technique) revealed results of 82–85% good or very good. Krips and colleagues [31] compared the outcomes of 41 athletes undergoing anatomic repair using the Broström technique, and 36 patients undergoing a nonanatomical reconstruction (Evans or

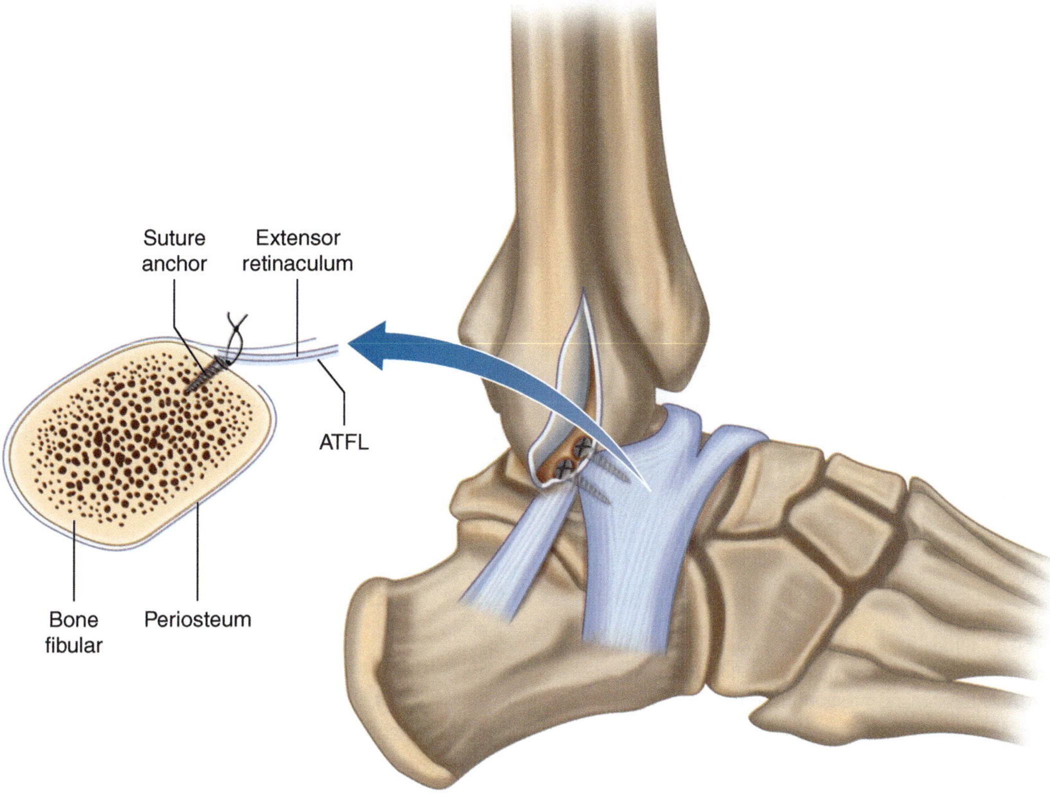

Fig. 14.4 Molloy modification of the Broström-Gould anatomical repair, raising of a periosteal flap from the anterior aspect of the fibular, allowing insertion of suture anchors into the ATFL and CFL fibular origin. The ATFL and CFL are shortened and sutured to the bone from these anchors, strengthened by the inferior extensor retinaculum and the periosteal sleeve

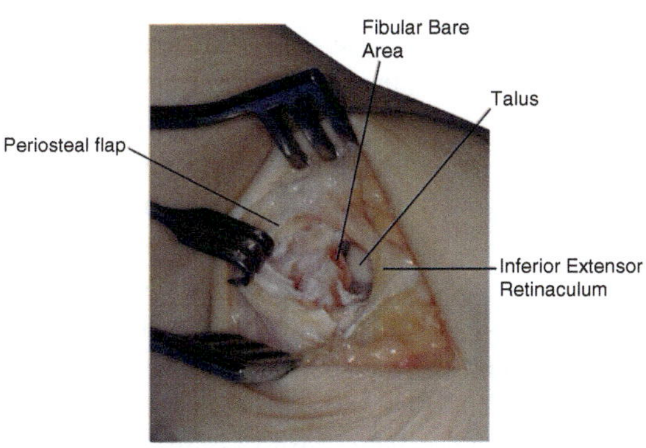

Fig. 14.5 Clinical photograph showing the elevation of the periosteal sheath and denuded fibular bare area

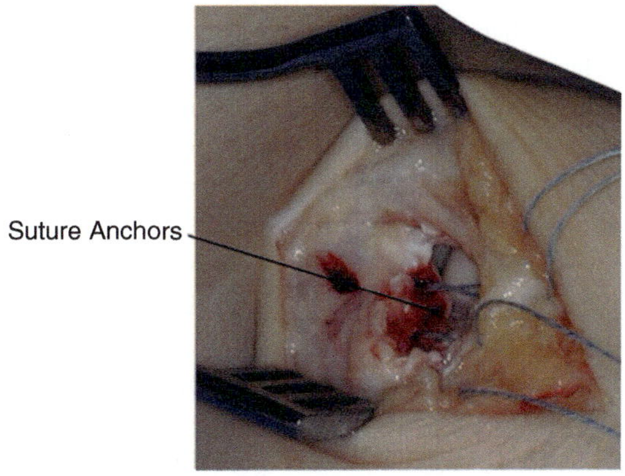

Fig. 14.6 Clinical photograph illustrating the anchor insertions and passing of the suture material through ATFL, CFL and inferior extensor retinaculum

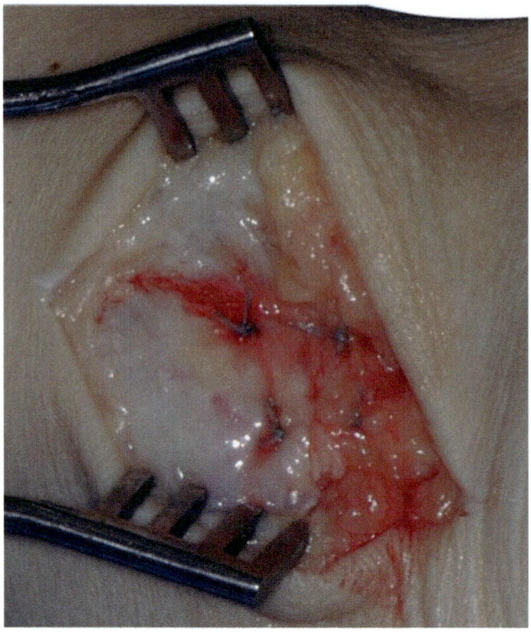

Fig. 14.7 Clinical photograph showing completion of the repair by suturing the periosteal flap over the ATFL/CFL/Inferior extensor retinaculum repair

Watson-Jones). They found that the athletes who had the nonanatomical reconstruction were more limited in their range of motion and had increased laxity, which resulted in a reduced activity level compared to the athletes who had the anatomical Broström repair. In 2016, Matheny compared activity level and function in patients who underwent either a Broström-Gould anatomical repair (61 patients) or an anatomical reconstruction using allograft (25 patients) and found no significant difference between the groups outcomes [32]. So and colleagues [33] performed a systematic review evaluating the recurrence rates and revision surgery rates in patients who had undergone a Broström-Gould repair. Eleven studies were included with 669 patients, with a mean follow-up of 8.4 years. The incidence rate of revision surgery in the included studies was 1.2%.

Other studies have also favourably reported on the modified Broström-Gould procedure, including work by Buerer and colleagues [34], who reported on 47 patients who underwent the procedure. Several outcome scores were used, including the AOFAS hindfoot score, the Foot and Ankle Ability Measurement (FAAM), the Cumberland Ankle Instability Tool (CAIT) and the Chronic Ankle Instability Scale (CAIS). With a minimum follow-up on 1 year, all outcomes demonstrated an improvement in mean scores.

More recently, Russo and colleagues presented their long-term results using the Broström-Gould procedure in athletes [35]. Included were 18 athletes involved in different competitive sports, with a follow-up of 10–15 years, the outcome of AOFAS scale improved from a mean of 67.6 preoperatively to a mean of 98.8. All athletes returned to their sports at the same competitive level, and imaging was performed in the form of plain radiographs, which demonstrated no radiographic features of arthritic degeneration.

14.5 Return to Sport

Most of the modern descriptions of surgical techniques for ankle instability include their postoperative protocol, which usually includes an initial short period of immobilisation, protected weight-bearing is allowed as tolerated in the first 2 weeks. At 4–6 weeks following surgery, physiotherapy is usually commenced and progress is enhanced with proprioceptive and strengthening exercises under supervision. Return to sport is most frequently described in the literature at approximately 16–20 weeks following surgery. In the series by White and colleagues [36], 42 elite level athletes underwent early surgical repair using the modified Broström-Gould repair, and all athletes returned to their pre-injury level of competition, with an expected return to play at 3 months. Despite these good results, a recent systematic review suggested that the overall evidence for reporting return to play in athletes following lateral ligament reconstruction was of low quality [37]. This review included 20 articles reviewing 489 athletes, with 13 of the studies calculating a return to play at 4.7 months. Important factors to consider in athletes returning to play from ankle sprains or ligament reconstruction may be their height and weight; an as yet unpublished study found increasing height and weight of athletes was a risk factor for recurrence of ankle injury following return to play [38] and these athletes may require a longer rehabilitation period following injury. The use of single limb balance training and neuromuscular training is advocated in the prevention and rehabilitation of ankle injuries and is most useful for those at risk of ankle injury or a history of previous injury [39]. The importance of ankle bracing or taping for athletes returning from ankle sprains has been studied. A systematic review in 2010 [40] demonstrated the use of an ankle brace or ankle taping amongst previously injured athletes significantly reduced the recurrence rate.

Fact Box 3

- Modern adaptations of surgery for lateral ankle instability promote early post-operative rehabilitation.
- Protected weight-bearing can be as early as 1–2 weeks.
- Sport-specific physiotherapy and proprioceptive exercises should be included in the rehabilitation.
- Return to high-level sport can take an average of 9–16 weeks post-surgery.

The author's current post-operative protocol is that patients are standardly placed in a below-knee non-weight-bearing cast for 2 weeks. This allows the incision to heal and the majority of swelling to settle.

At 2 weeks, the patient can fully weight bear in a locked hinged boot. The patient will commence physiotherapy at this point; this initially will be ankle range of motion exercises and soft tissue modalities. Early proprioceptive exercises can commence. A patient can use an exercise bike in the boot. The boot can gradually be unlocked as directed by the physiotherapist.

At 4 weeks, the patient can wean into a rigid ankle brace. Gentle inversion and eversion exercises can be commenced. More rigorous exercise can be undertaken in the brace and the patient can swim wearing fins. Running with reduced gravity (e.g., immersed in water) can also be started. At 6 weeks the patient can wean out of the brace and graduate up to sports-specific exercises as symptoms allow. Graduation through different elements of sports-specific exercise should be under the guidance of an experienced physiotherapist.

14.6 Conclusion

The Broström-Gould technique is an open technique with a proven track record of excellent reduction in symptoms, return to sport and a low level of recurrence of instability. With modern fixation techniques, patients can be rehabilitated in a more aggressive way, thereby reducing the morbidity of this common condition.

References

1. Molloy AP, Ajis A, Kazi H. The modified Broström-Gould procedure–early results using a newly described surgical technique. Foot Ankle Surg. 2014;20(3):224–8.
2. Shakked RJ, Karnovsky S, Drakos MC. Operative treatment of lateral ligament instability. Curr Rev Musculoskelet Med. 2017;10(1):113–21.
3. Jones RW. Fractures and other bone and joint injuries. Am J Phys Med Rehabil. 1942;21(1):54.
4. Evans DL. Recurrent instability of the ankle—a method of surgical treatment. Proc R Soc Med. 1953;46:343–4.
5. Chrisman OD, Snook GA. Reconstruction of lateral ligament tears of the ankle: an experimental study and clinical evaluation of seven patients treated by a new modification of the Elmslie procedure. J Bone Joint Surg. 1969;51(5):904–12.
6. Tourné Y, Mabit C. Lateral ligament reconstruction procedures for the ankle. Orthop Traumatol Surg Res. 2017;103(1):S171–81.
7. Brostrom L. Sprained ankles IV: Surgical treatment of "chronic" ligament ruptures. Acta Chir Scand. 1966;132:551–65.
8. Hamilton WG, Thompson FM, Snow SW. The modified Broström procedure for lateral ankle instability. Foot Ankle. 1993;14(1):1–7.
9. Javors JR, Violet JT. Correction of chronic lateral ligament instability of the ankle by use of the Broström procedure: a report of 15 cases. Clin Orthop Relat Res. 1985;198:201–7.
10. Bell SJ, Mologne TS, Sitler DF, Cox JS. Twenty-six-year results after Broström procedure for

chronic lateral ankle instability. Am J Sports Med. 2006;34(6):975–8.
11. Roos EM, Brandsson S, Karlsson J. Validation of the foot and ankle outcome score for ankle ligament reconstruction. Foot Ankle Int. 2001;22(10):788–94.
12. Good CJ, Jones MA, Livingstone BN. Reconstruction of the lateral ligament of the ankle. Injury. 1975;7(1):63–5.
13. Maffulli N, Del Buono A, Maffulli GD, Oliva F, Testa V, Capasso G, Denaro V. Isolated anterior talofibular ligament Broström repair for chronic lateral ankle instability: 9-year follow-up. Am J Sports Med. 2013;41(4):858–64.
14. Karlsson J, Bergsten T, Lansinger O, Peterson L. Surgical treatment of chronic lateral instability of the ankle joint: a new procedure. Am J Sports Med. 1989;17(2):268–74.
15. Duquennoy A, Létendard J, Loock P. Chronic instability of the ankle treated by reefing of the lateral ligament (author's transl). Rev Chir Orthop Reparatrice Appar Mot. 1980;66(5):311–6.
16. Ahlgren OL, Larsson SU. Reconstruction for lateral ligament injuries of the ankle. Bone Joint J. 1989;71(2):300–3.
17. Gould N, Seligson D, Gassman J. Early and late repair of lateral ligament of the ankle. Foot Ankle. 1980;1(2):84–9.
18. Aydogan U, Glisson RR, Nunley JA. Extensor retinaculum augmentation reinforces anterior talofibular ligament repair. Clin Orthop Relat Res. 2006;442:210–5.
19. Behrens SB, Drakos M, Lee BJ, Paller D, Hoffman E, Koruprolu S, DiGiovanni CW. Biomechanical analysis of Broström versus Broström-Gould lateral ankle instability repairs. Foot Ankle Int. 2013;34(4):587–92.
20. Keller M, Grossman J, Caron M, Mendicino RW. Lateral ankle instability and the Broström-Gould procedure. J Foot Ankle Surg. 1996;35(6):513–20.
21. Karlsson J, Eriksson BI, Bergsten T, Rudholm O, Swärd L. Comparison of two anatomic reconstructions for chronic lateral instability of the ankle joint. Am J Sports Med. 1997;25(1):48–53.
22. Messer TM, Cummins CA, Ahn J, Kelikian AS. Outcome of the modified Broström procedure for chronic lateral ankle instability using suture anchors. Foot Ankle Int. 2000;21(12):996–1003.
23. Angirasa AK, Barrett MJ. Talar anchor placement for modified Broström lateral ankle stabilization procedure. J Am Podiatr Med Assoc. 2008;98(6):473–6.
24. Li X, Killie H, Guerrero P, Busconi BD. Anatomical reconstruction for chronic lateral ankle instability in the high-demand athlete. Am J Sports Med. 2009;37(3):488–94.
25. Tegner Y, Lysholm J. Rating systems in the evaluation of knee ligament injuries. Clin Orthop Relat Res. 1985;(198):42–9.
26. Karlsson J, Peterson L. Evaluation of ankle joint function: the use of a scoring scale. Foot. 1991;1(1):15–9.
27. Lubowitz JH, MacKay G, Gilmer B. Knee medial collateral ligament and posteromedial corner anatomic repair with internal bracing. Arthrosc Tech. 2014;3(4):e505–8.
28. Schuh R, Benca E, Willegger M, Hirtler L, Zandieh S, Holinka J, Windhager R. Comparison of Broström technique, suture anchor repair, and tape augmentation for reconstruction of the anterior talofibular ligament. Knee Surg Sports Traumatol Arthrosc. 2016;24(4):1101–7.
29. Yoo JS, Yang EA. Clinical results of an arthroscopic modified Broström operation with and without an internal brace. J Orthop Traumatol. 2016;17(4):353–60.
30. Mabit C, Tourné Y, Besse JL, Bonnel F, Toullec E, Giraud F, Proust J, Khiami F, Chaussard C, Genty C. Chronic lateral ankle instability surgical repairs: the long term prospective. Orthop Traumatol Surg Res. 2010;96(4):417–23.
31. Krips R, van Dijk CN, Lehtonen H, Halasi T, Moyen B, Karlsson J. Sports activity level after surgical treatment for chronic anterolateral ankle instability. Am J Sports Med. 2002;30(1):13–9.
32. Matheny LM, Johnson NS, Liechti DJ, Clanton TO. Activity level and function after lateral ankle ligament repair versus reconstruction. Am J Sports Med. 2016;44(5):1301–8.
33. So E, Preston N, Holmes T. Intermediate-to long-term longevity and incidence of revision of the modified broström-gould procedure for lateral ankle ligament repair: a systematic review. J Foot Ankle Surg. 2017;56(5):1076–80.
34. Buerer Y, Winkler M, Burn A, Chopra S, Crevoisier X. Evaluation of a modified Broström–Gould procedure for treatment of chronic lateral ankle instability: a retrospective study with critical analysis of outcome scoring. Foot Ankle Surg. 2013;19(1):36–41.
35. Russo A, Giacchè P, Marcantoni E, Arrighi A, Molfetta L. Treatment of chronic lateral ankle instability using the Broström-Gould procedure in athletes: long-term results. Joints. 2016;4(2):94.
36. White WJ, McCollum GA, Calder JD. Return to sport following acute lateral ligament repair of the ankle in professional athletes. Knee Surg Sports Traumatol Arthrosc. 2016;24(4):1124–9.
37. Hunt KJ, Fuld RS, Sutphin BS, Pereira H, D'Hooghe P. Return to sport following lateral ankle ligament repair is under-reported: a systematic review. J ISAKOS. 2017;2(5):234–40.
38. McCann RS, Kosik KB, Terada M, Gribble PA. O12 prediction of recurrent injury following return-to-play from an ankle sprain. Br J Sports Med. 2017;51(Suppl 1):A5.1–A5.
39. Shawen SB, Dworak T, Anderson RB. Return to play following ankle sprain and lateral ligament reconstruction. Clin Sports Med. 2016;35(4):697–709.
40. Dizon JM, Reyes JJ. A systematic review on the effectiveness of external ankle supports in the prevention of inversion ankle sprains among elite and recreational players. J Sci Med Sport. 2010;13(3):309–17.

15 Reinforcement of the Broström Technique: When and How to Do It?

Tekin Kerem Ülkü, Barış Kocaoğlu, and Jón Karlsson

15.1 Introduction

The ankle joint is the most congruent joint of the human body. Joint stability is reinforced by bony configuration of the ankle mortise, talar dome, and strong ligamentous structures. Despite this stable nature ankle sprains are among the most common athletic injuries brought to the attention of the orthopedic surgeon, especially in athletes [1, 2]. Majority of these injuries involve lateral ligamentous complex. Despite mounting evidence about the effectiveness of nonsurgical treatment, approximately 20% of these injuries eventually evolve to chronic ankle instability [3].

When chronic ankle instability remains despite adequate rehabilitation, surgical intervention becomes inevitable. For these patients, a multitude of surgical techniques has been described. Basically, these methods can be classified as anatomic and nonanatomic procedures. Among the anatomic procedures, Broström technique and its modifications are currently accepted as the gold standard. Different modifications have been added to the original technique; the Gould procedure being the most popular and most studied one [4–8] .

The Broström technique involves direct repair, imbrication, and reinsertion of injured ankle ligaments. Even though excellent clinical and functional outcomes have been reported, some limitations have been reported.

It has been shown in previous studies that the reconstruction of the anterior talofibular ligament (ATFL) may not restore the full strength of the native ligament even using suture anchors or the Broström technique. Moreover, a restriction in postoperative rehabilitation is a concern especially for elite athletes [9]. Also although rare, in some specific patient groups Broström technique and its modifications appear to be unsatisfactory. However, data are still limited [10].

These concerns have caused new techniques to evolve. Recently tape augmentation techniques for traditional Broström are described to improve the laxity of the reconstructed ATFL. The aims are to improve laxity restoration at time zero, faster recovery, and faster rehabilitation.

15.2 Biomechanics

In the loaded ankle joint bony configuration of the mortise provides most of the stability of the joint [11, 12]. However, in unloaded state

T. K. Ülkü · B. Kocaoğlu (✉)
Department of Orthopedics and Traumatology, Acibadem University School of Medicine, Istanbul, Turkey

J. Karlsson
Department of Orthopedics, University of Gothenburg, Goteborg, Sweden
e-mail: jon.karlsson@telia.com

H. Pereira et al. (eds.), *Lateral Ankle Instability*, https://doi.org/10.1007/978-3-662-62763-1_15

ligaments are more critical. According to the position of ankle and subtalar joins all ligaments have a stabilizing role. ATFL is taut in plantarflexion and loose in dorsiflexion whereas calcaneofibular ligament (CFL) is taut in dorsiflexion and loose in plantarflexion. Lateral ankle ligament injury usually involves an inversion and plantarflexion. Rotational trauma leads to injury of ATFL than CFL and PTFL sequentially.

Biomechanical studies have shown that the ATFL has a lower load to failure compared with the CFL [13]. Meanwhile, it is capable of undergoing greater strain compared to CFL [14]. Native ATFL has a maximum load to failure of 139 ± 23.5 Newton, whereas native CFL has about 346 ± 55.2 Newton [15].

Several studies have been performed to evaluate the biomechanical status of ankle joint comparing sectioned and intact ATFL and biomechanical evaluation after Broström-Gould procedure [16–18]. In a cadaver study by Behrens et al., it was shown that the ATFL has highest translation in sectioned state; however, there was no difference between intact and surgically repaired ligaments [17]. Shuh et al. investigated the angle and torque at the failure of ATFL after traditional Broström and Broström with tape augmentation techniques [19]. These researchers concluded that Broström including tape augmentation technique had superior mechanical results compared with traditional Broström technique. Both the angle of failure and failure torque were higher than after traditional Broström technique at time zero. When Broström technique including tape augmentation was compared with native ATFL biomechanical study showed no differences at time zero [18].

15.3 Proprioception

The foot and ankle complex is the entire surface of the body in contact with the ground during ambulation. They act as the sixth sense of the body and have an important role in proprioception. Two anatomical structures around the foot and ankle have major importance in terms of proprioception. They are the superior and inferior extensor ankle retinaculum. Zheng described the ankle retinacula as pulleys only preserving tendons close to bony structures [20]. However, in histological studies Vidalot et al. [21] and in 2006 Kynsburg [22] showed that the retinacula are more than just mechanical stabilizers. Stecco et al. also showed that their histological features resemble a network of receptors rather than a pulley [23]. It is also suggested that the peroneal retinaculum is stretched during inversion maneuver thus inducing peroneal stretch reflex [23].

The lateral ankle ligament complex is the second important anatomical structure for ankle proprioceptive function. Freeman stated that the injured lateral ligament complex and capsule causes deafferentation due to damaged mechanoreceptors [24]. More recent studies have shown that individuals with chronic ankle instability have depressed levels of alpha motor neuron activity in the quadriceps and hamstring muscles [25, 26].

The effect of surgical lateral ligament complex repair has been studied by Li et al., who showed that postural sway and proprioceptive control were improved at 6 months after ATFL repair using the Broström-Gould technique [20]. Further studies are needed to evaluate the effects of tape augmentation techniques on proprioception.

15.4 Ligamentous Laxity

Because of the inherent connective tissue deficiency, generalized ligamentous laxity is commonly considered a risk factor for failure of the anatomic ligament repair for chronic ankle instability. The prevalence of generalized ligamentous laxity has been reported 36.7% in females and 13.7% in males with an overall prevalence of 26.2% [27]. Karlsson et al. have previously reported inferior outcomes in patients with ligamentous laxity after lateral ankle ligament reconstruction compared with patients without generalized ligamentous laxity [28]. Matsui et al. and Petrera et al. reported that several patients with failure after Broström-Gould procedure had signs of generalized ligamentous laxity [29, 30]. Recently, Park et al. stated that rates of clinical failure after the modified Broström procedure were 45.2% in the ligamentous laxity group whereas it was only 10.8% in non-laxity group [31].

All these data suggest that surgical results may not be satisfactory in all patients after the Broström-Gould technique ATFL repair. Recent studies compared the clinical outcomes after suture-tape augmentation with modified Broström technique in patients with ligamentous laxity, concluding that suture-tape augmentation is an effective alternative for this group [16].

15.5 Professional Athletes

Ankle sprains account for up to 40% of all sports injuries. Therefore, professional athletes are a patient group in need of a specific treatment approach. Treatment of this high-demand patient group is challenging both because of extreme physical demands of the patients (weight, height, etc.), and the need for faster and aggressive rehabilitation and faster return to play. This caused the augmentation of the modified Broström technique to be popular for high-demand athletes. However, scientific data is still limited. Li et al. showed good clinical results using suture anchor augmentation of modified Broström technique in elite athletes [32]. Accelerated postoperative physical therapy regimens can allow patients return to cycling at 2 weeks and running at 8 weeks [33].

15.6 Other Specific Patient Groups

Since anatomical ligament repair or reconstruction is the primary goal, patients lacking strong ligament remnants are always challenging. This can be caused either by failed previous surgery, long-standing ligamentous insufficiency, or obesity. Previous studies have shown that these patient groups often sustain poor outcomes after ankle ligament reconstruction surgery and accordingly suture-tape augmentation appears to be a sound option which is named as "internal bracing" [10].

15.7 Surgical Techniques

15.7.1 Broström with Tape Augmentation (Open)

1. After skin preparation and tourniquet application, a J shaped skin anterior-lateral incision is performed to allow easy exposure to the anterolateral capsule, the ATFL, and CFL ligaments (Fig. 15.1).
2. The dissection is then carried out to the level of periosteum by protecting the lateral branch of superficial peroneal nerve and sural nerve. The fascia of the peroneus tertius is incised longitudinally and the muscle is retracted medially exposing the joint capsule.
3. The joint capsule is opened longitudinally. ATFL is identified and a curved hemostat is placed under the anterolateral joint capsule and exited distally in the soft spot over the anterior-inferior extensor retinaculum.
4. After division of the capsule, the remnant of the ATFL embedded in the capsule is exposed. For tape augmentation technique, division of

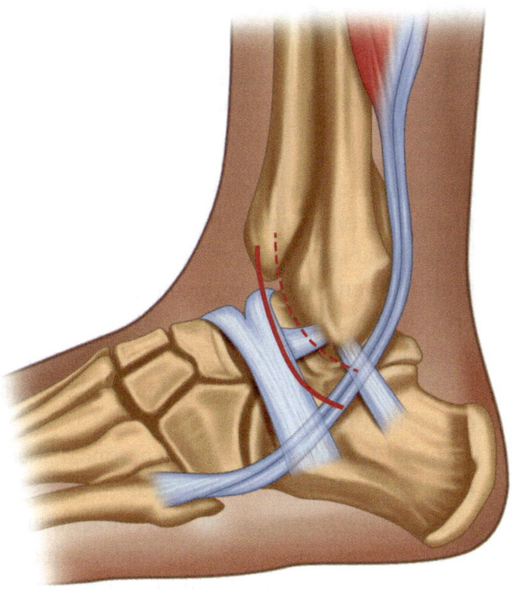

Fig. 15.1 J shaped skin incision over the anterior border of the fibula to the peroneal tendons

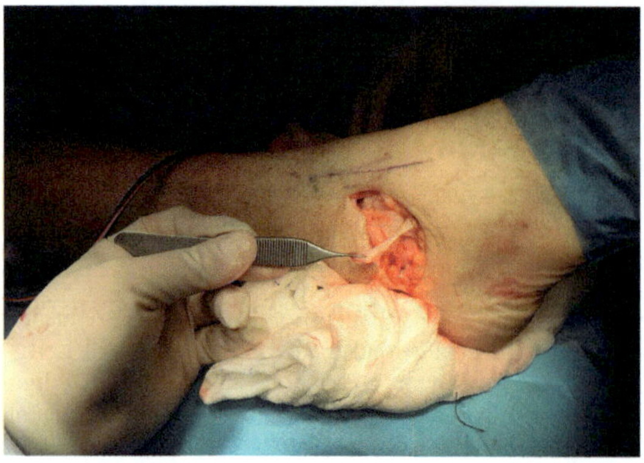

Fig. 15.2 After the division of capsule Remnants ATFL is exposed

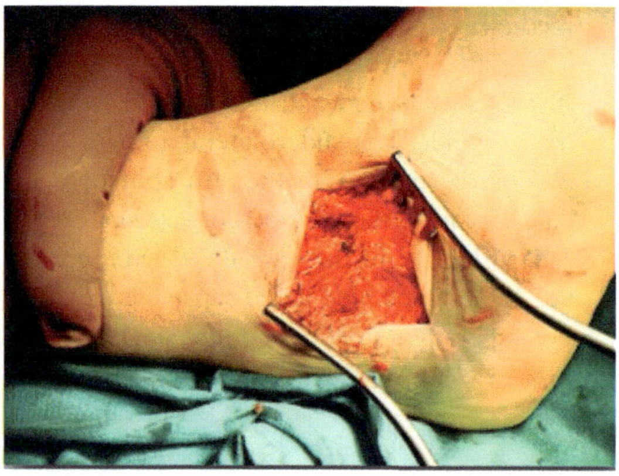

Fig. 15.3 Two Korakow sutures are imbricated and tied while the foot is plantarflexed and everted

the capsule closer to midsubstance of the ligament is recommended (Fig. 15.2).

5. Two non-absorbable No: 0 continuous braided multifilament ultra high molecular weight polyethylene sutures using Krakow technique are placed and tied in an imbricated position, with the foot held in slight plantarflexion and eversion (Fig. 15.3).
6. If the CFL is also injured, the peroneal sheath is opened. When the peroneal tendons are retracted, CFL is exposed. CFL attachment to fibula should be carefully evaluated, as it commonly detaches from the fibular anchor. Once the CFL is located it can be imbricated or

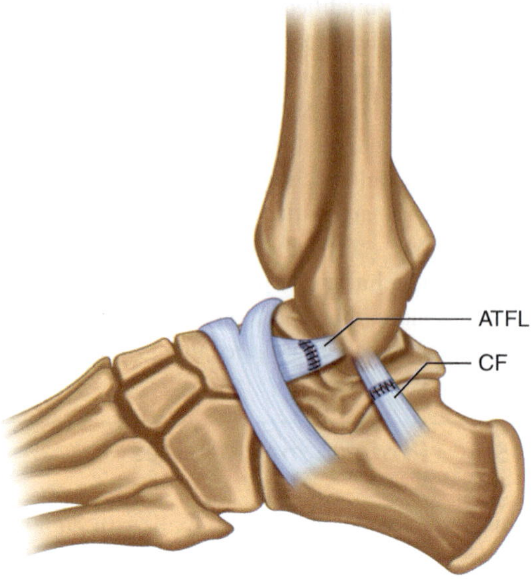

Fig. 15.4 Position of ATFL and CFL is anatomically secured or imbricated

repaired in the same fashion as ATFL using Krakow technique (Fig. 15.4).

7. After application of standard Broström repair, abony area 1.5 cm proximal to the tip of the fibula is prepared. A hole is drilled with a 2.7 mm drill angling slightly proximally in line with the lateral border of the foot. No: 2, braided multifilament ultra high molecular weight polyethylene suture is loaded to a 3.5 mm Anchor and inserted into the drill hole.
8. The lateral aspect of the talus close to the insertion site of the ATFL is prepared and drilled with a 2.7 mm drill. Both legs of the No: 5, braided multifilament ultra high molecular weight polyethylene tape is inserted into the 3.5 mm anchor. After assessment of the range of motion, a hemostat clamp is placed to avoid over-tensioning and an anchor is placed (Fig. 15.5).
9. The inferior extensor retinaculum is sutured over the periosteum over the fibula border before closure (Fig. 15.6). Subcutaneous tissue is closed with absorbable sutures and the skin is closed in a subcuticular technique. A posterior splint or a walking boot is applied.

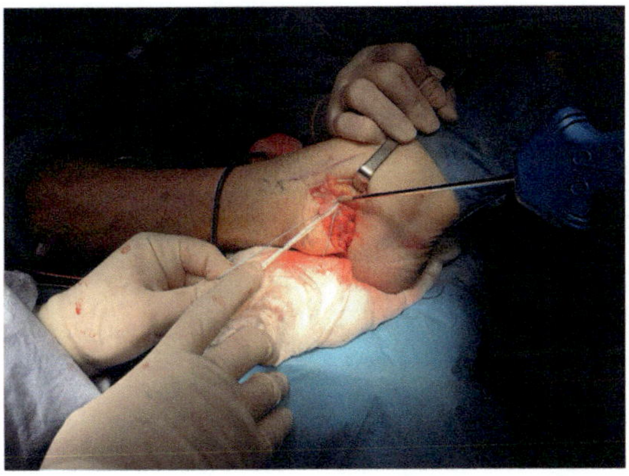

Fig. 15.5 The insertion of suture tape to the hole in talus

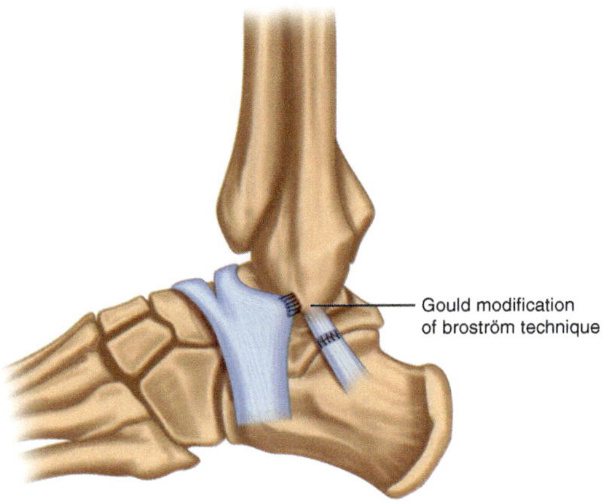

Fig. 15.6 Gould modification of suture-tape augmentation with extensor retinaculum repair

15.7.2 Broström with Tape Augmentation (Arthroscopic)

1. After skin preparation and tourniquet application standard anteromedial and anterolateral portals are created. After careful intra-articular examination and if no other pathologies are found lateral compartment is visualized.
2. Ruptured or fibrotic remnants of ATFL are dissected and identified. The attachment site of the ATFL at the fibula is prepared with a radiofrequency device and a cortical abrasion is carefully done with a shaver and burr, taking care of not excising too much bone, especially in older patients (Fig. 15.7).

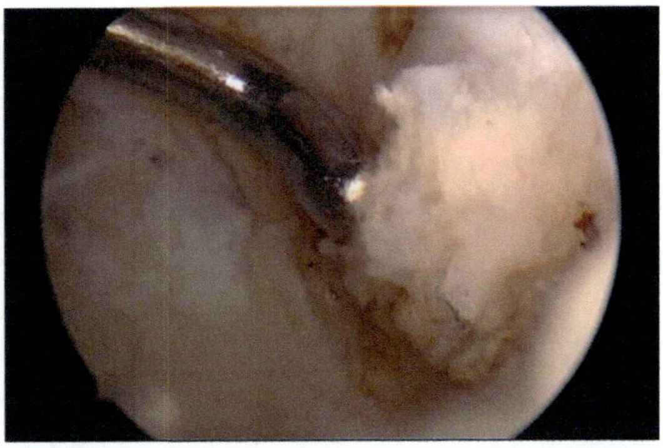

Fig. 15.7 Arthroscopic preparation of the fibular site and ATFL remnant

3. With the camera in the medial portal, a curved suture passer device is inserted through the lateral portal to the ATFL. No: 2, braided multifilament ultra high molecular weight polyethylene suture is passed from the ATFL in a looped fashion and the ligament is secured.
4. A hole is drilled with a 2.0 mm drill, angling slightly proximally in line with the lateral border of the foot. No: 2, braided multifilament ultra high molecular weight polyethylene suture along with ATFL stump is thereafter inserted to a 2.4 mm anchor and secured to the fibula.
5. After securing the ATFL at second drill a 2.7 mm hole is created angling slightly proximally in line with the lateral border of the foot. No: 5, braided multifilament ultra high molecular weight polyethylene tape is loaded to a 3.5 mm anchor and inserted tightly.
6. To prepare the talar hole an inferolateral accessory portal is created and the free end of the Tape is shuttled. The lateral aspect of the talus close to the insertion site of the ATFL is prepared and drilled with a 2.7 mm drill. Both legs of the No: 5, braided multifilament ultra high molecular weight polyethylene tapes are inserted into the 3.5 mm anchor. The anchor is inserted into the talus with appropriate tensioning (Fig. 15.8a–c).

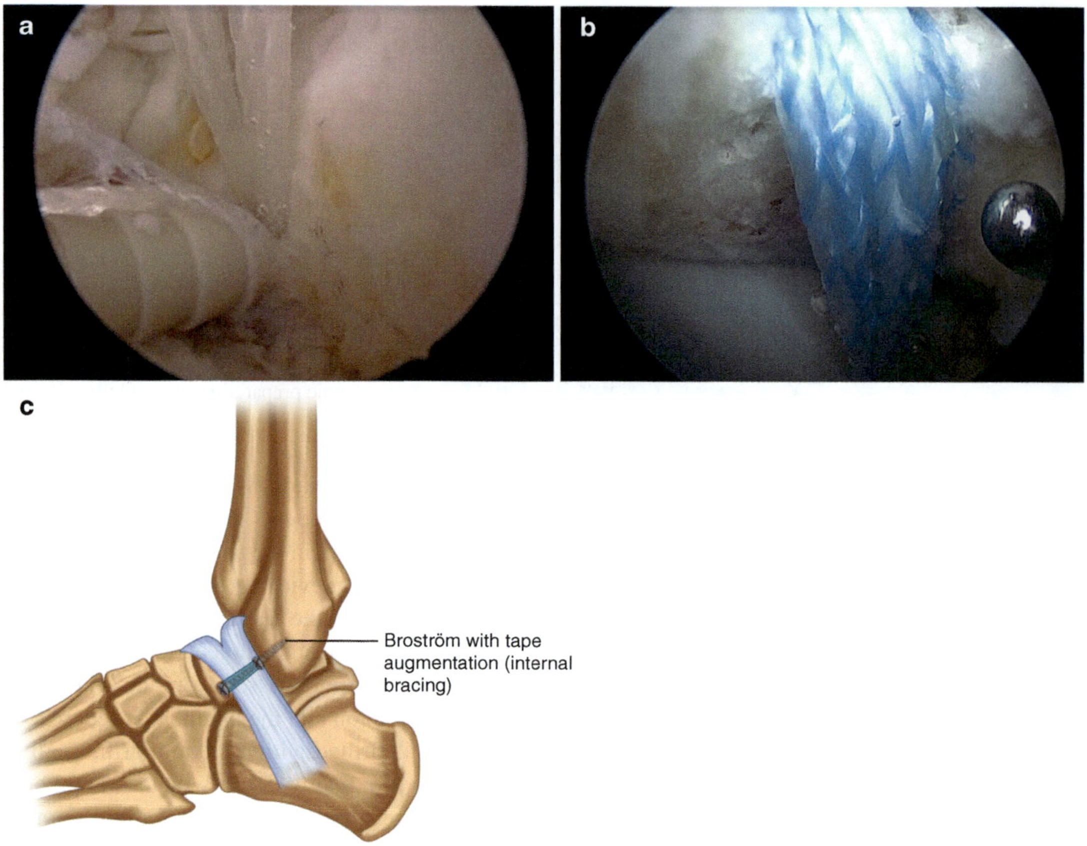

Fig. 15.8 (**a**) Inserting the suture-tape loaded talar anchor. (**b**) After tightening of the suture tape. (**c**) Schematic representation of Broström with tape augmentation

15.8 Postoperative Rehabilitation

After surgery, a short-leg splint and non-weight-bearing ambulation using crutches for 2 weeks is maintained. Thereafter range of motion exercises together with partial weight-bearing are encouraged. Full active weight-bearing is permitted after 6–8 weeks together with peroneal strengthening exercises and proprioceptive training. After confirming the restoration of ankle laxity approximately 4–6 months after the reconstruction, the pre-injury activity level can be resumed.

15.9 Conclusion

After an acute ankle sprain, approximately 20% of patients develop chronic recurrent ankle instability and nearly half of these patients need surgery despite extensive proprioceptive training. The Broström procedure is an effective method for surgical treatment, with good and excellent results in 90% of patients. However, the remaining 10% of patients remain symptomatic. The reason for this appears to be related to patient-specific problems. These are ligamentous laxity, obesity, low quality of the remaining ligamentous tissue, and early return to play. To overcome these problems reinforcement techniques with tape or suture augmentations were introduced. Although the traditional Broström technique is generally successful, reinforcement techniques like Gould modification can be used in these specific patient groups. Further studies are needed to investigate the mechanical and proprioceptive properties of reinforcement techniques.

References

1. Colville MR. Surgical treatment of the unstable ankle. J Am Acad Orthop Surg. 1998;6(6):368–77.
2. DiGiovanni CW, Brodsky A. Current concepts: lateral ankle instability. Foot Ankle Int. 2006;27(10):854–66.
3. Karlsson J, Lansinger O. Chronic lateral instability of the ankle in athletes. Sports Med. 1993;16(5):355–65.
4. Broström L. Sprained ankles. VI. Surgical treatment of "chronic" ligament ruptures. Acta Chir Scand. 1966;132:551–65.
5. Gould N, Seligson D, Gassman J. Early and late repair of lateral ligament of the ankle. Foot Ankle. 1980;1:84–9.
6. Grönmark T, Johnsen O, Kogstad O. Rupture of the lateral ligaments of the ankle: a controlled clinical trial. Injury. 1980;11:215–8.
7. Hamilton WG, Thompson FM, Snow SW. The modified Broström procedure for lateral ankle instability. Foot Ankle. 1993;14:1–7.
8. Karlsson J, Bergsten T, Lansinger O, Peterson L. Reconstruction of the lateral ligaments of the ankle for chronic lateral instability. J Bone Joint Surg Am. 1988;70-A:581–8.
9. Waldrop NE, Wijdicks CA, Jansson KS, Laprade RF, Clanton TO. Anatomic suture anchor versus the Broström technique for anterior talofibular ligament repair: a biomechanical comparison. Am J Sports Med. 2012;40:2590–6.
10. Park JS, Kim BS. Risk factors for failure after lateral ankle ligament repair. J Korean Foot Ankle Soc. 2016;20(2):62–6.
11. McCullough CJ, Burge PD. Rotatory stability of the load-bearing ankle: an experimental study. J Bone Joint Surg Am. 1980;62-A:460–4.
12. Stormont DM, Morrey BF, An KN, Cass JR. Stability of the loaded ankle: relation between articular restraint and primary and secondary static restraints. Am J Sports Med. 1985;13:295–300.
13. Siegler S, Block J, Schneck CD. The mechanical characteristics of the collateral ligaments of the human ankle joint. Foot Ankle. 1988;8:234–42.
14. Colville MR, Grondel RJ. Anatomic reconstruction of the lateral ankle ligaments using a split peroneus brevis tendon graft. Am J Sports Med. 1995;23:210–3.
15. Attarian DE, McCrackin HJ, DeVito DP, McElhaney JH, Garrett WE Jr. Biomechanical characteristics of human ankle ligaments. Foot Ankle. 1985;6:54–8.
16. Cho BK, Park KJ, Park JK, SooHoo NF. Outcomes of modified Broström procedure augmented with suture-tape for ankle instability in patients with generalized ligamentous laxity. Foot Ankle Int. 2017;38(4):405–11.
17. Behrens SB, Drakos M, Lee BJ, Paller D, Hoffman E, Koruprolu S, DiGiovanni CW. Biomechanical analysis of Brostrom versus Brostrom-Gould lateral ankle instability repairs. Foot Ankle Int. 2013;34(4):587–92.
18. Viens NA, Wijdicks CA, Campbell KJ, LaPrade RF, Clanton TO. Anterior talofibular ligament ruptures, part 1: biomechanical comparison of augmented Broström repair techniques with the intact anterior talofibular ligament. Am J Sports Med. 2014;42(2):405–11.
19. Schuh R, Benca E, Willegger M, Hirtler L, Zandieh S, Holinka J, Windhager R. Comparison of Broström technique, suture anchor repair, and tape augmentation for reconstruction of the anterior talofibular ligament. Knee Surg Sports Traumatol Arthrosc. 2016;24(4):1101–7.
20. Li HY, Zheng JJ, Zhang J, Cai YH, Hua YH, Chen SY. The improvement of postural control in patients with mechanical ankle instability after lateral ankle ligaments reconstruction. Knee Surg Sports Traumatol Arthrosc. 2016;24(4):1081–5.
21. Viladot A, Lorenzo JC, Salazar J, Rodríguez A. The subtalar joint: embryology and morphology. Foot Ankle Int. 1984;5:54–66.
22. Kynsburg A, Halasi T, Tállay A, Berkes I. Changes in joint position sense after conservatively treated chronic lateral ankle instability. Knee Surg Sports Traumatol Arthrosc. 2006;14(12):1299–306.
23. Stecco C, Macchi V, Porzionato A, Morra A, Parenti A. The ankle retinacula: morphological evidence of the proprioceptive role of the fascial system. Cells Tissues Organs. 2010;192:200–10.
24. Hertel J. Sensorimotor de cits with ankle sprains and chronic ankle instability. Clin Sports Med. 2008;27:353–70.
25. McVey ED, Palmieri RM, Docherty CL, Zinder SM, Ingersoll CD. Arthrogenic muscle inhibition in the leg muscles of subjects exhibiting functional ankle instability. Foot Ankle Int. 2005;26:1055–61.
26. Sedory EJ, McVey ED, Cross KM, Ingersoll CD, Hertel J. Arthrogenic muscle response of the quadriceps and hamstrings with chronic ankle instability. J Athl Train. 2007;42:355–60.
27. Russek LN, Errico DM. Prevalence, injury rate and, symptom frequency in generalized joint laxity and joint hypermobility syndrome in a "healthy" college population. Clin Rheumatol. 2016;35(4):1029–39.
28. Karlsson J, Eriksson BI, Bergsten T, Rudholm O, Swärd L. Comparison of two anatomic reconstructions for chronic lateral instability of the ankle joint. Am J Sports Med. 1997;25(1):48–53.
29. Matsui K, Takao M, Miyamoto W, Matsushita T. Early recovery after arthroscopic repair compared to open repair of the anterior talofibular ligament for lateral instability of the ankle. Arch Orthop Trauma Surg. 2016;136(1):93–100.
30. Petrera M, Dwyer T, Theodoropoulos JS, Ogilvie-Harris DJ. Short- to medium-term outcomes after a modified Broström repair for lateral ankle instability with immediate post-operative weight-bearing. Am J Sports Med. 2014;42(7):1542–8.
31. Park KH, Lee JW, Suh JW, Shin MH, Choi WJ. Generalized ligamentous laxity is an independent predictor of poor outcomes after the modified broström procedure for chronic lateral ankle instability. Am J Sports Med. 2016;44(11):2975–83.

32. Li X, Killie H, Guerrero P, Busconi BD. Anatomical reconstruction for chronic lateral ankle instability in the high-demand athlete: functional outcomes after the modified Broström repair using suture anchors. Am J Sports Med. 2009;37(3):488–94.
33. Mackay GM, Ribbans WJ. The addition of an "internal brace" to augment the Broström technique for lateral ankle ligament instability. Tech Foot Ankle Surg. 2016;15(1):47–56.

16 Collateral Lateral Ligament Repair: Anatomic Ligaments Reinsertion with Augmentation Using an Extensor Retinaculum Flap

Yves Tourné

16.1 Introduction

The aims of any surgical repair/reconstruction technique are to restore the capsuloligamentous structure, and thus articular stability while preserving the mobility of the talocrural and subtalar joints and avoiding secondary arthrosis [1, 2].

The surgical technique we report combines re-tensioning of the incompetent lateral collateral ligament (ATFL and CFL) with reinforcement by a neoligament harvested from the extensor retinaculum. While the re-tensioning of the capsuloligamentous structures resembles the techniques described by Broström [3] or Duquennoy [4], the reinforcement using the extensor retinaculum described by Saragaglia [5] and modified by Tourné [2], and reported in his work, is different to that reported by Blanchet [6] or Gould [7] (Figs. 16.1 and 16.2).

The retinaculum flap works as an actual neoligament, providing not only reinforcement and collagen input but also peripheral stabilization of the subtalar joint by its calcaneal insertion, reinforcing the CFL.

Y. Tourné (✉)
Foot and Ankle Institute of Grenoble, Centre Ostéo Articulaire des Cèdres, rue des Tropiques, Parc Sud Galaxie, Echirolles, France

16.2 Surgical Technique

16.2.1 Settling

The patient is secured in a lateral decubitus position, with a thigh-level pneumatic tourniquet and the lower limb in internal rotation (Fig. 16.3).

16.2.2 Approach and Ankle Arthrotomy

The skin incision is anterolateral, curvilinear, and centered on the lateral malleolus. It runs over the sinus tarsi to the dorsal aspect of the midfoot (Fig. 16.4).

A periosteal flap is developed posteriorly towards the sulcus for the peroneal tendons (Fig. 16.5). It will reinforce the capsular shift at the end stage of the procedure.

An L-shaped arthrotomy is performed along the course of the peroneus tertius (Fig. 16.6a), creating a residual capsuloligamentous flap, attached to the neck of the talus and the lateral border of the calcaneus (Fig. 16.6b). This arthrotomy allows the talar dome cartilage, mainly on the lateral side, the anterior edge of the tibia, and talar neck to be checked.

H. Pereira et al. (eds.), *Lateral Ankle Instability*, https://doi.org/10.1007/978-3-662-62763-1_16

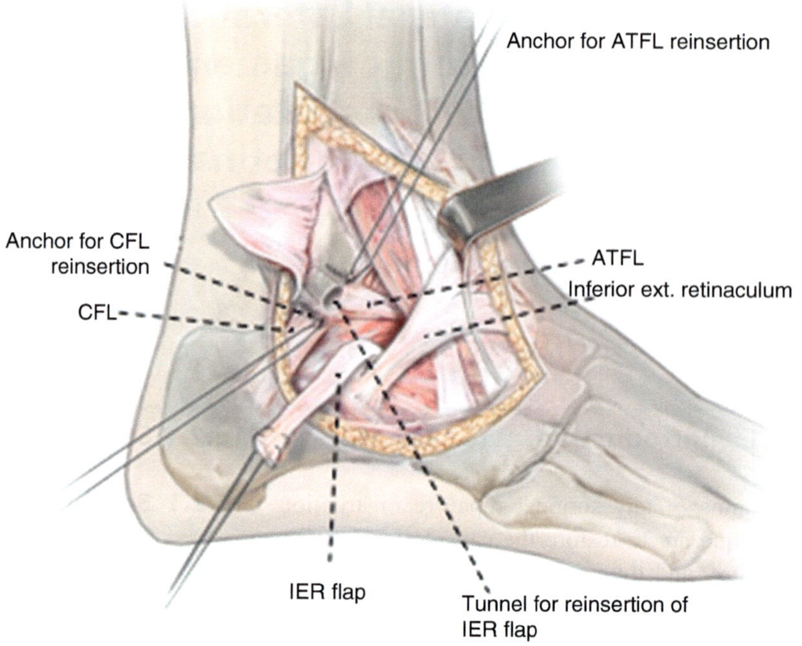

Fig. 16.1 Anterior tibiofibular ligament (ATFL) and calcaneofibular ligament (CFL) ready for reinsertion and flap harvested from the inferior extensor retinaculum (IER) before its reinsertion. The flap remains attached to the lateral aspect of the calcaneus

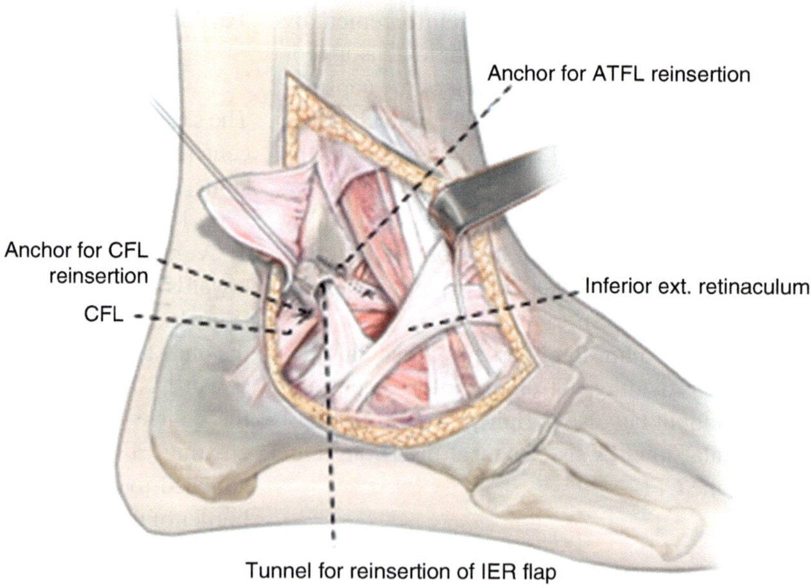

Fig. 16.2 Overall reinsertion, using anchors for anterior tibiofibular ligament (ATFL) and calcaneofibular ligament (CFL) and a tunnel with an interference screw for the flap

The residual anterior tibiofibular and calcaneofibular ligaments are located and the possibility of reinsertion is assessed (Fig. 16.6c).

Synovial, bone, and osteochondral procedures may be associated as necessary, depending on the preoperative lesion assessment.

16.2.3 Anchors Fixation

Fixation of two 3 × 14 mm Biocomposite SutureTak anchors is performed for the reinsertion at a later stage of the procedure: one for the capsule and the ATFL-superior bundle at the upper anterior part of the fibular malleolus

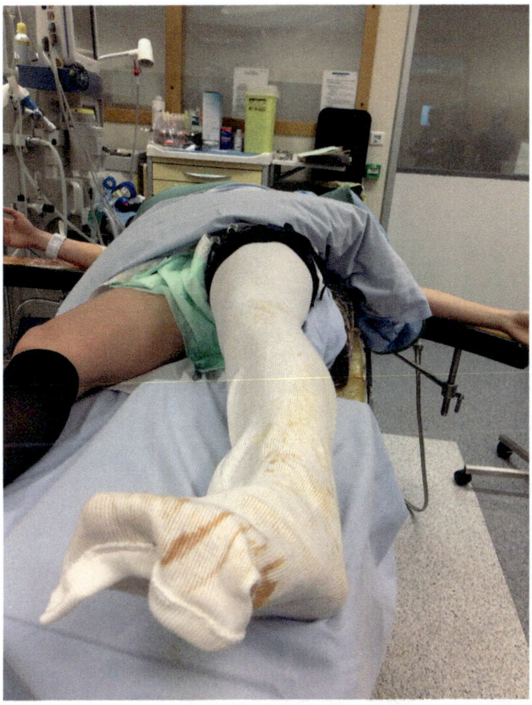

Fig. 16.3 The patient is secured in a supine position, with a thigh-level pneumatic tourniquet and the lower limb maintained in internal rotation by a buttress under the ipsilateral buttock

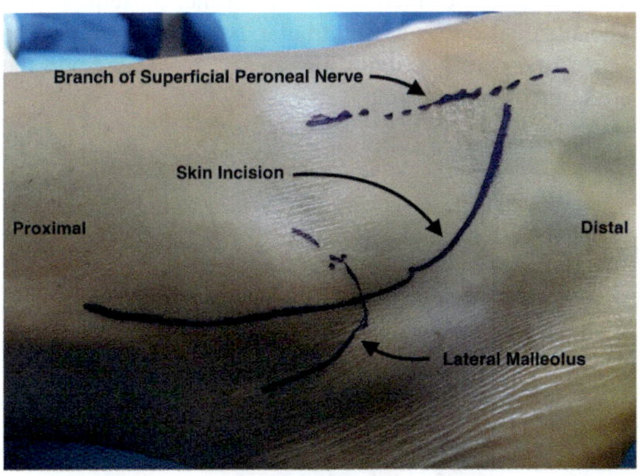

Fig. 16.4 The skin incision is anterolateral, curvilinear, and centered on the lateral malleolus. It runs over the sinus tarsi to the dorsal aspect of midfoot

(Fig. 16.7a) (footprint of the ATFL, inferior insertion of the Bassett ligament, resected at the same time), one at the obscure tubercule, medial to the tip of the fibular malleolus for the ATFL-inferior bundle and the calcaneofibular ligaments (Fig. 16.7b).

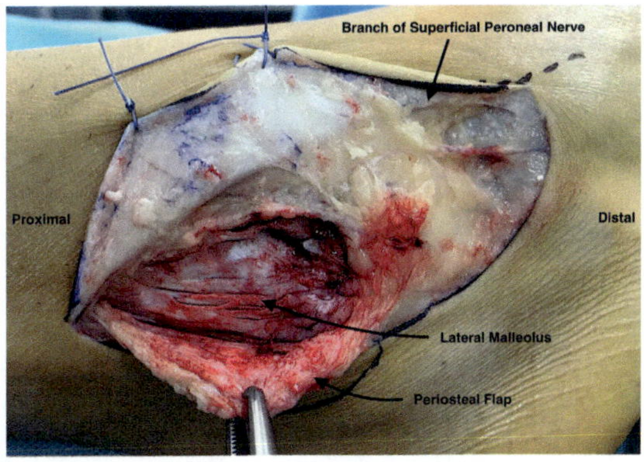

Fig. 16.5 A periosteal flap is developed posteriorly towards the sulcus for the peroneal tendons. It will reinforce the capsular shift at the end stage of the procedure

16.2.4 Extensor Retinaculum Flap (EFR) Elevation and Preparation

Subcutaneous release isolates the distal extensor retinaculum, from which a rectangular flap, about 1 cm by 3–4 cm, is harvested from the superior bundle (Fig. 16.8a).

It is mandatory to pay attention to the superficial branches of the peroneal and sural nerves (Fig. 16.8b).

The flap remains inserted on the calcaneus at the entry to the sinus tarsi. The neoligament is reinforced using a 2-0 non-absorbable looped suture: fiber loop (Fig. 16.8c). Its size is checked (Fig. 16.8d).

Because it remains attached to the calcaneus, this flap stabilizes the subtalar joint at the end of procedure.

16.2.5 EFR Reinsertion

A 2.4 mm pin is inserted between the two anchors, from the anterior margin of the lateral malleolus to its posterior aspect (Fig. 16.9a). A retractor protects the fibular tendons. The orientation is 45° to the plantar aspect of the foot. It represents the bissectrix between the ATL and CFL ligaments orientation.

The pin is overdrilled according to the previous sizing of the neoligament (diameter between 4.5 and 5.0 mm) (Fig. 16.9b).

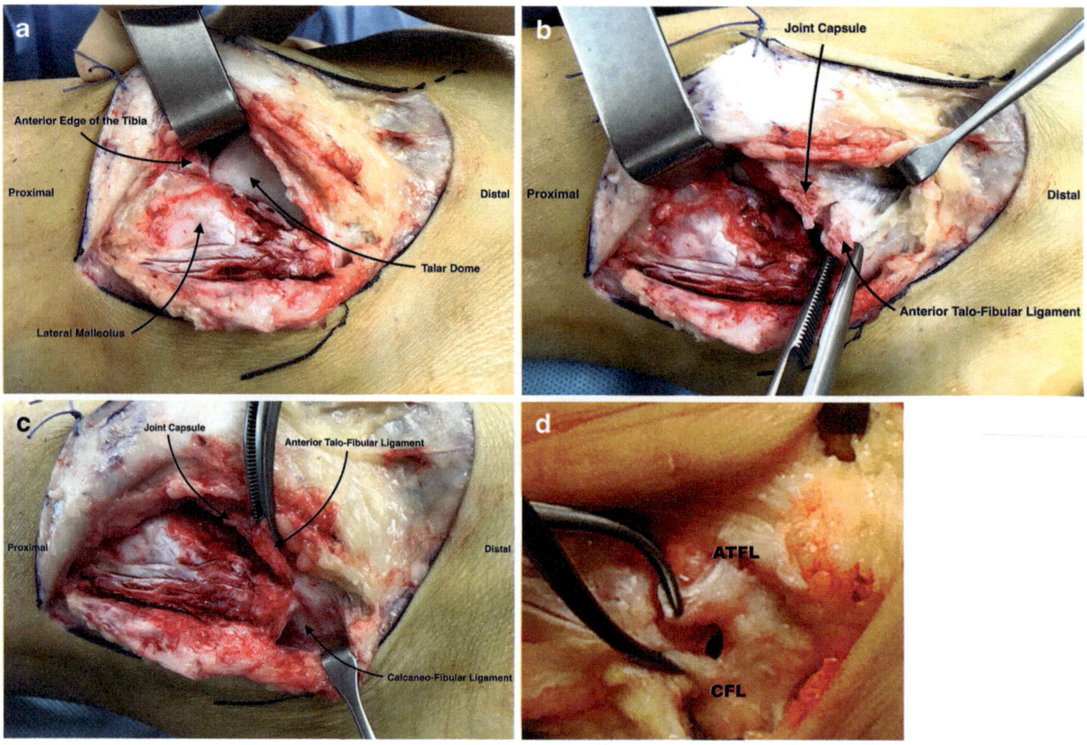

Fig. 16.6 Arthrotomy. (**a**) An L-shaped arthrotomy is then performed along the course of the peroneus tertius. This arthrotomy allows the talar dome cartilage, mainly on the lateral side, the anterior edge of the tibia and talar neck to be checked. Synovial, bone, and osteochondral procedures may be associated as necessary, depending on the preoperative lesion assessment. (**b**) Thus, a residual capsuloligamentous flap is created, attached to the neck of the talus (Capsule + ATFL). (**c**) The fibular tendons sheet is open at the anterior aspect of the tip of the fibular malleolus. The condition of the CFL is assessed properly (status, tension) and the peroneal tendons too. Peroneal tendons tears are fixed in the meantime, on request. (**d**) The residual anterior tibiofibular (with its two components) and calcaneofibular ligaments are located and the possibility of reinsertion is assessed

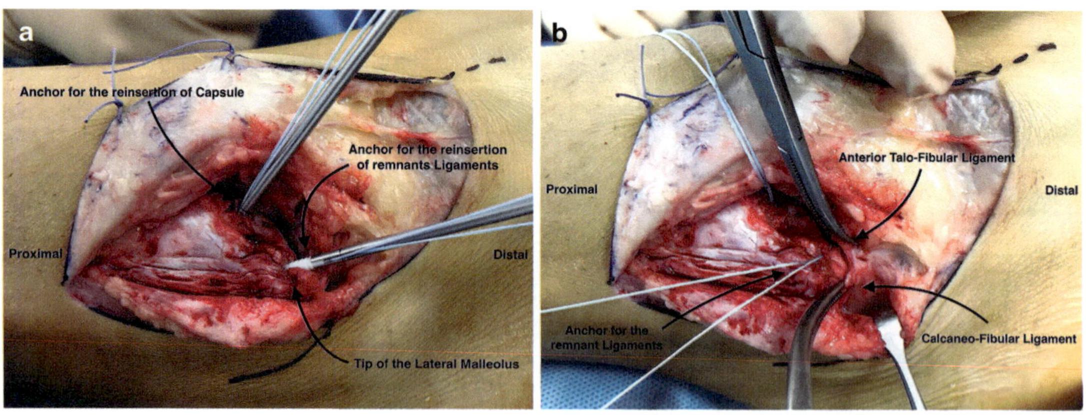

Fig. 16.7 Anchors fixation. (**a**) Fixation of two 3 × 14 mm anchors is performed for the reinsertion at a later stage of the procedure: one for the capsule and the ATFL-superior bundle at the upper anterior part of the fibular malleolus. (**b**) And one at the fibular obscure tubercule of the fibular malleolus for the ATFL-inferior bundle calcaneofibular ligament (one needle per ligament)

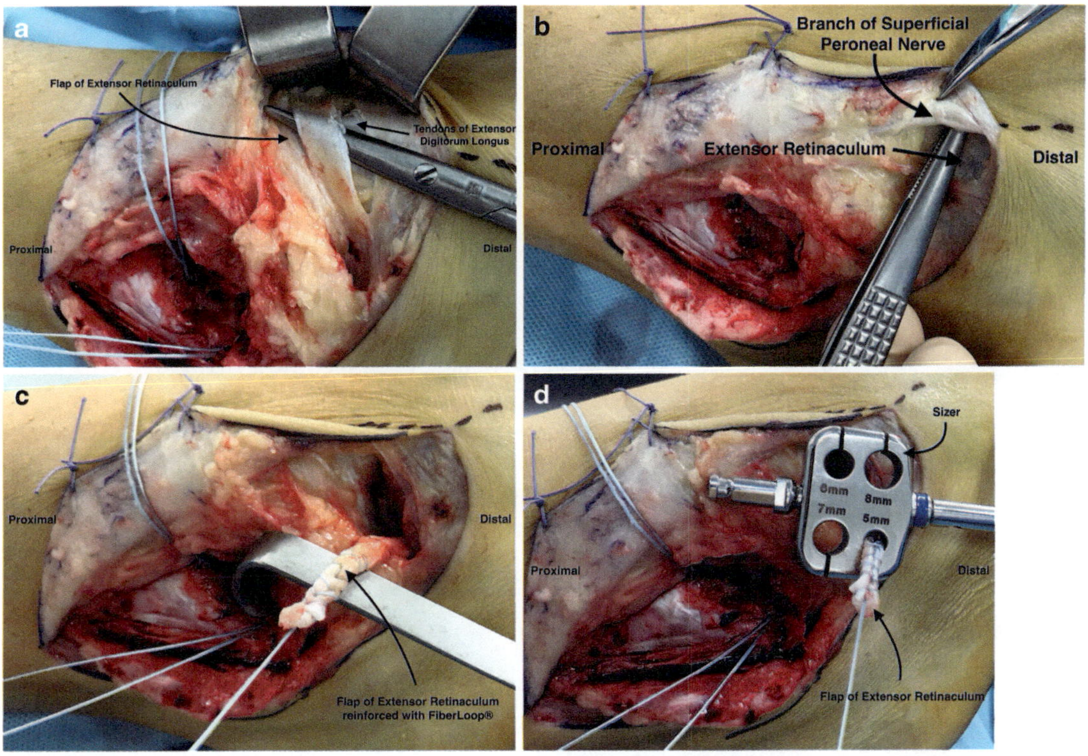

Fig. 16.8 Inferior Extensor retinaculum flap (IERF) elevation and preparation. (**a**) Subcutaneous release isolates the IER, from which a rectangular flap, about 1 cm width by 3–4 cm length, is harvested. Depending on the shape of the IER (X or Y, sometimes H), the bulkier part, so-called stem of frondiform ligament, is used. (**b**) It is mandatory to pay attention to the superficial branches of the peroneal and sural nerves. (**c**) The flap remains inserted on the calcaneus at the entry to the sinus tarsi. The neoligament is reinforced using a 2–0 non-absorbable looped suture: fiber loop. (**d**) Its size is checked. Because it remains attached to the calcaneus, this flap stabilizes the subtalar joint at the end of the procedure

The flap is passed through a short gap into the capsule, and then into the tunnel, using a Nitinol suture passing wire (Fig. 16.9c).

The unhindered sliding of this flap is checked prior to the final fixation.

16.2.6 Overall Fixations

The ATFL-inferior bundle with CFL first, then the ATFL-superior bundle with the capsule are secured to the previously placed anchors and so reinserted onto the anterior part of the lateral malleolus (Fig. 16.10a).

The sutures are tied to the ankle in a neutral position (Fig. 16.10b).

The extensor retinaculum flap is fixed by a Biotenodesis interference screw of 4.75 mm (Fig. 16.10c).

Its tension is checked.

16.2.7 Additional Procedures

The periosteal flap is repositioned on the lateral side of the fibular malleolus, reinforcing the reconstruction (Fig. 16.11a).

Further sutures, placed over the extensor digitorum brevis muscle, completely close the sinus tarsi entry, and reinforce the subtalar joint ligaments (Fig. 16.11b).

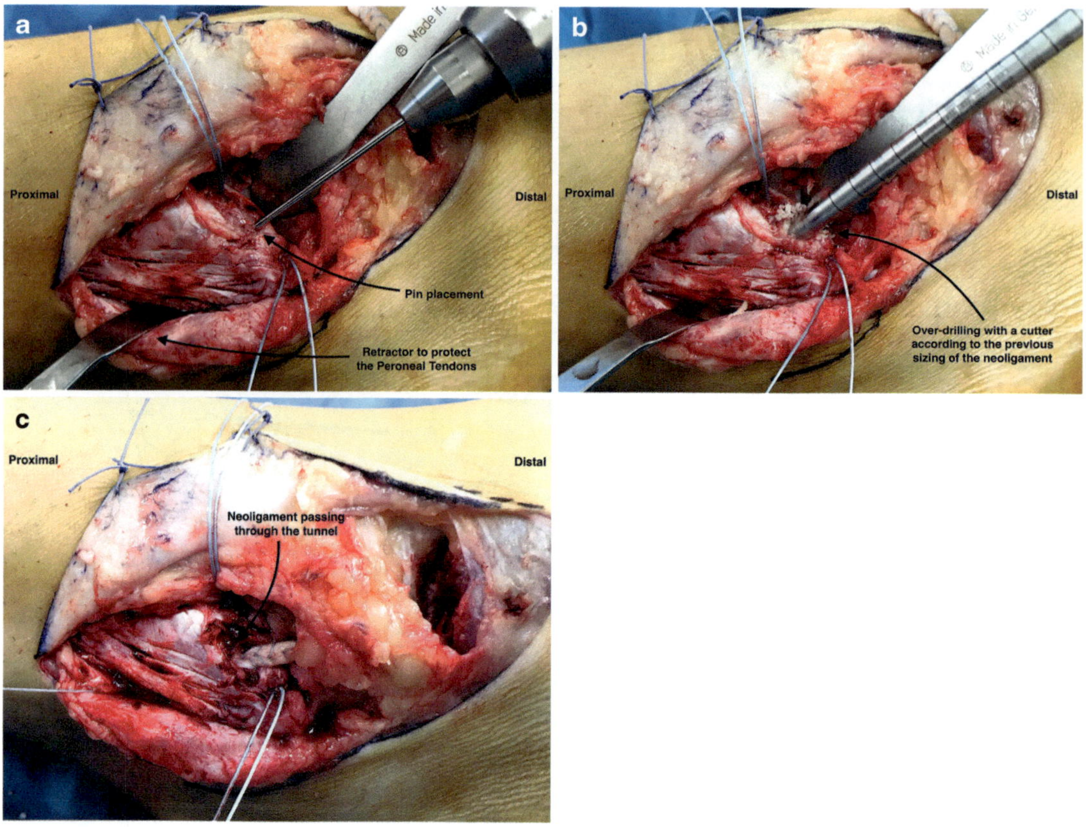

Fig. 16.9 Inferior Extensor retinaculum flap (IERF) reinsertion. (**a**) A 2.5 mm pin is inserted between the two anchors, from the anterior margin of the lateral malleolus to its posterior aspect. A retractor protects the fibular tendons. The orientation is 45° to the plantar aspect of the foot. (**b**) The pin is overdrilled according to the previous sizing of the neoligament (diameter between 4.5 and 5.0 mm). (**c**) The flap is passed through a short gap into the capsule and then into the tunnel, using a Nitinol suture passing wire. The unhindered sliding of this flap is checked prior to the final fixation

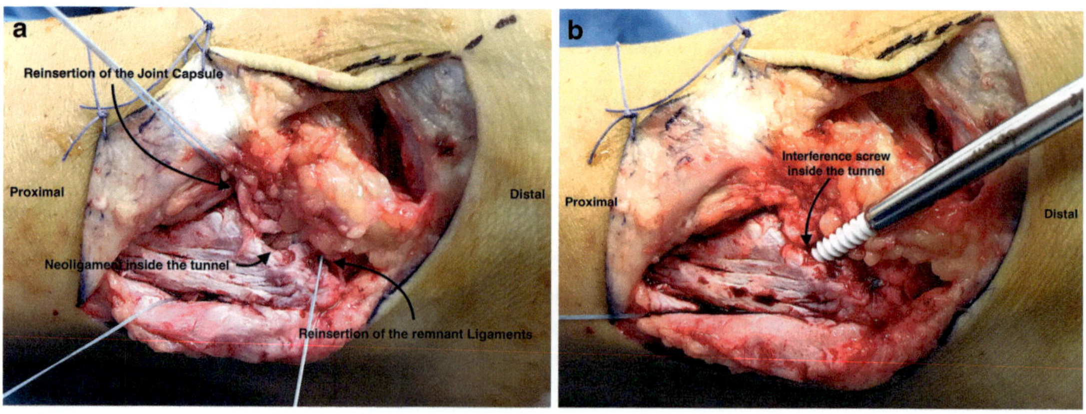

Fig. 16.10 Overall fixations. (**a**) The ATFL-inferior bundle with CFL first, then the ATFL-superior bundle with the capsule are secured to the previously placed anchors and so reinserted onto the anterior part of the lateral malleolus. The sutures are tied to the ankle in a neutral position. (**b**) The inferior extensor retinaculum flap is fixed by an interference screw of 4.75 mm. Its tension is checked

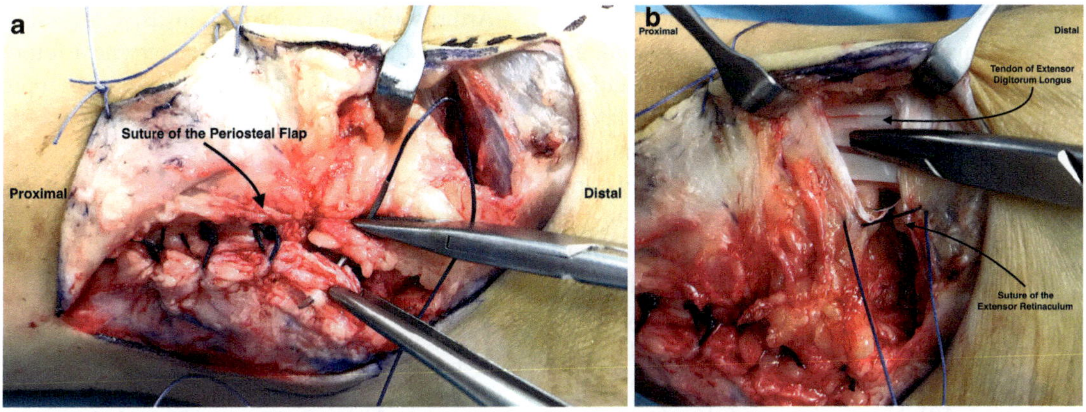

Fig. 16.11 Additional procedures. (**a**) The periosteal flap is repositioned on the lateral side of the fibular malleolus, reinforcing the reconstruction. (**b**) Further sutures, placed over the extensor digitorum brevis muscle, completely close the sinus tarsi entry and reinforce the subtalar joint ligaments. Subcutaneous and skin closures are performed

16.2.8 End Stage

Subcutaneous and skin closures are performed.

Immobilization is initiated for 3 weeks in a non-weight-bearing below-knee cast, followed, for 3 weeks, by a removable weight-bearing plastic boot to allow early rehabilitation.

Postoperative proprioceptive physiotherapy is routinely prescribed and completed [8].

16.3 Why to Use this Procedure?

1. The first step of this technique consists of an **anatomical repair**, as the Brostrom procedure, by repairing ATFL and CFL, on request. The preop assessments [1], but also intraoperative findings will validate the anatomic conditions of the remnant ligaments suitable for reinsertion. Nevertheless, this first step is rarely performed as a stand-alone procedure, regarding recurrence of laxity at long-term follow-up results, especially for high laxities [8].
2. So, **augmentation** is mandatory, using anatomical structures close to the collateral lateral ligament, such as peroneus brevis, periosteum, and, obviously, the extensor retinaculum [2, 9].
   (a) Furthermore, the literature findings recommend to avoid the use of the peroneus brevis entirely, muscle evertor, so essential to recover the proprioception after surgery. It leads to worse long-term results, with stiffness, lack of proprioception, and osteoarthritis at the ankle and the subtalar joints [1, 10–13]. Even partially, its use remains debated, with poor results also, at long-term follow-up [14]. So the use of the extensor retinaculum seems to be worldwide consensual [15]. The Gould technique [7], which consists of a proximal advancement of the extensor retinaculum, provides an enhanced proprioceptive environment, more than a mechanical support. This is correlated to the poor anatomical structure of the very proximal retinaculum. The inferior extensor retinaculum (IER) is an aponeurotic structure in continuation with the sural fascia. It could be a Y- or X-shaped structure with strong correlations to an intermediate dorsal cutaneous nerve (superficial peroneal nerve). To pay attention to those dorsal neurological structures is mandatory before using the IER. Furthermore, the X-shaped structure means a superolateral band very thin and so, not so powerful to increase the strength of the remnant ligaments reinsertion. These anatomical findings could advise against the use of the Gould augmentation [16, 17]. Furthermore, the restriction of the plantarflexion at the ankle has been reported [1, 18].

3. Thus, to perform a flap from the extensor retinaculum seems the best option. It remains independent from the extensor retinaculum but vascularized because fixed on the lateral aspect of the calcaneus. Its reinsertion into the lateral malleolus is closed to the ATFL and CFL footprints, at the anterior aspect of the distal end of the fibula. It works as a new ligament but stabilizes both the ankle and the subtalar joint. This is a very accurate key point while the literature reports over 65% of cervical ligament rupture combined with an ATFL one [12, 19]. No restriction of the plantarflexion was reported at the ankle joint [2].
4. The effectiveness of such a procedure was well established in the literature [2]. At long-term follow-up (medium 11 years) revision of 150 cases reported 95.2% of stable ankles, 3% only of ankle osteoarthritis (G2 of VanDijk staging) [20], with no subtalar joint stiffness. A recent publication confirmed those results [21].
5. Complimentary examinations such as CT arthrogram and MRI allow surgeons to identify preoperatively and correct, from the outset, multiple ligamentous injuries (lateral and medial talocrural, subtalar), associated lesions (osteochondral lesions of the talus, anterior and posterior impingement), and the morphotype of the hindfoot through calcaneal realignment osteotomy. Only a comprehensive clinical and radiographic assessment will yield the best possible outcomes [1].
6. Neuro-muscular balance reprogramming is mandatory to improve the reults of this technique [22].

16.4 Conclusions

The technique of repairing the collateral ligament bundles, using an extensor retinaculum flap as an augmentation, is the best option when the remnant ligaments (ATFL, CFL) are suitable for reinsertion.

The technique reported, with very satisfactory results at long-term follow-up, is an open one.

Arthroscopic or minimal invasive developments must be considered in the very next future and would be an alternative to arthroscopic reconstruction using (and scarifying) the Gracilis tendon.

References

1. Tourné Y, Besse JL, Mabit C. Chronic ankle instability. Which tests to assess the lesions? Which therapeutic options? Orthop Traumatol Surg Res. 2010;96:433–46.
2. Tourné Y, Mabit C, Moroney P, et al. Long-term follow-up of lateral reconstruction with extensor retinaculum flap for chronic ankle instability. Foot Ankle Int. 2012;33(12):1079–86.
3. Brostrom L. Sprained ankles. V. Treatment and prognosis in recent ligament ruptures. Acta Chir Scand. 1966;132:537–50.
4. Duquennoy A, Letendard J, Loock P. Remise en tension ligamentaire externe dans les instabilitès chroniques de la cheville. Apropos de 22 cas. Rev Chir Orthop. 1980;66:311–6.
5. Saragaglia D, Fontanel F, Montbarbon E, et al. Reconstruction for the lateral ankle ligaments using an inferior extensor retinaculum flap. Foot Ankle Int. 1997;18:723–5.
6. Blanchet A. La réfection capsuloligamentaire dans les instabilités chroniques de la tibiotarsienne. Rev Chir Orthop. 1975;61(suppl II):175–6.
7. Gould N, Seligson D, Gassman J. Early and late repair of the lateral ligament of the ankle. Foot Ankle. 1980;1:354–8.
8. Mabit C, Tourné Y, Besse J-L, et al. Chronic lateral ankle instability surgical repairs: the long-term prospective. Orthop Traumatol Surg Res. 2010;96:417–23.
9. Tourné Y, Mabit C. Lateral ligament reconstruction procedures for the ankle. Orthop Traumatol Surg Res. 2017;103(1):S171–81.
10. Krips R, Brandsson S, Swensson C. Anatomical reconstruction and Evans tenodesis of the lateral ligaments of the ankle: clinical and radiological findings after follow up for 15 to 30 years. J Bone Joint Surg Am. 2002;84:232–6.
11. Krips R, Van Dijk CN, Halasi PT. Long-term outcome of anatomical reconstruction versus tenodesis for the treatment of chronic anterolateral instability of the ankle joint: a multicenter study. Foot Ankle Int. 2001;22(5):415–21.
12. Mabit C, Chaudruc JM, Fiorenza F. Lateral ligament reconstruction of the ankle: comparative study of peroneus brevis tenodesis versus periostal ligamentoplasty. Foot Ankle Surg. 1998;4:71–6.

13. Van der Rijt A, Evans GA. The long term results of Watson Jones tenodesis. J Bone Joint Surg Br. 1984;66:371–5.
14. Schepers T, Vogels LMM, van Lieshout EMM. Hemi-Castaing ligamentoplasty for the treatment of chronic lateral ankle instability: a retrospective assessment and outcome. Int Orthop. 2011;35:1805–12.
15. Guillo T, Bauer JW, Lee M, Takao SW, Kong JW, Stone PG, Mangone A, Molloy A, Perera CJ, Pearce F, Michels Y, Tourné A, Ghorbani J. Calder consensus in chronic ankle instability: aetiology, assessment, surgical indications and place for arthroscopy. Orthop Traumatol Surg Res. 2013;99S:S411–9.
16. Dalmau-Pastor M, Yasui Y, Calder JD, Karlsson J, Kerkhoffs GM, Kennedy JG. Anatomy of the inferior extensor retinaculum and its role in lateral ankle ligament reconstruction: a pictorial essay. Knee Surg Sports Traumatol Arthrosc. 2016;24(4):957–62.
17. Dalmau-Pastor M, Malagelada F, Kerkhoffs GMMJ, Manzanares MC. Vega J. X-shaped inferior extensor retinaculum and its doubtful use in the Bröstrom-Gould procedure. Knee Surg Sports Traumatol Arthrosc. 2018;26(7):2171–6.
18. Muijs SP, Dijkstra PD, Bos CF. Clinical outcome after anatomical reconstruction of the lateral ankle ligaments using the Duquennoy technique in chronic lateral instability of the ankle: a long-term follow-up study. J Bone Joint Surg. 2008;90(1):50–6.
19. Bonnel F, Toullec E, Mabit C, Tourné Y. Chronic ankle instability: biomechanics and pathomechanics of ligaments injury and associated lesions. Orthop Traumatol Surg Res. 2010;96:424–32.
20. Van Dijk CN, Tol JL, Verheyen CC. A prospective study of prognostic factors concerning the outcome of arthroscopic surgery for anterior ankle impingement. Am J Sports Med. 1997;25:737–45.
21. Trichine F, Friha T, Boukabou A, Belaid L, Bouzidi T, Bouzitouna M. Surgical treatment of chronic lateral ankle instability using an inferior extensor retinaculum flap: a retrospective study. J Foot Ankle Surg. 2018;57(2):226–31.
22. Pearce CJ, Tourné Y, Zellers J, Terrier R, Toschi P, Silbernagel KG. ESKKA-AFAS ankle instability group rehabilitation after anatomical ankle ligament repair or reconstruction. Knee Surg Sports Traumatol Arthrosc. 2016;24(4):1130–9.

17 Anatomical Reconstruction: Open Procedure to Percutaneous Procedure (P-AntiRoLL)

Masato Takao, James Stone, and Mark Glazebrook

In 2014, Dr. Glazebrook devised a percutaneous procedure for the reconstruction of the lateral ligaments of the ankle. We developed this technique and reached clinical application [1]. This procedure is superior in many respects compared to open surgery [2], so we left open surgery and shifted to percutaneous anatomical reconstruction of the lateral ligaments of the ankle (P-AntiRoLL, see Chap. 31).

In this chapter, we would like to describe P-AntiRoLL technique.

17.1 Indication

Choice of a surgical procedure is performed by evaluating the quality of the residual ligament with stress ultrasonography before surgery (see Chap. 26). P-AntiRoLL is selected if there is no ligament fiber on stress ultrasonography, and there are no intra-articular comorbid lesions including osteochondral lesions and/or anterior ankle impingement on MRI or CT scan before surgery. If there were intra-articular lesions, it may be better to perform A-AntiRoLL [3] (see Chap. 31).

There are five steps for P-Antiroll; step 1 as to make the portals, step 2 as to make a Y-shaped graft, step 3 as to make the bone tunnels at each attachment to fibula, talus, and calcaneus, step 4 as to collect the guide threads inserted from each portal into one portal, and step 5 as to introduce a Y-shaped graft into the bone tunnels and fix with the interference screw.

17.2 Surgical Procedure

17.2.1 Position

The position is supine, and the lower leg is held with a leg holder (see Chap. 26). The tourniquet is not normally used, but it should be worn on the thigh for use when the field of vision is hindered by bleeding. Fluoroscopy is useful for correctly positioning the bone tunnels.

17.2.1.1 Step 1: Make Portals

Fibular, talar, and calcaneal portals are used (Fig. 17.1).

M. Takao (✉)
Clinical and Research Institute for Foot and Ankle Surgery, Jujo Hospital, Kisarazu, Chiba, Japan
e-mail: m.takao@carifas.com

J. Stone
Medical College of Wisconsin, Milwaukee, WI, USA

M. Glazebrook
Department of Orthopaedic Surgery, Dalhousie University, Halifax, NS, Canada

H. Pereira et al. (eds.), *Lateral Ankle Instability*, https://doi.org/10.1007/978-3-662-62763-1_17

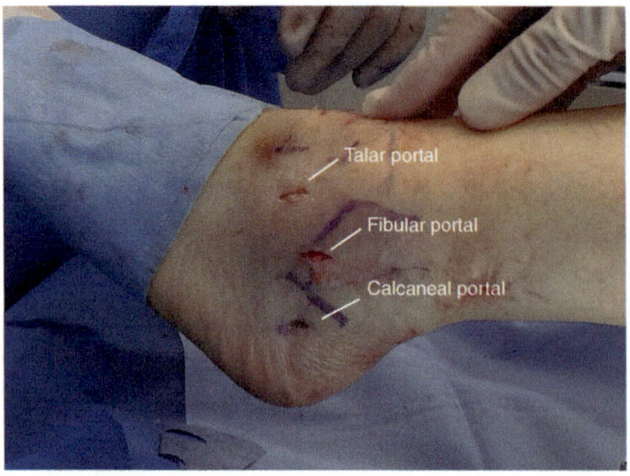

Fig. 17.1 Portals

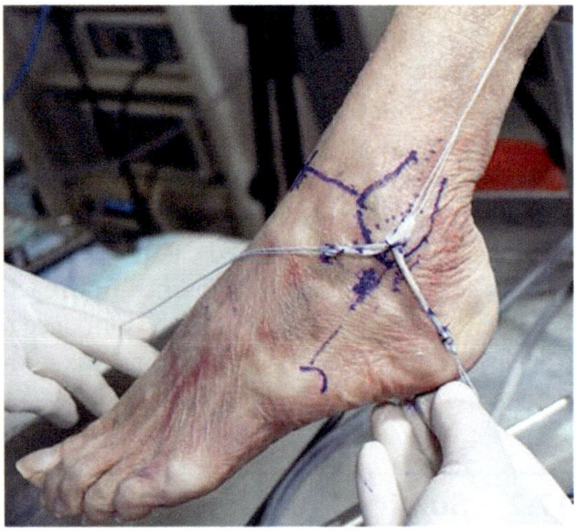

Fig. 17.2 Y-shaped tendon graft

17.2.1.2 Step 2: Make a Y-Shaped Graft

An autologous gracilis tendon is harvested from ipsilateral knee and it is formed to Y-shaped tendon graft [2] (Fig. 17.2, see Chap. 26).

17.2.1.3 Step 3: Make the Bone Tunnels at Each Attachment to Fibula, Talus, and Calcaneus

Positioning of each fibular, talar, and calcaneal bone tunnels are made by using the landmarks existing on the bone surface [4] (see Chap. 26).

A landmark for fibular bone tunnel is fibular obscure tubercle (FOT) which exists at the border of the footprints of the ATFL and the CFL, and it is easy to palpate over the skin and easy to clarify fluoroscopically [4]. After blunt dissection and palpate a FOT with mosquito Pean (Fig. 17.3a), a guide wire for cannulated drill is inserted via fibular portal and penetrates the center of the fibula at FOT toward the direction of proximal-posterior fibular cortex as 30° to the axis of fibula (Fig. 17.3b), and finally penetrates the posterior leg skin (Fig. 17.3c). Next, an overdrilling 6 mm in diameter and 20 mm in depth is done using cannulated drill (Fig. 17.3c). Finally, a guide wire is replaced to guide thread (Fig. 17.3d).

A landmark for talar bone tunnel is anterolateral and posterolateral corners of the talar body (see Chap. 26). Under fluoroscopy, on the line to connect the anterolateral and posterolateral corners of the talar body, about 40% inferior point from anterolateral corner of the talar body is the center of the footprint of the ATFL [4]. A guide wire for cannulated drill is inserted via talar portal and penetrates the talus (Fig. 17.3d) toward the direction to the tip of the medial malleolus (Fig. 17.3e), and finally penetrates the skin (Fig. 17.3f). Next, an overdrilling 6 mm in diameter and 20 mm in depth is done using a cannulated drill (Fig. 17.3g). Finally, a guide wire is replaced to guide thread (Fig. 17.3h).

A landmark for calcaneal bone tunnel is the posterior facet of the talocalcaneal joint (see Chap. 26). On the line perpendicular bisector of the posterior facet, 17 mm inferior point from the posterior facet is the center of the footprint of the CFL [4]. But in actual cases, peroneal tendons run just over the insertion of the CFL. To avoid damage to the peroneal tendons, the authors make a calcaneal bone tunnel proximal to the peroneal tendon sheath, about 10 mm inferior point from the posterior facet. A guide wire for cannulated drill is inserted via calcaneal portal (Fig. 17.3i) and penetrates the calcaneus in

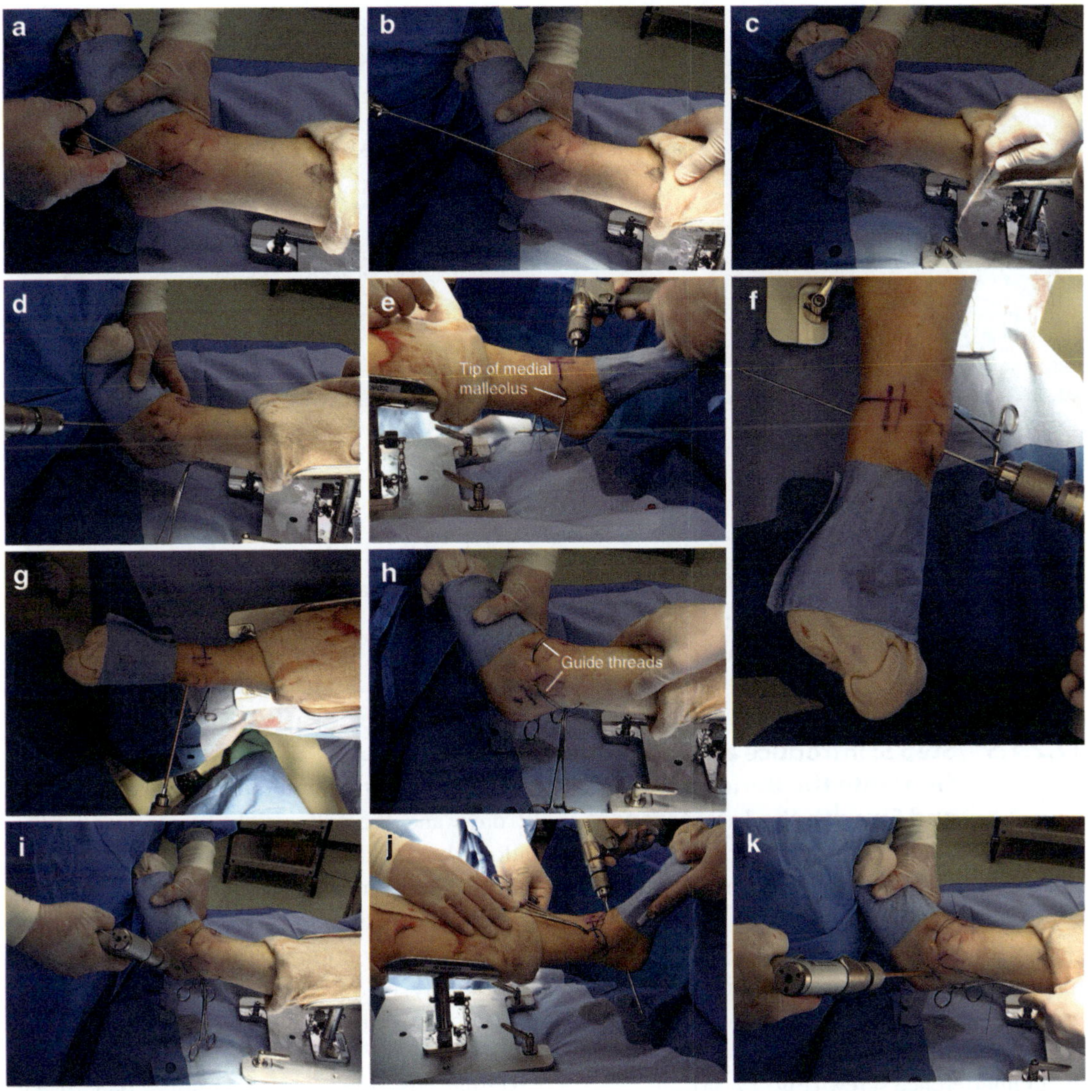

Fig. 17.3 Make the bone tunnels at each attachment to fibula, talus, and calcaneus. (**a**) Blunt dissection and palpate a FOT with mosquito Pean. (**b**) A guide wire for cannulated drill is inserted via fibular portal and penetrates the center of the fibula at FOT toward the direction of proximal-posterior fibular cortex as 30° to the axis of fibula, and finally penetrates the posterior leg skin. (**c**) An over-drilling 6 mm in diameter and 20 mm in depth is done using cannulated drill. (**d**) A guide wire for cannulated drill is inserted via talar portal and penetrates the talus. (**e**) A direction of talar guide wire is toward the direction to tip of the medial malleolus. (**f**) Finally penetrates the skin. (**g**) Next an over-drilling 6 mm in diameter and 20 mm in depth is done using cannulated drill. (**h**) A guide wire is replaced to guide thread. (**i**) A guide wire for cannulated drill is inserted via calcaneal portal. (**j**) Penetrate the calcaneus as the direction of the center of the posterior corner of the calcaneus and finally penetrate the posterior heel skin. (**k**) An over-drilling 6 mm in diameter and 20 mm in depth is done using cannulated drill

the direction of the center of the posterior corner of the calcaneus, and finally penetrates the posterior heel skin (Fig. 17.3j). Next, an over-drilling 6 mm in diameter and 20 mm in depth is done using cannulated drill (Fig. 17.3k). Finally, a guide wire is replaced to guide thread.

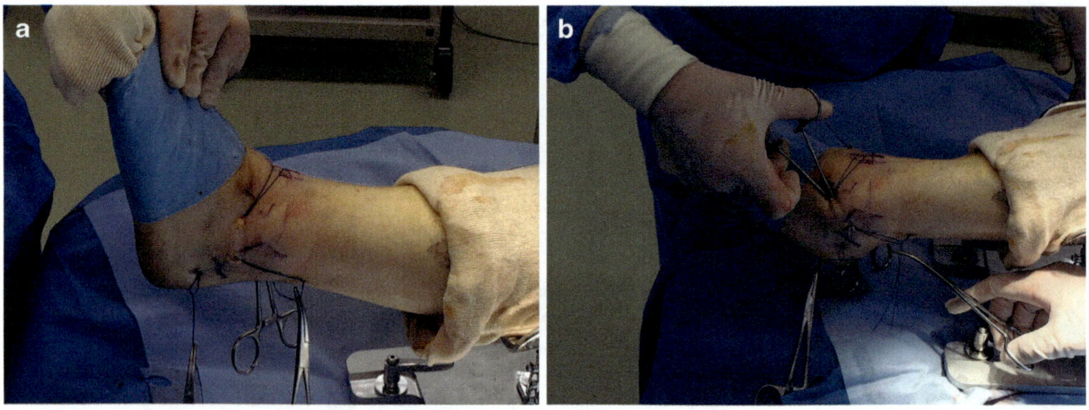

Fig. 17.4 Collect the guide threads into one portal. (**a**) In this time, guide threads are inserted from all three portals. (**b**) Each guide threads are collected into one portal. In this case, the guide threads were collected in talar portal

17.2.1.4 Step 4: Collect the Guide Threads into One Portal

In this time, guide threads are inserted from all three portals (Fig. 17.4a). Each guide threads are collected into one portal (Fig. 17.4b).

17.2.1.5 Step 5: Introduce a Y-Shaped Graft into the Bone Tunnels and Fix with the Interference Screw

A Y-shaped graft is introduced and fixed into the bone tunnels firstly fibula, next talus, and finally calcaneus. It is important to insert a guide wire for the interference screw before introducing a graft into the bone tunnels to prevent penetrating the graft by a guide wire following graft damage by an interference screw (Fig. 17.5a).

A fibular end of a Y-shaped graft is introduced into the fibular bone tunnel using guide thread with inside-out technique at the level of the suture which ties the graft at the position 15 mm from the turning point (Fig. 17.5b). A graft is fixed into the bone tunnel with an interference screw 6 mm in diameter and 15 or 20 mm in length (Fig. 17.5c).

Then, the talar and calcaneal ends of a Y-shaped graft are introduced into each bone tunnel using guide thread with inside-out technique (Fig. 17.5d). As ankle is positioned in 0° neutral position and to tensile the tendon graft pulling a guide thread manually, a graft is fixed into the bone tunnel with an interference screw 6 mm in diameter and 15 or 20 mm in length.

All guide threads can be removed easily to cut the one end near the skin and pull the other end manually.

17.3 Postoperative Management

After surgery, the elastic bandage is applied for 2 days and the full weight-bearing walking is allowed according to pain from a day after surgery. The bone tendon attachment gradually increases the strength of biological bonding and becomes nearly normal strength at 4 weeks postoperatively [4]. Accordingly, jogging and proprioceptive training will be from 4 weeks postoperatively and return to sports without external fixation shall be after 6–8 weeks postoperative.

17.4 Summary

Arthroscopic AntiRoLL (A-AntiRoLL) is an anatomical reconstruction of the lateral ligaments of the ankle performing all arthroscopically with minor invasion. It is superior in many respects compared to open surgery, so the authors left open surgery and shifted to P-AntiRoLL. The author recommends it for surgical treatment of lateral instability of the ankle if there is no ligament fiber and there are no intra-articular comorbid lesions including osteochondral lesions and/

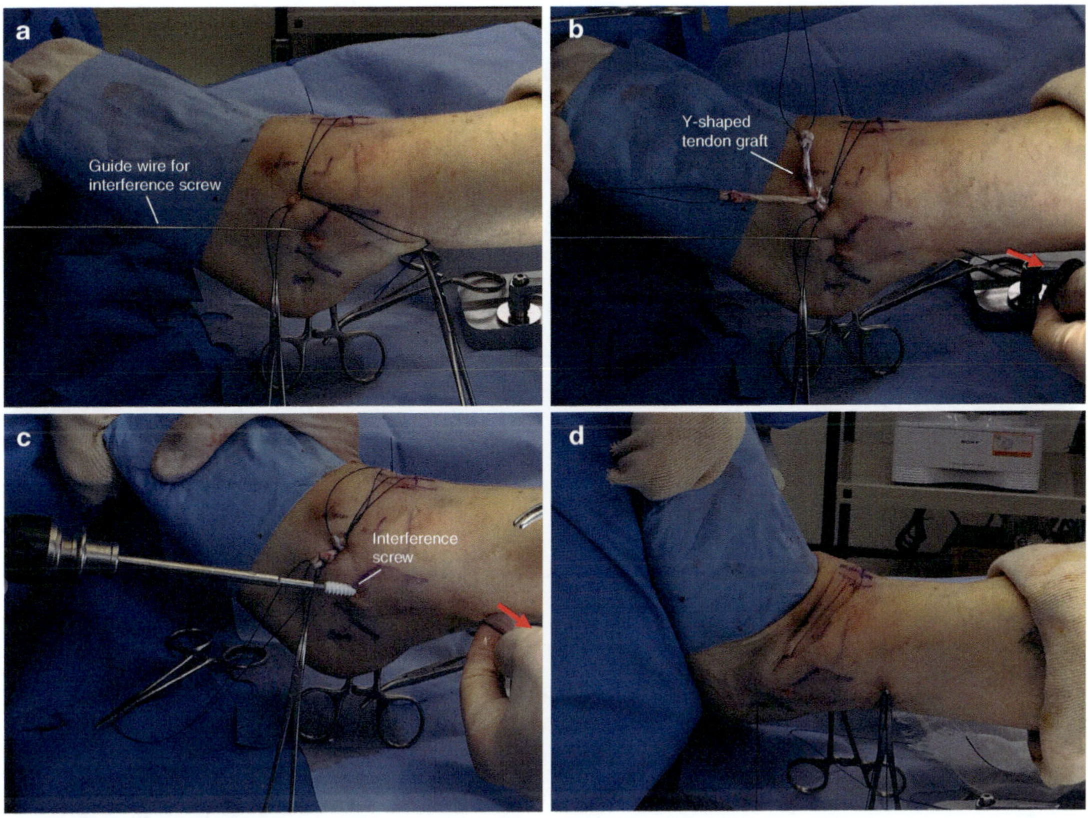

Fig. 17.5 Introduce a Y-shaped graft into the bone tunnels and fix with the interference screw. (**a**) A guide wire for interference screw is inserted into the fibular bone tunnel via fibular portal. (**b**) A fibular end of a Y-shaped graft is introduced into the fibular bone tunnel using a guide thread with inside-out technique. (**c**) A graft is fixed into the bone tunnel with an interference screw 6 mm in diameter and 15 or 20 mm in length. (**d**) Then, a talar and calcaneal ends of a Y-shaped graft are introduced into each bone tunnel and fixed into the bone tunnel with an interference screw

or anterior ankle impingement on MRI or CT scan before surgery. If there were intra-articular lesions, it may be better to perform A-AntiRoLL which can be used to treat the intra-articular lesions simultaneously (see Chap. 31).

References

1. Glazebrook M, Stone J, Matsui K, Guillo S, Takao M, ESSKA-AFAS Ankle Instability Group. Percutaneous ankle reconstruction of lateral ligaments (Perc-Anti RoLL). Foot Ankle Int. 2016;37:659–64.
2. Takao M, Oae K, Uchio Y, Ochi M, Yamamoto H. Anatomical reconstruction of the lateral ligaments of the ankle with a gracilis autograft: a new technique using an interference-fit anchoring system. Am J Sports Med. 2005;33:814–23.
3. Takao M, Glazebrook MA, Stone JW, Guillo S, Ankle Instability Group. Ankle arthroscopic reconstruction of lateral ligaments (Ankle Anti-ROLL). Arthrosc Tech. 2015;4:e595–600.
4. Matsui K, Oliva XM, Takao M, Pereira BS, Gomes TM, Lozano JM; ESSKA AFAS Ankle Instability Group, Glazebrook M. Bony landmarks available for minimally invasive lateral ankle stabilization surgery: a cadaveric anatomical study. Knee Surg Sports Traumatol Arthrosc. 2017;25:1916–24.

Open Surgical Treatment: Nonanatomic Reconstruction

18

Kwang Hwan Park, Gwen Vuurberg,
Hélder Pereira, Mike Carmont, and Jin Woo Lee

18.1 History of Nonanatomic Reconstruction

There have been more than 80 surgical procedures in previous literature for the treatment of the chronic lateral ankle instability [1]. The surgical procedures are divided into two broad categories: anatomic procedures and nonanatomic procedures. Nonanatomic procedures include nonanatomic tendon transfer and tenodesis for the substitution of the injured ligaments and the correction of the pathological ankle mobility [2]. Most of these procedures have utilized the peroneal tendons to restore ankle stability through restraint of inversion and anterior translation by placing graft tendon perpendicular to the line of instability (Fig. 18.1). These procedures required harvesting all or part of the peroneus brevis tendon as proximally as possible, conserving the distal insertion onto the fifth metatarsal styloid process and rerouting the tendon through bone tunnels [3–8]. We considered these historical value procedures due to in nature problems of nonanatomic procedure.

Historically, surgical treatment of lateral ligament instability was first described in 1932 involving a nonanatomic peroneus brevis transfer based on the work of Gallie in 1913 in the paralytic clubfoot [9, 10]. Thereafter, many peroneal tendon sacrificing procedures were introduced and were used widely [11]. In 1952, Watson-Jones described ATFL reconstruction using the entire peroneus brevis, through two horizontal fibular tunnels and one tunnel in the neck of talus [12]. This procedure effectively reinforced the weak anterior drawer but less effectively corrected the lateral talocrural opening due to lack of CFL reconstruction [12]. In 1953, Evans reported a rerouting procedure of peroneus brevis tendon through an oblique fibular tunnel. This tenodesis procedure reconstructed neither the ATFL nor the CFL but functioned as a sum of the two vectors

K. H. Park · J. W. Lee (✉)
Yonsei University College of Medicine, Seoul, Republic of Korea
e-mail: khpark@yuhs.ac; LJWOS@yuhs.ac

G. Vuurberg
Department of Orthopedic Surgery, Academic Medical Center, University of Amsterdam, Amsterdam Movement Sciences, Amsterdam, The Netherlands
e-mail: g.vuurberg@amc.uva.nl

H. Pereira
Orthopedic Department, Centro Hospitalar Póvoa de Varzim, Vila do Conde, Portugal

Ripoll y De Prado Sports Clinic: FIFA Medical Centre of Excellence, Murcia-Madrid, Spain

International Sports Traumatology Centre of the Ave, Vila do Conde, Portugal

M. Carmont
The Princess Royal Hospital, Shrewsbury & Telford NHS Trust and the Northern General Hospital, Sheffield Teaching Hospitals NHS Foundation Trust, Sheffield, UK

H. Pereira et al. (eds.), *Lateral Ankle Instability*, https://doi.org/10.1007/978-3-662-62763-1_18

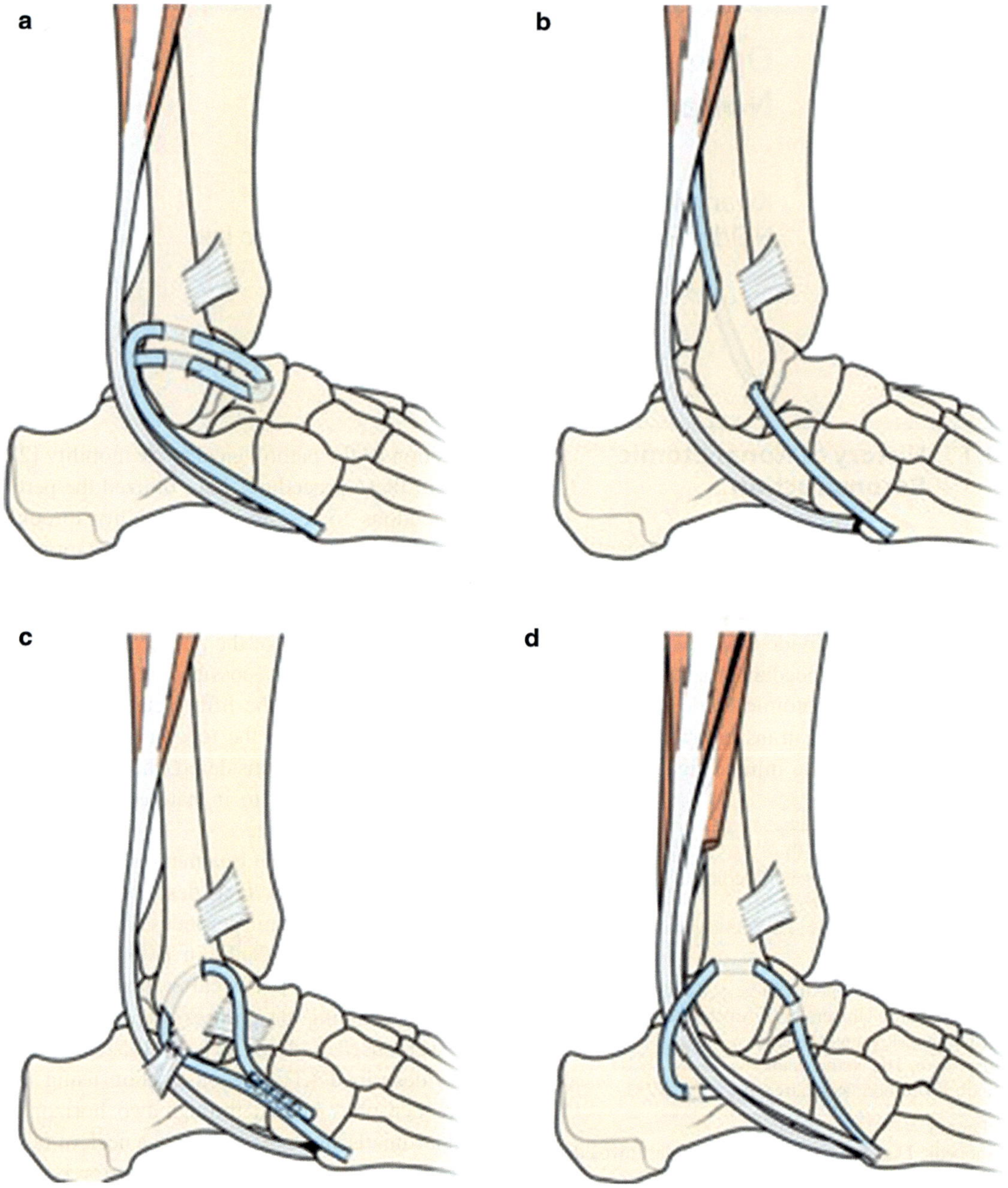

Fig. 18.1 Nonanatomic reconstruction using peroneal brevis tendon. (**a**) Watson-Jones procedure, (**b**) Evans procedure, (**c**) Castaing procedure, (**d**) Chrisman–Snook procedure

[6]. In 1961, Castaing described a ligamentoplasty technique using the entire peroneus brevis tendon. Later it was shown that the hemi-Castaing procedure by using a split tendon in 1978 provides a better outcome [13]. In 1969, Chrisman–Snook reported a modification of the Elmslie procedure (anatomical reconstruction using fascia lata) with the tenodesis to fibula and calcaneus using a split peroneus brevis for the reconstruction of the ATFL and CFL [3].

Table 18.1 Results of nonanatomic reconstruction techniques

	Follow-up	Good/very good	Residual instability	Osteoarthritis
Watson-Jones /Evans	>10 years	50/70%	15/44%	20/40%
Castaing	>10 years	71–80%	32%	Unknown
Hemi-Castaing	>10 years	91/92%	4/20%	4%

Reference: Tourné Y, Mabit C. Lateral ligament reconstruction procedures for the ankle. Orthop Traumatol Surg Res. 2017;103(1S):S171–S181

18.2 Outcomes and Complications of Nonanatomic Reconstruction

Stability and long-term control of progression towards osteoarthritis are the two main criterias referred in the literature and should guide the choice of reconstruction technique (Table 18.1) [12–14]. About 88% of patients revealed good-to-excellent results in Watson-Jones reconstruction procedure after 13-year follow-up [15]. The Watson-Jones technique, with 50–70% good and very good results, which is more than Evans procedure, showed stability loss and induced osteoarthritis in the long term [13, 16–18]. Also, the Watson-Jones technique was not as good as anatomic repair with reinforcement [16, 17]. Long-term results with the Castaing technique vary between 71 and 80% good and very good results [18]. Reconstruction with the whole peroneal tendon gives poorer long-term results than reconstruction using a hemi-tendon but, even using a hemi-tendon, reconstruction with the peroneal tendon gives poorer results than other techniques [12, 13, 18, 19]. In the Chrisman–Snook reconstruction procedure, the peroneus brevis tendon is the first split and then driven into the fibula and then into the calcaneus [3]. This procedure supports anatomic reconstruction, but some patients were reported to experience nonphysiological kinematics and subtalar stiffness [20].

Long-term outcomes of nonanatomic reconstructions are hindered by alterations in ankle and hindfoot kinematics and often result in loss of subtalar motion [17, 21–27]. Although initial reports were promising, comparison studies with longer follow-up, generally favor anatomic repair over nonanatomic tenodesis reconstructions [28]. Mabit et al. were the first to compare anatomic repair with nonanatomic reconstruction, showing superior short-term results for anatomic repair [29]. Other studies confirmed these results [30–34]. Krips et al. published a series of comparison studies, including more than 300 patients, with up to 30 years of follow-up data [17, 27]. These authors ultimately concluded that long-term, nonanatomic tenodesis lead to decreased function, increased pain, limited range of motion, instability, increased need for revision procedures, and greater degrees of osteoarthritis compared to anatomic reconstructions [28].

Several studies reported an increased rate of complications in nonanatomic techniques as compared with anatomic procedures. Abnormal ankle kinematics and restricted subtalar motion are the major drawbacks encountered with nonanatomic reconstruction [35–37]. Also, these techniques often result in joint stiffness and limited range of motion of the ankle and subtalar joints [2, 15, 17, 38–40]. In addition, splitting the peroneus brevis tendon for use of the reconstruction may weaken or affect the performance of the main tendon responsible for dynamic stabilization of the lateral ankle complex [41].

18.3 Conclusion

The ankle joint is a complex anatomic structure in which stability and mobility depend on accurate ligamentous balancing and support. The goal of surgery is to restore the isometricity of the torn ligaments thus obtaining ankle kinematics as similar as possible to the contralateral healthy side. However, most studies have shown restricted ankle and subtalar motion as well as arthritic changes associated with these procedures. For these reasons, the various nonanatomic reconstructions should be thought of as historical in nature and the author should not endorse them.

References

1. Bauer GR. New method for reconstruction in lateral ankle instability. J Am Podiatr Med Assoc. 1995;85(9):459–63. https://doi.org/10.7547/87507315-85-9-459.
2. Giannini S, Ruffilli A, Pagliazzi G, Mazzotti A, Evangelisti G, Buda R, Faldini C. Treatment algorithm for chronic lateral ankle instability. Muscles Ligaments Tendons J. 2014;4(4):455–60.
3. Chrisman OD, Snook GA. Reconstruction of lateral ligament tears of the ankle. An experimental study and clinical evaluation of seven patients treated by a new modification of the Elmslie procedure. J Bone Joint Surg Am. 1969;51(5):904–12.
4. Clanton TO. Athletic injuries to the soft tissues of the foot and ankle. In: Coughlin MJ, Saltzman C, Anderson RB, editors. Mann's surgery of the foot and ankle. 9th ed. Philadelphia, PA: Elsevier; 2014. p. 1570–9.
5. Colville MR, Grondel RJ. Anatomic reconstruction of the lateral ankle ligaments using a split peroneus brevis tendon graft. Am J Sports Med. 1995;23(2):210–3. https://doi.org/10.1177/036354659502300214.
6. Evans DL. Recurrent instability of the ankle; a method of surgical treatment. Proc R Soc Med. 1953;46(5):343–4.
7. Girard P, Anderson RB, Davis WH, Isear JA, Kiebzak GM. Clinical evaluation of the modified Brostrom-Evans procedure to restore ankle stability. Foot Ankle Int. 1999;20(4):246–52. https://doi.org/10.1177/107110079902000407.
8. Snook GA, Chrisman OD, Wilson TC. Long-term results of the Chrisman-Snook operation for reconstruction of the lateral ligaments of the ankle. J Bone Joint Surg Am. 1985;67(1):1–7.
9. Gallie WE. VIII. Tendon fixation: a preliminary report of a simple operation for the prevention of deformity in paralytic talipes. Ann Surg. 1913;57(3):427–9.
10. Shakked RJ, Karnovsky S, Drakos MC. Operative treatment of lateral ligament instability. Curr Rev Musculoskelet Med. 2017;10(1):113–21. https://doi.org/10.1007/s12178-017-9391-x.
11. Bonnin JG. Injuries to the ankle. Darien, CT: Hafner; 1970. p. 109–18.
12. Tourne Y, Mabit C. Lateral ligament reconstruction procedures for the ankle. Orthop Traumatol Surg Res. 2017;103(1S):S171–81. https://doi.org/10.1016/j.otsr.2016.06.026.
13. Tourne Y, Besse JL, Mabit C, Sofcot. Chronic ankle instability. Which tests to assess the lesions? Which therapeutic options? Orthop Traumatol Surg Res. 2010;96(4):433–46. https://doi.org/10.1016/j.otsr.2010.04.005.
14. Guillo S, Bauer T, Lee JW, Takao M, Kong SW, Stone JW, Mangone PG, Molloy A, Perera A, Pearce CJ, Michels F, Tourne Y, Ghorbani A, Calder J. Consensus in chronic ankle instability: aetiology, assessment, surgical indications and place for arthroscopy. Orthop Traumatol Surg Res. 2013;99(8 Suppl):S411–9. https://doi.org/10.1016/j.otsr.2013.10.009.
15. Sugimoto K, Takakura Y, Akiyama K, Kamei S, Kitada C, Kumai T. Long-term results of Watson-Jones tenodesis of the ankle. Clinical and radiographic findings after ten to eighteen years of follow-up. J Bone Joint Surg Am. 1998;80(11):1587–96.
16. Krips R, Brandsson S, Swensson C, van Dijk CN, Karlsson J. Anatomical reconstruction and Evans tenodesis of the lateral ligaments of the ankle. Clinical and radiological findings after follow-up for 15 to 30 years. J Bone Joint Surg Br. 2002;84(2):232–6.
17. Krips R, van Dijk CN, Halasi PT, Lehtonen H, Corradini C, Moyen B, Karlsson J. Long-term outcome of anatomical reconstruction versus tenodesis for the treatment of chronic anterolateral instability of the ankle joint: a multicenter study. Foot Ankle Int. 2001;22(5):415–21. https://doi.org/10.1177/107110070102200510.
18. Mabit C, Tourne Y, Besse JL, Bonnel F, Toullec E, Giraud F, Proust J, Khiami F, Chaussard C, Genty C, Sofcot. Chronic lateral ankle instability surgical repairs: the long term prospective. Orthop Traumatol Surg Res. 2010;96(4):417–23. https://doi.org/10.1016/j.otsr.2010.04.004.
19. Schepers T, Vogels LM, Van Lieshout EM. Hemi-Castaing ligamentoplasty for the treatment of chronic lateral ankle instability: a retrospective assessment of outcome. Int Orthop. 2011;35(12):1805–12. https://doi.org/10.1007/s00264-011-1284-9.
20. Al-Mohrej OA, Al-Kenani NS. Chronic ankle instability: current perspectives. Avicenna J Med. 2016;6(4):103–8. https://doi.org/10.4103/2231-0770.191446.
21. Bahr R, Pena F, Shine J, Lew WD, Tyrdal S, Engebretsen L. Biomechanics of ankle ligament reconstruction. An in vitro comparison of the Brostrom repair, Watson-Jones reconstruction, and a new anatomic reconstruction technique. Am J Sports Med. 1997;25(4):424–32. https://doi.org/10.1177/036354659702500402.
22. de Vries JS, Krips R, Sierevelt IN, Blankevoort L. Interventions for treating chronic ankle instability. Cochrane Database Syst Rev. 2006;(4):CD004124. https://doi.org/10.1002/14651858.CD004124.pub2.
23. de Vries JS, Krips R, Sierevelt IN, Blankevoort L, van Dijk CN. Interventions for treating chronic ankle instability. Cochrane Database Syst Rev. 2011;(8):CD004124. https://doi.org/10.1002/14651858.CD004124.pub3.
24. Hennrikus WL, Mapes RC, Lyons PM, Lapoint JM. Outcomes of the Chrisman-Snook and modified-Brostrom procedures for chronic lateral ankle insta-

bility. A prospective, randomized comparison. Am J Sports Med. 1996;24(4):400–4. https://doi.org/10.1177/036354659602400402.
25. Korkala O, Sorvali T, Niskanen R, Haapala J, Tanskanen P, Kuokkanen H. Twenty-year results of the Evans operation for lateral instability of the ankle. Clin Orthop Relat Res. 2002;405:195–8.
26. Korkala O, Tanskanen P, Makijarvi J, Sorvali T, Ylikoski M, Haapala J. Long-term results of the Evans procedure for lateral instability of the ankle. J Bone Joint Surg Br. 1991;73(1):96–9.
27. Krips R, van Dijk CN, Halasi T, Lehtonen H, Moyen B, Lanzetta A, Farkas T, Karlsson J. Anatomical reconstruction versus tenodesis for the treatment of chronic anterolateral instability of the ankle joint: a 2- to 10-year follow-up, multicenter study. Knee Surg Sports Traumatol Arthrosc. 2000;8(3):173–9. https://doi.org/10.1007/s001670050210.
28. McCriskin BJ, Cameron KL, Orr JD, Waterman BR. Management and prevention of acute and chronic lateral ankle instability in athletic patient populations. World J Orthop. 2015;6(2):161–71. https://doi.org/10.5312/wjo.v6.i2.161.
29. Pijnenburg AC, Bogaard K, Krips R, Marti RK, Bossuyt PM, van Dijk CN. Operative and functional treatment of rupture of the lateral ligament of the ankle. A randomised, prospective trial. J Bone Joint Surg Br. 2003;85(4):525–30.
30. Kerkhoffs GM, Handoll HH, de Bie R, Rowe BH, Struijs PA. Surgical versus conservative treatment for acute injuries of the lateral ligament complex of the ankle in adults. Cochrane Database Syst Rev. 2007;(2):CD000380. https://doi.org/10.1002/14651858.CD000380.pub2.
31. Matsui K, Takao M, Miyamoto W, Innami K, Matsushita T. Arthroscopic Brostrom repair with Gould augmentation via an accessory anterolateral port for lateral instability of the ankle. Arch Orthop Trauma Surg. 2014;134(10):1461–7. https://doi.org/10.1007/s00402-014-2049-x.
32. Moher D, Liberati A, Tetzlaff J, Altman DG, Group P. Preferred reporting items for systematic reviews and meta-analyses: the PRISMA statement. PLoS Med. 2009;6(7):e1000097. https://doi.org/10.1371/journal.pmed.1000097.
33. Nery C, Raduan F, Del Buono A, Asaumi ID, Cohen M, Maffulli N. Arthroscopic-assisted Brostrom-Gould for chronic ankle instability: a long-term follow-up. Am J Sports Med. 2011;39(11):2381–8. https://doi.org/10.1177/0363546511416069.
34. Vuurberg G, Pereira H, Blankevoort L, van Dijk CN (2017) Anatomic stabilization techniques provide superior results in terms of functional outcome in patients suffering from chronic ankle instability compared to non-anatomic techniques. Knee Surg Sports Traumatol Arthrosc https://doi.org/10.1007/s00167-017-4730-4
35. Becker HP, Ebner S, Ebner D, Benesch S, Frossler H, Hayes A, Gritze G, Rosenbaum D. 12-year outcome after modified Watson-Jones tenodesis for ankle instability. Clin Orthop Relat Res. 1999;358:194–204.
36. Hoy GA, Henderson IJ. Results of Watson-Jones ankle reconstruction for instability. The influence of articular damage. J Bone Joint Surg Br. 1994;76(4):610–3.
37. Sammarco VJ. Complications of lateral ankle ligament reconstruction. Clin Orthop Relat Res. 2001;391:123–32.
38. Coughlin MJ, Schenck RC Jr, Grebing BR, Treme G. Comprehensive reconstruction of the lateral ankle for chronic instability using a free gracilis graft. Foot Ankle Int. 2004;25(4):231–41. https://doi.org/10.1177/107110070402500407.
39. Lee MS, Hofbauer MH. Evaluation and management of lateral ankle injuries. Clin Podiatr Med Surg. 1999;16(4):659–78.
40. Liu SH, Baker CL. Comparison of lateral ankle ligamentous reconstruction procedures. Am J Sports Med. 1994;22(3):313–7. https://doi.org/10.1177/036354659402200303.
41. Miller AG, Raikin SM, Ahmad J. Near-anatomic allograft tenodesis of chronic lateral ankle instability. Foot Ankle Int. 2013;34(11):1501–7. https://doi.org/10.1177/1071100713494377.

19 Anatomic Open Repair Procedures: Periosteal Flap

João Lobo, Pedro L. Ripoll, Mariano de Prado, and Hélder Pereira

19.1 Introduction

Ankle sprains are responsible for 4–7% of emergency department admissions [1, 2]. These types of injuries are common at any age, but they mainly affect younger people between 15 and 35 years old [1, 2]. The majority of these patients will achieve favorable outcome with conservative management; however, up to 20% will develop symptoms of chronic ankle instability (CAI) and require surgical treatment [1–3]. Chronic instability occurs as inadequate healing of the torn ligament with poor fibrous tissue with lower biological and biomechanical features, sometimes as an elongated structure [1, 2, 4]. Moreover, proprioceptive deficit and/or peroneal muscle weakness might play a role in symptomatic CAI requiring surgery [1, 2, 5]. Moreover, imaging is not always feasible in the assessment of the extent of the injury or in predicting the properties of the remnant tissue, particularly in children [6].

Although the incidence of chronic lateral ankle instability has increased, its management remains poorly clarified. Therefore, the literature dedicated to its treatment is fundamentally important [1]. Chronic lateral ankle instability is rare in children and teenagers. However, its incidence has been increasing because of the lowering age of sports involvement and heightened level of practice. However, it has also increased because of the inappropriate early approach in the treatment of the skeletally immature or adolescent patients [7].

Surgical management of chronic instability remains somewhat controversial given the use of various different techniques. In fact, over 80 distinct methods of repair have been described, which can be categorized into two groups, anatomic and nonanatomic reconstructions [8]. In the anatomic reconstruction, local tissue is used for reconstruction as in the Brostrom technique further modified by Gould in 1980 [3, 8]. The nonanatomic reconstruction uses tissue grafts harvested at a distance to reconstruct the disrupted ligaments. Examples include the Evans, Chrisman-Snook, and the Watson-Jones procedures [8].

J. Lobo
Centro Hospitalar Universitário de S. João, EPE, Porto, Portugal

P. L. Ripoll · M. de Prado
Ripoll y De Prado Sports Clinic: FIFA Medical Centre of Excellence, Murcia-Madrid, Spain

H. Pereira (✉)
Ripoll y De Prado Sports Clinic: FIFA Medical Centre of Excellence, Murcia-Madrid, Spain

Orthopaedic Department, Centro Hospitalar Póvoa de Varzim, Vila do Conde, Portugal

ICVS/3B's—PT Government Associate Laboratory, University of Minho, Braga/Guimarães, Portugal

H. Pereira et al. (eds.), *Lateral Ankle Instability*, https://doi.org/10.1007/978-3-662-62763-1_19

Several grafts have been used for CAI surgical management; however, increased morbidity must be considered [9].

It has recently been demonstrated that these nonanatomic options provide poorer outcome and higher risk of complications when compared to anatomical repair or reconstruction; however this discussion is considered out of the scope of this text [10].

In contrast to adults, literature concerning CAI management in pediatric and teenager populations are less frequent [7]; however, valid options are required and currently depend also on availability of some adequate surgical devices which permit repair while preserving the anatomy and growth plate (if that is the case) [5].

Fibular periosteal flaps have been used to address chronic lateral ankle instability [7, 11, 12].

It has been used as a single procedure [7, 11] or as augmentation [12] in cases where the quality of the torn remnant tissue is considered to be poor. Augmentation is more frequently considered in patients with very frequent recurrent ankle sprains or in obese or high demand athletes [11, 12].

19.2 Operative Technique

A tourniquet is used during the procedure to control bleeding.

An L-shaped skin incision with an anterior concavity starting 6 cm proximally from the tip of the lateral malleolus is performed. The incision passes slightly posterior to the malleolus and ends about 3 cm distally from its tip to provide good exposure for adequate graft fixation in the talus.

The periosteal flap is isolated proximally to distally for about 5 cm (Figs. 19.1 and 19.2) and the maximum width possible to split it in two if CFL ligament reconstruction is needed.

The fibular flap is turned (Fig. 19.2), and at the two distal angles (in the fibular attachment), two 2–0 or 3–0 Vicryl sutures are placed to reinforce the insertion and avoid stripping from the fibula when the neoligament is tensioned.

ATFL reconstruction varies according to whether or not a residual ligament is present. If so, it can be overlapped by the periosteal flap, with the foot in eversion, and sutured with 3–0 Vicryl separated stitches after anchoring it to the talus with an anchor. If there is no residual ATFL, the fibular flap will aim to replace it.

The length of the periosteal flap is confirmed (Fig. 19.3) to enable both proper tension and efficient fixation in case of tunnel creation or any other means of distal fixation in the talus.

Ligament fixation on the talus must be performed with the foot in slight eversion. Minor variations of the technique can be used according to the pathology found during surgery.

A lesion of the CFL ligament is usually complete and the ligament difficult to recognize. The posterior half of the doubled flap can be also fixed distally and slightly posteriorly from the tip of the malleolus on the calcaneum with an anchor.

During reconstructive maneuvers, the foot is kept in eversion to maintain a slight overcorrection to retain tension in the reconstructed structures. When a capsular lesion is found, repair with reabsorbable 2–0 Vicryl sutures can be performed.

The postoperative protocol comprises several phases:

- Immobilization in a plaster cast with no weight-bearing for 3 weeks.
- Weight-bearing in a plaster or walker boot for 3 weeks.
- Progressive ROM recovery starting from cast removal.
- Proprioceptive rehabilitation, muscle strengthening with isometric exercises and progressively isotonic work, from day 50 postoperatively.
- Eccentric muscle strengthening from day 65 postoperatively.
- Beginning sports activity no earlier than 4 months postoperatively.

The biggest issue surrounding the actual surgical technique is to obtain a good flap and to protect it from stripping of the distal end before overlapping it. Another important phase of the

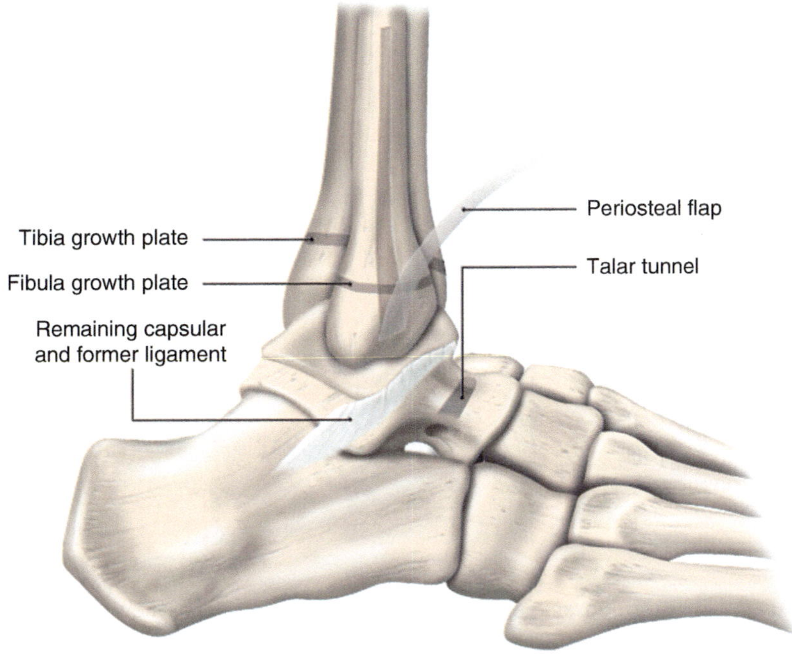

Fig. 19.1 Schematic representation of fibular periosteal flap harvesting in skeletally immature children; growth plates are visible; the remnant of the anterior talofibular ligament is represented. The periosteal flap is harvested and the place for a talar tunnel for distal fixation of the repair

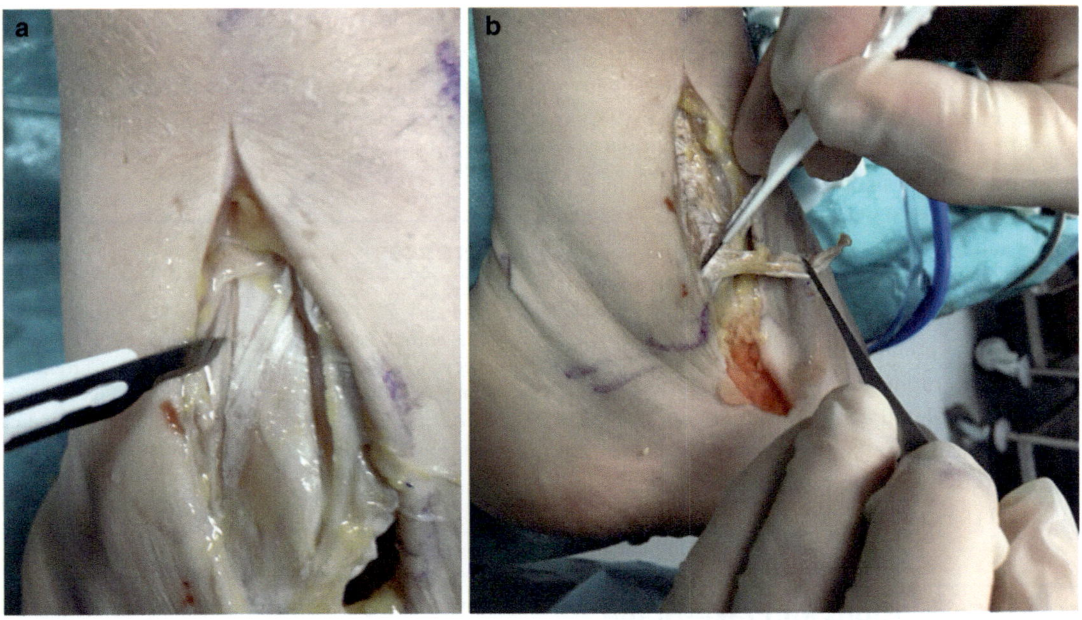

Fig. 19.2 (**a**) Cadaveric demonstration of the surgical approach and periosteal identification and cut by means of bisturi blade for subsequent detachment; (**b**) Detachment and flipping (turning) of the periosteal flap

procedure is flap fixation and tensioning, which must be performed in a slight overcorrection.

The possible advantages of a periosteal flap are that it is relatively simple to harvest the flap, it needs only a small 5 cm incision and it does not require any costly special devices or implants. It does not cause harm to any local tendon and it enables anatomic with resultant close to normal ankle and subtalar kinematics. A periosteal flap has also shown to provide adequate biomechanical

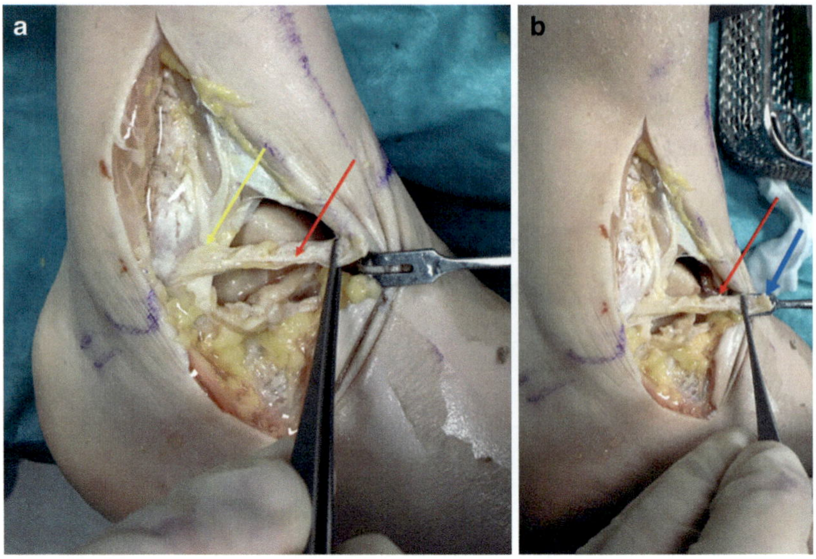

Fig. 19.3 (**a**) Fibular attachment of the periosteal flap (yellow arrow) and testing the proper length for the distal attachment site of the flap (red arrow); (**b**) Testing the adequate tension of the graft identifying the attachment site to the talus (red arrow) and measuring the remaining graft which can be introduced in a tunnel or used for reinforcement by reversing it proximally in a pants over-vest way

resistance [9]. Bohnsack et al. reported on the biomechanical properties of various autogenous transplants commonly used for the reconstruction of lateral ankle ligaments [9]. The authors found no significant difference in the biomechanical stability between the periosteal flap and the native ATFL. Furthermore, periosteal tissue serves as a scaffold for the formation of fibroblastic tissue and subsequent transformation into ligament [9].

There are some disadvantages of this technique, which are basically related to the postoperative protocol, which requires 6 weeks of immobilization to allow the process of fixation and early ligamentization of the periosteal flap. The risk of epiphysiodesis of the lateral malleolus in the skeletally immature patients or transplant ossification resulting from this procedure remains possible, although these theoretical complications have never been described so far.

19.3 Conclusions and Take-Home Message

When surgical repair is required for treatment of chronic ankle instability, a periosteal fibular flap technique remains a possibility enabling favorable outcome either in children and adolescents or high-level athletes.

The "key to success" is to obtain a good flap and avoid that it detaches from the distal fibula before flipping it and tensioning. Adequate fixation is critical and usually is done in slight overcorrection.

As a major drawback, this technique requires a period of 6 weeks of protection of the construct by immobilization.

References

1. Michels F, Pereira H, Calder J, Matricali G, Glazebrook M, Guillo S, Karlsson J, Group E-AAI, Acevedo J, Batista J, Bauer T, Calder J, Carreira D, Choi W, Corte-Real N, Glazebrook M, Ghorbani A, Giza E, Guillo S, Hunt K, Karlsson J, Kong SW, Lee JW, Michels F, Molloy A, Mangone P, Matsui K, Nery C, Ozeki S, Pearce C, Pereira H, Perera A, Pijnenburg B, Raduan F, Stone J, Takao M, Tourne Y, Vega J. Searching for consensus in the approach to patients with chronic lateral ankle instability: ask the expert. Knee Surg Sports Traumatol Arthrosc. 2017;26:2095. https://doi.org/10.1007/s00167-017-4556-0.
2. Pereira H, Vuurberg G, Spennacchio P, Batista J, D'Hooghe P, Hunt K, Van Dijk N. Surgical treatment paradigms of ankle lateral instability, osteochondral defects and impingement. Adv Exp Med Biol. 2018;1059:85–108. https://doi.org/10.1007/978-3-319-76735-2_4.
3. Colville MR. Surgical treatment of the unstable ankle. J Am Acad Orthop Surg. 1998;6(6):368–77. https://doi.org/10.5435/00124635-199811000-00005.

4. Kirk KL, Campbell JT, Guyton GP, Parks BG, Schon LC. ATFL elongation after Brostrom procedure: a biomechanical investigation. Foot Ankle Int. 2008;29(11):1126–30. https://doi.org/10.3113/FAI.2008.1126.
5. Pereira H, Vuurberg G, Gomes N, Oliveira JM, Ripoll PL, Reis RL, Espregueira-Mendes J, Niek van Dijk C. Arthroscopic repair of ankle instability with all-soft knotless anchors. Arthrosc Tech. 2016;5(1):e99–e107. https://doi.org/10.1016/j.eats.2015.10.010.
6. Endele D, Jung C, Bauer G, Mauch F. Value of MRI in diagnosing injuries after ankle sprains in children. Foot Ankle Int. 2012;33(12):1063–8. https://doi.org/10.3113/FAI.2012.1063.
7. Mathieu PA, Marcheix PS, Vacquerie V, Dijoux P, Mabit C, Fourcade L. Reconstruction of the lateral ligaments of the ankle using a periosteal flap in children and teenagers: a midterm follow-up survey. J Pediatr Orthop. 2015;35(5):511–5. https://doi.org/10.1097/BPO.0000000000000303.
8. Vuurberg G, Pereira H, Blankevoort L, van Dijk CN. Anatomic stabilization techniques provide superior results in terms of functional outcome in patients suffering from chronic ankle instability compared to non-anatomic techniques. Knee Surg Sports Traumatol Arthrosc. 2018;26(7):2183–95. https://doi.org/10.1007/s00167-017-4730-4.
9. Bohnsack M, Surie B, Kirsch IL, Wulker N. Biomechanical properties of commonly used autogenous transplants in the surgical treatment of chronic lateral ankle instability. Foot Ankle Int. 2002;23(7):661–4. https://doi.org/10.1177/107110070202300714.
10. Vuurberg G, Veen OC, Pereira H, Blankevoort L, van Dijk CN. Tenodesis reconstruction in patients with chronic lateral ankle instability is associated with a high risk of complications compared with anatomic repair and reconstruction: a systematic review and meta-analysis. J ISAKOS. 2017; https://doi.org/10.1136/jisakos-2016-000121.
11. Benazzo F, Zanon G, Marullo M, Rossi SM. Lateral ankle instability in high-demand athletes: reconstruction with fibular periosteal flap. Int Orthop. 2013;37(9):1839–44. https://doi.org/10.1007/s00264-013-2049-4.
12. Chew CP, Koo KOT, Lie DTT. Periosteal flap augmentation of the modified Brostrom-Gould procedure for chronic lateral ankle instability. J Orthop Surg (Hong Kong). 2018;26(1):2309499018757530. https://doi.org/10.1177/2309499018757530.

Ankle Ligament Injuries: Long-Term Outcomes After Stabilizing Surgery

20

Jón Karlsson, Louise Karlsson, Eleonor Svantesson, and Eric Hamrin Senorski

20.1 Introduction

It is well known that acute ligament injuries are one of the main causes of visits to orthopedic emergency trauma units worldwide. An ankle sprain may result in rupture of the ankle's lateral collateral ligaments, especially the anterior talofibular ligament (ATFL) and calcaneofibular ligament (CFL) are at risk of rupture while the posterior talofibular ligament (PTFL) is seldom ruptured (Fig. 20.1). Ankle ligament injuries are also known as the most common sports-related injuries and these injuries represent a major socioeconomic burden due to their high frequency of occurrence [1–4]. The ATFL is the weakest of these three ligaments and is most vulnerable to injuries. Accordingly, it is the most frequently injured lateral ankle ligament. An initial nonsurgical treatment is recommended, based on activity modification, load management, cryotherapy, compression bandage, elevation, and functional rehabilitation starting after a few days [5, 6]. The rehabilitation is based on range of motion (ROM) exercises, full weight-bearing, balance/coordination training, and progressive strength training. This form of treatment is usually successful and return to sports is usually allowed after 1–2 weeks, sometimes with external support, such as athletic tape or a supporting brace to reduce recurrence. Following an acute ankle sprain and in chronic cases, deficits in postural control, proprioception, muscle reaction time, and strength typically occur, which when these symptoms are persistent is commonly believed to be the cause of chronic ankle instability [7–10]. For instance, an inability to complete jumping and landing tasks within 2 weeks of a primary lateral ankle sprain, poorer dynamic control, and lower self-reported function after 6 weeks were predictive of eventual chronic ankle instability outcome [11]. Chronic ankle instability is defined by mechanical instability, range of motion that exceeds normal physiological limits, and subjective feelings of instability of the ankle joint related to sensorimotor or neuromuscular deficit [12–15].

The patient history of chronic ankle instability reveals past recurrent ankle sprains, where patients commonly have precautions against weight-bearing and ankle-strenuous sport/activities [7–9]. The main causes of symptoms in chronic ankle instability are decreased proprioceptive abilities due to the loss of mechanoreceptors and decreased muscle strength of invertor and evertor muscles [8, 11, 15]. Because of this,

J. Karlsson (✉) · L. Karlsson · E. Svantesson
E. Hamrin Senorski
Department of Orthopaedics, Sahlgrenska University Hospital, Sahlgrenska Academy, Gothenburg University, Gothenburg, Sweden
e-mail: jon.karlsson@vgregion.se; louise.karlsson0628@gmail.com; eleonor.svantesson@outlook.com; eric.hamrin.senorski@gu.se

H. Pereira et al. (eds.), *Lateral Ankle Instability*, https://doi.org/10.1007/978-3-662-62763-1_20

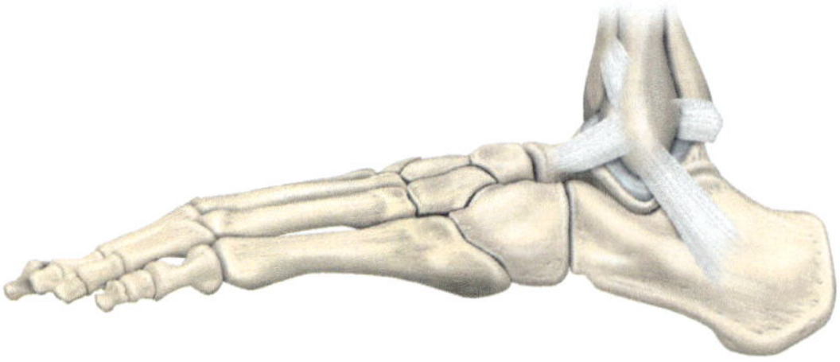

Fig. 20.1 The anatomy of the lateral ankle ligaments; anterior talofibular ligament, calcaneofibular ligament, and posterior talofibular ligament

isotonic strength training is the foundation of rehabilitation in chronic cases of ankle instability and has been associated with a positive effect on the functional stability, muscle strength, and proprioception of the ankle. In addition, balance training is an important part of the current rehabilitation protocols, stimulating sensorimotor deficits typical for chronic ankle instability, postural control, dynamic balance, and joint position sense [16, 17].

The treatment is also a matter of debate [3, 4, 18–20]. When a recurrent sprain occurs, chronic lateral ankle instability develops in approximately 10–30% of cases [12–15, 21, 22]. This will result in recurrent pain, increasing insecurity, and giving way episodes of the ankle. A chronic instability and recurrent injuries may also be associated with loss of integrity of the lateral ankle ligaments, proprioceptive deficit, peroneal muscle weakness/peroneal tendon (partial) rupture, tibiofibular sprain, and recurrent laxity of the subtalar joint, which are all factors that contribute to the development of chronic ankle instability. Patients who develop chronic ankle instability will not regain function and stability of the ankle by nonoperative treatment and, in these cases, surgical treatment is indicated. This is important since it has been reported that chronic ankle instability is correlated with an increased risk of osteoarthritis of the ankle [14, 23]. Thus, in contrast to an acute rupture, where most researchers agree that surgical intervention with sutures of the torn ligaments is not needed due to the high self-healing capacity of the lateral ligaments, stability should be restored surgically in case of chronic functional ankle instability [18, 24]. The aims of the surgical intervention are to stabilize the ankle ligament, prevent further giving way, treat associated injuries (such as cartilage injuries), and possibly to reduce the risk of long-term osteoarthritis (OA). The last indication is, however, not well stated in the literature.

When it comes to treating chronic lateral ankle instability, more than 60 different procedures have been described [3, 4, 13, 14]. Originally, the most commonly used procedure was tenodesis, using one of the peroneal tendons, in most cases the peroneus brevis tendon [24–26]. The augmentation is usually performed with an autograft, while allograft options are also available. The different procedures can be divided into anatomic repair, anatomic reconstruction, and nonanatomic reconstruction [27, 28] (Figs. 20.2, 20.3, 20.4, 20.5).

Of the many surgical techniques proposed for treating chronic ankle instability, the first proposed procedures were nonanatomic, like the Evans, Watson-Jones, and Castaing procedures [24–26]. All of these procedures utilized either the peroneus brevis or the peroneus longus tendons in various configurations to restore function, however, without any repair of the ligament remnants. All of the techniques sacrificed local tissue on the lateral side of the ankle, including partial or total tenodesis from the Achilles tendon or peroneus tendon(s). They were all related to extensive surgical exposure, were technically demanding, and all required prolonged immobilization. Due to extensive surgical exposure, the risk of surgical complications is also high. In addition, the sacrifice of normal lateral ankle tissue, like the peroneal tendons will lead to the development of nonanatomical forces over the ankle, with an increased risk of ankle degeneration and OA in the medium- to long-term [29, 30].

Due to the possible limitations of the nonanatomic procedures, anatomic procedures were proposed. Broström described in 1966 a procedure using the remnants of the ATFL [18]. His procedure was a simple suture of the ligament remnants. This procedure has been modified, for instance by Gould et al., [31] in 1980 (Fig. 20.6), who proposed reinforcement using the inferior extensor retinaculum (originally proposed for subtalar

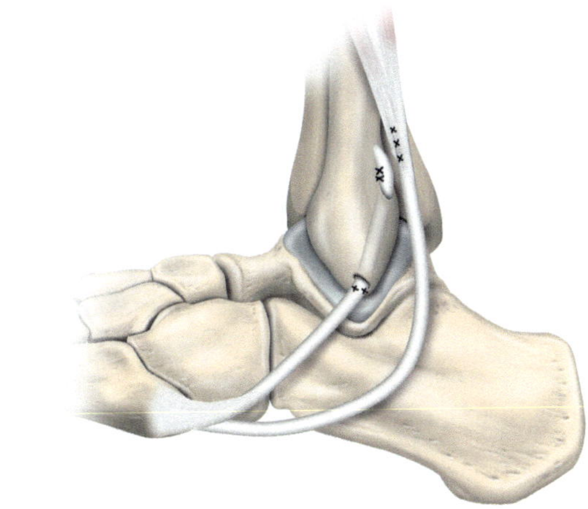

Fig. 20.2 Nonanatomic reconstruction using tenodesis; the Evans technique is nonanatomical tenodesis, utilizing the peroneus brevis tendon. The tendon is routed through a drill hole in the fibula and sutured back to itself

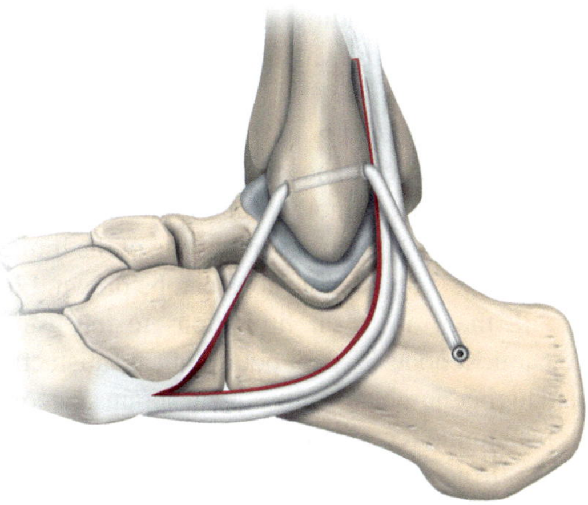

Fig. 20.3 Anatomic reconstruction using tenodesis; Chrisman-Snook technique is an anatomic tenodesis. Either half or all of the peroneus brevis tendon is used. The tendon is routed through drill holes in the fibula and finally secured with an interference screw in the calcaneus

instability) and Karlsson et al. (Fig. 20.5), who recommended reattachment of the ATFL and CFL to the fibula using drill holes at the ligament's original anatomical origin [13–15]. The last researchers recommended to always reconstruct both the ATFL and CFL in order to restore the laxity of the lateral ankle ligaments [13]. The goal is to restore the normal anatomy and ankle joint mechanics by the in situ repair of the injured ligaments, by either shortening them with fixation to the anatomic location of the bone surface and/or augmenting them with local structures to enhance the repair [13, 29, 30]. There are several advantages of the anatomical procedures, like the simplicity of the surgical procedure, with less risk of surgical complications, the restoration of normal physiological ankle anatomy and thereby normal kinematics and finally preservation of subtalar joint mobility [13, 15]. In fact, the Broström procedure or modifications of the Broström procedure are, more than 50 years after first being reported, still considered "gold" standard for the treatment of chronic lateral ankle instability [18].

More recently the use of autologous or synthetic grafts has been reported. This type of reconstruction uses tendon grafts in a similar fashion as other nonanatomical procedures, but the advantage is that they preserve local tissue, especially the peroneal tendons as anatomical procedures. These kinds of procedures are indicated in cases of recurrence after a modified Broström procedure/repair, generalized ligament laxity, high body mass index, and probably in high-demand athletes [13, 32, 33].

Even more recently several surgeons have developed all-arthroscopic procedures aimed at restoring ankle instability [34]. These procedures all mimic Broström-like procedures and their use is rapidly increasing. The common nominator for all these procedures is that they repair/reconstruct the ATFL and anterior joint capsule to the anatomical origin of the distal fibula, utilizing suture anchors. Some of these procedures also repair the CFL and even reinforce the repair with the inferior extensor retinaculum, like the Gould modified technique [31]. Generally, the short- and mid-term outcomes after both anatomic and nonanatomic ligament reconstructions are satisfactory. However, long-term outcomes are less known [35, 36].

20.2 Long-Term Follow-Up

The Broström technique (Fig. 20.4) is the original anatomical repair of the lateral ligaments of the ankle [18]. Several researchers have sug-

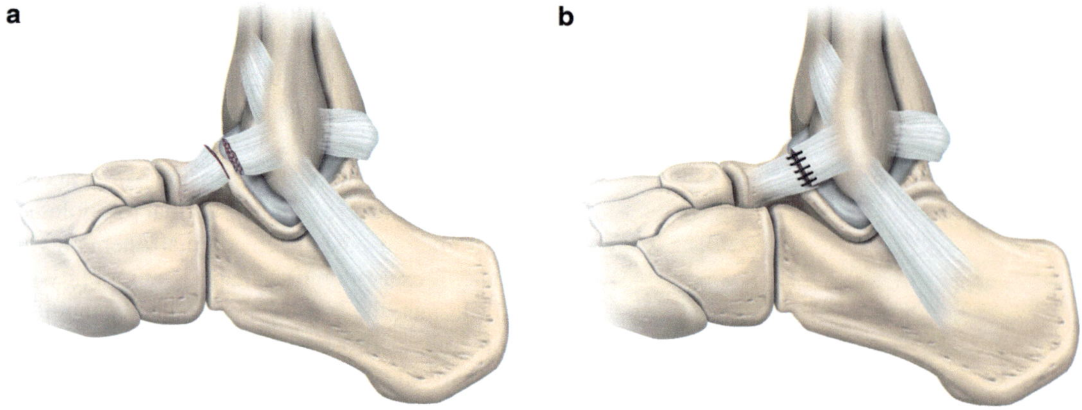

Fig. 20.4 Direct repair of the anterior talofibular ligament; the original Broström technique

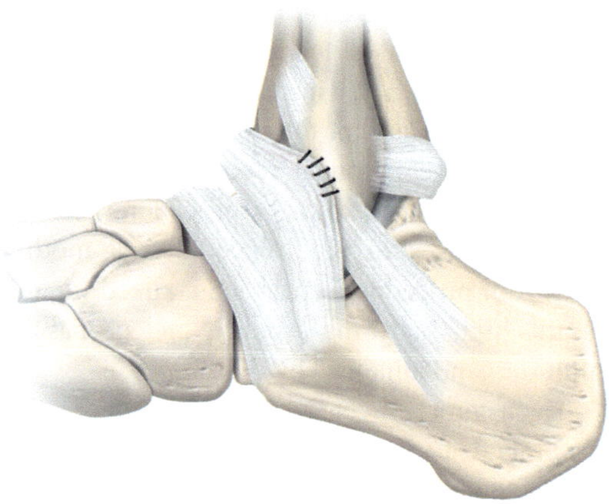

Fig. 20.5 Direct repair of the anterior talofibular ligament and reinforcement using the inferior extensor retinaculum; i.e., the Gould modification of the Broström technique. This procedure was originally designed for the reconstruction of subtalar instability

gested that long-term results may be improved with an anatomical repair, due to the loss of subtalar motion, sacrifice of peroneal tendons (loss of ankle eversion strength), and, not least, concern raised for subsequent deterioration of the ankle joint function, including increased risk of OA that may occur with nonanatomical repair. For instance, the long-term results of the Watson-Jones procedure (peroneus longus tenodesis) have shown signs of early OA changes. Bell et al. [22] followed 22/31 patients who underwent the Broström procedure for chronic ankle instability from the US Naval Academy. The follow-up period was 26.3 (24.6–27.9) years. Taken together, 91% of the patients reported their ankle function as good or excellent at long-term. In this cohort, the anterior talofibular ligament was always repaired and the calcaneofibular ligament was repaired as well in some cases (unknown how many). No radiographs were taken at follow-up and the prevalence of OA is therefore unknown.

At this point, it should be borne in mind that there is limited evidence to support any one surgical technique over another for chronic ankle instability [13, 14, 21]. However, in spite of the limited evidence, several conclusions can be drawn. First of all, there are clear limitations to the use of dynamic tenodesis, with poor clinical satisfaction and higher number of subsequent sprains. Second, nonanatomic reconstruction(s) increase the inversion stiffness of the subtalar joint(s) compared with the anatomic procedures, at least when using the ligament remnants [14]. Anatomic reconstruction is preferred by most patients and there are several modifications of the original Broström reconstruction that have been shown to produce good-to-excellent results [13, 18].

Noailles et al. [37] followed 181 patients for more than 15 years. They divided their cohort into direct anatomical repair (Broström, Duquennoy) and nonanatomical repair (Watson-Jones, Evans, and Castaing). They found that the functional outcome was better after anatomical repair, but with the presence of recurrent instability. Contrarily, loss of range of motion and secondary OA were more frequent after nonanatomical repair. Grade I–II (van Dijk clas-

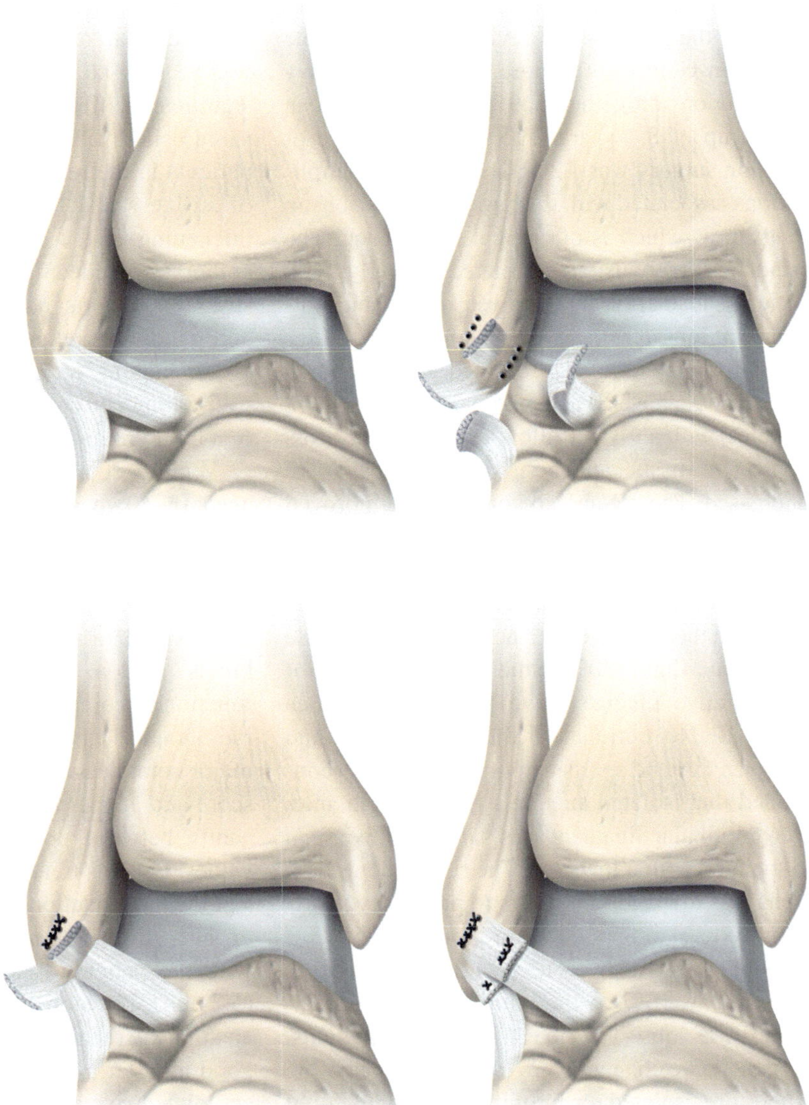

Fig. 20.6 Anatomic reconstruction, using the remnants of the injured ligaments, with shortening, imbrication, and reinsertion to bone (fibula) of the anterior talofibular ligament and calcaneofibular ligament. This specific modification of the Broström technique was originally described by Karlsson et al.

sification) OA was found in between 7 and 100% of operated ankles in the nonanatomical group. Van der Rijt reported 100% Grade I OA 22 years after Watson-Jones procedure [38, 39]. The clinical functional outcome was 33% good and excellent, meaning that only one-third of the patients were free of symptoms at the 22-year follow-up. The presence of osteophytes (Grade I OA) was directly related to recurrent instability, especially sagittal laxity and positive drawer test.

Karlsson et al. [14] reported on the long-term outcomes after Evans peroneus brevis tenodesis at 14 years in 42 patients. They found only 50% good and excellent results and 13 reinterventions, while 32/37 patients had Grade I OA. Less than 50% of the patients reported good or excellent functional outcome after a mean follow-up of 14 years and more than 80% had signs of OA. Reoperations were frequent. These researchers concluded that the long-term outcome after Evans tenodesis was far from satisfactory. Therefore, tenodesis of this kind should not be considered as a first-line treatment selection.

So et al. [40] performed a systematic review to evaluate the incidence of revision surgery of the Broström-Gould procedure [18, 24]. They reported on altogether 669 patients at a mean follow-up of 8.4 years. The mean incidence of revision surgery was 1.2%. The reported complications associated with this procedure are consistently low, which is of clinical importance. The incidence of revision correlated strongly with patient satisfaction and showed acceptable outcomes at long-term.

Maffulli et al. [41] reported on combined Broström repair [18] and ankle arthroscopy in 42 athletes, with a 9-year follow-up. During arthroscopy, soft tissue and bony impingement were addressed. The mean Kaikkonen score improved from 45 to 90 points; however, there were 9 failures and only 22 (58%) returned to the pre-injury activity level. Six of the nine failures did not feel safe with their ankle due to new episodes of ankle instability. Eight (30%) patients showed signs of degenerative changes; five grade I and three grade II. No correlation was, however, found between OA and sports activity. The authors concluded that isolated anatomic repair of the anterior talofibular ligament was safe, effective, and associated with a low cost. The risk of complications was low and safe return to pre-injury sports activity level was possible in more than 50% of the patients. However, recurrent instability occurred in 16% of the patients and poor outcome was observed in 24% of the patients. Degenerative changes were found in almost 40%. Therefore, isolated repair of the ATFL only might be questioned, at least after this study. Several previous researchers have recommended combined/simultaneous repair of the ATFL and CFL.

Li et al. [6] reported on 5–10 year outcomes after either anatomical repair or reconstruction. They followed 45 patients, with assessment using the Karlsson score and Tegner activity level for activity assessment. The repair group ($n = 25$) underwent modified Broström repair and the reconstruction group was treated with a semitendinosus allograft ($n = 20$) through drill tunnels in the fibula and calcaneus. Bioabsorbable screws were used for fixation. At follow-up examination, no patient had recurrent ankle instability. Moreover, there were no differences in functional outcome scores; Karlsson score was 93 vs 90.6 points [42]. There were also no significant differences in activity level as measured using the Tegner activity level score. Five patients in the reconstruction group complained of stiffness and ultrasonography showed some thickening of the reconstructed ligaments. The authors concluded that both the repair and reconstruction cohorts had high patient satisfaction and good to excellent function and activity levels, indicating recreational sports participation over a long period of time (Tegner activity score 6 in both groups).

Ventura et al. [43] reported on 40 patients aged 18–40 years who underwent surgical treatment for chronic lateral ankle instability; 20 patients underwent direct anatomical repair using the Broström-Gould technique and 20 patients underwent lateral tenodesis with a split peroneus brevis tendon. Follow-up included Karlsson functional score, Tegner activity level, and stress radiographs, using Telos stress equipment. No major complication occurred; the mean Karlsson score and Tegner activity level improved significantly between preoperative and postoperative values. Patients treated with tenodesis reported a significant reduction in the radiographic values of anterior talar translation (1.4 mm) compared with the patients treated with Broström repair (5.7 mm). The authors concluded that both direct anatomical repair and lateral tenodesis provide good long-term outcomes in terms of functional and objective parameters in a 15-year follow-up. There were no significant OA changes. It is noteworthy that the tenodesis improved restoration of laxity more effectively, while the reduced range of motion that was reported in 20% of the patients (tenodesis) did not affect the overall functional outcome.

Mabit et al. [44] in a French multicenter study investigated the clinical and radiological results and long-term impact of different surgical techniques of lateral ankle ligament reconstruction. Altogether, 310 patients were included and the mean follow-up was 13 years (minimum 5 years). They studied four groups of patients, (a) direct ligament complex reattachment, (b) augmented repair, (c) ligament reconstruction using a part of the peroneus brevis tendon, and finally (d) ligament reconstruction using the whole peroneus brevis tendon. Clinical and functional outcome was performed using the Karlsson score and radiographic evaluation included dynamic views, including Telos or self-imposed varus. The majority of the results were satisfactory, with a mean Karlsson score of 90 (19–100) points, and 87% of patients claimed good or excellent results. Postoperative complications (20%) were correlated with poorer outcomes. The progression of degenerative changes was minor over time. However, there was no correlation between functional results and residual laxity on radiographs. In terms of comparisons, the functional results were less good with ligament reconstruction using the whole peroneus brevis tendon and the laxity restoration control was poorest with direct ligament complex reattachment. The authors concluded that surgery generally yielded good results, and should be adapted to the ligamentous and associated lesions.

De Vries et al. [3] followed 37 patients over 20–30 years after the Weber operation (Fig. 20.7). This is an anatomic tenodesis that only reconstructs the anterior talofibular ligament. At the long-term follow-up, approximately half of the patients had symptoms, but 32/37 claimed to be satisfied with the final outcome. According to the Karlsson score, approximately two-thirds had a good and excellent result. The authors concluded that the Weber procedure was a good alternative for the treatment of chronic anterolateral instability when direct anatomical repair is not feasible or has failed. However, this technique is rather invasive and utilizes the plantaris tendon as a free graft.

Cao et al. [19] performed a meta-analysis related to surgical management of chronic lateral instability. They were able to include seven (all randomized or quasi-randomized) studies in order to compare different surgical techniques. They concluded that there was limited evidence to support any one surgical technique over another for chronic lateral instability. However, they claimed that there are definitive limitations to the use of dynamic tenodesis, which obtained

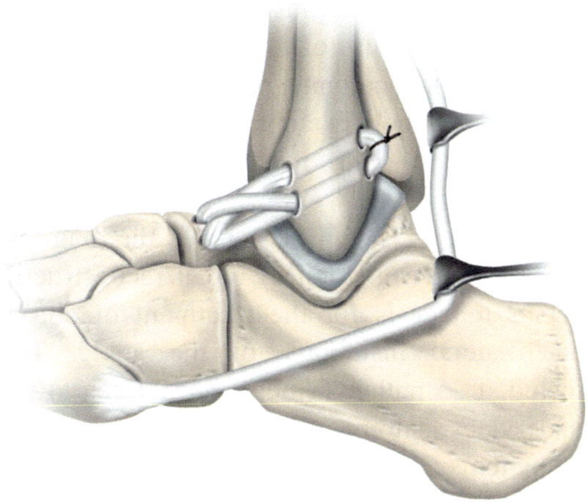

Fig. 20.7 Weber plantaris tenodesis technique. This technique utilizes the free plantaris tendon but reconstructs only the anterior talofibular ligament

poorer clinical satisfaction and an increased number of subsequent sprains. Moreover, nonanatomic reconstruction abnormally increased inversion stiffness at the subtalar level as compared with anatomic repair and multiple types of modified Broström procedures acquired good clinical results [13, 18]. The overall conclusion was that anatomic reconstruction is a better procedure for many specific patients.

Vuurberg et al. [45] performed a systematic review and included 882 patients. The modified Coleman Methodology Score ranged from 30 to 73 points (max 90 points), indicating fair to good methodological strength. The Karlsson score was the most commonly used patient-reported outcome score after surgery. They compared the functional outcomes between anatomic repair, anatomic reconstruction, and tenodesis (nonanatomic reconstruction). They concluded that anatomic repair and anatomic reconstruction provided better functional outcome in patients with chronic lateral instability compared with tenodesis (nonanatomic) reconstruction. Also, anatomic reconstruction showed the highest score increase after surgery. These researchers concluded that anatomic reconstruction produced the best results, but may, however, be more invasive than nonanatomic repair. This also needs to be kept in mind when choosing between anatomic repair and reconstruction in the treatment of chronic ankle instability. This study also discourages the use of tenodesis reconstruction and other nonanatomic procedures. Moreover, the risk of the development of degenerative changes and OA needs to be carefully considered.

Krips et al. [29, 30] compared the long-term outcome after anatomical repair/reconstruction versus tenodesis for the treatment of chronic anterolateral instability of the ankle. They included 25 patients (mean age 22 years) who underwent anatomical repair/reconstruction and 29 patients (mean age 23 years) who underwent tenodesis. For both groups, the mean follow-up period was 12.3 years. At follow-up, there were significantly more patients in the tenodesis group who had positive anterior drawer sign and medially located osteophytes as seen on standard radiographs. The mean talar tilt was 4.7° in the anatomic repair group and 6.9° in the tenodesis group. The anterior talar translation was also significantly higher in the tenodesis group; 4.3 mm versus 2.9 mm (mean values). These researchers concluded that the tenodesis procedure did not restore the normal anatomy of the lateral ankle ligaments and when compared with anatomical repair or reconstruction, a tenodesis leads to inferior results in terms of functional stability and restoration of laxity, as well as overall satisfaction at long-term and increased risk of OA [46].

Fact Box 1
- Ankle ligament injuries are common, especially in sports.
- Approximately 10–30% of patients who sustain ankle ligament injury report medium- to long-term functional problems, with recurrent instability.
- The first line of treatment is nonsurgical with a structured rehabilitation program.
- If rehabilitation fails, and the patients still complain of functional instability, surgical stabilization may be considered.

Fact Box 2
- More than 60 different surgical procedures have been described to restore laxity and improve function.
- The surgical procedures are either repair or reconstruction. They are either anatomical or nonanatomical.
- The most common procedure is anatomical repair, i.e., Broström ligament repair and was described more than 50 years ago.
- Today, most ligament procedures are modifications of the original Broström ligament repair, e.g., the Karlsson procedure.
- The medium- to long-term results after anatomical repair or reconstruction are satisfactory in the majority of patients. There is evidence that both the anterior talofibular and calcaneofibular ligaments should be reconstructed simultaneously for an improved result.
- Anatomical procedures will generally produce better functional results in the long run and at the same time, the risk of osteoarthrosis is lower than after nonanatomical procedures.

Take-Home Message
Anatomical repair or anatomical reconstruction are the preferred surgical methods for the treatment of functional lateral ankle instability. There are more than 60 surgical methods, and the evidence to choose between many of these methods is limited. The original Broström method is a direct repair of the anterior talofibular ligament only. There is at least some evidence that both the anterior talofibular and calcaneofibular ligaments should be repaired/reconstructed at the same time. Anatomic reconstruction is the preferred procedure in many specific patients over nonanatomical reconstructions or tenodesis. The risk of osteoarthrosis after nonanatomical reconstruction is increased.

References

1. Ajis A, Maffulli N. Conservative management of chronic ankle instability. Foot Ankle Clin. 2006;11:539–45.
2. Castaing J. Apropos of severe sprains of the ankle. Sem Hop Ther Paris. 1962;38:535–7.
3. De Vries JS, Krips R, Sierevelt IN, Blankevoort L. Interventions for treating chronic ankle instability. Cochrane Database Syst Rev. 2006;4:CD004124.
4. De Vries JS, Krips R, Sierevelt IN, Blankevoort L, van Dijk CN. Interventions for treating chronic ankle instability. Cochrane Database Syst Rev. 2013;8:CD004124.
5. Konradsen L, Hölmer P, Söndergaard L. Early mobilizing treatment for grade III ankle ligament injuries. Foot Ankle. 1991;12:69–73.
6. Li H, Hua Y, Li H, Chen S. Anatomical reconstruction produced similarly favourable outcomes as repair procedures for the treatment of chronic lateral ankle instability at long-term follow-up. Knee Surg Sports Traumatol Arthrosc. 2018; https://doi.org/10.1007/s00167-018-5176-z.
7. Ferran NA, Maffulli N. Epidemiology of sprains of the lateral ankle ligament complex. Foot Ankle Clin. 2006;11:659–62.
8. Genthon N, Bouvat E, Banihachemi JJ, Bergeau J, Abdellaoui A, Rougier PR. Lateral ankle sprain alters postural control in bipedal stance: part 2 sensorial and mechanical effects induced by wearing an ankle orthosis. Scand J Med Sci Sports. 2010;20(2):255–61.
9. Holme E, Magnusson SP, Becher K, Bieler T, Aagaard P, Kjaer M. The effect of supervised rehabilitation on strength, postural sway, position sense and re-injury risk after acute ankle ligament sprain. Scand J Med Sci Sports. 1999;9(2):104–9.
10. Soboroff SH, Pappies EM, Komaroff AL. Benefits, risks and costs of alternative approaches to the evaluation and treatment of severe ankle sprain. Clin Orthop Relat Res. 1984;183:160–8.
11. Doherty C, Bleakley C, Hertel J, Caulfield B, Ryan J, Delahunt E. Recovery from a first-time lateral ankle sprain and the predictors of chronic ankle instability: a prospective cohort analysis. Am J Sports Med. 2016;44(4):995–1003.
12. Holmer P, Söndergaard L, Konradsen L, Nielsen PT, Jörgensen LN. Epidemiology of sprains in the lateral ankel and foot. Foot Ankle Int. 1994;15(2):72–4.
13. Karlsson J, Bergsten T, Lansinger O, Peterson L. Reconstruction of the lateral ligaments of the ankle for chronic lateral instability. J Bone Joint Surg. 1988;70-A:581–8.
14. Karlsson J, Bergsten T, Lansinger O, Peterson L. Lateral instability of the ankle treated by the Evans procedure: a long-term clinical and radiological follow-up. J Bone Joint Surg. 1988;70-B:476–80.
15. Karlsson J, Eriksson BI, Bergsten T, Rudholm O, Swärd L. Comparison of two anatomic reconstructions for chronic lateral instability of the ankle joint. Am J Sports Med. 1997;25:48–53.
16. Sefton JM, Hicks-Little CA, Hubbard TJ, Clemens MG, Yengo CM, Koceja DM. Sensorimotor function as a predictor of chronic ankle instability. Clin Biomech (Bristol, Avon). 2009;24(5):451–8.
17. Urguden M, Kizilay F, Sekban H, Samanci N, Ozkaynak S, Ozdemir H. Evaluation of the lateral instability of the ankle by inversion simulation device and assessment of the rehabilitation program. Acta Orthop Traumatol Turc. 2010;44(5):365–77.
18. Broström L. Sprained ankles VI. Surgical treatment of "chronic" ligament rupture. Acta Chir Scand. 1966;132:551–65.
19. Cao Y, Hong Y, Xu Y, Zhu Y, Xu Y. Surgical management of chronic lateral ankle instability: a meta-analysis. J Orthop Surg Res. 2018;13:159.
20. Porter M, Shadbolt B, Stuart R. Primary ankle ligament augmentation versus modified Broström-Gould procedure: a 2-year randomized controlled trial. ANZ J Surg. 2015;85:44–8.
21. Becker HP, Ebner S, Ebner D, Benesch S, Frössler H, Hayes A. 12-year outcome after modified Watson-Jones tenodesis for ankle instability. Clin Orthop Relat Res. 1999;(358):194–204.
22. Bell SJ, Mologne TS, Sitler DF, Cox JS. Twenty-six year results after Broström procedure for chronic lateral ankle instability. Am J Sports Med. 2006;34(6):975–9.
23. De Vries JS, Struijs PAA, Raaymakers ELFB, Marti RK. Long-term results of the weber operation for chronic ankle instability. Acta Orthop. 2005;76(6):891–8.
24. Evans DL. Recurrent instability of the ankle; a method of surgical treatment. Proc R Soc Med. 1953;46:343–4.
25. Chrisman OD, Snook GA. Reconstruction of lateral ligament tears of the ankle: an experimental study and clinical evaluation of seven patients treated by a new modification of the Elmslie procedure. J Bone Joint Surg. 1969;51-A:904–12.
26. Watson-Jones R. Recurrent forward dislocation of the ankle joint. J Bone Joint Surg. 1952;34-B:519.
27. Ellis SJ, Williams BR, Pavlov H, Deland J. Results of anatomic lateral ankle ligament reconstruction with tendon allograft. HSS J. 2011;7(2):134–40.
28. Snook GA, Chrisman OD, Wilson TC. Long-term results of the Chrisman-Snook operation for reconstruction of the lateral ligaments of the ankle. J Bone Joint Surg. 1985;67-A:1–7.
29. Krips R, van Dijk CN, Halasi T, Lehtonen H, Corradini C, Moyen B, Karlsson J. Long-term outcome of anatomical reconstruction versus tenodesis for the treatment of chronic anterolateral instability of the ankle joint: a multicenter study. Foot Ankle Int. 2001;22:415–21.
30. Krips R, van Dijk CN, Lehtonen H, Halasi T, Moyen B, Karlsson J. Sports activity level after surgical treat-

ment for chronic anterolateral ankle instability. A multicenter study. Am J Sports Med. 2002;30(1):13–9.
31. Gould N, Seligson D, Gassman J. Early and late repair of lateral ankle ligament of the ankle. Foot Ankle. 1980;1:84–9.
32. Larsen E. Static or dynamic repair of chronic lateral ankle instability. Clin Orthop Relat Res. 1990;257:184–92.
33. Lee K, Jegal H, Chung H, Park Y. Return to play after modified Broström-operation for chronic ankle instability in elite athletes. Clin Orthop Surg. 2019;11(1):126–30.
34. Guelfi M, Zamperetti M, Pantalone A, Usuelli FG, Salini V, Oliva M. Open and arthroscopic lateral ligament repair for treatment of chronic ankle instability: a systematic review. Foot Ankle Surg. 2018;24:11–8.
35. Guillo S, Bauer T, Lee JW, Takao M, Kong SW, Stone JW, Mangone PG, Molloy A, Perera A, Pearce CJ. Consensus in chronic ankle instability: aetiology, assessment, surgical indications and place for arthroscopy. Orthop Traumatol Surg Res. 2013;99:411–9.
36. Hennrikus WL, Mapes RC, Lyons PM, Lapoint JM. Outcomes of the Chrisman-Snook and modified Broström procedures for chronic lateral ankle instability: a prospective, randomized comparison. Am J Sports Med. 1996;24:400–4.
37. Noailles T, Lopes R, Padiolleau G, Gouin F, Brilhault J. Non-anatomical or direct anatomical repair of chronic lateral instability of the ankle: a systematic review of the literature after at least 10 years follow-up. Foot Ankle Surg. 2018;24:80–5.
38. Sugimoto K, Takakura Y, Akiyama K, Kamei S, Kitada C, Kumai T. Long-term results of Watson-Jones tenodesis of the ankle: clinical and radiographic findings after ten to eighteen years of follow-up. J Bone Joint Surg. 1998;80-A:1587–96.
39. Van der Rijt AJ, Evans GA. The long-term results of Watson-Jones tenodesis. J Bone Joint Surg. 1984;66-B:371–5.
40. So E, Preston N, Holmes T. Intermediate- to long-term longevity and incidence of revision of the modified Broström-Gould procedure for lateral ankle ligament repair: a systematic review. J Foot Ankle Surg. 2017;56:1076–80.
41. Maffulli N, Del Buono A, Maffulli GD, Oliva F, Testa V, Capasso G, Denaro V. Isolated anterior talofibular ligament Broström repair for chronis lateral ankle instability. Am J Sports Med. 2013;41(4):858–64.
42. Roos EM, Brandsson S, Karlsson J. Validation of the foot and ankle outcome score for ankle ligament reconstruction. Foto Ankle Int. 2001;22:788–94.
43. Ventura A, Legnai C, Corradini C, Borgo E. Lateral ligament reconstruction and augmented direct anatomical repair restore ligament laxity in patients suffering from chronic ankle instability up to 15 years from surgery. Knee Surg Sports Traumatol Arthrosc. 2018; https://doi.org/10.1007/s00167-018-5244-4.
44. Mabit C, Tourne Y, Besse J-L, Bonnel F, Toullec E, Giraud F, Proust J, Khiami F, Chaussard C, Genty C. SOFCOT (French Society of Orthopaedic and Traumatologic Surgery). Orthop Traumatol. 2019;96:417–23.
45. Vuurberg G, Pereira H, Blanevoort L, van Dijk CN. Anatomic stabilization techniques provide superior results in terms of functional outcome in patients suffering from chronic ankle instability compared to non-anatomic techniques. Knee Surg Sports Traumatol Arthrosc. 2018;26:2183–95.
46. Rosenbaum D, Becker HP, Sterk J, Gerngross H, Claes L. Functional evaluation of the 10-year outcome after modified Evans repair for chronic ankle instability. Foot Ankle Int. 1997;18:765–71.

21 Level of Evidence for Mini-Invasive Treatment of Chronic Ankle Instability

Kentaro Matsui, Haruki Odagiri, and Mark Glazebrook

21.1 Introduction

The current literature for open surgical procedures on anatomic repair or reconstruction of the Anterior talofibular ligament (ATFL) and/or Calcaneofibular ligament (CFL) provides good clinical results [1]. There has been a recent advent of published descriptions on minimally invasive surgeries (MIS) for chronic ankle instability (CAI) [2–37]. In this chapter, an evidence-based review of the literature published on MIS for the treatment of CAI has been summarized.

K. Matsui (✉)
Department of Orthopaedic Surgery, Trauma Center, Teikyo University Hospital, Tokyo, Japan
e-mail: kenor@med.teikyo-u.ac.jp

H. Odagiri
Department of Orthopaedic Surgery, Hotakubo Orthopedic Hospital, Kumamoto, Japan

M. Glazebrook
Queen Elizabeth II Health Sciences Center Halifax Infirmary (Suite 4867), Dalhousie University, Halifax, NS, Canada

21.2 Classification of Mini-Invasive Treatment of Chronic Ankle Instability

The MIS for CAI can be classified into four categories based on the adopted surgical technique. This includes two major categories: anatomic repair or reconstruction of the ATFL and/or CFL. Both categories embrace arthroscopic or non-arthroscopic minimally invasive techniques. Percutaneous techniques or mini-open techniques were included in non-arthroscopic minimally invasive approach [38]. In this review, we have used the following four classification categories.

1. Arthroscopic repair
2. Non-arthroscopic minimally invasive repair
3. Arthroscopic reconstruction
4. Non-arthroscopic minimally invasive reconstruction

21.3 Literature Search, Level of Evidence and Grade of Recommendation for Each Category of Mini-Invasive Treatment

A comprehensive review of the literature was conducted on March 4, 2016, using PubMed, EMBASE, Cochrane databases, Web of Science,

H. Pereira et al. (eds.), *Lateral Ankle Instability*, https://doi.org/10.1007/978-3-662-62763-1_21

and a thorough hand searching of references in narrative and systematic reviews. All published and unpublished clinical studies regarding MIS for CIA written in English were included. The reconstruction techniques were defined as the use of grafts to reconstruct the new connections between bones to replace ligaments. Conversely, the repair techniques were defined as reattachment or shortening of torn or damaged ligaments. This systematic review excluded biomechanical studies, review articles, and studies about non-repair or non-reconstruction MIS procedures such as tenodesis or tape augmentation procedure. Each article was classified according to research method quality of evidence into Level I to V by use of the Level of Evidence criteria described by Wright et al. [39]. Based on the Level of Evidence, Level I: high-quality randomized trial with no statistically significant difference but narrow confidence intervals or systematic reviews of Level I RCTs (and study results were homogenous); Level II: lesser quality RCT (e.g., 80% follow-up, no blinding, or improper randomization), prospective comparative studies or systematic reviews of Level II studies or Level I studies with inconsistent results; Level III: case-control studies, retrospective comparative studies or systematic reviews of Level III studies; Level IV: case series; and Level V: expert opinion [39]. Series with fewer than five patients or those that had poor data correction were classified as Level of Evidence V. Studies in which the retrospective or prospective nature was not apparent were classified as retrospective. After the assignment of the quality of evidence for each paper, analysis of all studies combined was then conducted to provide a Grade of recommendation for each MIS category using four grades of recommendation (A, B, C, or I) according to Wright et al. in 2005 [40]. Based on the Grade of recommendation, Grade A: Good evidence (Level I studies with consistent findings) for or against recommending intervention; Grade B: Fair evidence (Level II or III studies with consistent findings) for or against recommending intervention; Grade C: Poor quality evidence (Level IV or V studies with consistent findings) for or against recommending intervention; and Grade I: There is insufficient or conflicting evidence not allowing a recommendation for or against intervention [40].

21.4 Summary of Level of Evidence and Grade of Recommendation

The systematic comprehensive literature searches of electronic databases and gray literature identified 491 non-duplicate records, of which 52 articles were selected for full-text review and 38 of these studies [2–37] met the inclusion criteria. Of the included studies, 34 studies were published after 2000. Twenty three studies [2–7, 12–17, 19, 21–34, 41] were classified into Arthroscopic repair category, eight studies [9, 10, 20, 28–30, 38] were classified into Arthroscopic reconstruction category, no papers were classified into non-arthroscopic minimally invasive repair category and seven papers [8, 11, 18, 26, 35–37, 42] were classified into Non-arthroscopic minimally invasive reconstruction category (Table 21.1).

21.4.1 Arthroscopic Repair

Twenty-three studies were published on arthroscopic repair [2–7, 12–17, 19, 21–23, 25, 31, 33, 34, 43], almost all of the studies repair only the ATFL but there was variety of surgical techniques. The most common technique was the repair with suture anchor [2, 3, 5, 6, 14, 15, 17, 19, 24, 32, 33, 43] followed by thermal shrinkage [4, 7, 13, 16, 22, 25, 34]. Arthroscopic repair with suture anchor [2, 3, 5, 6, 14, 15, 17, 19, 24, 32, 33, 43] techniques were varied. The most commonly utilized procedure was Arthroscopic Brostrom procedure: one or two anchors introduced from accessory anterolateral portal to the fibula footprint of the ATFL under arthroscopic view, then grasped and sutured the ATFL. Some techniques added the reinforcement with Inferior Extensor Retinaculum.

The first arthroscopic repair technique was reported in 1987 [11]. Suture anchor fixation of the ligaments was adopted in 14 papers [2, 3, 5, 6, 14, 15, 17, 19, 24, 32, 33, 43], thermal shrinkage

Table 21.1 Summary of the current literature and for or against surgical treatment of ankle instability using minimally invasive surgical approach

Surgical Technique category	No. of studies	Level I	Level II	Level III	Level IV	Level V	Grade of recommendation	Recommendation
Arthroscopic repair	23	0	0	1	13	9	C	For
Non-arthroscopic[a] repair	0	0	0	0	0	0	I	NA
Arthroscopic reconstruction	8	0	0	0	1	7	C	For
Non-arthroscopic[a] reconstruction	7	0	0	2	1	4	C	For

NA Not applicable
[a]Non-arthroscopic minimally invasive

Table 21.2 Summary of the current literature for or against surgical treatment of ankle instability using arthroscopic repair

Surgical Technique	No. of studies	Level I	Level II	Level III	Level IV	Level V	Grade of recommendation	Recommendation
Suture anchor	14	0	0	1	7	6	C	For
Thermal shrinkage	7	0	0	0	6	1	C	For
Other	2	0	0	0	0	2	I	For

NA Not applicable

in seven [4, 7, 13, 16, 22, 25, 34], and others included stapling [11] and bone tunnel [21] (Table 21.2). The first arthroscopic suture anchor repair technique was reported in 1994 by Kashuk et al. [15] and the following 13 studies [2, 3, 5, 6, 14, 17, 19, 24, 32, 33, 43] were published after 2009. However, only one Level III [23], seven Level IV [2, 5, 6, 17, 19, 33, 43], and six Level V studies [3, 14, 16, 24, 32] were available and variety of surgical techniques were reported using this approach (Table 21.2).

21.4.1.1 Suture Anchor Technique

One comparative study showed that this technique allows earlier return to activities of daily life with significantly lower pain score using visual analog pain scores at 3 days after surgery compared to the open surgery. The arthroscopic techniques in six Level V studies [3, 14, 15, 24, 32] has demonstrated the arthroscopic suture anchor technique to be relatively simple to perform if the surgeon has sufficient ankle arthroscopy experience, and results in shorter surgical time comparing to the open procedure. There were seven Level IV studies on arthroscopic repair using suture anchor reporting good functional result [2, 5, 6, 17, 19, 33, 43]. However, the complication rate in this category was reported as high (0–29%) including nerve injury, subcutaneous suture prominence, and wound infection [31]. There was one comparative study to the open procedure [23] which favored the arthroscopic technique showing lower VAS score at 3 days after surgery, earlier recovery to activities of daily living, and shorter surgical time [23].

21.4.1.2 Thermal Shrinkage Technique and Others

Seven studies [4, 7, 13, 16, 22, 25, 33] included in this review focused on thermal shrinkage of the ATFL or thermal assist capsular shrinkage, with six Level IV [4, 7, 16, 22, 25, 34] and one Level V [13] study available. These procedures seem to offer many of the same advantages as the arthroscopic Brostrom procedure and were technically simple with a short convalescence when compared to other techniques. Some of these studies suggested further studies would be needed to confirm the long-term efficacy of these procedures. Mechanical instability with complete ligament rupture was cited as a relative contraindication to this procedure in many of these studies [4, 7]. Other arthroscopic repair techniques included stapling [12] the use of bone tunnel [21] to avoid the complications of suture anchors were Level V studies.

Grade of Recommendation

On the basis of the current literature available a Grade C recommendation (poor quality evidence with Level IV and V studies recommending for the use of this intervention) is assigned to arthroscopic repair using suture anchors or thermal shrinkage (in the absence of mechanical disruption of ligaments) surgery for treatment of CAI. The literature available to support the use of staples or bone tunnels during arthroscopic repair deserves Grade I (incomplete) recommendation due to the lack of published evidence on each surgical approach.

21.4.2 Arthroscopic Reconstruction

Only one Level IV [28] study and seven Level V [9, 10, 20, 27, 30, 31, 44] studies were published on arthroscopic reconstruction surgery for CAI. One level IV [28] and a Level V [30] study reconstructed only ATFL and other six Level V [9, 10, 20, 27, 31, 44] studies reconstructed both ATFL and CFL using arthroscopy. The first report of the arthroscopic reconstruction of the ATFL came from Priano et al. [28] in 1994. In this retrospective case series, 10 patients were treated with a pedicle flap of fibular periosteum lowered like a drawbridge from the lateral malleolus to the anterolateral surface of the talus, and fixed with anchors set between the remaining ligament fibers. This technique was free from risks or substantial drawbacks compared with open surgery. However, it required a long learning curve and there are poor quality studies to provide support.

The first report on the arthroscopic anatomical reconstruction of both the ATFL and the CFL was by Lui [20]. The calcaneal insertion of the CFL could be identified arthroscopically through the anterolateral portal with the peroneal tendon sheath stripped through the middle subtalar portal. Two bone tunnels were constructed in the fibula to reconstruct ATFL and CFL anatomically. Guillo et al. [9, 10, 44] described a novel arthroscopic ATFL and CFL reconstruction technique in 2014 that utilized peroneal endoscopy to provide a better view of ATFL and CFL. This endoscopic technique made it possible to carry out anatomical reconstruction with greater accuracy of the tunnel positioning and the view obtained using this technique was suggested to be superior to that seen in open surgery [10]. It was also noted that the procedure especially endoscopic dissection was technically demanding [9]. Prissel et al. [30] reported arthroscopic stabilization reinforced with synthetic ligament for revision or complex primary lateral ankle stabilization and Piraino et al. [29] also reported their arthroscopic "recreation" of the ATFL technique with two suture anchors. Takao et al. advanced his open ATFL and CFL reconstruction technique with the core concept of "Anatomic Y-graft" and "Inside-out technique" to the Arthroscopic "Anti-RoLL" technique [31]. The same concept was adopted in the Percutaneous "Anti-RoLL" technique [11].

Grade of Recommendation

On the basis of the previously mentioned literature of this category, arthroscopic reconstruction for CAI would clearly warrant a Grade C recommendation (poor quality evidence Level IV and V studies recommending for the use of this intervention). Further, there is no evidence that shows one technique is superior to another for arthroscopic ATFL and CFL reconstruction.

21.4.3 Non-Arthroscopic Repair

There was no literature published on this approach.

The Grade of recommendation regarding the non-arthroscopic minimally invasive repair surgery is Grade I (incomplete) recommendation due to the lack of published evidence on this surgical approach.

21.4.4 Non-Arthroscopic Reconstruction

Seven studies (two Level III [36, 37], one Level IV [35], and four level V [8, 18, 26]) were found in this review for this category: minimally invasive reconstruction without using arthroscopy. All the included studies reconstructing both ATFL and CFL using auto or allograft by percutaneous technique with three to six small incisions.

Xu et al. [36] conducted a Level III retrospective comparative case series in 2014 that compared the therapeutic effect between semitendinosus autograft and allograft for ATFL and CFL reconstruction. The study involved 68 patients of which 32 had received the autograft and 36 the allograft, both via a percutaneous technique. They concluded that the clinical outcomes of the two grafts were both excellent with no significant difference identified for graft type. They also reported a relatively short recovery time for healing with minimal donor site problems in the autograft group (Table 21.1).

Another Level III study by Youn et al. [37] reviewed the outcomes of their percutaneous ATFL and CFL reconstruction with a peroneal or hamstring tendon allograft and compared results with and without tenodesis screw in fibular bone tunnel. They described their inclusion criteria as a previously failed reconstruction surgery, severe ankle instability (more than 15° of talar tilt, more than 10 mm of anterior drawer), general laxity of ligaments, and body mass index (BMI) higher than 25. They concluded that percutaneous reconstruction with allograft was effective as a salvage procedure for the treatment of severe and complicated types of CAI (Table 21.1).

Wang et al. [35] published a Level IV retrospective case series to evaluate the efficacy of their percutaneous ATFL and CFL reconstruction using a semitendinosus autograft. They concluded that the use of this technique in a minimally invasive approach could achieve ankle stability while avoiding extensive exposure and risk of nerve injury (Table 21.1). Three Level V studies [8, 18, 26] described percutaneous techniques of ATFL and CFL reconstruction. M Glazebrook published a fairly simple percutaneous reconstruction technique (Percutaneous "Anti-RoLL") adopting the same method with Arthroscopic "Anti-RoLL".

Grade of Recommendation
On the basis of the current literature, non-arthroscopic minimally invasive reconstruction approaches to treat CAI deserve a Grade C recommendation (poor quality evidence Level III, IV, and V studies recommending for the use of this intervention).

A comprehensive review of the literature has identified predominantly Level IV and V with few level III studies on MIS and arthroscopic surgery for the treatment for CAI. This literature provides poor quality evidence to support the use of MIS and arthroscopic approaches in treating CAI. This may have more to do with lack of evidence than ineffectiveness of these approaches. It is recommended that surgeons currently using MIS and arthroscopic techniques for the treatment of CAI should do this in the confines of prospective case series, comparative or randomized controlled trials to provide a higher quality of evidence on safety and efficacy.

References

1. Guillo S, Bauer T, Lee JW, Takao M, Kong SW, Stone JW, Mangone PG, Molloy A, Perera A, Pearce CJ, Michels F, Tourne Y, Ghorbani A, Calder J. Consensus in chronic ankle instability: aetiology, assessment, surgical indications and place for arthroscopy. Orthop Traumatol Surg Res. 2013;99:S411–9.
2. Acevedo JI, Mangone PG. Arthroscopic lateral ankle ligament reconstruction. Tech Foot Ankle Surg. 2011;10:111–6.
3. Acevedo JI, Mangone P. Arthroscopic Brostrom technique. Foot Ankle Int. 2015;36:465–73.
4. Berlet GC, Saar WE, Ryan A, Lee TH. Thermal-assisted capsular modification for functional ankle instability. Foot Ankle Clin. 2002;7:567–76.
5. Corte-Real NM, Moreira RM. Arthroscopic repair of chronic lateral ankle instability. Foot Ankle Int. 2009;30:213–7.
6. Cottom JM, Rigby RB. The "all inside" arthroscopic brostrom procedure: a prospective study of 40 Consecutive Patients. J Foot Ankle Surg. 2013;52:568–74.
7. de Vries JS, Krips R, Blankevoort L, Fievez AW, van Dijk CN. Arthroscopic capsular shrinkage for chronic ankle instability with thermal radiofrequency: prospective multicenter trial. Orthopedics. 2008;31:655.
8. Espinosa N, Smerek J, Kadakia AR, Myerson MS. Operative management of ankle instability:

reconstruction with open and percutaneous methods. Foot Ankle Clin. 2006;11:547–65.
9. Guillo S, Archbold P, Perera A, Bauer T, Sonnery-Cottet B. Arthroscopic anatomic reconstruction of the lateral ligaments of the ankle with gracilis autograft. Arthrosc Tech. 2014;3:e593–8.
10. Guillo S, Cordier G, Sonnery-Cottet B, Bauer T. Anatomical reconstruction of the anterior talofibular and calcaneofibular ligaments with an all-arthroscopic surgical technique. Orthop Traumatol Surg Res. 2014;100:S413–7.
11. Glazebrook M, Stone J, Matsui K, Guillo S, Takao M, ESSKA AFAS Ankle Instability Group. Percutaneous ankle reconstruction of lateral ligaments (Perc-Anti RoLL). Foot Ankle Int. 2016;37:659–64.
12. Hawkins RB. Arthroscopic stapling repair for chronic lateral instability. Clin Podiatr Med Surg. 1987;4:875–83.
13. Hyer CF, Vancourt R. Arthroscopic repair of lateral ankle instability by using the thermal-assisted capsular shift procedure: a review of 4 cases. J Foot Ankle Surg. 2004;43:104–9.
14. Kashuk KB, Carbonell JA, Blum JA. Arthroscopic stabilization of the ankle. Clin Podiatr Med Surg. 1997;14:459–78.
15. Kashuk KB, Landsman AS, Werd MB, Hanft JR, Roberts M. Arthroscopic lateral ankle stabilization. Clin Podiatr Med Surg. 1994;11:407–23.
16. Khan A, Fanton G. Use of thermal energy in treatment of ankle disorders. Sports Med Arthrosc Rev. 2000;8:354–64.
17. Kim ES, Lee KT, Park JS, Lee YK. Arthroscopic anterior talofibular ligament repair for chronic ankle instability with a suture anchor technique. Orthopedics. 2011;34(4) https://doi.org/10.3928/01477447-20110228-03.
18. Kim HN, Dong Q, Hong DY, Yoon YH, Park YW. Percutaneous lateral ankle ligament reconstruction using a split peroneus longus tendon free graft: technical tip. Foot Ankle Int. 2014;35:1082–6.
19. Labib SA, Slone HS. Ankle arthroscopy for lateral ankle instability. Tech Foot Ankle Surg. 2015;14:25–7.
20. Lui TH. Modified arthroscopic Brostrom procedure. Foot Ankle Surg. 2015;21:216–9.
21. Lui TH. Arthroscopic-assisted lateral ligamentous reconstruction in combined ankle and subtalar instability. Arthroscopy. 2007;23:554.e1–5.
22. Maiotti M, Massoni C, Tarantino U. The use of arthroscopic thermal shrinkage to treat chronic lateral ankle instability in young athletes. Arthroscopy. 2005;21:751–7.
23. Matsui K, Takao M, Miyamoto W, Matsushita T. Early recovery after arthroscopic repair compared to open repair of the anterior talofibular ligament for lateral instability of the ankle. Arch Orthop Trauma Surg. 2016;136:93–100.
24. Matsui K, Takao M, Miyamoto W, Innami K, Matsushita T. Arthroscopic Brostrom repair with Gould augmentation via an accessory anterolateral port for lateral instability of the ankle. Arch Orthop Trauma Surg. 2014;134:1461–7.
25. Oloff LM, Bocko AP, Fanton G. Arthroscopic monopolar radiofrequency thermal stabilization for chronic lateral ankle instability: a preliminary report on 10 cases. J Foot Ankle Surg. 2000;39:144–53.
26. Panchbhavi VK. Minimally invasive allograft lateral ankle ligament reconstruction. Tech Foot Ankle Surg. 2011;10:117–21.
27. Pijnenburg AC, Bogaard K, Krips R, Marti RK, Bossuyt PM, Dijk CN. Operative and functional treatment of rupture of the lateral ligament of the ankle. J Bone Joint Surg Br. 2003;85:525–30.
28. Piraino JA, Busch EL, Sansosti LE, Pettineo SJ, Creech C. Use of an all-suture anchor for re-creation of the anterior talofibular ligament: a case report. J Foot Ankle Surg. 2015;54:126–9.
29. Priano F, Gatto P. Arthroscopic reconstruction of inveterate anterior talofibular ligament tears. Notes on the technique employed and the short-term results. J Sports Traumatol Relat Res. 1994;16:97–104.
30. Prissel MA, Roukis TS. All-inside, anatomical lateral ankle stabilization for revision and complex primary lateral ankle stabilization: a technique guide. Foot Ankle Spec. 2014;7:484–91.
31. Takao M, Glazebrook M, Stone J, Guillo S. Ankle arthroscopic reconstruction of lateral ligaments (ankle anti-ROLL). Arthrosc Tech. 2015;23:e595–600.
32. Takao M, Matsui K, Stone JW, Glazebrook MA, Kennedy JG, Guillo S, Calder JD, Karlsson J, Ankle Instability Group. Arthroscopic anterior talofibular ligament repair for lateral instability of the ankle. Knee Surg Sports Traumatol Arthrosc. 2015; https://doi.org/10.1007/s00167-015-3638-0.
33. Vega J, Golano P, Pellegrino A, Rabat E, Pena F. All-inside arthroscopic lateral collateral ligament repair for ankle instability with a knotless suture anchor technique. Foot Ankle Int. 2013;34:1701–9.
34. Ventura A, Terzaghi C, Legnani C, Borgo E. Arthroscopic four-step treatment for chronic ankle instability. Foot Ankle Int. 2012;33:29–36.
35. Wang B, Xu X. Minimally invasive reconstruction of lateral ligaments of the ankle using semitendinosus autograft. Foot Ankle Int. 2013;34:711–5.
36. Xu X, Hu M, Liu J, Zhu Y, Wang B. Minimally invasive reconstruction of the lateral ankle ligaments using semitendinosus autograft or tendon allograft. Foot Ankle Int. 2014;35:1015–21.
37. Youn H, Kim YS, Lee J, Choi WJ, Lee JW. Percutaneous lateral ligament reconstruction with allograft for chronic lateral ankle instability. Foot Ankle Int. 2012;33:99–104.
38. Matsui K, Burgesson B, Takao M, Stone J, Guillo S, Glazebrook M, ESSKA AFAS Ankle Instability Group. Minimally invasive surgical treatment for chronic ankle instability: a systematic review. Knee Surg Sports Traumatol Arthrosc. 2016;24:1040–8.
39. Wright JG, Swiontkowski MF, Heckman JD. Introducing levels of evidence to the journal. J Bone Joint Surg Am. 2003;85-A:1–3.

40. Wright JG, Einhorn TA, Heckman JD. Grades of recommendation. J Bone Joint Surg Am. 2005;87:1909–10.
41. Pereira H, Vuurberg G, Gomes N, Oliveira JM, Ripoll PL, Reis RL, Espregueira-Mendes J, Niek van Dijk C. Arthroscopic repair of ankle instability with all-soft knotless anchors. Arthrosc Tech. 2016;5:e99–e107.
42. Wang J, Hua Y, Chen S, Li H, Zhang J, Li Y. Arthroscopic repair of lateral ankle ligament complex by suture anchor. Arthroscopy. 2014;30:766–73.
43. Nery C, Raduan F, Del Buono A, Asaumi ID, Cohen M, Maffulli N. Arthroscopic-assisted Brostrom-Gould for chronic ankle instability: a long-term follow-up. Am J Sports Med. 2011;39:2381–8.
44. Guillo S, Takao M, Calder J, Karlson J, Michels F, Bauer T, Ankle Instability Group. Arthroscopic anatomical reconstruction of the lateral ankle ligaments. Knee Surg Sports Traumatol Arthrosc. 2016;4:998–1002.

22 Arthroscopic Capsular Shrinkage

Gwendolyn Vuurberg and Niek Van Dijk

22.1 Objective and Technical Details

Arthroscopic capsular shrinkage is an arthroscopic technique that may be used in the treatment of chronic lateral ankle instability (CAI) (Fig. 22.1). This technique is mainly performed as an outpatient procedure with the patient in the supine position. After introduction of a 4.0-mm arthroscope through the anteromedial portal, the lateral portal is created under direct vision. First additional pathology such as osteophytes or a synovitis may be treated. Subsequently the capsular shrinkage is performed (Fig. 22.2). Radiofrequent energy is applied to the capsular-ligamentous tissue of the lateral ankle joint to induce shrinkage of collagenous structures. Inducing heat to these collagenous structures results in structure shrinkage and with that tightening of the lateral ankle ligaments and joint capsule [1, 2].

22.2 Patient Reported Outcomes

Overall postoperative improvement is seen in studies on capsular shrinkage. Only six studies so far have been published on capsular shrinkage of the ankle with publication dates between 2000 and 2012 [1, 3–7]. A wide range in sample sizes has been reported (range 4–90 patients per study) as did the mean follow-up term (range 6–48 months). Results after surgery were mainly assessed using patient reported outcome measures (PROMs). The main advantage of PROM usage is the fact scores reflect the patients' perceptions of complaints and recovery. However, many PROMs have been developed over time, leading to heterogeneity in outcome assessment. In the case of capsular shrinkage, results have been evaluated using five different PROM scores, all showing significant improvement postoperatively compared to the preoperative assessment. PROMs used were the Karlsson score (improvement 58.8 ± 8.1 to 88.2 ± 6.3) [1, 5, 7], the AOFAS score (63.0 ± 3.1 to 91.9 ± 3.6) [4, 6, 7], the SF-36 physical (44.4 ± 7.7 to 51.0 ± 9.2) [1], Tegner (3.4 ± 1.2 to 4.8 ± 1.1) [1, 7] and Sefton scale (4.0 ± 0.0 to 1.8 ± 0.8) [7].

G. Vuurberg (✉) · N. Van Dijk
Department of Orthopedic Surgery, Amsterdam UMC, Amsterdam Movement Sciences, University of Amsterdam, Amsterdam, The Netherlands

Academic Center for Evidence Based Sports Medicine (ACES), Amsterdam, The Netherlands

Amsterdam Collaboration for Health and Safety in Sports (ACHSS), Academic Medical Center/VU University Medical Center, Amsterdam, The Netherlands
e-mail: g.vuurberg@amsterdamumc.nl; c.n.vandijk@amsterdamumc.nl

H. Pereira et al. (eds.), *Lateral Ankle Instability*, https://doi.org/10.1007/978-3-662-62763-1_22

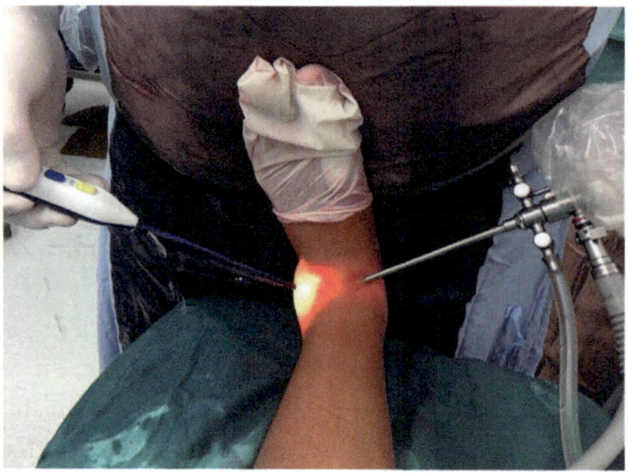

Fig. 22.1 Outside view of arthroscopic shrinkage technique

22.3 Satisfaction

De Vries et al. [1] reported that despite high satisfaction rates, the capsular shrinkage technique failed to improve mechanical joint laxity [4]. Improvement and satisfaction may therefore be related to an improved proprioception and coordination of the ankle, possibly caused by a combination of joint debridement and capsule tightening.

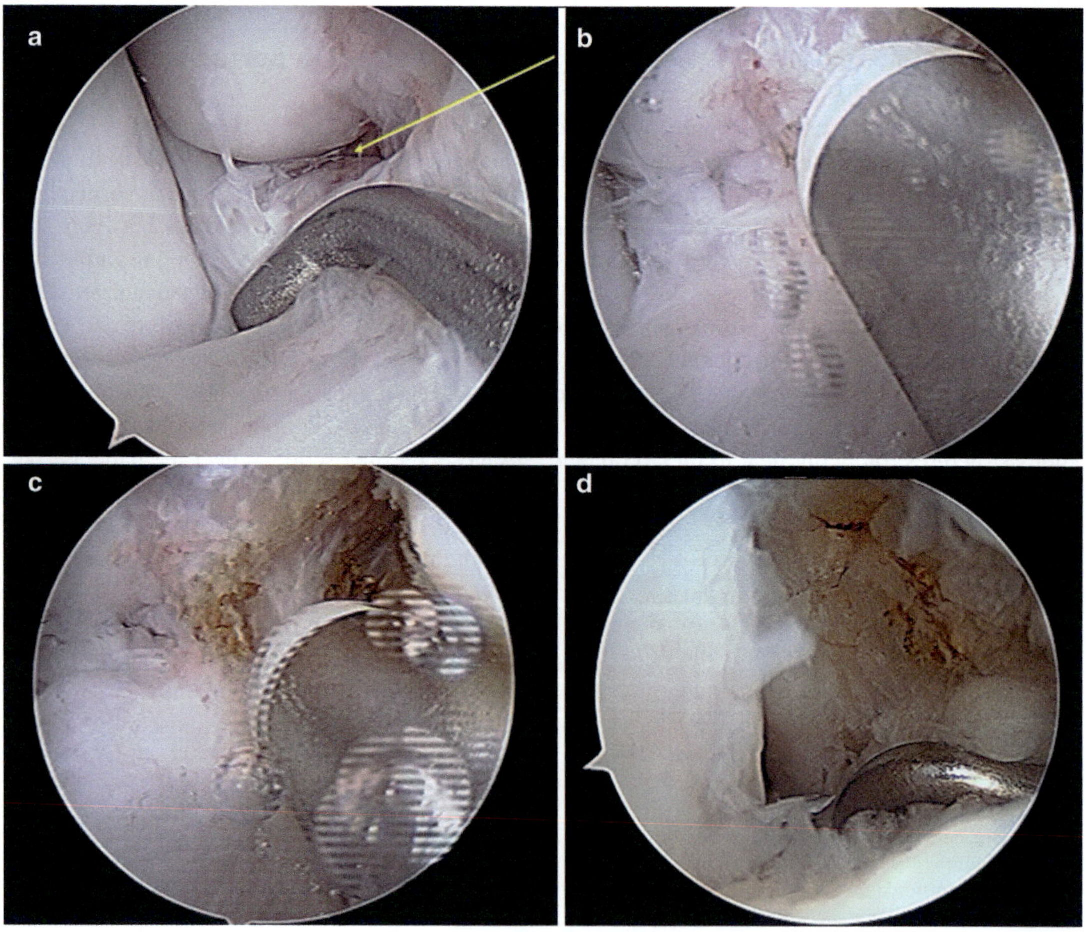

Fig. 22.2 (**a**) Anterior tibiofibular ligament (ATFL) detachment from the fibula with elongation of ATFL; (**b** and **c**) use of radiofrequency probe for tissue shrinkage; (**d**) increased tissue tension after the procedure as tested by the hook probe

22.4 Complications

For the total of 165 patients reported complications included numbness (0.6%), altered sensation (3%), reoperation (2%), tape allergy (1%), ROM restriction (2%) and persistent postoperative pain (0.6%) [1, 3, 5, 7].

22.5 Conclusion

Despite high satisfaction rates and a low number of reported complications, capsular shrinkage does not resolve mechanical joint laxity.

Take-Home Message

- With a maximum assessed follow-up of 4 years, an overall low population size apart from Ventura et al. [7] and a lack of analyses on factors that may be correlated to recurrence of instability and low treatment satisfaction, it is not possible to identify for which patients capsular shrinkage is indicated.

References

1. de Vries JS, Krips R, Blankevoort L, Fievez AW, van Dijk CN. Arthroscopic capsular shrinkage for chronic ankle instability with thermal radiofrequency: prospective multicenter trial. Orthopedics. 2008;31:655.
2. Liu SH, Jacobson KE. A new operation for chronic lateral ankle instability. J Bone Joint Surg Br. 1995;77:55–9.
3. Berlet GC, Saar WE, Ryan A, Lee TH. Thermal-assisted capsular modification for functional ankle instability. Foot Ankle Clin. 2002;7:567–576, ix.
4. Hyer CF, Vancourt R. Arthroscopic repair of lateral ankle instability by using the thermal-assisted capsular shift procedure: a review of 4 cases. J Foot Ankle Surg. 2004;43:104–9.
5. Maiotti M, Massoni C, Tarantino U. The use of arthroscopic thermal shrinkage to treat chronic lateral ankle instability in young athletes. Arthroscopy. 2005;21:751–7.
6. Oloff LM, Bocko AP, Fanton G. Arthroscopic monopolar radiofrequency thermal stabilization for chronic lateral ankle instability: a preliminary report on 10 cases. J Foot Ankle Surg. 2000;39:144–53.
7. Ventura A, Terzaghi C, Legnani C, Borgo E. Arthroscopic four-step treatment for chronic ankle instability. Foot Ankle Int. 2012;33:29–36.

Arthroscopic-Assisted Repair of Chronic Lateral Ankle Instability

23

Nuno Côrte-Real, Caio Nery, Fernando C. Raduan, and Francisco Guerra-Pinto

23.1 Introduction

Chronic lateral ankle instability (CLAI) is closely related to inversion trauma of the ankle ("ankle sprain"). This type of trauma is extremely frequent, making the prevalence of ankle instability relatively high, as previously discussed. Therefore, most of the cases of CLAI have a traumatic onset [1–6].

Ankle sprains are also the cause of a numerous group of lesions, either intra-articular lesions, such as osteochondral defect, ankle impingements, synovitis, loose bodies, or extra-articular lesions such as peroneal tendons ruptures and tenosynovitis [1]. Since CLAI and several intra-articular pathologies have the same ethiopathological origin (one acute or several chronic supination traumas of the ankle), it is common to find these types of intra-articular lesions simultaneously with CLAI [2, 3, 6–9].

Some of these situations can be underdiagnosed preoperatively, even with modern diagnostic tools [10, 11].

N. Côrte-Real (✉)
Hospital de Cascais, Alcabideche, Portugal

C. Nery · F. C. Raduan
Hospital Israelita Albert Einstein, São Paulo, Brazil
e-mail: fernando@raduan.com.br

F. Guerra-Pinto
Hospital de Sant'Ana, Parede, Portugal

The standard surgical treatment of CLAI should respect same principles of open surgery, frequently an anatomic and physiologic repair like the Broström-Gould procedure [3, 4, 6, 12–14].

Due to the high incidence of concomitant lesions, which can be underdiagnosed preoperatively, several authors recommend an arthroscopic exploration of the ankle joint before a lateral ligament repair. Usually the recommendation is to perform an ankle arthroscopy followed by an open repair of the lateral ligament complex [2, 7, 10, 11, 13, 15, 16].

On the other hand, there is clear trend in all fields of Orthopedics toward less invasive surgeries with some advantages for the patients (less morbidity, faster recovery, lower wound complication rate). So, whenever possible, the open procedures have been progressively replaced by arthroscopic surgery.

For these reasons (the necessity of doing an arthroscopic inspection of the joint and desire of a less invasive surgery) arthroscopic-assisted repair of CLAI a useful technique avoiding the need of switching from an arthroscopic to an open procedure during the operation, especially because the open repair can be more demanding after arthroscopic exploration due joint infusion with saline solution and consequent soft tissue infiltration.

H. Pereira et al. (eds.), *Lateral Ankle Instability*, https://doi.org/10.1007/978-3-662-62763-1_23

The main issue is to find an arthroscopic procedure for CLAI that can produce a strong and durable repair in a reproducible manner.

For more than 15 years, we have been using a method of arthroscopic-assisted repair for CLAI which has shown good results [17–19].

23.2 Surgical Technique

23.2.1 The Surgical Procedure as Performed by Corte-Real

The procedure is done under spinal or general anesthesia.

The patient is positioned supine with the foot on the distal edge of the table and with a small beam bag under the ipsilateral buttock. The tourniquet is placed on the thigh. The extremity is draped in the regular manner. An arthroscopic pump is used to maintain the fluid pressure constant inside the joint, regulated to 40/50 mmHg. A non-invasive distraction strap rapped around the surgeon waist may be used, allowing intermittent distraction and full mobilization of the joint.

Anatomic landmarks are identified and referenced, especially the superficial peroneal nerve (when visible). This nerve can be more easily evident by doing supination of the foot by pushing the fourth toe.

The anteromedial portal is made first, and the location of the anterolateral portal is defined using trans illumination, avoiding the superficial peroneal nerve. The location of the lateral portal must be defined carefully. If we are planinig to do a lateral ligament repair, it should be placed lateraly to the superficial peroneal nerve (and not medially as usaly describded) to avoid damaging the nerve when doing the suture (as discussed below).

A full arthroscopic inspection of the ankle joint is performed, and any concomitant intra-articular lesions are treated accordingly. These gestures must be done before the ligament repair because instability favors visualization (allows greater separation of tibia and talus), and the maneuvers necessary for the treatment of these lesions can put the ligament repair in risk.

Mechanical instability is confirmed under direct vision; a supination force is manually applied to the foot, and a significant separation of tibia and talus can be observed on the lateral side of the joint. This instability is more evident reproducing the supination direction of force that produce the lesion, rather than talar tilt or anterior drawer done isolated, highlighting the rotational characteristic of this instability.

The lateral gutter is cleaned of all fibrous tissue using shaver and radiofrequency wand alternatively, especially the periosteal tissue on the fibula's anterior face (immediately distal from the anterior tibio-fibular ligament), corresponding roughly to the higher part of the anterior talofibular ligament (ATFL) footprint.

A bone anchor larger than 5 mm with four sutures (with needles) is introduced through the anterolateral portal. It must be placed perpendicular to the bone, into the fibula, to avoid slippage and allowed better visual control of its insertion. We can use titanium, PEEK, or bioabsorbable anchors (Fig. 23.1).

When the anchor is fully seated into the fibula, the anchor driver is removed, and we will have four sutures exiting the anterolateral portal (Fig. 23.2a).

An accessory anterolateral portal is made 2 cm anteriorly and 1 cm distally of the tip of the lateral malleolus. This portal is located over the position where the retracted end of the ATFL (the peroneal insertion) is expected to be and on the superior edge of the extensor retinaculum, and must be located lateral to superficial peroneal nerve. Both anterolateral portals (the regular and the accessory) must be lateral to the nerve; if not, the nerve will be impinged when passing the sutures or be trapped by the knot (Fig. 23.2b, c).

A suture retriever is passed through the accessory anterolateral portal, and three of the four sutures are retrieved, resulting in one suture exiting the superior regular anterolateral portal and three sutures exiting inferior accessory anterolateral portal (Fig. 23.3a, b).

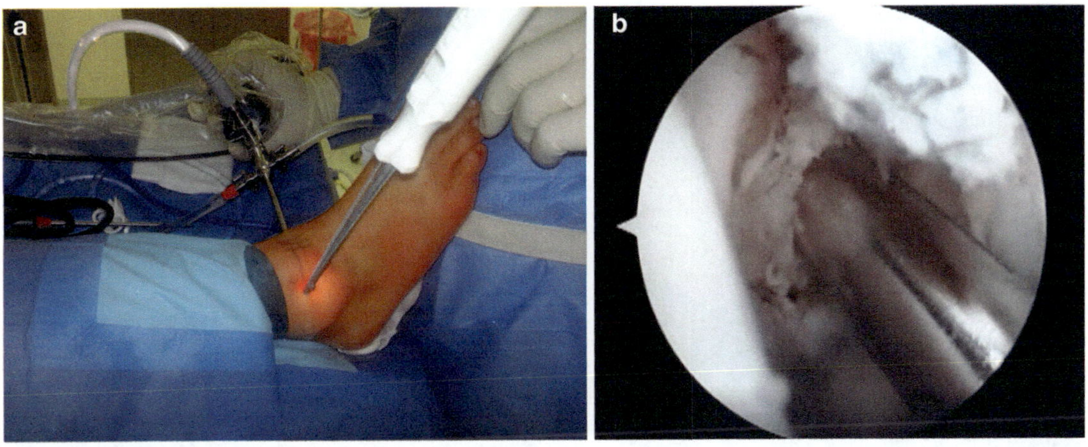

Fig. 23.1 Placement of the anchor through the anterolateral portal on the anterior face of the fibular on the upper part of the ATFL footprint (**a**) Exterior view showing the placement of the anchor through the regular lateral portal. (**b**) Intra-articular view

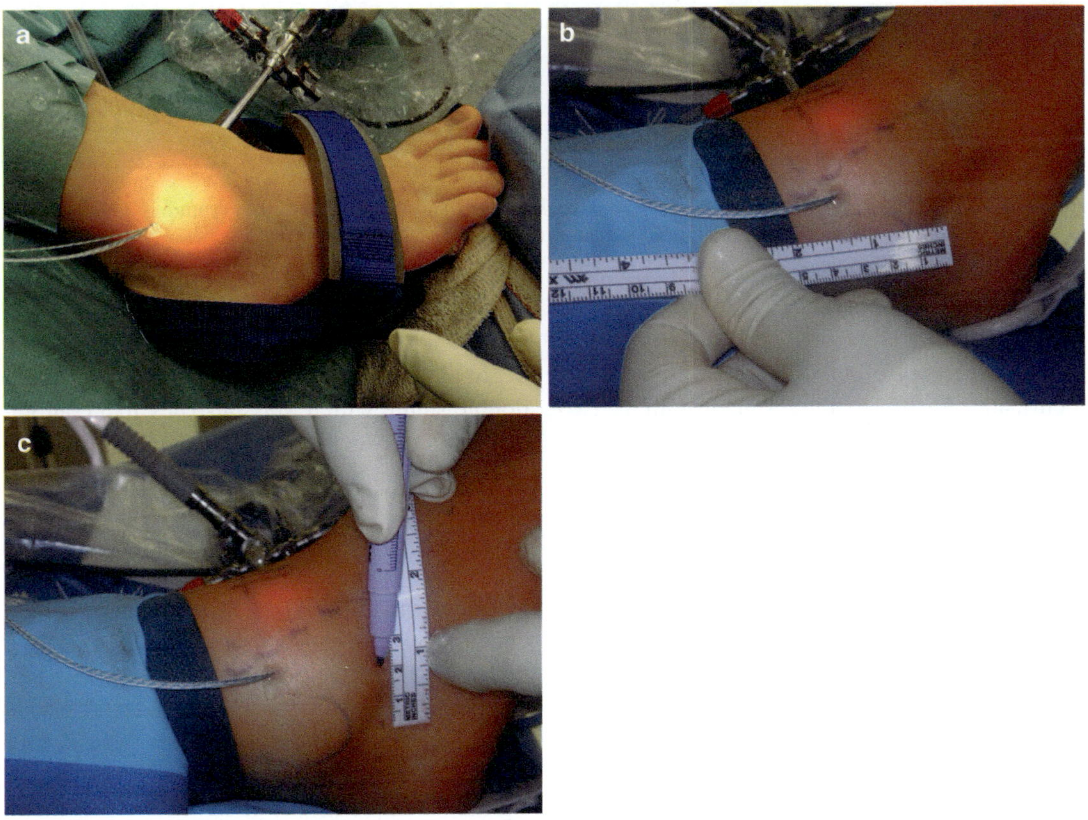

Fig. 23.2 (**a**) Four sutures exiting the anterolateral portal. (**b**, **c**) The location of the accessory portal

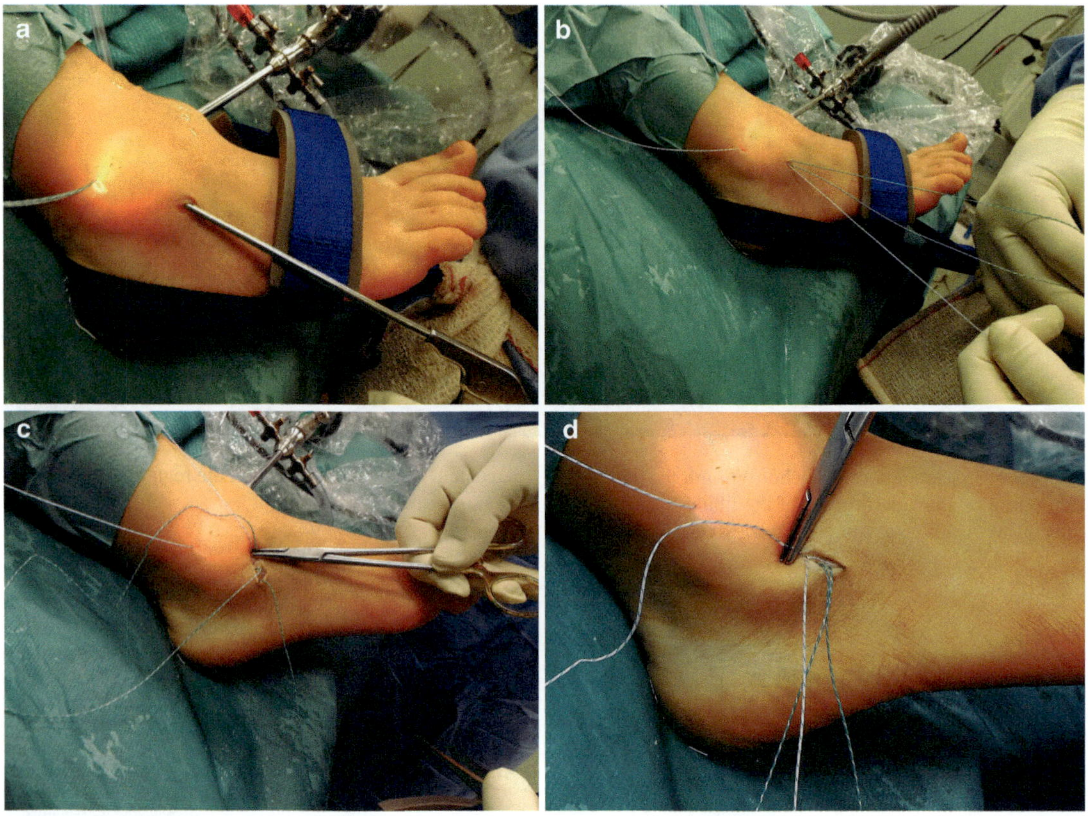

Fig. 23.3 (**a**, **b**) Retrieving three sutures through the accessory lateral portal. (**c**, **d**) A mattress suture is done, reaching as deep as possible on the accessory portal, reaching the extensor retinaculum

The arthroscope can be removed from the joint.

The accessory portal is slightly enlarged (to 1 cm), and a mattress suture is made with the two sutures of the same color. The sutures are passed as deep as possible, trying to reach the remnant ATFL and the extensor retinaculum. The third suture is passed more profound than the first two on a longitudinal way, making a Masson-Alley effect. Then the first knot is tied with the foot held in pronation and dorsiflexion (Fig. 23.3c, d).

A subcutaneous tunnel is made with the suture retriever from the accessory portal to the antero-lateral portal, and the last suture is retrieved to the accessory portal. A sliding knot is performed maintaining the foot in maximal pronation and dorsiflexion (Fig. 23.4).

The first knot will reattach the retracted ATFL to the fibula, but it will produce a point fixation of that ligament. The second suture, which has an intra-articular limb and an extra-articular limb, will compress the "body" of the ligament against the fibula, filling the "footprint" of ligament. This double suture with a Masson-Alley like configuration is self-locking and produces a stronger construct then simple sutures. It also compress the remanant ligament against the foot-print because it has a intra-articular limb tyed to an extra-articular one.

The normal foot in the rest position (as seen in an anesthetized patient lying on the operating table) is slightly supinated. After tightening of the knots, we can observe that the foot losses that typical rest position and becomes pronated or neutral (evidence of the tightening of the lateral ligament complex).

The arthroscope is reintroduced in the joint, and stability is confirmed with direct vision doing a gentle manual supination of the foot. Usually no separation of the tibia and the talus is observed.

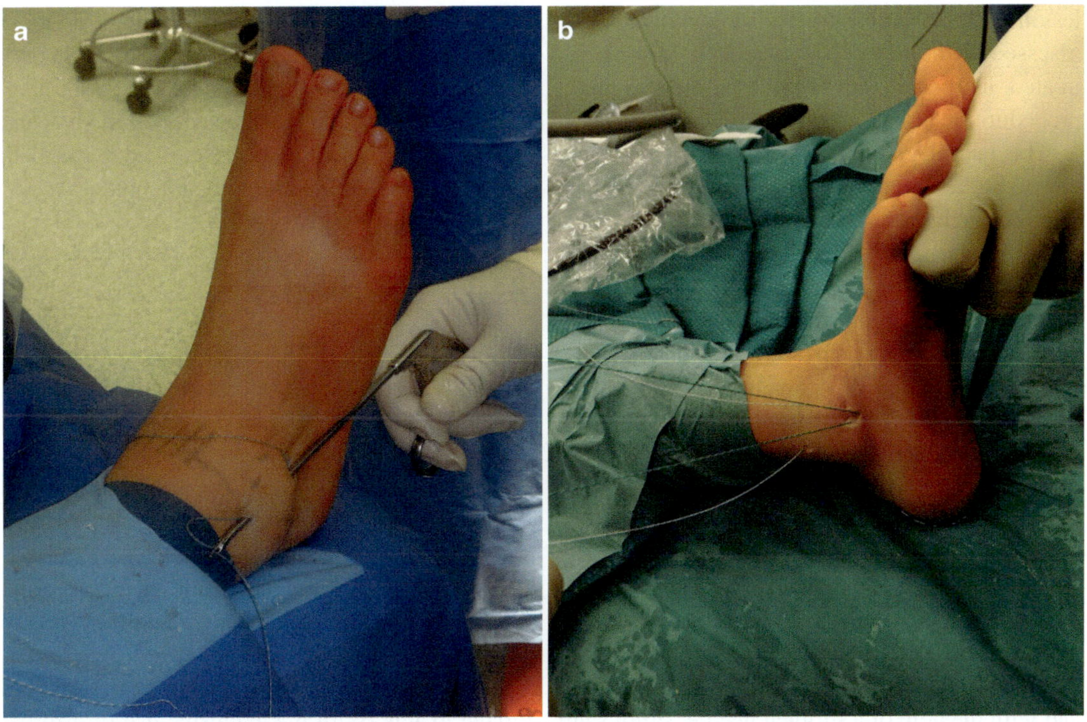

Fig. 23.4 (**a**) Retrieving the fourth suture through a subcutaneous tunnel. (**b**) A sliding knot is tied with the foot in maximum pronation and dorsiflexion

The portals are sutured in the regular manner, and a soft dressing (forcing the foot on pronation) is made. No rigid immobilization is used.

The sutures are removed on the second week. The patient is instructed not to bear weight for 3 weeks and start physiotherapy on the second post-op week (physiotherapy is usually helpful during 3 months).

One month after surgery, walking with no limitations is allowed, and the patient can return to sports and heavy work on the fourth month.

23.2.2 The Surgical Procedure as Performed by Nery

The procedure is done under spinal anesthesia and sedation with the patient in supine position and the ankle in neutral position. Sometimes, it is necessary to use a small round silicone support under the buttock to obtain the correct positioning of the foot and ankle. The pneumatic tourniquet is placed as high as possible on the thigh, and the extremity is draped in the usual manner. A 20-cm-diameter rounded support is placed under the ankle to be operated to permit full access and free mobility of the joints. After exsanguination with Esmarch bands, the tourniquet is inflated to 280 mmHg. No joint distraction is needed to perform the lateral ligament repair.

Using the classical anatomic landmarks of the ankle, three portals—anteromedial, anterolateral, and accessory anterolateral portals are demarked with a surgical pen. The superficial peroneal nerve is visible and palpable on most patients by putting the foot in full invertion with the lesser toes kept in plantar flexion, and it is also marked with the surgical pen. A 2.7 mm, 30° angled arthroscope is introduced in the ankle joint through the anteromedial portal and an arthroscopic probe through the lateral portal. During the different steps of the procedure, one can alternate the arthroscope allowing the better visualization of the entire joint.

A complete inventory of the joint is performed in order to identify soft tissue or bone impingements, loose bodies, and possible osteochondral lesions. Medial ankle instability should also be assessed. All diagnosed associated lesions are treated in the classic manner before the main procedure.

The lateral gutter is carefully inspected and cleaned to assess all the ligament lesions and to remove the hypertrophic fibrous tissue and ATFL remnants. With the help of the shaver, radiofrequency wands or small curettes, the anterior inferior border of the fibula is debrided to the bleeding bone creating a rough surface that will help in the healing of the repaired ligaments.

Under direct arthroscopic vision, a CorkScrew® anchor (Arthrex Inc., Naples, FL) double-loaded with #2 FiberWire® sutures is introduced through an anterolateral accessory portal right on the foot print of the ATFL at the anteroinferior aspect of the lateral malleolus. All the sutures are exteriorized through the accessory anterolateral portal.

The accessory portal is extended to 1.5 cm, and with the help of a surgical needle, sutures are passed through the lateral capsular and ligament remnants.

A blind knot between arms of each suture is performed. Applying a firm traction on the other arms of the sutures will strain and push the articular capsule and ligaments over the anterior aspect of the fibula. Some other knots performed with the aid of a knot-pusher will stabilize the construct attaching soft tissues over the anatomic footprint.

After manual assessment of the joint stability, the proximal aspect of the inferior extensor retinaculum (IER) is exposed. Then, to augment the repair, the IER is mobilized proximally and sutured to the soft tissue already repaired using the same sutures as described by Gould et al. Before ending the procedure, it is advisable to take a look at the suture site to be sure that the soft tissue was securely fixed to the anterior surface of the fibula and test the tension of the construct and the clinical stability with the ankle in slight eversion, at 90°.

After the operation, the ankle is immobilized in a short leg cast, and no weight bearing is allowed for 2 weeks. Patients submitted to treatment of other intra-articular lesions can have their non-weight-bearing period extended. At 4 weeks, physical therapy, including proprioceptive training, eversion exercises, and active ankle extension, is started, with the ankle in a semi-rigid brace. Swimming, running, and cycling are allowed by 3 months and return to high-contact sports (soccer, basketball, volleyball, handball) is allowed at 6 months.

23.3 Discussion

Arthroscopic surgery has progressively gained, over the last decades, an irreplaceable role on dealing with articular lesions, being, nowadays, the gold standard for those pathologies. It has several advantages over the open surgery like less morbidity, faster recovery, and lower risk of wound complications, among others.

Arthroscopy is also important as a diagnostic tool. It is possible to not only visualize but also palpate and stress structures testing their integrity, which could be missed even in the modern image exams. With the extensive use of arthroscopy and the crescent experience of surgeons on that field, some groups of pathology, previously unknown, are now being identified and treated.

Ankle arthroscopy, first labeled as impossible because of its tight space, gained extreme relevance and is a consensual method for treatment of several conditions with excellent results published like many other joints [20]. It is an important diagnostic and therapeutic tool for the foot and ankle surgeon [20].

There is a close relation between supination trauma and ankle instability, as seen before, and ankle sprains are extremely frequent. This type of trauma can also cause other traumatic pathologies in and around the joint as intra-articular lesions and tendinopathies. For that reason, the association of CLAI with other conditions (also consequence of multiple ankle sprains) is extremely frequent. Pereira et al., analyzing a group of our patients, reported this association in 88% of the patients [19]. Hintermann found cartilage damage in 66% of patients treated for lateral ankle instability [2]. Taga et al. performed arthroscopic examination before ligament reconstruction and found that 95% of the chronic injury group and 89% of the acute injury group had cartilage lesions [16].

Sugimoto et al. described 77% of osteochondral lesions in a group of 99 arthroscopies performed on patients with long-standing ankle instability. They also found those injuries more frequently on the medial aspect of the talus and related the presence of osteochondral lesions with the progression to ankle osteoarthritis [8]. Komenda and Ferkel reported, on 55 ankles treated for instability, 93% of intra-articular abnormalities including loose bodies, synovitis, osteochondral lesions of the talus, ossicles, osteophytes, adhesions, and chondromalacia. They concluded that ankle arthroscopy was mandatory before ankle instability treatment [3]. Nery et al. reported that, on a series of 38 patients submitted arthroscopic-assisted Broström-Gould, 10 patients had osteochondral talar defects. These osteochondral defects were treated at the same time that the arthroscopic-assisted Broström-Gould was done and the presence and treatment of the defects didn't influnce the final results on these patients (compared with the patients with intact cartilage) [18].

Preoperative exams (namely MRI) can miss some simultaneous lesions. They can be unidentified either by radiologist or by orthopedic surgeon. O'Neill reviewed 127 arthroscopies (previous to ligament repair) which had 64 concomitant lesions, and both the radiologist and attending surgeon only identified on the MRI a part of the existing lesions, 39% and 47% of the chondral injuries, 56% and 71% of the peroneous brevis tears, and 57% and 89% of the loose bodies, respectively. The attending surgeon achieved a better sensitivity than the radiologist (63% versus 45%) [11]. Cha et al. reviewed 65 MRI performed on patients that subsequently were operated for CLAI (ankle arthroscopy followed by open ligament repair) and concluded that the MRI sensitivity and inter-observer reliability were low for the identification of concomitant lesion [10]. Nery et al. series showed that only 71% of MRI findings were fully confirmed on arthroscopies performed to treat their ankle instability [18].

The failure to recognize and treat these simultaneous lesions can be the cause for persistent pain on an otherwise well-performed ligament repair [6, 7, 21]. Van Dijk related the persistence of medial pain after ankle sprain with the presence of osteochondral lesion. In arthroscopies made after acute supination trauma, in elite athletes, he found in 67% of cases a fresh chondral lesion, more frequently on the medial side. Adhesion, synovitis, and loose bodies were also a frequent finding [7].

Due to the high incidence of concomitant articular lesions, several authors recommend an arthroscopic inspection prior to the ligament repair (usually an open Broström-Gould procedure or similar) [2, 3, 7, 13, 15]. Considering ankle arthroscopy is mandatory on the treatment of CLAI (for the concomitant lesions confirmation and treatment), the arthroscopic repair methods become even more interesting.

Some arthroscopic methods have been tried. The first technique proposed, as far as we know, was by Hawkins in 1987, which implied the application of a staple on the talus. This gesture would result in a tensioning of lax scar tissue that replaced the torn ligament and was unable to fully restore the mechanical proprieties of lateral ligament complex. The author reported good results, but the method failed to achieve general acceptance [22].

Thermal shrinkage of the scared and distended lateral ligaments using a radiofrequency was proposed by some authors, following the initial enthusiasm produced by its use in shoulder arthroscopies [23, 24]. Nowadays, this method is almost abandoned due to its catastrophic results, mainly in shoulder arthroscopy, and its use has been relatively abandoned.

On ankle instability treatment, experience showed that thermal shrinkage was unable to correct mechanical instability.

Nevertheless, radiofrequency can be useful treating functional instability, probably due to its action on nerve endings and neurological receptors.

The "Arthroscopic Broström," like the technique that we present above, has been discussed by some authors, reporting good results. It is an anatomic and physiologic repair [9, 17–19, 25, 26]. In 2009 Corte-Real and Moreira reported a series of 28 patients operated using the technique described above with the average follow-up of 27 months. They presented good functional results and satisfaction rate. Seven patients had complications, but only two were persistent (one superficial peroneal nerve injury and one deep venous thrombosis) [17]. Nery et al. presented in 2011 his experience using a technique which he named as "arthroscopic-assisted Broström-Gould." On a series of 38 patients, with an average follow-up of 10 years, 94.7% of cases were rated as good or excellent, with only two bad results. One patient was reoperated for anterolateral impingement syndrome [18]. Kim et al. reported good results with arthroscopic repair using a single anchor on 28 patients. After a mean follow-up of 16 months, the AOFAS score was 92 with a complication rate of 14% [26].

Following these early reports, several other authors reported arthroscopic solutions for CLAI that will be addressed in other section of this book [9, 25, 27].

The double stich used in the technique described above can provide a stronger fixation than several points fixation compressing the torn end of the ligament against the fibula, filling the "footprint." Its configuration, like a Masson-Allen stich (used on rotator cuff repair), has more tensile strength than simple knots [28].

The technique presented was able to produce a strong repair that lasts several years. This clinical impression was confirmed in a cadaveric study published by Giza et al. They compared open and arthroscopic Broström and could not find any statistical difference in terms of repair strength or stiffness between both techniques [27].

None of our patients needed a second procedure to treat persistent instability. Some patients came back reporting an additional ankle sprain with minor trauma, but none of them showed stress radiographs with mechanical instability. They were then classified as functional instability. All these patients recovered after a short period and a few physical therapy sessions.

On the series presented by the authors of this chapter, there was only one reoperation for ankle anterolateral impingement, and the results were rated as good or excellent. These results are comparable to the outcomes of "open" Broström-Gould (or Broström like) series presented by several authors.

The worst results reported after a Broström-Gould procedure was in a population with workers compensation incidence as high as 21%, close to open technique numbers [6, 12, 13]. Most complications resolved after conservative means and only one case had persistent pain (a superficial peroneal nerve neuritis). This nerve is the greatest enemy of the ankle arthroscopist and can be damaged in this technique. Four complications (8%) related to the superficial peroneal nerve (one persistent) were reported in that paper, but this rate is similar to the rate registered after open surgeries like Broström-Gould procedure [6, 12–14].

Drakos et al. published an anatomic study and determined what structures would be in risk with an arthroscopic repair of the lateral ligaments. They placed the anterolateral portals on usual position (in the interval between the extensor tendons and superficial peroneal nerve). They concluded that several structures were at risk like the peroneus tertius, the extensors digitorum longus tendons, and superficial peroneal nerve [29]. That is why extreme care is recommended when determining the lateral portals positions. Both must be lateral and not medial to the superficial peroneal nerve to diminish the risk of lesion.

Based on available data on this surgical technique for the treatment of CLAI, we are convinced that this is a safe and reproducible method that can be considered as the first line of surgical treatment for the vast majority of patients regardless the age, gender, or level of activity. However, its use in specific groups of patients with changes in ligamentous elasticity, patients with morbid obesity, extremely high-demand athletes, or heavy-duty workers should be considered judiciously and with extreme discretion.

23.4 Conclusion

Arthroscopic repair of chronic lateral ankle instability is a desirable technique. The challenge is to create a procedure that is solid, reproducible, feasible, and easy to perform.

The technique described showed good clinical results, and satisfaction rate was achieved.

No recurrences of mechanical instability were reported after surgery. The risk to superficial peroneal nerve is the main concern.

In our practice, the primary correction of ankle instability is always arthroscopic.

We are convinced that the future of ankle instability will have an arthroscopic repair that will gather consensual approval.

References

1. Garrick JG. The frequency of injury, mechanism of injury, and epidemiology of ankle sprains. Am J Sports Med. 1977;5:241–2.
2. Hintermann B, Boss A, Schafer D. Arthroscopic findings in patients with chronic ankle instability. Am J Sports Med. 2002;30:402–9.
3. Komenda GA, Ferkel RD. Arthroscopic findings associated with unstable ankle. Foot Ankle Int. 1999;20:708–13.
4. Maffulli N, Ferran N. Management of acute and chronic ankle instability. J Am Acad Orthop Surg. 2008;16:606–15.
5. van Rijn RM, van Os AG, Bernsen RM, Luijsterburg PA, Koes BW, Bierma-Zeinstra SM. What is the clinical course of acute ankle sprains? A systematic literature review. Am J Med. 2008;121(4):324–31.
6. Tourné Y, Mabit C, Moroney PJ, Chaussard C, Saragaglia D. Long-term follow-up of lateral reconstruction with extensor retinaculum flap for chronic ankle instability. Foot Ankle Int. 2012;33(12):1079–86.
7. van Dijk CN, Bossuyt PM, Marti RK. Medial ankle pain after lateral ligament rupture. J Bone Joint Surg Br. 1996;78(4):562–7.
8. Sugimoto K, Takakura Y, Okahashi K, Samoto N, Kawate K, Iwai M. Chondral injuries of the ankle with recurrent lateral instability: an arthroscopic study. J Bone Joint Surg Am. 2009;91(1):99–106.
9. Vega J, Golanó P, Pellegrino A, Rabat E, Peña F. All-inside arthroscopic lateral collateral ligament repair for ankle instability with a knotless suture anchor technique. Foot Ankle Int. 2013;34:1701.
10. Cha SD, Kim HS, Chung ST, Yoo JH, Park JH, Kim JH, Hyung JW. Intra-articular lesions in chronic lateral ankle instability: comparison of arthroscopy with magnetic resonance imaging findings. Clin Orthop Surg. 2012;4(4):293–9.
11. O'Neill PJ, van Aman SE, Guyton GP. Is MRI adequate to detect lesions in patients with ankle instability? Clin Orthop Relat Res. 2010;468(4):1115–9.
12. Bell SJ, Mologne TS, Sitler DF, et al. Twenty-six-year results after Broström procedure for chronic lateral ankle instability. Am J Sports Med. 2006;34:975–8.
13. Hua Y, Chen S, Li Y, et al. Combination of modified Broström procedure with ankle arthroscopy for chronic ankle instability accompanied by intra-articular symptoms. Arthroscopy. 2011;26:524–8.
14. Messer TM, Cummings CA, Ahn J, Kelikian AS. Outcome of the modified Brostrom procedure for chronic lateral ankle instability using suture anchors. Foot Ankle Int. 2000;21:996–1003.
15. Buchhorn T, Sabeti-Aschraf M, Dlaska CE, Wenzel F, Graf A, Ziai P. Combined medial and lateral anatomic ligament reconstruction for chronic rotational instability of the ankle. Foot Ankle Int. 2011;32(12):1122–6.
16. Taga I, Shino K, Inoue M, Nakata K, Maeda A. Articular cartilage lesions in ankles with lateral ligament injury. An arthroscopic study. Am J Sports Med. 1993;21(1):120–6.
17. Corte-Real NM, Moreira RM. Arthroscopic repair of chronic lateral ankle instability. Foot Ankle Int. 2009;30:213–7.
18. Nery C, Raduan F, Del Buono A, Asaumi ID, Cohen M, Maffulli N. Arthroscopic-assisted Brostrom-Gould for chronic ankle instability: a long-term follow-up. Am J Sports Med. 2011;39:2381–8.
19. Pereira R, Constantino H, Moreira R, Corte-Real N. Ligamentoplastia artroscópica na instabilidade crónica do tornozelo. Paper presented on XXXII Congresso Nacional de Ortopedia e Traumatologia, Vilamoura; 2012 (Portuguese).
20. van Dijk CN, von Bergen CJ. Advancements in ankle arthroscopy. J Am Acad Orthop Surg. 2008;16(11):635–46.
21. Strauss JE, Forsberg JA, Lippert FG. Chronic lateral ankle instability and associated conditions: a rationale for treatment. Foot Ankle Int. 2007;28:1041–4.
22. Hawkins RB. Arthroscopic stapling repair for chronic lateral instability. Clin Podiatr Med Surg. 1987;4:875–83.
23. Maiotti M, Massoni C, Tarantino U. The use of arthroscopic thermal shrinkage to treat chronic lateral ankle instability in young athletes. Arthroscopy. 2005;21:751–7.
24. Olof LM, Bocko AP, Fanton G. Arthroscopic monopolar radiofrequency thermal stabilization for chronic lateral ankle instability: a preliminary report of 10 cases. J Foot Ankle Surg. 2000;39:144–53.
25. Cottom JM, Rigby RB. The "all inside" arthroscopic Brostrom procedure: a prospective study of 40 consecutive patients. J Foot Ankle Surg. 2013;52(5):568–74.
26. Kim ES, Lee KT, Park JS, Lee YK. Arthroscopic anterior talofibular ligament repair for chronic ankle instability with a suture anchor technique. Orthopedics 2011;34(4).
27. Giza E, Shin EC, Wong SE, Acevedo JI, Mangone PG, Olson K, Anderson MJ. Arthroscpic suture anchor repair of the lateral ligament ankle complex: a cadaveric study. Am J Sports Med. 2013; https://doi.org/10.1177/0363546513500639.
28. Gerber C, Schneeberger AG, Beck M, Schlegel U. Mechanical strength of repairs of the rotator cuff. J Bone Joint Surg Br. 1994;76(3):371–80.
29. Drakos M, Behrens SB, Mulcahey MK, Paller D, Hoffman E, DiGiovanni CW. Proximity of arthroscopic ankle stabilization procedures to surrounding structures: an anatomic study. Arthroscopy. 2013;29(6):1089–94.

24 Arthroscopic ATFL Repair with Percutaneous Gould Augmentation

Pedro Diniz, Peter G. Mangone, Eric Giza, Jorge Acevedo, and Hélder Pereira

Required Equipment

- Standard 4 mm 30° arthroscope and instruments
- Two 3 mm bone anchors
- Curved suture passer

Fact Box

- The Broström-Gould operation is currently considered the gold standard [1].
- The Gould augmentation significantly increases the strength of the repair [2].
- Arthroscopic techniques have shown less surgical morbidity [3], and faster recovery [4] compared to open surgery.
- This technique is contraindicated in patients with hyperlaxity syndromes, morbid obesity, severely frayed or degenerated ligament remnants, isolated subtalar instability, prior failed reconstruction, severe and longstanding instability, paralysis, or large high-demand athletes [5].

P. Diniz (✉)
Department of Orthopaedic Surgery, Hospital de Sant'Ana, Parede, Portugal

Institute for Bioengineering and Biosciences, Instituto Superior Técnico, Universidade de Lisboa, Lisbon, Portugal

Fisiogaspar, Lisbon, Portugal

P. G. Mangone
Department of Orthopedics, Blue Ridge Division of EmergeOrtho, Foot and Ankle Center, Arden, NC, USA

E. Giza
University of California, Davis, Sacramento, CA, USA

J. Acevedo
Department of Orthopedics, Southeast Orthopedic Specialists, Jacksonville, FL, USA

H. Pereira
Knee and Ankle Orthopaedic Department, Centro Hospitalar Póvoa de Varzim, Vila do Conde, Portugal

Ripoll y De Prado Sports Clinic: FIFA Medical Centre of Excellence, Murcia-Madrid, Spain

ICVS/3B's – PT Government Associate Laboratory, University of Minho, Braga/Guimarães, Portugal

24.1 Introduction

Surgical treatment of chronic ankle instability (CAI) is indicated when conservative treatment fails [6]. Surgical options include anatomical repairs and reconstructions, and non-anatomical reconstructions.

The Broström-Gould operation is currently considered the gold standard [1]. It has been shown to be a reproducible surgical procedure with good results [7]. The Gould augmentation [8] is an important adjunction to the repair. First, it significantly increases its strength [2]. Second, because

H. Pereira et al. (eds.), *Lateral Ankle Instability*, https://doi.org/10.1007/978-3-662-62763-1_24

inferior extensor retinaculum inserts in the calcaneus near the peroneal tubercle, it may be of special interest in cases where the calcaneofibular ligament (CFL) is not repaired [5].

There is a trend toward lesser invasive procedures, with several arthroscopic techniques having been developed in recent years [9–12]. Studies have shown less surgical morbidity in the postoperative period [3], and faster recovery [4] with arthroscopic techniques when compared with open surgery.

Furthermore, arthroscopy is a useful tool in the management of CAI patients [13] since it can be used to assess and treat concurrent pathology [6]. However, one should be aware of a somewhat demanding learning curve compared to open procedures, which may be overcome with proper training [14].

24.2 Surgical Technique

This technique has been previously described by Jorge I. Acevedo and Peter G. Mangone [15].

24.2.1 Indications and Contraindications

Lateral ligament reconstruction should be considered in patients in whom conservative treatment for chronic ankle instability has failed [13].

Arthroscopic repair should not be done in patients with hyperlaxity syndromes, morbid obesity, severely frayed or degenerated ligament remnants, isolated subtalar instability, prior failed reconstruction, severe and longstanding instability, paralysis, or large high-demand athletes.

24.2.2 Preoperative Planning

A thorough history collection and physical exam is required, with special attention to the presence of hyperlaxity, concurrent pathology, or limb alignment issues.

Although magnetic resonance imaging may not be determinant to the assessment of ligament function, it is a useful adjunct in the diagnosis of associated pathology, such as impingement lesions, osteochondral defects, and peroneal tears [16].

24.2.3 Positioning and Required Equipment

A 4.0-mm, 30° arthroscope is used. This technique requires two anchors, of which size and type are a matter of surgeon preference. Commonly used sizes are 3.0 mm anchors with a No. 2 suture. A curved suture passer is also required.

The patient is positioned supine with a leg bolster under the ipsilateral hip. The plantar border of the calcaneal region should be aligned with the end of the operations table. A tourniquet is applied at the thigh and inflated. The ankle is prepped and draped in the usual fashion, and important anatomical landmarks are drawn with a surgical pen.

24.2.4 Approach

A standard two-portal anterior arthroscopic approach is used [17]. Distraction is optional. Not using distraction is preferable because there is less risk of iatrogenic damage to the neurovascular structures [18]. The lateral portal should be made using a 18-gauge needle as pointer, making sure that the fibula is easily accessible for anchor placement. Arthroscopic examination of the ankle is performed, and associated pathology is treated as needed.

An appropriate debridement of the lateral gutter needs to be performed. This can be done with a shaver, biters, and/or radiofrequency probe. Afterwards, the probe should be able to touch the tip of the fibula, and with no soft tissues impairing visualization of the anchors, sutures, and ligament repair.

24.2.5 Arthroscopic ATFL Reconstruction and Percutaneous Gould Augmentation

After all necessary preparations have been made, the next step is placing the first anchor. It should be positioned 1 cm above the tip of the lateral malleolus. Fluoroscopy can be used to help determine the correct location of the anchor insertion site.

The first two sutures should then be retrieved, passing through the inferior capsule, inferior extensor retinaculum, subcutaneous tissue, and exiting the skin 1.5–2 cm anteriorly to the inferior half of the lateral malleolus, with approximately 1 cm between them.

Two methods of passing the suture have been described by the authors: outside-in and inside-out. In the outside-in technique (Fig. 24.1), the curved suture passer pierces the skin first, in the intended position, a nitinol loop is introduced, and one of the sutures is retrieved. This step is repeated for the other sutures and exit sites. In the inside-out technique, the curved suture passer is introduced through the antero-lateral portal and exists through the skin at the intended position. The nitinol loop is passed through the suture passer, and the suture passer is then removed. The nitinol loop is then used to pass the suture outwards through the skin.

The second anchor is then placed 1 cm above the first (Figs. 24.2 and 24.3), and the two sutures are passed through, using the methods explained above, but making sure that the ATFL remnant is adequately catch.

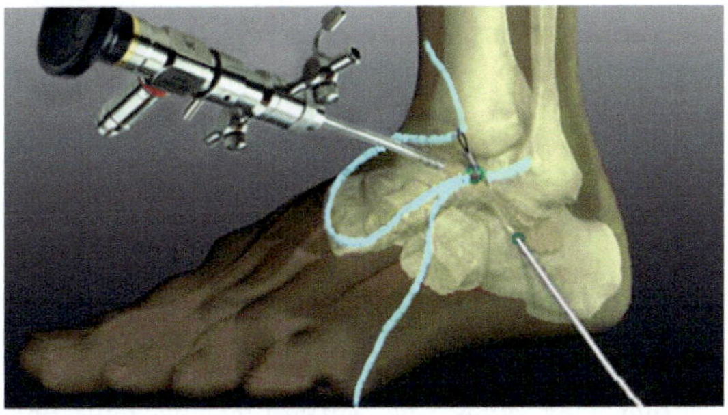

Fig. 24.1 The first anchor is in place, curved suture passer pierces the skin; a nitinol loop is used to retrieve the sutures

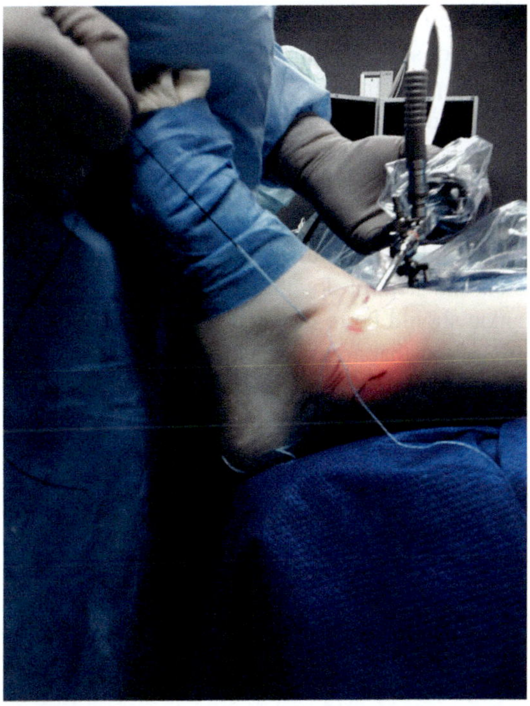

Fig. 24.2 Outside view of the retrieval of sutures through the skin by using the nitinol loop

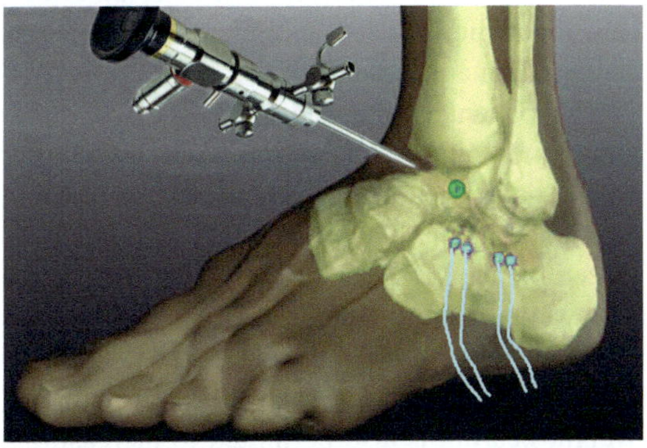

Fig. 24.3 Both anchors are in place and sutures retrieved through the skin; In green one sees the lateral portal

Two oblique, 0.5 cm, skin incisions are then made, locating them between the two most inferior and two most superior sutures. Another option is to do a single 1 cm incision between the two sets of sutures. The sutures are pulled through these incisions using a hemostat. This is done to minimize the risk of entrapment of subcutaneous nerves or skin dimpling after tying of the sutures.

Using the arthroscope, the lateral gutter is then inspected to make sure that there are no impinging soft tissues, loose debris, or suture entanglement. If being used, distraction should be removed at this stage. A simulation of knot tying is then employed, after putting the ankle in slight eversion and neutral dorsiflexion/plantarflexion. The ankle should be re-checked with the arthroscope to confirm that no tissue is impinging in the ankle. Sutures are then tied, starting with the most superior set. Anterior drawer and talar tilt tests are then performed. If residual instability is of concern, conversion to an open procedure can be done.

The arthroscopic portals and the small incisions are then closed with a nylon 4-0 suture. Sterile dressings and a posterior splint in the neutral position are applied.

24.3 Postoperative Care

Patients can be discharged on the same day, except if other procedures, such as osteotomies, have been performed, and there are concerns about pain management.

The patient is checked after 7–10 days, for removal of sutures. These can be removed after 14–20 days, if concerns about wound healing exist. The splint is removed, and the patient is placed on a cast or walker boot. Fifty-percent of bodyweight weight-bearing is permitted.

At 4 weeks the cast, or walker boot, is removed and the patient is placed in an ankle stirrup brace. Weight-bearing is also permitted to increasingly progress to full weight-bearing. Formal physical therapy is started around 6 weeks after surgery.

Patients may wean out of the brace at 3 months, but its use is recommended for vigorous physical activity, or any activity on uneven ground, until 6 months after surgery.

24.4 Outcomes

Acevedo and Mangone have reported the results of this procedure in 23 patients (24 ankles), with an age average of 39 (15–55) years. There were 14 males and 9 females. Average follow-up was 10.9 (range: 1.5–24) months. All patients stated a subjective improvement of ankle stability. No surgeries had to be revised. In one patient, a 1+ talar tilt positive test was found, but no evident anterior drawer. This patient had no complaints of ankle instability. In their report, another patient developed a neurological issue 12 months after surgery, which was deemed to be unrelated to the surgical procedure, with the ankle remaining stable on talar tilt and anterior drawer tests. Another patient sustained a new injury 9 months after surgery, and although the repair was considered intact, the patient underwent another surgery due to persistent residual pain. In this patient, a peroneal tendon exploration and repair was performed, but the authors consider that this injury was not present at the time of the ATFL repair. Two other patients reported complications: one complained of peroneal tendonitis and another of sural nerve neuritis, with both having resolved [5]. The authors reported no other complications.

Take-Home Messages

- The anterior talofibular repair and Gould augmentation can be done safely using an arthroscopic approach. The anchors should be placed 1 cm from the tip of the fibula, and 1 cm above the first anchor. Care should be taken to confirm that no soft tissues are impinging in the ankle joint before and after suture tying. If residual instability is of concern, the surgeon can always convert to an open procedure. Good outcomes can be expected with this technique, with no major complications having been reported.

References

1. Michels F, Cordier G, Guillo S, Stockmans F, ESKKA-AFAS Ankle Instability Group. Endoscopic ankle lateral ligament graft anatomic reconstruction. Foot Ankle Clin. 2016;21:665–80. https://doi.org/10.1016/j.fcl.2016.04.010.
2. Aydogan U, Glisson RR, Nunley JA. Extensor retinaculum augmentation reinforces anterior talofibular ligament repair. Clin Orthop. 2006;442:210–5. https://doi.org/10.1097/01.blo.0000183737.43245.26.

3. Yeo ED, Lee K-T, Sung I, Lee SG, Lee YK. Comparison of all-inside arthroscopic and open techniques for the modified Broström procedure for ankle instability. Foot Ankle Int. 2016;37:1037–45. https://doi.org/10.1177/1071100716666508.
4. Matsui K, Takao M, Miyamoto W, Matsushita T. Early recovery after arthroscopic repair compared to open repair of the anterior talofibular ligament for lateral instability of the ankle. Arch Orthop Trauma Surg. 2016;136:93–100. https://doi.org/10.1007/s00402-015-2342-3.
5. Acevedo JI, Mangone PG. Arthroscopic lateral ankle ligament reconstruction. Tech Foot Ankle Surg. 2011;10:111–6. https://doi.org/10.1097/BTF.0b013e318229bdb8.
6. Pereira H, Vuurberg G, Spennacchio P, Batista J, D'Hooghe P, Hunt K, van Dijk N. Surgical treatment paradigms of ankle lateral instability, osteochondral defects and impingement. Adv Exp Med Biol. 2018;1059:85–108. https://doi.org/10.1007/978-3-319-76735-2_4.
7. Vuurberg G, Pereira H, Blankevoort L, van Dijk CN. Anatomic stabilization techniques provide superior results in terms of functional outcome in patients suffering from chronic ankle instability compared to non-anatomic techniques. Knee Surg Sports Traumatol Arthrosc. 2018;26:2183–95. https://doi.org/10.1007/s00167-017-4730-4.
8. Gould N, Seligson D, Gassman J. Early and late repair of lateral ligament of the ankle. Foot Ankle. 1980;1:84–9. https://doi.org/10.1177/107110078000100206.
9. Corte-Real NM, Moreira RM. Arthroscopic repair of chronic lateral ankle instability. Foot Ankle Int. 2009;30:213–7. https://doi.org/10.3113/FAI.2009.0213.
10. Pereira H, Vuurberg G, Gomes N, Oliveira JM, Ripoll PL, Reis RL, Espregueira-Mendes J, Niek van Dijk C. Arthroscopic repair of ankle instability with all-soft knotless anchors. Arthrosc Tech. 2016;5:e99–e107. https://doi.org/10.1016/j.eats.2015.10.010.
11. Guillo S, Archbold P, Perera A, Bauer T, Sonnery-Cottet B. Arthroscopic anatomic reconstruction of the lateral ligaments of the ankle with gracilis autograft. Arthrosc Tech. 2014;3:e593–8. https://doi.org/10.1016/j.eats.2014.06.018.
12. Nery C, Raduan F, Del Buono A, Asaumi ID, Cohen M, Maffulli N. Arthroscopic-assisted Brostrom-Gould for chronic ankle instability: a long-term follow-up. Am J Sports Med. 2011;39:2381–8. https://doi.org/10.1177/0363546511416069.
13. Michels F, Pereira H, Calder J, Matricali G, Glazebrook M, Guillo S, Karlsson J, ESSKA-AFAS Ankle Instability Group, Acevedo J, Batista J, Bauer T, Calder J, Carreira D, Choi W, Corte-Real N, Glazebrook M, Ghorbani A, Giza E, Guillo S, Hunt K, Karlsson J, Kong SW, Lee JW, Michels F, Molloy A, Mangone P, Matsui K, Nery C, Ozeki S, Pearce C, Pereira H, Perera A, Pijnenburg B, Raduan F, Stone J, Takao M, Tourné Y, Vega J. Searching for consensus in the approach to patients with chronic lateral ankle instability: ask the expert. Knee Surg Sports Traumatol Arthrosc. 2018;26:2095–102. https://doi.org/10.1007/s00167-017-4556-0.
14. Zwiers R, Wiegerinck JI, Murawski CD, Smyth NA, Kennedy JG, van Dijk CN. Surgical treatment for posterior ankle impingement. Arthrosc J Arthrosc Relat Surg. 2013;29:1263–70. https://doi.org/10.1016/j.arthro.2013.01.029.
15. Acevedo JI, Mangone P. Ankle instability and arthroscopic lateral ligament repair. Foot Ankle Clin. 2015;20:59–69. https://doi.org/10.1016/j.fcl.2014.10.002.
16. Salat P, Le V, Veljkovic A, Cresswell ME. Imaging in foot and ankle instability. Foot Ankle Clin. 2018;23:499–522.e28. https://doi.org/10.1016/j.fcl.2018.07.011.
17. van Dijk CN. Ankle arthroscopy techniques developed by the Amsterdam Foot and Ankle School. Berlin: Springer; 2014.
18. de Leeuw PAJ, Golanó P, Clavero JA, van Dijk CN. Anterior ankle arthroscopy, distraction or dorsiflexion? Knee Surg Sports Traumatol Arthrosc. 2010;18:594–600. https://doi.org/10.1007/s00167-010-1089-1.

The Arthroscopic All Inside Knotless Option

25

Jordi Vega, Jorge Batista, Hélder Pereira, Francesc Malagelada, and Miki Dalmau-Pastor

25.1 Introduction

Ankle arthroscopy is an emerging field and some of its indications, concepts, and techniques have significantly evolved during the last few years. The potential for addressing both the instability and the associated pathology makes ankle arthroscopy the technique of choice when treating ankle instability [1–5].

Similarly to open techniques, several arthroscopic options to restore ankle stability have been proposed, and both the mechanical and histological characteristics of the ligament should be considered. The native histological characteristics of the injured ligament can only be maintained through its repair. Thus, anatomic repair under direct arthroscopic visualization is preferred over other arthroscopic techniques.

The all-inside arthroscopic lateral collateral ligament repair with a knotless-suture-anchor described by Vega et al. was the first all-arthroscopic technique described in 2013 [6]. Variations of this procedure include ligament repair through a knot-anchor or a soft-anchor, modification of the portals location, or a two-portal technique [7–9]. These technique modifications reflect differences in terms of surgeon preferences.

J. Vega (✉)
Foot and Ankle Unit, iMove Traumatology-Clinica Tres Torres, and Hospital Quirón Barcelona, Barcelona, Spain

Laboratory of Arthroscopic and Surgical Anatomy, Department of Pathology and Experimental Therapeutics (Human Anatomy Unit), University of Barcelona, Barcelona, Spain

Groupe de Recherche et Etude de la Chirurgie Miniinvasive du Pied-Cheville (GRECMIP) soon Minimally Invasive Foot and Ankle Society (MIFAS), Bordeaux, France
e-mail: jordivega@hotmail.com

J. Batista
Centro Artroscópico Jorge Batista (CAJB), Buenos Aires, Argentina

H. Pereira
Ripoll-DePrado Sports Clinic, FIFA Medical Centre of Excellence, Madrid, Spain

F. Malagelada
Foot and Ankle Unit, Department of Trauma and Orthopaedic Surgery, Royal London Hospital, Barts Health NHS Trust, London, UK

M. Dalmau-Pastor
Laboratory of Arthroscopic and Surgical Anatomy, Department of Pathology and Experimental Therapeutics (Human Anatomy Unit), University of Barcelona, Barcelona, Spain

Groupe de Recherche et Etude de la Chirurgie Miniinvasive du Pied-Cheville (GRECMIP) soon Minimally Invasive Foot and Ankle Society (MIFAS), Bordeaux, France

H. Pereira et al. (eds.), *Lateral Ankle Instability*, https://doi.org/10.1007/978-3-662-62763-1_25

25.2 Indications/Contraindications

Patients with chronic ankle instability and isolated ATFL injury are excellent candidates to the all-inside arthroscopic ligament repair. Concomitant intra-articular pathology can be treated arthroscopically before the ligament tear repair.

Symptomatic ankle microinstability due to partial ATFL injury is also a candidate to an arthroscopic ligament repair.

Quality of the remnant ligament-tissue should be assessed during the procedure, and it can be subjectively categorized as poor, moderate, or excellent ligament-tissue quality. Moderate or excellent ligament-tissue quality remnant is the most common finding, allowing for a ligament repair as the optimal technique. Poor ligament-tissue quality is a very uncommon scenario according to the author's experience. Poor ligament-tissue quality can limit repair techniques, and reconstruction should be considered in these cases.

25.3 Operative Setup

A laminar flow operating theatre is preferable. Although popliteal peripheral nerve blockade or general anesthesia is a possible anesthetic option, spinal anesthesia is routinely used.

The patient is positioned in supine position, with the operated side placed in a thigh holder optionally. Plantar and dorsiflexion of the ankle joint has to be free and easy to be performed.

A thigh tourniquet is applied and inflated after exsanguination of the leg. Application of chlorhexidine skin preparation is used up to the tourniquet. A knee arthroscopy drape with a fluid collection bag can be applied with one sleeve around the calf.

No inflow pump system is required.

General instruments include a 4.0-mm 30° scope, arthroscopic 3.5–4.5 mm motorized shaver and burr plus the standard arthroscopic instruments. Specific instruments are required for this technique. An automatic suture passer (MiniScorpion, Arthrex, Naples, FL) or non-automatic (Microsuture lasso curved 70°, Arthrex, Naples, FL) is used to penetrate the ligament. Once the ligament is penetrated, it should be grasped with a 2:0 or 0 high-resistance and non-absorbable suture (FiberWire, Arthrex, Naples, FL; Hi-Fi, Conmed, Largo, FL). Finally, a knotless anchor (Pushlock 2.9 mm × 15 mm, Arthrex, Naples, FL; SwiveLock 3.5 mm × 12.5 mm; PopLok 3.3 mm × 11 mm, ConMed, Largo, FL; ReelX STT 4.5, Stryker, San Jose, CA) is used for ligament reattachment. The use of a cannula introduced in the anterolateral portal or working portal (PassPort Button cannula, 6 mm ID × 2 cm, Arthrex, Naples, FL) will minimize the risk of injuries to the superficial peroneal nerve during instruments, sutures and anchors passing.

25.4 Surgical Technique

Cutaneous landmarks of the anterior aspect of the ankle are marked. As the working portal is located close to the superficial peroneal nerve, ankle maneuvers to identify the nerve are recommended (Fig. 25.1). The nerve moves with ankle motion [10] and its subcutaneous course becomes evident with inversion of the ankle and plantarflexion of the fourth toe [11, 12].

Distraction of the ankle is not used, and dorsiflexion of the ankle without distraction technique is mandatory. A no-distraction arthroscopic technique provides good visualization and easy access to the anterior compartment as well as the lateral and medial gutters of the ankle [13].

Arthroscopic portals for the ankle joint are performed in a systematic way. Distension of the capsular joint with saline is not performed routinely. Use of a needle is useful for correct placement of the portals. The skin incision is made with a number 11 surgical blade. A vertical incision through only the skin followed by blunt dissection up to the capsule with a mosquito clamp contributes to decreasing the risk of nerve, vascular, and tendinous injuries. Next, the capsule joint is opened with the mosquito clamp. This step is critical because the ankle joint must be in maximum dorsiflexion to avoid cartilage injury. This

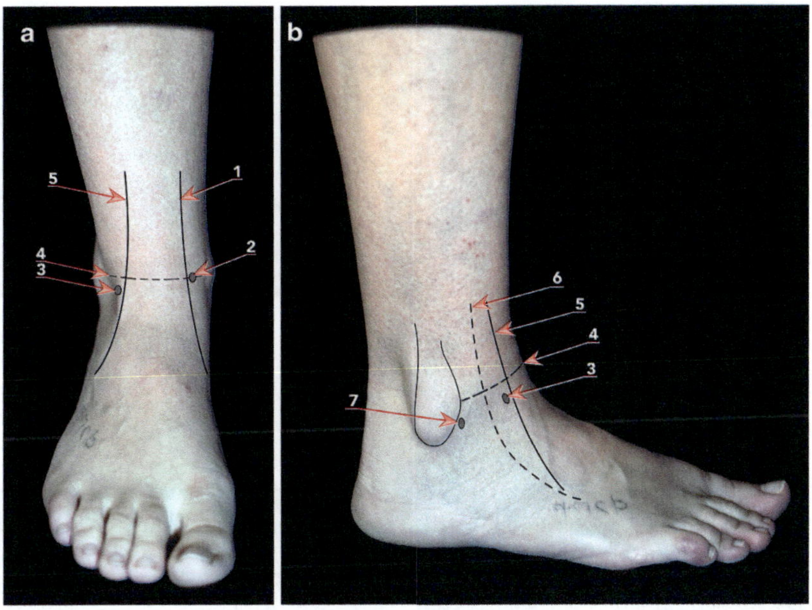

Fig. 25.1 Anatomical landmarks and location of arthroscopic portals. (**a**) Anterior view. (**b**) Lateral view. (1) Anterior tibialis tendon. (2) Anteromedial portal. (3) Anterolateral portal. (4) Ankle joint line. (5) Peroneus tertius tendon or in its absence extensor digitorum longus tendon. (6) Superficial peroneal nerve. (7) Accessory anterolateral portal

technique is applied for both anteromedial and anterolateral portals.

The anteromedial portal (visualization portal) is the first to be performed. It is established just medial to the anterior tibialis tendon at the level of the ankle joint line. The scope cannula with a blunt obturator is inserted into the joint through the anteromedial portal with the ankle joint in dorsiflexion. This cannula is first directed towards the joint firstly and after passing the joint capsule the direction of the cannula is modified, moving towards the lateral region of the ankle, to end in the anterior compartment of the joint. Inflow is connected to the scope cannula. Once the anteromedial portal is created, the anterolateral portal is made in a similar way through direct arthroscopic visualization.

Location of the anterolateral portal (working portal) is variable. Classically, it is created just lateral to the peroneus tertius tendon or, in its absence, lateral to the extensor digitorum longus tendon, and at the level of the ankle joint line. However, modifications have been described when all-inside ligament repair, and some surgeons create the working portal about 0.5 cm distal to the anterior joint line, or more lateral and distal, just proximal to the sinus tarsi. When a three portals technique, an accessory anterolateral portal is created just anterior to the fibula, and about 1 cm proximal to the tip of the lateral malleolus.

A probe is used during the initial ankle exploration. Lateral gutter examination is mandatory. The scope is introduced through the anteromedial portal and directed to the lateral gutter. Examination of the anterior talofibular ligament (ATFL) is performed with the ankle in dorsiflexion. In this position, the ATFL is lax. Arthroscopic criteria of ATFL injury is defined as partial or complete desinsertion of the fibular attachment with visualization of the ATFL footprint. In addition, the ATFL remnant quality can be evaluated.

After a full arthroscopic examination, the ATFL is repaired under direct arthroscopic view. In the presence of synovitis or scar tissue, the procedure is started with a synovectomy or lysis of adhesions with shaver.

When non-automatic suture passer, it is introduced through the working portal, and under direct arthroscopic visualization, the ligament is penetrated. Then, the nitinol loop wire is pulled out through the accessory portal with the help of an arthroscopic grasper (Fig. 25.2). A folded-in-half high-resistance suture is placed through the loop, and pulled back. The double suture runs from the accessory portal through the ligament

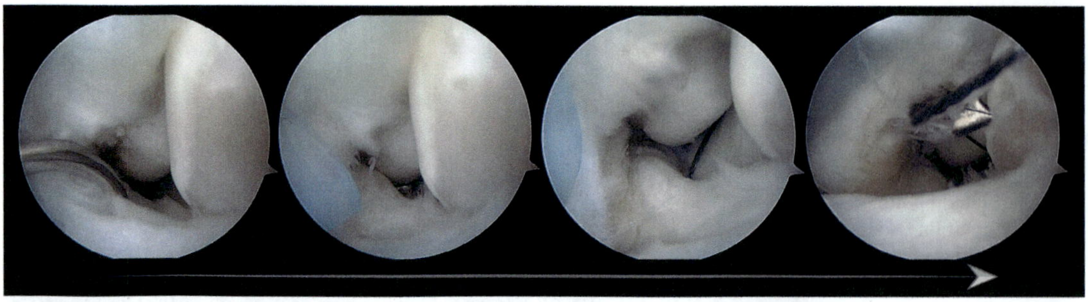

Fig. 25.2 Arthroscopic vision showing the use of a non-automatic suture passer to grasp the ATFL (right ankle). Scope introduced through the anteromedial portal and directed to the lateral gutter. Non-automatic suture passer introduced through the anterolateral portal. The nitinol wire is pulled out through the accessory portal with the help of an arthroscopic grasper

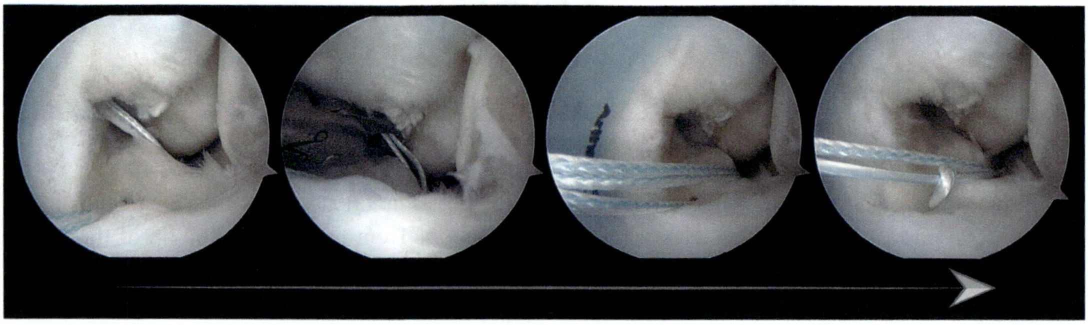

Fig. 25.3 The nitinol loop wire is changed by a folded-in-half high-resistance suture. The limbs of the suture located in the accessory portal are passed through the anterolateral portal with the help of an arthroscopic grasper. Next, one limb of the suture is passed through the loop suture, and by pulling the suture limbs, the loop is introduced into the joint and the ligament is grasped

and to the anterolateral portal. The two limbs of the suture are located in the accessory portal while the loop of the suture is in the anterolateral portal. The limbs of the suture located in the accessory portal are passed through the anterolateral portal. An arthroscopic grasper is helpful for this suture passage. Next, one or both limbs of the suture are passed through the loop suture. By pulling the suture limbs, the loop is introduced into the joint and the ligament is grasped by the suture (Fig. 25.3). Some surgeons penetrate the ligament percutaneously. If so, the accessory portal is not required, and the nitinol is pulled out through the working portal.

Alternatively, an automatic suture passer can be used to penetrate the ligament. No accessory portal is required. The high-resistance suture is placed first into the automatic clamp. The suture thread is folded in half, a loop and two ends are obtained. Then, the automatic suture passer is introduced through the anterolateral portal, and the ligament is penetrated as the suture is passed through it. Once the clamp is removed, the loop and the ends of the suture are in the same portal, the anterolateral. Next, one or both limbs of the suture are introduced into the loop, and by pulling the ends, the loop is introduced into the joint and the ligaments are grasped by the suture.

Then, the footprint for the fibular attachment of the ATFL is debrided with a shaver or a curette introduced through the working portal (Fig. 25.4).

The location for the bone anchor is identified. The fibular attachment of the ATFL is located just distal to the fibular insertion of the

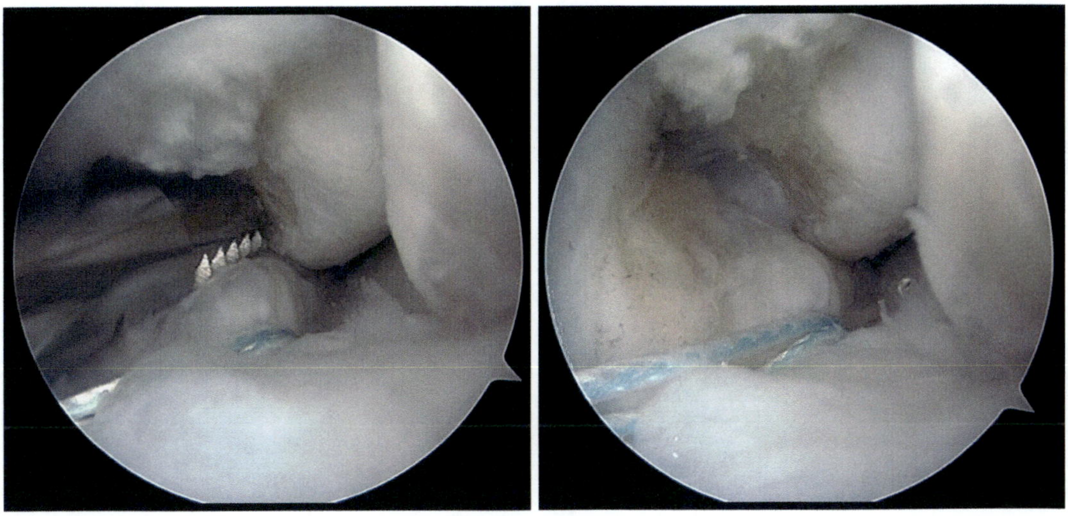

Fig. 25.4 The fibular footprint for the ATFL is debrided with a shaver introduced through the anterolateral portal

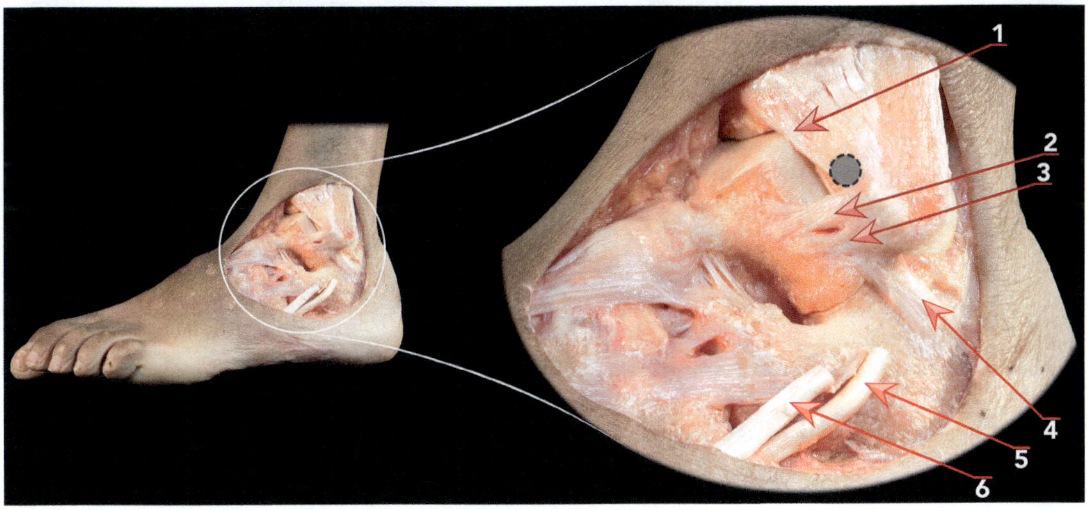

Fig. 25.5 Anatomic location for the bone anchor on the anterior aspect of the lateral malleolus, just distal to the fibular insertion distal fascicle of the ATiFL (indicated with a gray circle). (1) Distal fascicle of the ATiFL. (2) Superior fascicle ATFL. (3) Inferior fascicle ATFL. (4) Calcaneofibular ligament. (5) Peroneus longus tendon cut. (6) Peroneus brevis tendon cut

distal fascicle of anterior tibiofibular ligament (ATiFL). To reproduce the native insertion of the ATFL, the anchor must be located right on the fibular attachment of the ATiFL distal fascicle or just distal to it (Fig. 25.5). The drill is placed through the anterolateral portal and centered over this location. The drill is directed from anterior to posterior, and parallel to the plantar plane as well as the plane of the talar lateral wall (Fig. 25.6). The hole is drilled and the bone anchor with the suture are passed through the portal and then introduced into the hole by impaction (Fig. 25.7). Tension of the suture can be modulated before introducing the

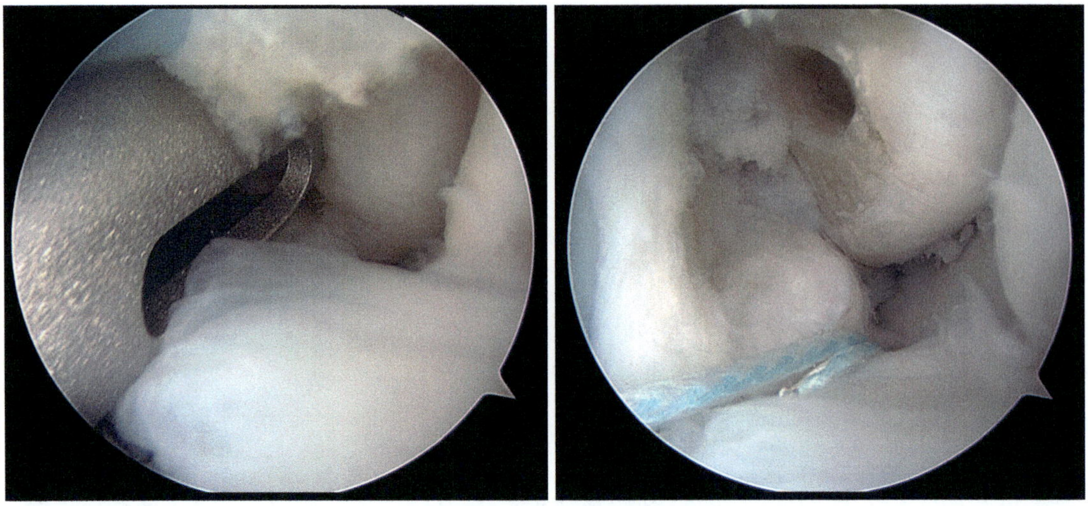

Fig. 25.6 Arthroscopic location for the bone anchor. Drill with its guide is introduced through the anterolateral portal

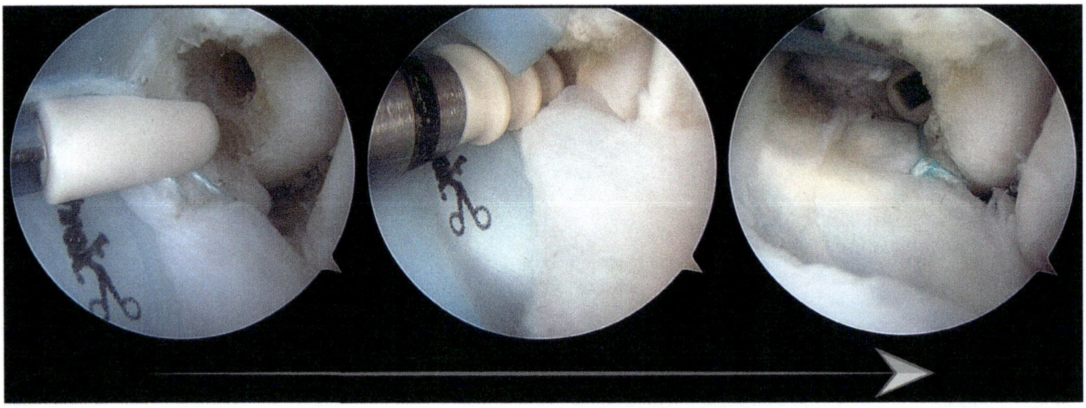

Fig. 25.7 Bone anchor with suture is introduced into the hole, and the ATFL is reattached

anchor. Once the anchor is introduced, the tension of the suture cannot be further modified. The ATFL is reattached with the ankle in dorsiflexion and valgus. Once the anchor is introduced, and the ligament is repaired, the remnants of the suture are cut (Fig. 25.8). Finally, the portals are sutured, and no suction drain is used.

25.5 Postoperative Care

A removable walking boot is used at all times for the first 3–4 weeks. Partial weight-bearing is permitted as tolerated by pain. Crutches are required. Antithrombotic prophylaxis is used for 10–15 days.

Once the walking boot is removed, the patient can undergo rehabilitation. Physical therapy includes active and passive range of motion, gait training, strengthening in ankle dorsiflexion and plantarflexion, eversion and inversion balance, and weight-bearing proprioception.

A return to non-contact sports can be expected at 6–8 weeks. Non-contact sports include swimming, biking, and running in a flat floor. Patients may return to sports without limitations at approximately 3 months from the operation.

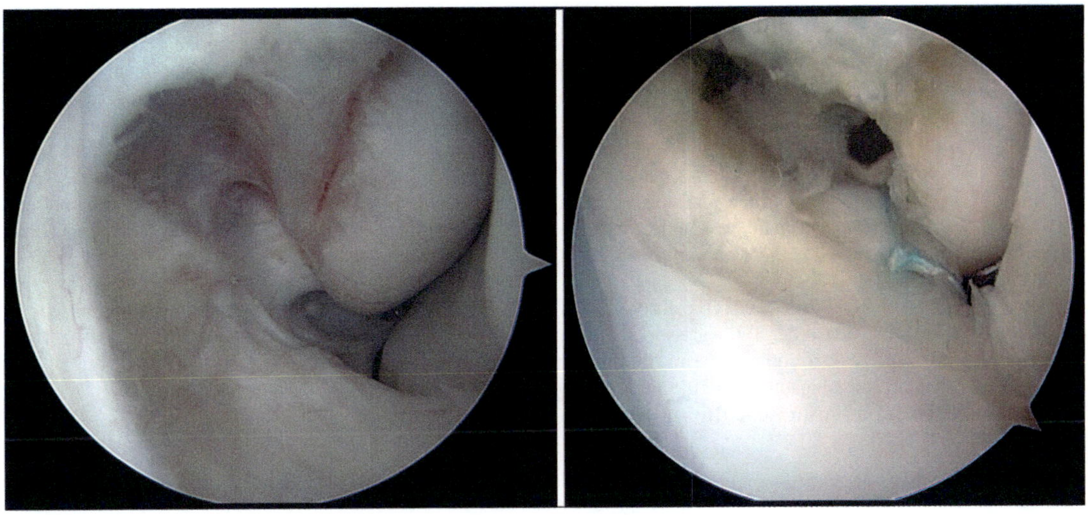

Fig. 25.8 Arthroscopic vision of a partial ATFL injury, before (**a**) and after arthroscopic all-inside ligament repair (**b**)

25.6 Pearls, Tips, and Pitfalls

When synovitis or scar tissue in the lateral recess, locate first the distal fascicle of the ATiFL at the syndesmotic level, and follow distally while debridement the pathological tissue. To avoid ligament injury with shaver, never enface the shaver window to the pathological tissue, and be careful with the motorized suction.

The ligament remnant needs to be defined before penetrated. Careful ligament cleaning with arthroscopic vaporizer instead of the shaver is recommended.

Once the ligament is grasped by the suture, and before to repair, the ligament remnant needs to be free, and adhesiolysis with osteotome is helpful.

A protector drill cannula is recommended to avoid soft-tissue damage during drilling.

25.7 Conclusions: Take-Home Message

The arthroscopic technique described has the advantage of its minimally invasive approach and the potential to treat concomitant intra-articular pathology.

In addition, the all-inside arthroscopic ATFL repair offers the benefit of maintaining the native ligament, and both the mechanical and histological ligament characteristics are also maintained. The ligament is repaired with a knotless-suture-anchor, uses knotless anchor allowing for reduced surgical time by minimizing the complexities of suture management and avoiding the presence of intra-articular knots when compared to other anchor types.

References

1. Cannon LB, Slater HK. The role of ankle arthroscopy and surgical approach in lateral ankle ligament repair. J Foot Ankle Surg. 2005;11(1):1–4.
2. Ferkel RD, Chams RN. Chronic lateral ankle instability: arthroscopic findings and long-term results. Foot Ankle Int. 2007;28(1):24–31.
3. Hintermann B, Boss A, Schäfer D. Arthroscopic findings in patients with chronic ankle instability. Am J Sports Med. 2002;30(3):402–9.
4. Hua Y, Chen S, Li Y, Chen J, Li H. Combination of modified Broström procedure with ankle arthroscopy for chronic ankle instability accompanied by intra-articular symptoms. Arthroscopy. 2010;26(4):524–8.
5. Komenda GA, Ferkel RD. Arthroscopic findings associated with the unstable ankle. Foot Ankle Int. 1999;20(11):708–13.
6. Vega J, Golanó P, Pellegrino A, Rabat E, Peña F. All-inside arthroscopic lateral collateral ligament repair

for ankle instability with a knotless suture anchor technique. Foot Ankle Int. 2013;34(12):1701–9.

7. Batista JP, del Vecchio JJ, Patthauer L, Ocampo M. Arthroscopic lateral ligament repair through two portals in chronic ankle instability. Open Orthop J. 2017;11:3–17.
8. Pereira H, Vuurberg G, Gomes N, Oliveira JM, Ripoll PL, Reis RL, Espregueira-Mendes J, van Dijk CN. Arthroscopic repair of ankle instability with all-soft knotless anchors. Arthrosc Tech. 2016;5(1):e99–e107.
9. Takao M, Matsui K, Stone JW, Glazebrook MA, Kennedy JG, Guillo S, Calder JD, Karlsson J, Ankle Instability Group. Arthroscopic anterior talofibular ligament repair for lateral instability of the ankle. Knee Surg Sports Traumatol Arthrosc. 2016;24(4):1003–6.
10. De Leeuw PAJ, Golanó P, Sierevelt IN, van Dijk CN. The course of the superficial peroneal nerve in relation to the ankle position: anatomical study with ankle arthroscopic implications. Knee Surg Sports Traumatol Arthrosc. 2010;18:612–7.
11. Ferkel RD. Arthroscopic surgery. The foot and ankle. Philadelphia, PA: Lippincott-Raven; 1996.
12. Stephens MM, Kelly PM. Fourth toe in flexion sign: a new clinical sign for identification of the superficial nerve. Foot Ankle Int. 2000;21:860–3.
13. Vega J, Marimón J, Golanó P, Pérez-Carro L, Salmerón J, Aguilera JM. True submalleolar accessory ossicles causing impingement of the ankle. Knee Surg Sports Traumatol Arthrosc. 2010;18(2):254–7.

Arthroscopic All Inside ATFL Repair

26

Masato Takao

Lateral instability of the ankle does not cause serious obstacles to sports activities like anterior cruciate ligament injury in the knee, and can demonstrate some performance by using taping or soft ankle brace. Therefore, many athletes continue to compete with ankle instability remaining. On the other hand, articular cartilage damage occurs at a high rate if ankle instability remains over a long period [1]. In addition, ankle lateral instability is considered to be one of the causes of osteoarthritis [2], and it is much more frequent that cases of osteoarthritis develop after ankle lateral ligament injury than previously believed [3]. In addition, while static stability cannot be obtained in the toe off phase during running, it is forced to rely on dynamic stability due to contraction of the peroneal muscle. It may have a negative effect on athlete's performance. Accordingly lateral instability of the ankle should be treated as long as there are no special circumstances.

In this chapter, I describe about the technique of all inside arthroscopic repair and reinforcement by inferior extensor retinaculum [4–6].

M. Takao (✉)
Clinical and Research Institute for Foot and Ankle Surgery, Jujo Hospital, Chiba, Japan
e-mail: m.takao@carifas.com

26.1 Indication

Choice of a surgical procedure is performed by evaluating the quality of the residual ligament with stress ultrasonography before surgery (Fig. 26.1a, b), and determined with arthroscopic evaluation during surgery. Arthroscopic Broström repair with/without reinforcement by inferior extensor retinaculum (Gould augmentation) is selected if the ligament fibers remain, and anatomical reconstruction of the lateral ligament of the ankle (AntiRoLL) is selected if there is no ligament fiber (see Chap. 31). When large os subfibulare is involved, it is difficult to treat arthroscopically, so open Broström repair is performed.

26.2 Surgical Procedure

26.2.1 Position

The position is supine, and the lower leg is held with a leg holder (Fig. 26.2). The tourniquet is not normally used, but it should be worn on the thigh for use when the field of vision is hindered by bleeding.

26.2.2 Step 1: Making Portals

Medial midline (MML) portal as viewing portal and accessary anterolateral (AAL) portal as

H. Pereira et al. (eds.), *Lateral Ankle Instability*, https://doi.org/10.1007/978-3-662-62763-1_26

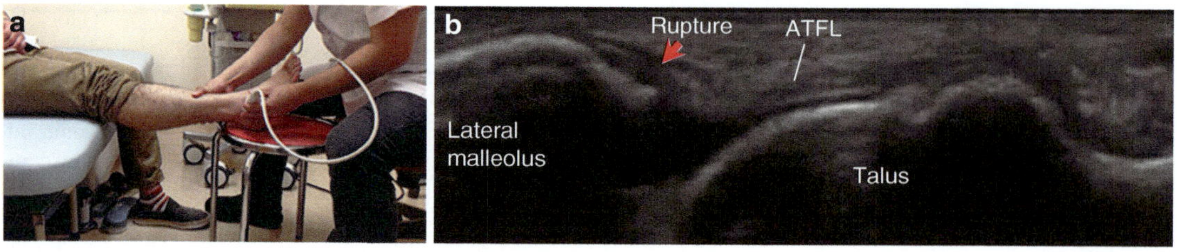

Fig. 26.1 Stress ultrasonography. (**a**) Position of the patient. (**b**) Ultrasonogram

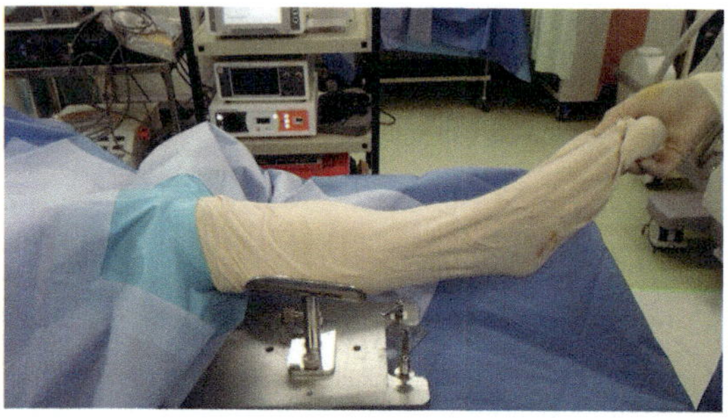

Fig. 26.2 Position

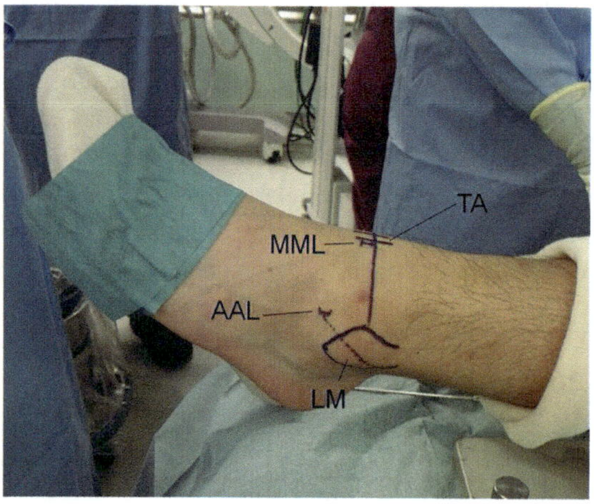

Fig. 26.3 Portals. *MML* medial midline, *AAL* accessary anterolateral, *AL* anterolateral portals

working portal are used. If it is needed to treat the intra-articular lesions, we add anterolateral (AL) portal (Fig. 26.3).

26.2.3 Step 2: View the Lesions

Insert the arthroscope (2.7 mm, 30° perspective scope) via the MML portal and view the lateral gutter. In this process, ankle should be slightly dorsiflexed position for extending the lateral pouch, turning the light cable upside to face the scope for directing the field of view of the arthroscope to the back (Fig. 26.4a) to be obtained a good field of view (Fig. 26.4b). If the field of vision is hindered by hypertrophic synovium, minimum resection is done using a 3.5-mm motorized shaver as not to damage the joint capsule and residual ligament.

26.2.4 Step 3: Insert a Suture Anchor

After confirming that the ligament fiber of ATFL remains, insert suture anchor for suturing the remaining ligament to fibula attachment. A drill hole is drilled about 5 mm proximally from the distal end of the articular surface of the lateral malleolus and about 5 mm outward from the lateral side of the articular surface. After inserting the anchor suture, it is confirmed that the thread slides (Fig. 26.5).

26.2.5 Step 4: Suture Relay Technique

Insert a 18 G needle through 2-0 nylon thread from AAL portal, and penetrate ATFL remnant fiber from front to back as deeply as possible (Fig. 26.6a). Rotating the needle forward for several times and reverse rotation the same number of times to enlarge the nylon loop (Fig. 26.6b). After that, insert a hook probe from the AAL portal and guide the nylon loop from the AAL portal to the outside (Fig. 26.6c).

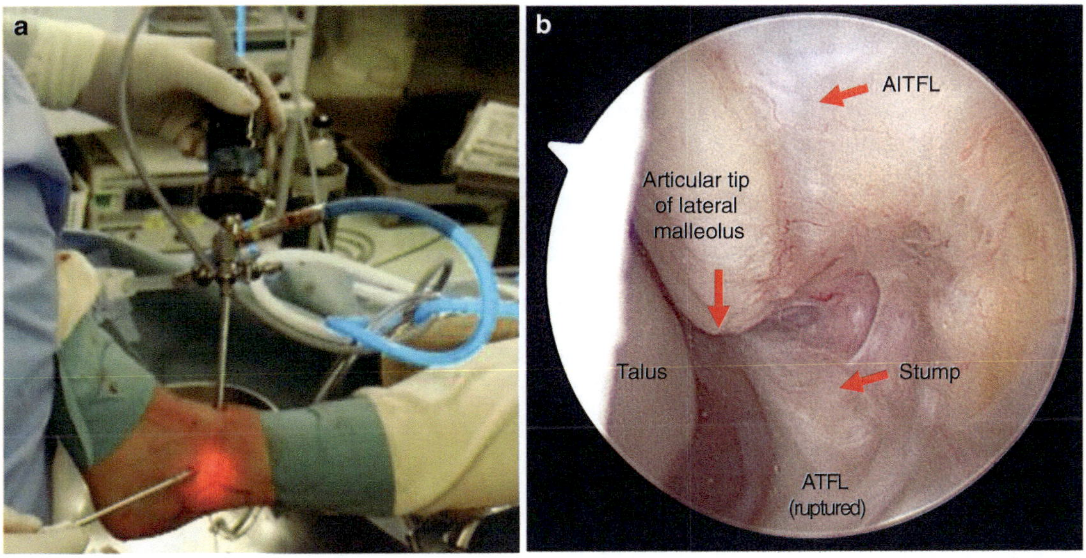

Fig. 26.4 View the lesions. (**a**) Position of the arthroscope. (**b**) Arthroscopic view of ATFL

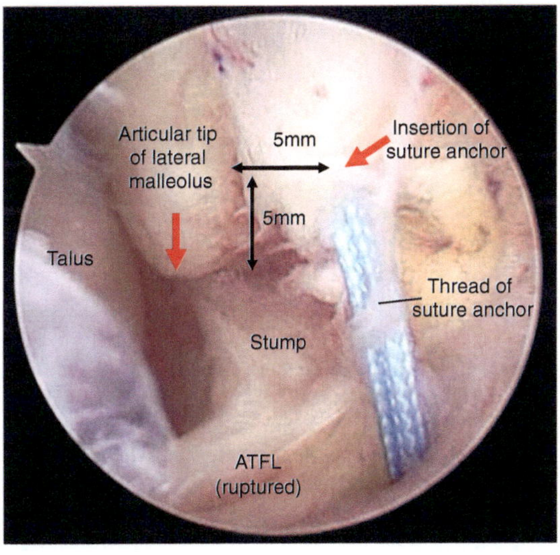

Fig. 26.5 Placement of the suture anchor for ATFL suture

26.2.6 Step 5: Suture the Remnant: Modified Lasso-Loop Stitch

Pass one thread of anchor suture to the nylon loop about 2/3 from the distal end (Fig. 26.7a). By pulling both ends of the nylon thread, the thread of anchor suture is looped through the remaining ligament (Fig. 26.7b). Rotate this loop half a turn, first pass the anchor suture thread on the opposite side (Fig. 26.7c). Then turn the loop again, pass the anchor suture thread on the same side through this second loop (Fig. 26.7d), and pull the end of the anchor suture thread on the same side as the loop and lightly tighten the loop (Fig. 26.7e). Finally, by making the ankle at 0° neutral position and strongly pulling the end of the anchor suture thread on the opposite side. Then the stump of the remaining ligament is crimped onto the fibular attachment, and at the same time the thread is appropriately slipped in the nodule and the knot is tighten strongly (Fig. 26.7f). After three more knot sutures are added, unnecessary threads are removed using a line cutter.

ATFL and CFL are connected with lateral talocalcaneal ligament [7] and attach together to fibula (Fig. 26.8a). And the rupture site in most cases of lateral instability of the ankle is close to fibular attachment [8] (Fig. 26.8b). Accordingly CFL is automatically moved to its fibular attachment and will recover to work well after ATFL suture alone (Fig. 26.8c).

26.2.7 Step 6: Gould Augmentation

If arthroscopic Broström method alone is concerned about the strength of the sutured ligament, Gould augmentation is added.

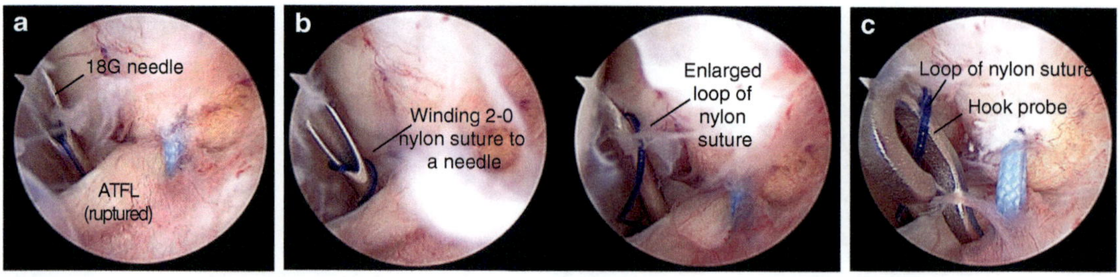

Fig. 26.6 Suture relay technique. (**a**) Insert a 18 G needle through 2-0 nylon thread from AAL portal and penetrate ATFL remnant fiber. (**b**) Rotating the needle forward for several times and reverse rotation the same number of times to enlarge the nylon loop. (**c**) Insert a hook probe from the AAL portal and guide the nylon loop from the AAL portal to the outside

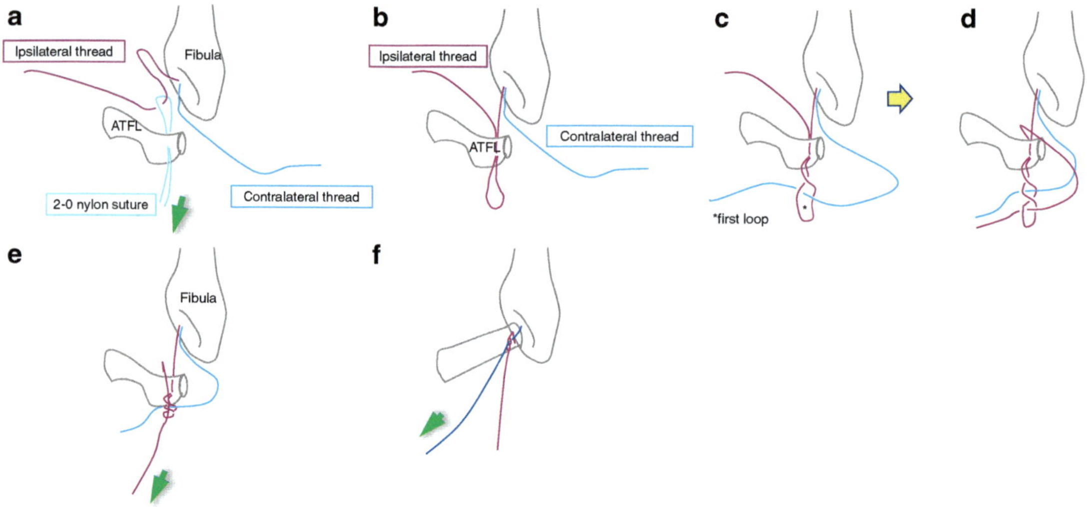

Fig. 26.7 Modified lasso-loop stitch. (**a**) Pass one thread of anchor suture to the nylon loop about 2/3 from the distal end. (**b**) By pulling both ends of the nylon thread, the thread of anchor suture is looped through the remaining ligament. (**c**) Rotate this loop half a turn, first pass the anchor suture thread on the opposite side. (**d**) Then turn the loop again, pass the anchor suture thread on the same side through this second loop. (**e**) Pull the end of the anchor suture thread on the same side as the loop and lightly tighten the loop. (**f**) Strongly pulling the end of the anchor suture thread on the opposite side. Then the stump of the remaining ligament is crimped onto the fibular attachment, and at the same time the thread is appropriately slipped in the nodule and the knot is tighten strongly

Insert second suture anchor about 5 mm proximal from the first suture anchor insertion. Since the upper edge of the inferior extensor retinaculum is close to the AAL portal, blunt dissection is performed on the surface layer and the deep layer of the inferior extensor retinaculum using mosquito Pean or a blunt rod (Fig. 26.9a). And after touching the upper edge of the inferior extensor retinaculum, it is grasped by mosquito Pean (Fig. 26.9b). After attaching the end of one thread of second suture anchor to a semicircular needle (Fig. 26.9b), insert the tip of the needle from the AAL portal and penetrate from the deep side of the inferior extensor retinaculum to the skin (Fig. 26.9c). Pull out the thread on the skin and remove the needle (Fig. 26.9d), then grip this thread with mosquito Pean inserted subcutaneously from the AAL portal and pull it out of the AAL portal (Fig. 26.9e). At this point, one thread of second suture anchor penetrates the inferior extensor retinaculum from the deep layer to the surface layer and is led out from the AAL portal. Then, a sliding knot technique is performed. It is desirable to use as small a sliding knot method as

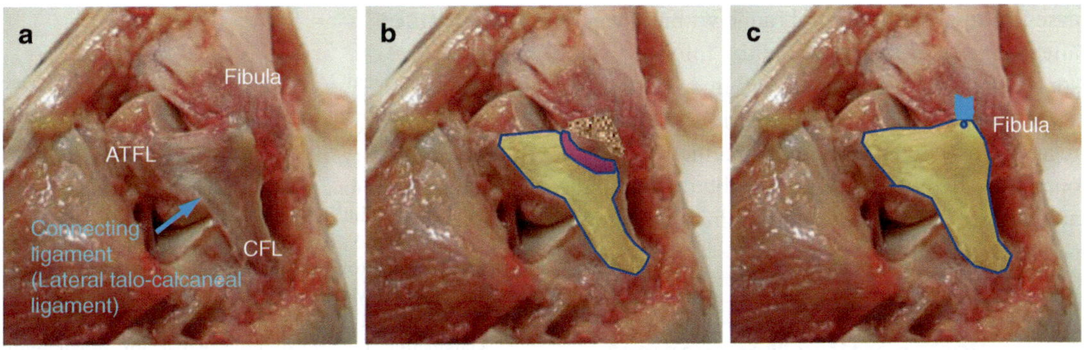

Fig. 26.8 Actual anatomy of the lateral ligament complex. (**a**) ATFL and CFL are connected with lateral talocalcaneal ligament and attach together to fibula. (**b**) The rupture site in most cases of lateral instability of the ankle is close to fibular attachment. (**c**) CFL is automatically moved to its fibular attachment and will recover to work well after ATFL suture alone

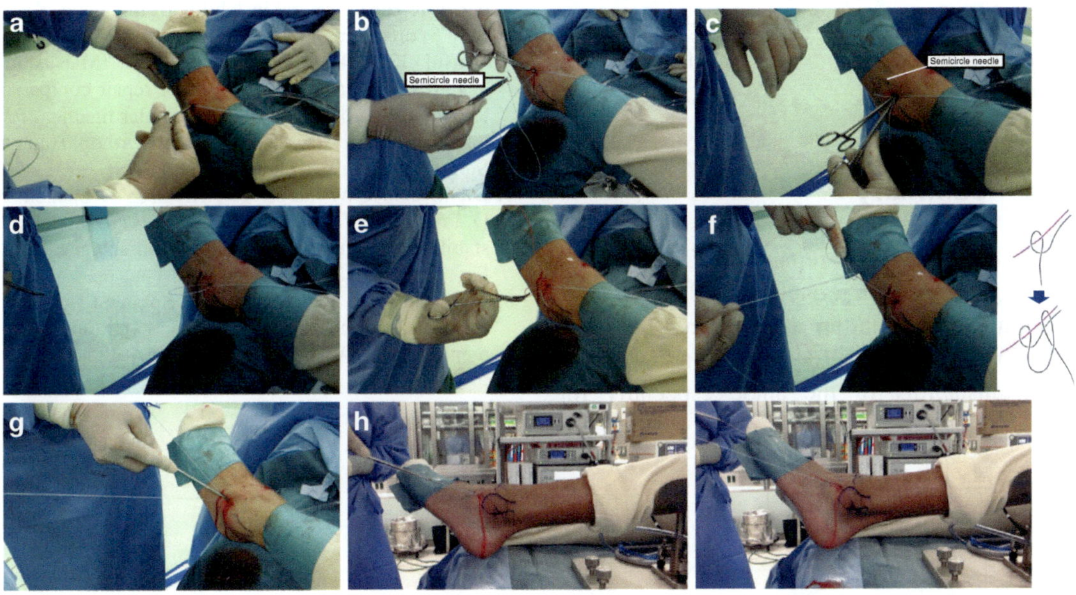

Fig. 26.9 Gould augmentation. (**a**) Blunt dissection is performed on the surface layer and the deep layer of the inferior extensor retinaculum using mosquito Pean or a blunt rod via AAL portal. (**b**) After touching the upper edge of the inferior extensor retinaculum, it is grasped by mosquito Pean. (**c**) After attaching the end of one thread of second suture anchor to a semicircular needle insert the tip of the needle from the AAL portal and penetrate from the deep side of the inferior extensor retinaculum to the skin. (**d**) Pull out the thread on the skin and remove the needle. (**e**) Grip the thread with mosquito Pean inserted subcutaneously from the AAL portal and pull it out of the AAL portal. (**f**) Sliding knot technique is performed. (**g**) Tighten the sliding knot and cut the thread with a knot cutter. (**h**) If the Gould augmentation is completed, the ankle moves about 10° in the dorsiflexion direction when knotting, and after tightening the maximum plantar flexion cannot be achieved passively

possible to prevent nodules touching subcutaneously after surgery (Fig. 26.9f). Tighten the sliding knot and cut the thread with a knot cutter (Fig. 26.9g). If the Gould augmentation is completed, the ankle moves about 10° in the dorsiflexion direction when knotting, and after tightening the maximum plantar flexion cannot be achieved passively (Fig. 26.9h). But in almost cases it improves to normal range within 4 weeks after surgery. This is because the inferior extensor retinaculum is loosened within 4 weeks after surgery. So Gould augmentation should be regarded as a temporary reinforcement after the operation. If enough stability is obtained with the arthroscopic Broström method, there is no need to add Gould augmentation.

26.3 Postoperative Management

After surgery, the elastic bandage is applied for 2 days, and the full weight-bearing walking is allowed according to pain from a day after surgery. Jogging and proprioceptive training will be from 2 weeks postoperatively and return to sports without external fixation shall be after 4 weeks postoperative.

26.4 Summary

All inside arthroscopic repair and reinforcement by inferior extensor retinaculum allows earlier returning to their initial athletic activities. The author recommends it for surgical treatment of lateral instability of the ankle especially for athletes.

References

1. Takao M, Ochi M, Uchio Y, Naito K, Kono T, Oae K. Osteochondral lesions of the talar dome associated with trauma. Arthroscopy. 2003;19(10):1060–6.
2. Harrington KD. Degenerative arthritis of the ankle secondary to long-standing lateral ligament instability. J Bone Joint Surg Am. 1979;61:354–61.
3. Valderrabano V, Hintermann B, Horisberger M, Fung TS. Ligamentous posttraumatic ankle osteoarthritis. Am J Sports Med. 2005;34:612–20.
4. Matsui K, Takao M, Miyamoto W, Innami K, Matsushita T. Arthroscopic Brostrom repair with Gould augumentation via an accessory anterolateral portal for lateral instability of the ankle. Arch Orthop Trauma Surg. 2014;134:1461–7.
5. Takao M, Matsui K, Stone JW, Glazebrook MA, Kennedy JG, Guillo S, Calder JD, Karlsson J. Ankle Instability Group: arthroscopic anterior talofibular ligament repair for lateral instability of the ankle. Knee Surg Sports Traumatol Arthrosc. 2016;24(4):1003–6.
6. Matsui K, Takao M, Miyamoto W, Matsushita T. Early recovery after arthroscopic repair compared to open repair of the anterior talofibular ligament for lateral instability of the ankle. Arch Orthop Trauma Surg. 2016;136:93–100.
7. DiGiovanni CW, Langer PR, Nickisch F, Spenciner D. Proximity of the lateral talar process to the lateral stabilizing ligaments of the ankle and subtalar joint. Foot Ankle Int. 2007;28:175–80.
8. Broström L, Sundelin P. Sprained ankles. IV. Histologic changes in recent and "chronic" ligament ruptures. Acta Chir Scand. 1966;132:248–53.

All Inside Endoscopic Brostrom-Gould Technique

27

Stéphane Guillo, Haruki Odagiri, and Thomas Bauer

27.1 Introduction

Ankle sprains are the most common sports injury, accounting for 45% and 31% of basketball and football injuries, respectively [1, 2]. With the exception of severe sprains in athletes who place heavy demands on their ankles [3], treatment is primarily medical and functional, and results in rehabilitation and a return to preinjury performance levels in 80% of cases. Surgical treatment is indicated in case of chronic instability following failure of medical treatment. The established surgical technique [4] consists of repairing the ligament (Brostrom [5]) and reinforcing the repair using the extensor retinaculum (Gould [6]). Over the past several years, arthroscopic alternatives have been proposed to treat ankle instability by thermal capsulorrhaphy, ligament repair and anatomical reconstruction [7]. However, no published endoscopic technique has actually reproduced the surgical ligament repair with retinacular reinforcement according to Brostrom-Gould. This technical note aims to describe Brostrom-Gould's procedure under complete endoscopic guidance.

27.2 Indications

As in open procedures, ligament repair is the first-line treatment and is recommended for young patients who still have an anterior talofibular ligament (ATFL). It may be contraindicated in revision surgery or on overweight patients and is technically impossible in patients with long-term instability whose ATFL has disappeared due to ligament degeneration [4].

27.3 Material

This technique requires a standard arthroscope (4 mm, 30°). Irrigation may be achieved by gravity or with an arthropump without exceeding 40 mmHg.

The arthroscopic dissection is performed using a 4-mm diameter shaver. An arthroscopic electric scalpel can be used. Ideally a suture passer is required, but a cathlon with a nylon suture can also be used. Other essential instruments include an arthroscopic forceps for the suture, a knot pusher and a knot cutter (Fig. 27.1).

S. Guillo (✉)
SOS Pied Cheville Bordeaux, Bordeaux-Mérignac, France

H. Odagiri
Kumamoto Foot and Ankle Center, Hotakubo Orthopedic Hospital, Kumamoto, Japan

T. Bauer
Hopital Ambroise Paré, Boulogne-Billancourt, France
e-mail: thomas.bauer@aphp.fr

H. Pereira et al. (eds.), *Lateral Ankle Instability*, https://doi.org/10.1007/978-3-662-62763-1_27

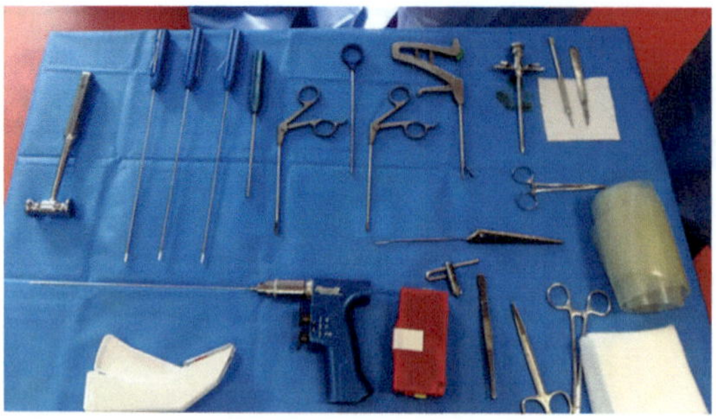

Fig. 27.1 Material needed for the surgery

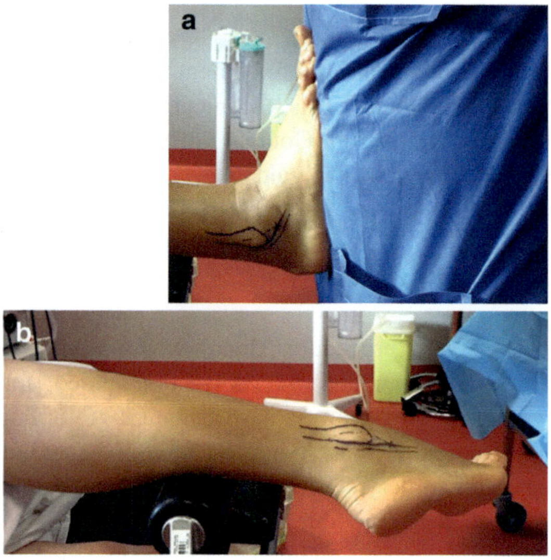

Fig. 27.2 Positions 1 (**a**) and 2 (**b**)

27.4 Positioning and Portals

27.4.1 Positioning

The patient is placed in the lateral decubitus position with the pelvis slightly tilted backwards, or in 3/4 position. A pneumatic tourniquet is applied at the top of the thigh. The procedure is performed under general or locoregional anaesthesia. Preoperatively, the surgeon should determine whether it is possible to perform an anterior arthroscopy (position 1) and a lateral endoscopy (position 2) (Fig. 27.2).

27.4.2 Landmark Identification and Portal Positioning

Three arthroscopic portals are established, incising only the skin with a scalpel and then dissecting the subcutaneous tissue using a Halsted forceps. The anteromedial portal (portal no. 1) is established in dorsal hyperflexion, as close as possible to the anterior tibial tendon. It is not necessary to give a serum injection before incising. The second portal is placed by transillumination. Once the arthroscope is perfectly positioned in the lateral gutter, portal no. 2 is positioned between the centre of this light spot and the anterior aspect of the lateral malleolus (Fig. 27.3). In practice, this portal is placed more distally than the anterolateral portal, which is generally used in anterior ankle arthroscopies. Portal no. 3 is established during the second-stage lateral endoscopy. It is placed 1 cm above the middle of the segment located between the tip of the malleolus and the tip of the base of the fifth metatarsal (Fig. 27.4).

27.5 Step 1: Anterior Arthroscopy, Ligament Repair (Broström)

The arthroscope is introduced through portal no. 1. The anteromedial portal must be established as close as possible to the anterior tibial tendon to give a clear view of the anterior tibiotalar recess, ankle joint line and lateral sulcus.

Once the arthroscope is perfectly centred over the lateral sulcus, the anterolateral portal is placed between the light spot and lateral malleolus. A needle may assist placement of this portal. It must arrive in the joint immediately in front of the malleolus in the lateral sulcus above the ATFL (Fig. 27.3). A Halsted forceps is introduced after performing the skin incision to prevent any injury to a cutaneous branch of the superficial fibular nerve. The procedure begins with cleaning the anterior site and performing an anterior synovectomy to resect scar and inflammatory tissue which may cause anterolateral impingement. The joint

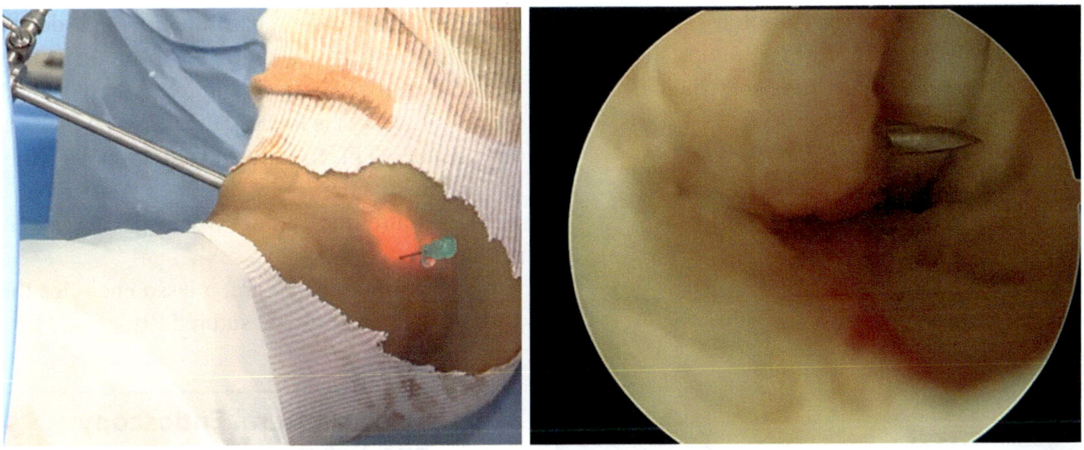

Fig. 27.3 Placement of the anterolateral portal

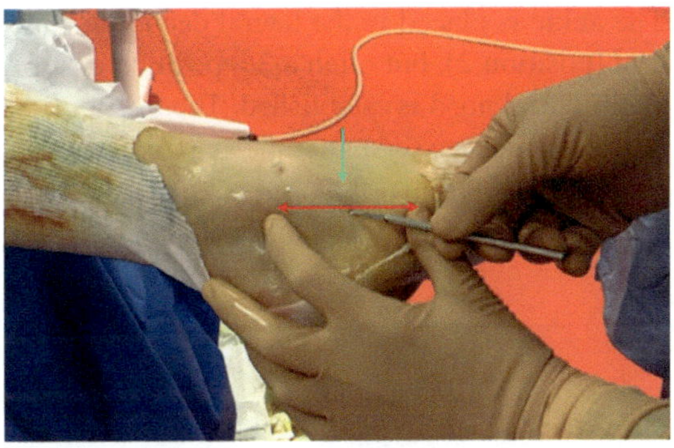

Fig. 27.4 Placement of the third portal

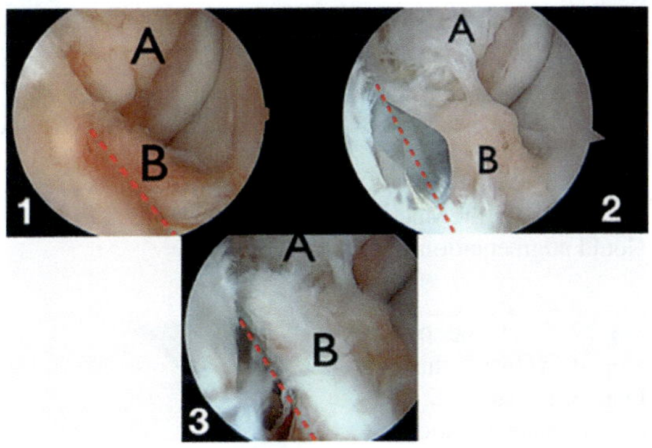

Fig. 27.5 Pic 1: (A) Basset ligament insertion. (B) Superior border of the ATFL. Pic 2: Red line shows the incision between the capsule and the ATFL. Pic 3: Vision of the ATFL (B) after complete dissection

line is explored to look for osteochondral lesions, foreign bodies and osteophytes (usually located on the medial side) [8]. After resecting the scar tissue which is often present at this site, the first landmark to be identified is the inferior edge of the anterior inferior tibiofibular ligament (AITFL or Basset's ligament) (Fig. 27.5.1A). By following this ligament from the inside to outside and from top to bottom, the malleolus is reached at the ATFL insertion located immediately below (Fig. 27.5.1B). At this stage, it is important to take a moment to visualise the talar neck and achieve a broad view of the operating site. A capsulotomy is then performed adjacent to the upper limit of the ATFL (Fig. 27.5.2). Using the shaver, dissection under arthroscopy should enable a perfect view of the ATFL from its talar to malleolar insertions (Fig. 27.5.3). The ATFL is then detached from its malleolar insertion, and the anterior aspect of the malleolus is prepared (scar tissue resection and shaver debridement). The upper portion of the ATFL should also be prepared by moving upwards towards the last insertion fibres of the AITFL.

Preparation is carried out using a burr to achieve complete debridement and preparation of the malleolar bone at the level of the ligament footprint. The inferior portion will receive the ATFL, and the superior portion will receive the retinaculum (Fig. 27.6). The first anchor is positioned at the ATFL insertion zone, with the arthroscope still placed in portal no. 1 and the instruments and anchor in portal no. 2. The second (and third if there is one) anchors are placed during lateral endoscopy. Before ATFL repair and reinsertion, the ATFL stump should be grasped with a forceps and stretched over the malleolus to assess repair quality and define where the suture should be placed in the ATFL. The Mini Scorpion suture passer (Arthrex, Naples FL, USA) is loaded (Fig. 27.7) and passes through the ATFL to form a suture loop, which is left on the outside.

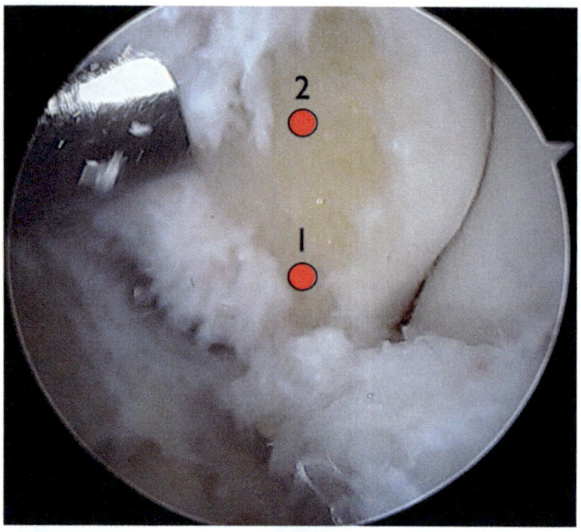

Fig. 27.6 Malleolus after preparation. Red spots are the placement of the anchors; 1, for the ATFL; 2, for the Gould augmentation

The suture protruding from the anchor is passed through the loop.

After pulling this suture, a lasso encircles the portion of ligament to be sutured [9].

27.6 Step 2: Lateral Endoscopy and Retinaculum Reinforcement (Gould)

The ankle is placed in the lateral decubitus position (position 2), but often a 3/4 position is sufficient. Portal no. 3 is established. The trocar of the arthroscope is passed under the skin to detach the retinaculum from the subcutaneous tissue (Fig. 27.8). During this manoeuvre, the subcuta-

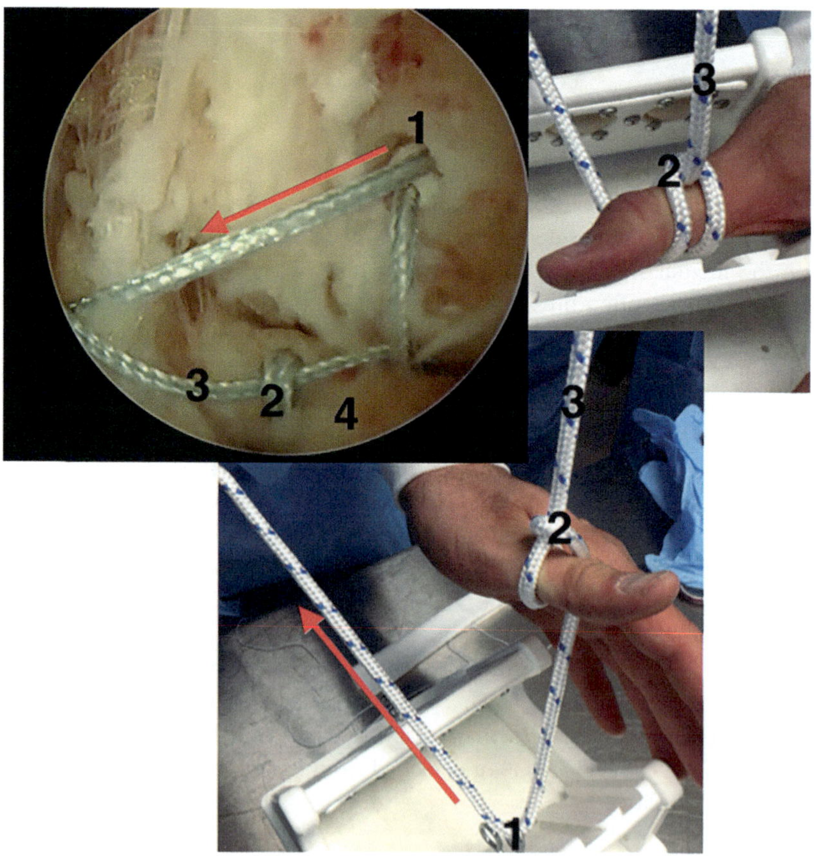

Fig. 27.7 The lasso loop. 4, ATFL; 2, the loop; 3, the suture passed inside the loop

neous nerve branches will remain at a distance and connected to the skin. The arthroscope is then introduced through portal 3, looking superiorly towards portal 2. Preparation ends after a shaver is introduced through portal no. 2. It is important to obtain a perfect view of the inferior reticulum and the key hole previously made by portal no. 2. The second (and the third if necessary) anchor is then introduced through portal no. 2 (Fig. 27.9). It is positioned at the anterior aspect of the malleolus just above the first anchor. The retinaculum, the four stands of suture, the malleolus and its preparation, and the lateral aspect of the talus deeper down should be perfectly visible.

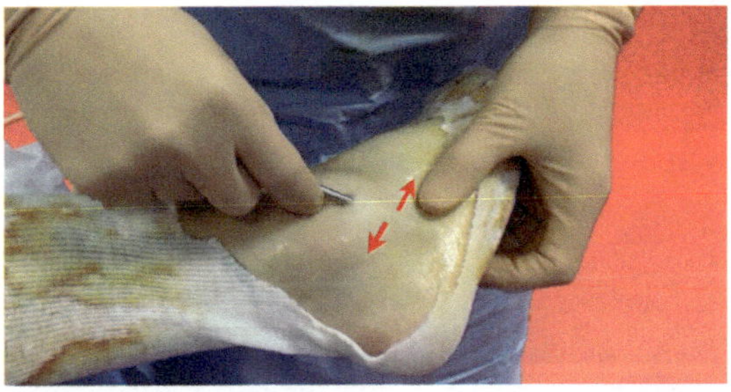

Fig. 27.8 Preparation of the space between the skin and the retinaculum

Using the Mini Scorpion forceps® (Arthrex, Naples FL, USA), the two strands (four if there is two anchors) of the anchors are passed through the retinaculum (Fig. 27.10) in order to achieve a mattress suture. If there is two anchors, the pulley technique may be used to increase the contact surface between the bone and ligament [10] (Fig. 27.10). The equivalent of two quilting

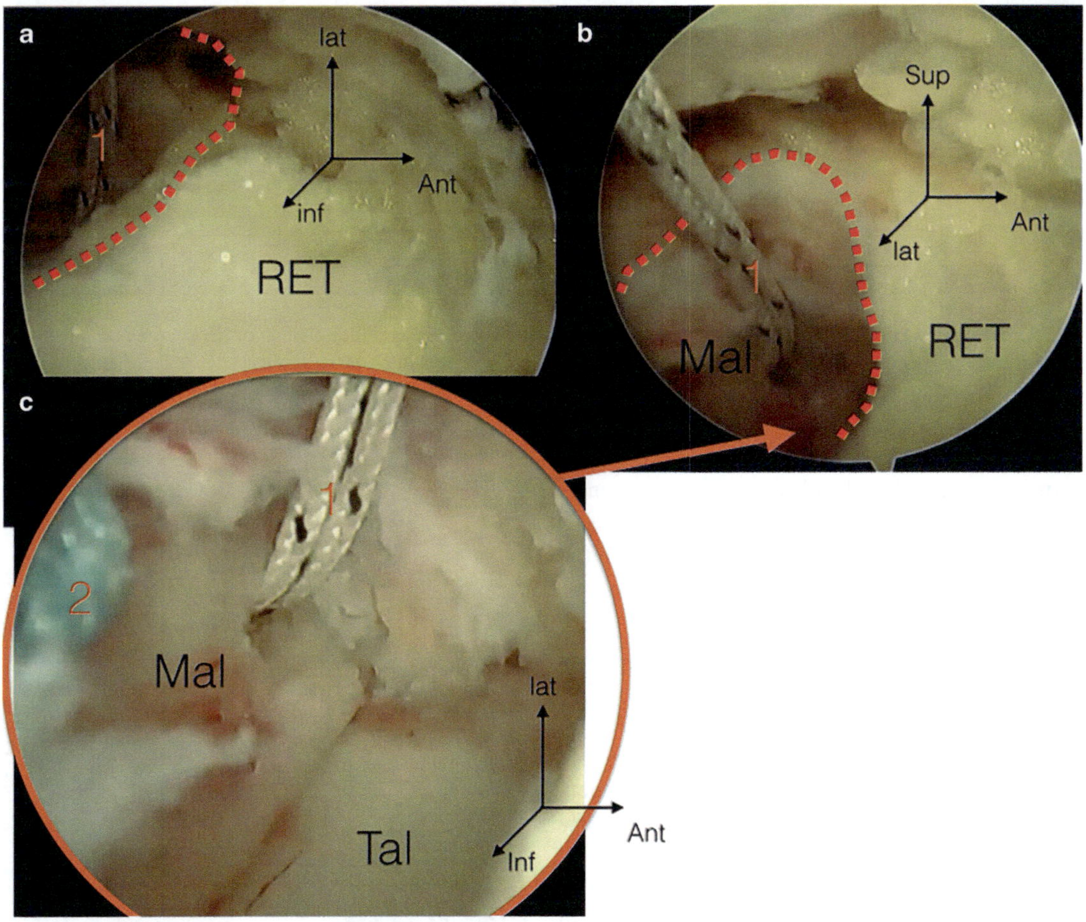

Fig. 27.9 Placement of the second anchor view from lateral endoscopic view (the scope is placed on the inferior). Vision of the retinaculum (RET), the anterior side of the malleolus (Mal) and the lateral side of the talus (TAL)

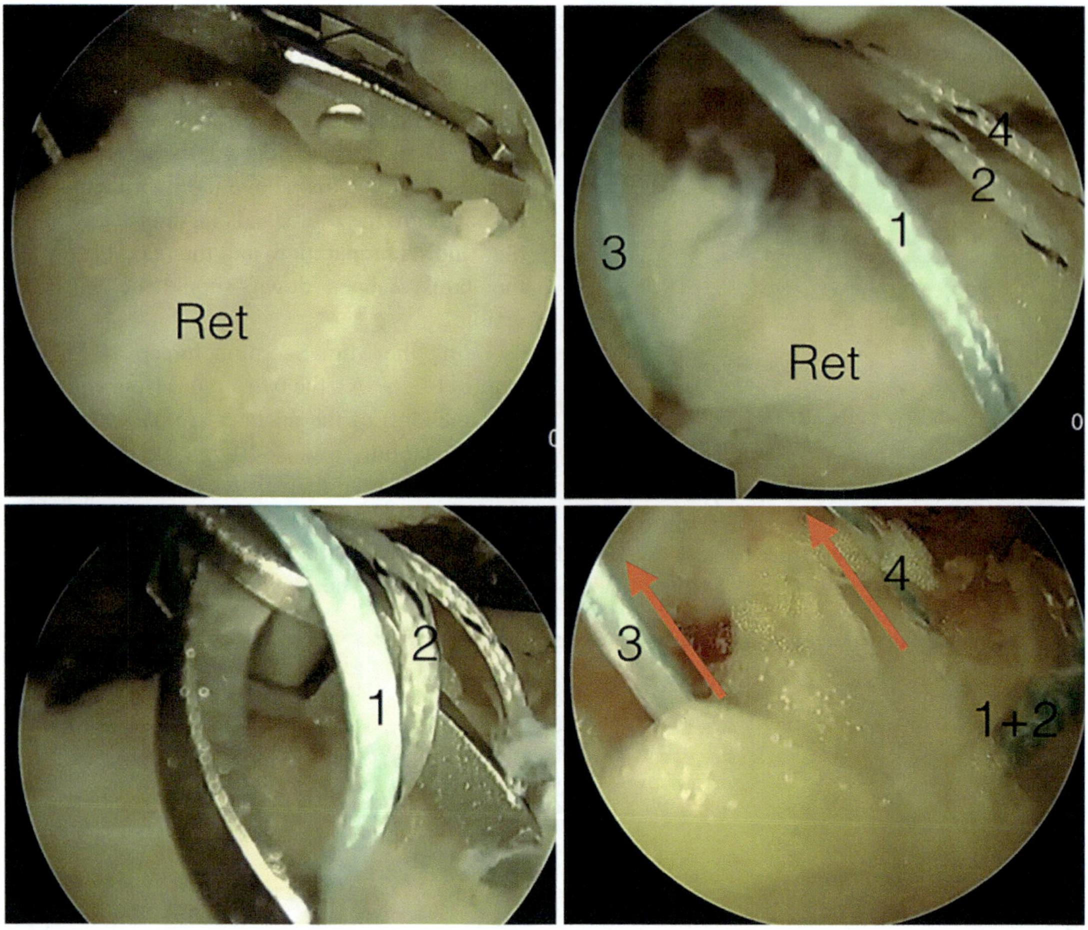

Fig. 27.10 The two-pulley technique: 1 is coming from one anchor; 2 is coming from the other anchor. 1 and 2 are tied outside and by pulling on 3 and 4, we are using the two anchors as pulley. The knot between 1 and 2 is going front of the anterior malleolus

sutures is thus placed, allowing for 'augmentation' of the initial repair (Fig. 27.11). The knots should be tightened in a neutral position with the ankle at 90°.

27.7 Postoperative Outcomes

The patient is immobilised, and a removable splint is used for 15 days. Load bearing is permitted depending on pain. Inflammatory responses and oedema should be prevented by icing and elevating the foot during the first 3 weeks, after which rehabilitation commences.

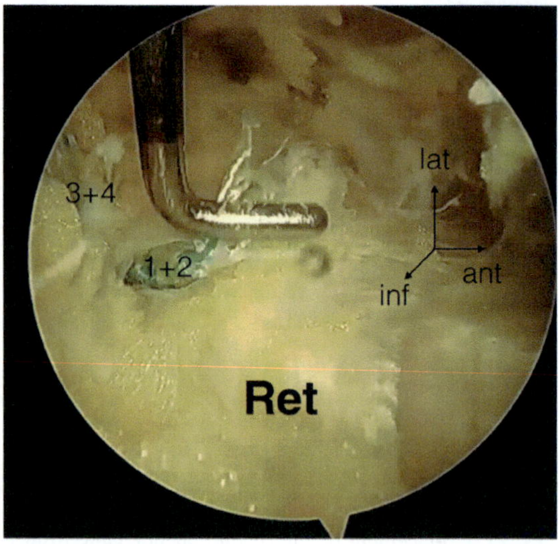

Fig. 27.11 Final aspect

27.8 Conclusion

Brostrom's anatomical repair technique [5] was described in the 1960s. It involves reattaching the ATFL and calcaneofibular ligament to the malleolus. However, it soon became evident that this procedure was insufficient, and modifications were subsequently described to tighten [11] and 'augment' the repair [6, 12–15]. This is why today, a Brostrom-type repair with Gould reinforcement is the recommended first-line procedure for ligament repair [4]. Arthroscopic techniques for repairing the ATFL have recently been described. Some of these provide only repair [16, 17], whereas others add retinacular reinforcement using a percutaneous or mini-approach, which can cause neurological damage [18–20]. We describe here a fully endoscopic Brostrom technique with retinaculum reinforcement (Gould), allowing direct endoscopic control of each step. It should also be noted that no published arthroscopic method mentions the requirement of bone debridement, which seems to us an essential element to achieve biological healing. We thus confirm that it is now possible to endoscopically perform endoscopically the same technique that has been described in open surgery and which is the recommended first-line treatment of chronic ankle instability. This reliable technique is enabled by lateral hind foot endoscopy. Studies should confirm the reliability, reproducibility and low morbidity of this Brostrom-Gould endoscopic technique.

References

1. Colville MR. Surgical treatment of the unstable ankle. J Am Acad Orthop Surg. 1998;6(6):368–77.
2. Garrick JG. The frequency of injury, mechanism of injury, and epidemiology of ankle sprains. Am J Sports Med. 1977;5(6):241–2.
3. van den Bekerom MP, Kerkhoffs GM, McCollum GA, Calder JD, van Dijk CN. Management of acute lateral ankle ligament injury in the athlete. Knee Surg Sports Traumatol Arthrosc. 2013;21(6):1390–5. https://doi.org/10.1007/s00167-012-2252-7.
4. Guillo S, Bauer T, Lee JW, Takao M, Kong SW, Stone JW, Mangone PG, Molloy A, Perera A, Pearce CJ, Michels F, Tourne Y, Ghorbani A, Calder J. Consensus in chronic ankle instability: aetiology, assessment, surgical indications and place for arthroscopy. Orthopaed Traumatol Surg Res. 2013;99(8 Suppl):S411–9. https://doi.org/10.1016/j.otsr.2013.10.009.
5. Brostrom L. Sprained ankles. VI. Surgical treatment of "chronic" ligament ruptures. Acta Chir Scand. 1966;132(5):551–65.
6. Gould N, Seligson D, Gassman J. Early and late repair of lateral ligament of the ankle. Foot Ankle. 1980;1:84–9.
7. Matsui K, Burgesson B, Takao M, Stone J, Guillo S, Glazebrook M, Group EAAI. Minimally invasive surgical treatment for chronic ankle instability: a systematic review. Knee Surg Sports Traumatol Arthrosc. 2016;24(4):1040–8. https://doi.org/10.1007/s00167-016-4041-1.
8. van Dijk CN, Wessel RN, Tol JL, Maas M. Oblique radiograph for the detection of bone spurs in anterior ankle impingement. Skelet Radiol. 2002;31(4):214–21. https://doi.org/10.1007/s00256-002-0477-0.
9. Lafosse L, Van Raebroeckx A, Brzoska R. A new technique to improve tissue grip: "the lasso-loop stitch". Arthroscopy. 2006;22(11):1246.e1241–3. https://doi.org/10.1016/j.arthro.2006.05.021.
10. Arrigoni P, Brady PC, Burkhart SS. The double-pulley technique for double-row rotator cuff repair. Arthroscopy. 2007;23(6):675.e671–4. https://doi.org/10.1016/j.arthro.2006.08.016.
11. Karlsson J, Bergsten T, Lansinger O, Peterson L. Reconstruction of the lateral ligaments of the ankle for chronic lateral instability. J Bone Joint Surg Am. 1988;70(4):581–8.
12. Boyer DS, Younger AS. Anatomic reconstruction of the lateral ligament complex of the ankle using a gracilis autograft. Foot Ankle Clin. 2006;11(3):585–95. https://doi.org/10.1016/j.fcl.2006.06.017.
13. Coughlin MJ, Schenck RC Jr, Grebing BR, Treme G. Comprehensive reconstruction of the lateral ankle for chronic instability using a free gracilis graft. Foot Ankle Int. 2004;25(4):231–41.
14. Jarvela T, Weitz H, Jarvela K, Alavaikko A. A novel reconstruction technique for chronic lateral ankle instability: comparison to primary repair. Int Orthop. 2002;26(5):314–7. https://doi.org/10.1007/s00264-002-0373-1.
15. Pagenstert GI, Hintermann B, Knupp M. Operative management of chronic ankle instability: plantaris graft. Foot Ankle Clin. 2006;11(3):567–83. https://doi.org/10.1016/j.fcl.2006.05.002.
16. Takao M, Matsui K, Stone JW, Glazebrook MA, Kennedy JG, Guillo S, Calder JD, Karlsson J, Ankle Instability Group. Arthroscopic anterior talofibular ligament repair for lateral instability of the ankle. Knee Surg Sports Traumatol Arthrosc. 2015;24:1003. https://doi.org/10.1007/s00167-015-3638-0.
17. Vega J, Golano P, Pellegrino A, Rabat E, Pena F. All-inside arthroscopic lateral collateral ligament repair for ankle instability with a knotless suture anchor

technique. Foot Ankle Int. 2013;34:1701. https://doi.org/10.1177/1071100713502322.
18. Acevedo J, Mangone PG. Arthroscopic lateral ankle ligament reconstruction. Tech Foot Ankle Surg. 2011;10(3):111–6.
19. Corte Real N, Moreira R. Arthroscopic repair of chronic lateral ankle instability. Foot Ankle Int. 2009;30(3):213–7.
20. Nery C, Raduan F, Del Buono A, Asaumi ID, Cohen M, Maffulli N. Arthroscopic-assisted Brostrom-Gould for chronic ankle instability: a long-term follow-up. Am J Sports Med. 2011;39(11):2381–8. https://doi.org/10.1177/0363546511416069.

Anatomical Reflections When Considering Tunnel Placement for Ankle Ligament Reconstruction

28

Frederick Michels, Kentaro Matsui, and Filip Stockmans

28.1 Introduction

In recent years there are two evolving shifts in lateral ligament surgery for ankle instability. First there is an evolution towards less invasive techniques as we see in other branches of surgery. This evolution emerges new endoscopic, endoscopically assisted, percutaneous and mini-open procedures [1–6]. The smaller incisions and dissection diminish the surgical soft tissue damage and also hamper the overview of the surgical site. In addition, there is an evolution towards the use of more anatomical procedures in an attempt to restore normal joint mechanics [7–10]. The non-anatomical techniques have fallen in disfavour since they tend to over-constrain the talocrural and subtalar joints, resulting in limitation of joint motion [11–13].

Both evolutions increase the need for additional knowledge about the normal anatomy and variations, but in particular the possible approaches, the endoscopic visualisation of the ligaments, the position of ligament insertions, the possible fixation techniques, the possible tunnel positions and the relationship with the surrounding anatomical structures. In this chapter, some of these aspects are discussed in an attempt to improve the surgical techniques.

28.2 Location of the Origins and Insertions of the ATFL and CFL Using Bony Landmarks

28.2.1 Introduction

Numerous techniques for open anatomical repair or reconstruction in treatment of chronic ankle instability (CAI) have reported good clinical results [13]. Most of these techniques use bone anchors or bone tunnels for fixation at the anatomical origins and insertions of the ATFL and CFL without open exposure. Therefore, these techniques require a more clear understanding of the ATFL and CFL anatomy to assure anatomical repair or reconstruction. The ATFL connects the fibula and talus, and consists of a single bundle or multiple bundles:

F. Michels (✉)
Orthopaedic Department AZ Groeninge, Kortrijk, Belgium

MIFAS by GRECMIP (Minimally Invasive Foot and Ankle Society), Merignac, France

K. Matsui
Department of Orthopaedic surgery, Trauma Center, Teikyo University Hospital, Tokyo, Japan

F. Stockmans
Orthopaedic Department AZ Groeninge, Kortrijk, Belgium

Department of Development and Regeneration, Faculty of Medicine, University of Leuven Campus Kortrijk, Kortrijk, Belgium
e-mail: filip.stockmans@kuleuven-kulak.be

H. Pereira et al. (eds.), *Lateral Ankle Instability*, https://doi.org/10.1007/978-3-662-62763-1_28

single bundle in 61.6%, double bundle in 35.7%, and triple bundle in 2.7% of the cadaveric specimens [14]. The superior band has been seen as the most important band in case of reconstruction [15]. The CFL connects the fibula and calcaneus, and has a solid, cord-like structure in 66% or a flat and fanning structure in 34%. The CFL was identified as an extra-capsular structure in 68% and as a capsular reinforcement in 32% [16].

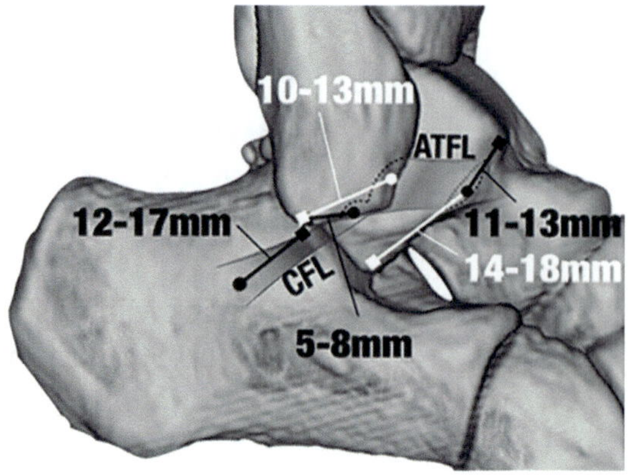

Fig. 28.2 Distances from the anatomic landmark (Square) to the footprint centre of the ATFL and CFL (dot)

28.2.2 The Talar Insertion of the ATFL

The ATFL inserts on the lateral side of the talar body just anterior to the lateral articular surface [17]. The insertion of the superior band of the ATFL is just below the triangular region of the talus [18]. In the study of Matsui, the talar obscure tubercle (TOT) was reported as the tubercle around the talar insertion (Fig. 28.1) [14]. This cadaveric study showed that the ATFL footprint centre on the talus was located 1.4 mm (range, 0.1–3.2 mm) from the TOT, but the TOT existed in 58.3% of the specimens, and it was detectable in 57.1% specimens by palpation or fluoroscopy in those specimens where it existed [14]. The tubercle was close to the ATFL insertion footprint centre on talus, and it may serve as a good reference point for the talar insertion of the ATFL, but sometimes it is not clinically relevant. In that case, an alternative method to define the footprint centre on the talus can be used. The footprint centre is at 11–13 mm from the anterolateral (AL) corner of the talar body or 14–18 mm from the inferolateral (IL) corner of the talar body, or the percentage of the distance from the IL corner to the ATFL insertion footprint centre on talus to the total length of anterolateral talar body (the distance from the IL to the AL corner of the talar body) was about 60% (Fig. 28.2) [14, 19].

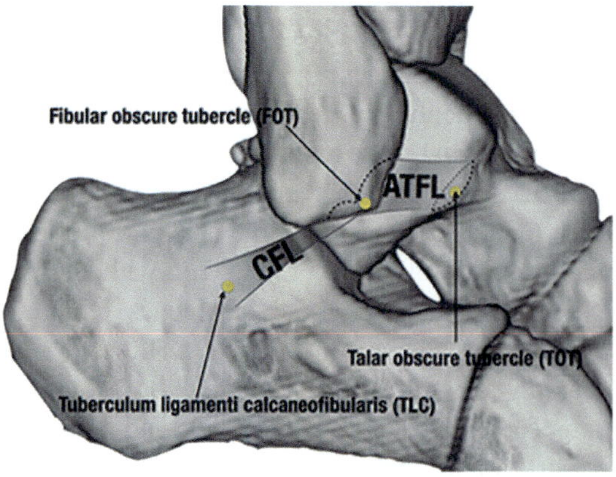

Fig. 28.1 Bony tubercles around the footprint of the ATFL and CFL

28.2.3 The Origin of ATFL and CFL

The ATFL and CFL originate on the inferior part of the anterior border of the distal fibula and just lateral to the articular cartilage of the fibula. The fibular origin of the CFL is just below the origin of the inferior band of the ATFL [20]. Buzzi et al. described that a rounded tubercle, the fibular obscure tubercle (FOT), can usually be found a few millimetres anterior to the apex of the fibula [21]. This obscure tubercle corresponded to the distally oriented apex of the articular facet of the distal fibula, while the apex of the fibula itself projected more distally and dorsally and corresponded to the apex of the retro-malleolar fossa [19]. This cadaveric study showed the FOT existed in all specimens and was detectable in 100% by palpation or fluoroscopy. The footprint centre of the ATFL and CFL origin on fibula was located 3.7 mm proximal to the FOT and 4.9 mm distal to the FOT, respectively [14]. The articular tip of the fibula (most distal part of the cartilage covering the fibula) is also a very helpful landmark during open or endoscopic surgery. This was located at 1.3 mm proximal from the FOT [14]. Subsequently, the FOT is a clinically relevant landmark, easily detectable by palpation or fluoroscopy, for the fibular tunnel. Alternatively, the tip of the fibula can be used as a landmark. The ATFL and CFL footprint centre is located 10–13 mm and 5–8 mm from the tip of the fibula, respectively [14, 19].

28.2.4 The Calcaneal Insertion of the CFL

The exact position of the calcaneal insertion of the CFL on the lateral surface of the calcaneus is difficult to locate. Laidlaw et al. reported that the CFL was inserted on a small tubercle, the tuberculum ligamenti calcaneofibularis (TLC), on the lateral surface of the calcaneus and posterior and superior to the posterior point of the peroneal process [22]. This tubercle was present as a well-defined tubercle in 43% [17]. The previous cadaveric study showed the TLC existed in 33.3% of the specimens and detectable on 25.0% of specimens by palpation or fluoroscopy [14]. When the tubercle exists, the CFL insertion footprint centre on the calcaneus was located 1.6 mm from the TLC, but the tubercle is not a clinically relevant landmark [19]. Alternatively, the posterior facet of the subtalar joint can be used as a landmark. The CFL insertion footprint is located on the perpendicular line from the midpoint of the subtalar joint at 12–17 mm [14].

28.3 Placement of the Tunnels in Reconstruction of ATFL and CFL

28.3.1 Introduction

There are several methods commonly used for fixation of a reconstructed ligament into bone. A curved bone tunnel was often used in the earlier techniques. However, this creates a bony bridge that may fracture. A tunnel with an interference screw or a bone anchor can help to avoid this risk. Interference screw fixation has demonstrated significantly greater fixation strength than bone anchors [23]. This technique is commonly used in ACL reconstruction. The development of newer, smaller, fixation devices facilitates the widespread use of this fixation technique.

28.3.2 The Talar Tunnel

The entry of the talar tunnel should be at the anatomical insertion point. The insertion site is situated just below the triangular region of the talus, immediately anterior to the joint surface occupied by the lateral malleolus. The tunnel can be oriented in several directions. The talus is a rather deeply located bone with an irregular form. When drilling a tunnel for graft fixation, one should take into account some guidelines. The tunnel should be as deep as safely possible and central in the bone to allow a good fixation. Cortical penetration should be avoided to avoid direct damage to or the joint or soft tissues. A tunnel close to the bone surface can cause fracture and presents a higher risk of graft pull-out. A recent study compared the different tunnel positions [18]. Virtual tunnels were generated in a 3D bone model, oriented towards different external landmarks: the talar neck, the most anterior point of the medial malleolus (MM), the most distal point of the MM, the most posterior point of the MM.

A tunnel towards the talar neck was discouraged because of the elevated risk of neck fracture even at small depth of the tunnel. In addition, the insertion of the ATFL is located on a convex surface just next to the sinus tarsi. An orientation towards the other side of the talar neck causes a sharp angle between the drill and the bony surface, increasing the risk of gliding of the drill or fracturing the tunnel entrance. A tunnel with a depth of 25 or 30 mm causes significant risk of perforation of the bone in any direction.

Two directions can be recommended (Fig. 28.3). A blind ended tunnel was found to be safest when directed to the posterior point of the medial malleolus. However, no perforation is permitted, in order to avoid damage to the pos-

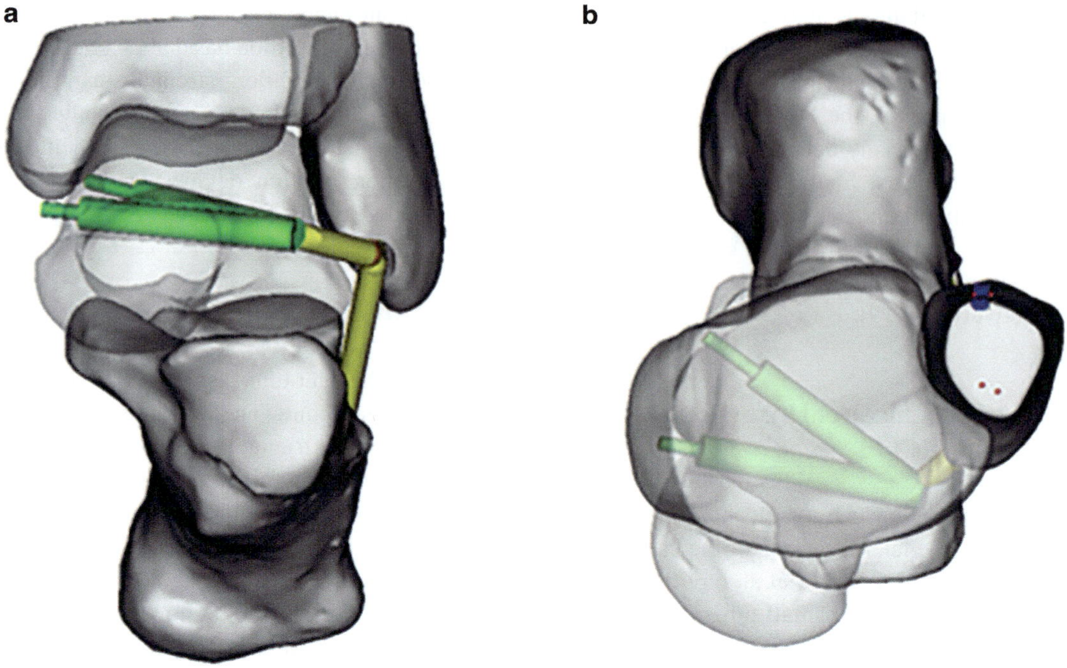

Fig. 28.3 Best talar tunnel options: a transosseous tunnel towards the most distal point of the medial malleolus or a blind ended tunnel towards the most posterior point of the medial malleolus. (**a**) Anterior view; (**b**) Superior view

teromedial neurovascular bundle. The tunnel should be limited to a diameter of 5 mm and a depth of 20 mm.

Alternatively, if a transosseous tunnel is preferred, the tunnel should be directed to the most distal part of the medial malleolus. In this case, a Beath pin is used to pull one end of a suture through the tunnel. The suture can be used to pull the end of the graft into the tunnel.

28.3.3 The Fibular Tunnel

As the insertion sites of the ATFL and CFL on the fibula are confluent, it is recommended to create only one common tunnel for fixation of both new ligaments in the fibula [15, 24]. In addition, two separate tunnels would increase the risk of fracture and fixation problems. The entry of the fibular tunnel should be at the anatomical insertion point. The correct insertion point is described earlier in this chapter. Different tunnel directions and diameters can be chosen (Fig. 28.4). A longer tunnel and a larger diameter favour a good fixation. As the fibula is rather small bone, maximal tunnel length and diameter are limited. In literature several directions and diameters are used. Some publications use a transverse tunnel [25], while others use a more oblique tunnel orientation [9, 10, 12]. Guillo et al. describe an oblique tunnel with a superior and posterior direction to reach the posterior cortex of the fibula 3–5 cm proximal and posterior to the distal tip [12].

We recently studied the different possible tunnel options and recommended the use of a more oblique tunnel [26]. An oblique tunnel safely allows a longer tunnel which corresponds with a better fixation. A perpendicular tunnel may cause an avulsion fracture of fibular tip. With the choice for a perpendicular tunnel, the surgeon would be tempted to opt for a more proximal (non-anatomical) insertion point to where the fibula becomes wider. In addition, posteromedial part of the lateral malleolus has a concave bone surface, the digital fossa [27]. The upper segment of that fossa is cribriform, with multiple vascular foramina. The lower segment gives origin to the posterior talofibular ligament. An oblique tunnel

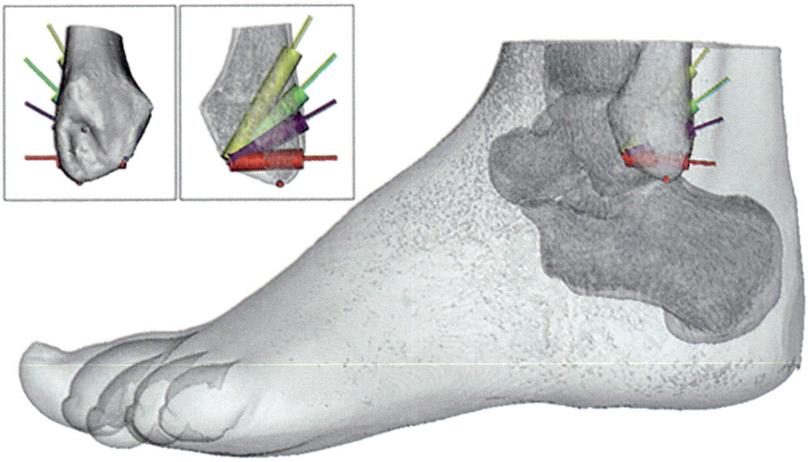

Fig. 28.4 Different tunnel positions and longitudinal axis of fibula

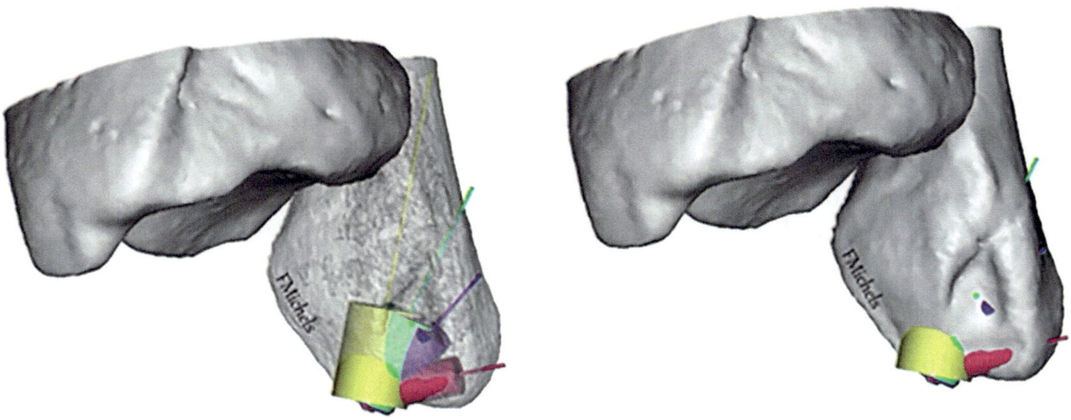

Fig. 28.5 Posteromedial view with digital fossa and relationship to different tunnel positions. The more obliquely directed tunnels allow a larger diameter before contact to the bone surface occurs

has less risk to damage the cribriform bone surface in this area (Fig. 28.5). Further studies are needed to provide more details.

28.3.4 The Calcaneal Tunnel

Tunnel length and diameter are usually not a problem when drilling the calcaneal tunnel. However, the exit of the tunnel may be very close to the neurovascular bundle (Fig. 28.6). We performed an anatomical study in 22 specimens and determined 4 squares related to the upper posterior edge and the lower anterior edge of the calcaneal tuberosity (Fig. 28.7) [28]. The lower posterior quadrant was found to be the safest

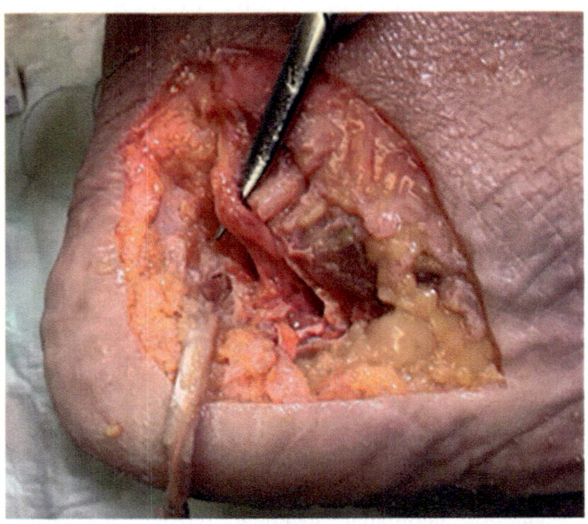

Fig. 28.6 Exit of the calcaneal tunnel on the medial side near the neurovascular bundle

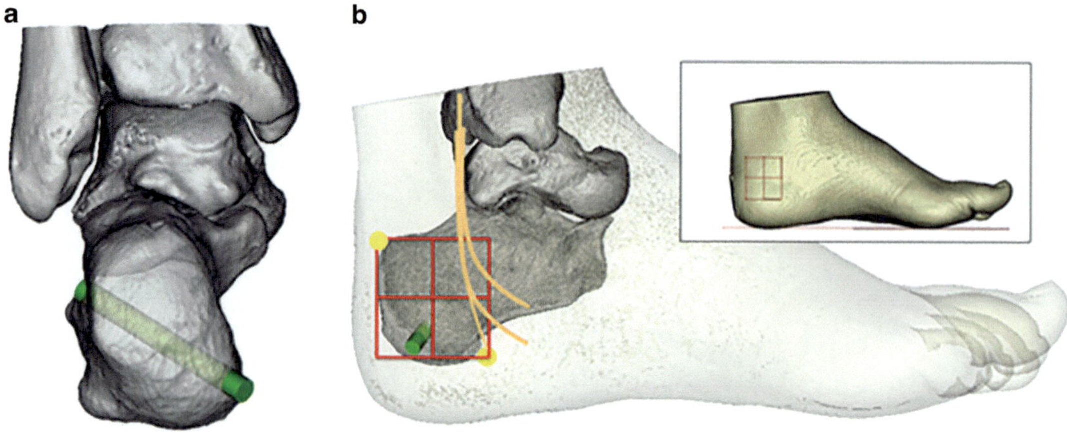

Fig. 28.7 (**a**) Posterior view of calcaneal tunnel. (**b**) Medial view of calcaneal tunnel

zone, most distant from the neurovascular bundle. So, the calcaneal tuberosity can be used as a landmark. According to these findings, this tunnel should be directed to the posterior medial edge of the calcaneal tuberosity.

The bone mineral density in the bone of the talus is higher than in the bone of the calcaneus [29]. This allows oversizing the interference screw in the calcaneal tunnel [30]. The screw should be placed under the level of the bone surface to avoid protrusion and irritation of the peroneal tendons. Good visualization during and after screw insertion is needed since the anatomical insertion of the CFL is behind the peroneal tendons. The peroneal tendons should be pushed aside during tunnel placement. A coloured screw can be checked more easily than a translucent screw.

References

1. Acevedo JI, Mangone PG. Arthroscopic lateral ligament reconstruction. Tech Foot Ankle. 2011;10:111–6.
2. Corte-Real NM, Moreira RM. Arthroscopic repair of chronic lateral ankle instability. Foot Ankle Int. 2009;30:213–7.
3. Giza E, Shin EC, Wong SE, et al. Arthroscopic suture anchor repair of the lateral ligament ankle complex: a cadaveric study. Am J Sports Med. 2013;41:2567–72.
4. Kim ES, Lee KT, Park JS et al. Arthroscopic anterior talofibular ligament repair for chronic ankle instability with a suture anchor technique. Orthopedics. 2011;34(4). https://doi.org/10.3928/01477447-20110228-03.
5. Nery C, Raduan F, Del Buono A, et al. Arthroscopic-assisted Broström-Gould for chronic ankle instability: a long-term follow-up. Am J Sports Med. 2011;39:2381–8.
6. Vega J, Golano P, Pellegrino A, et al. All-inside arthroscopic lateral collateral ligament repair for ankle instability with a knotless suture anchor technique. Foot Ankle Int. 2013;34:1701–9.
7. Guillo S, Takao M, Calder J, et al. Arthroscopic anatomical reconstruction of the lateral ankle ligaments. Knee Surg Sports Traumatol Arthrosc. 2016;24:998–1002.
8. Jung HG, Kim TH, Park JY, et al. Anatomic reconstruction of the anterior talofibular and calcaneofibular ligaments using a semitendinosus tendon allograft and interference screws. Knee Surg Sports Traumatol Arthrosc. 2012;20:1432–7.
9. Michels F, Cordier G, Burssens A, et al. Endoscopic reconstruction of CFL and the ATFL with a gracilis graft: a cadaveric study. Knee Surg Sports Traumatol Arthrosc. 2016;24(4):1007–14.
10. Takao M, Oae K, Uchio Y, et al. Anatomical reconstruction of the lateral ligaments of the ankle with a gracilis autograft: a new technique using an interference fit anchoring system. Am J Sports Med. 2005;33:814–23.
11. Bahr R, Pena F, Shine J, et al. Biomechanics of ankle ligament reconstruction. An in vitro comparison of the Broström repair, Watson-Jones reconstruction, and a new anatomic reconstruction technique. Am J Sports Med. 1997;25:424–32.
12. Guillo S, Archbold P, Perera A, et al. Arthroscopic anatomic reconstruction of the lateral ligaments of the ankle with gracilis autograft. Arthrosc Tech. 2014;3:e593–8.
13. Guillo S, Bauer T, Lee JW, et al. Consensus in chronic ankle instability: aetiology, assessment, surgical indi-

cations and place for arthroscopy. Orthop Traumatol Surg Res. 2013;99:411–9.
14. Matsui K, Oliva XM, Takao M, et al. Bony landmarks available for minimally invasive lateral ankle stabilization surgery: a cadaveric anatomical study. Knee Surg Sports Traumatol Arthrosc. 2017;25:1916–24.
15. Neuschwander T, Indressano A, Hughes T, et al. Footprint of the lateral ligament complex of the ankle. Foot Ankle Int. 2013;34:582–6.
16. Wiersma PH. Variations of three lateral ligaments of the ankle. A descriptive anatomical study. Foot. 1992;2:218–24.
17. Wenny R, Duscher D, Meytap E, Weninger P, Hirtler L. Dimensions and attachments of the ankle ligaments: evaluation for ligament reconstruction. Anat Sci Int. 2015;90:161–71.
18. Michels F, Guillo S, Vanrietvelde F, et al. How to drill the talar tunnel in ATFL reconstruction? Knee Surg Sports Traumatol Arthrosc. 2016;24:991–7.
19. Matsui K, Takao M, Tochigi Y, et al. Anatomy of anterior talofibular ligament and calcaneofibular ligament for minimally invasive surgery: a systematic review. Knee Surg Sports Traumatol Arthrosc. 2017;25:1892–902.
20. Taser F, Shafiq Q, Ebraheim NA. Anatomy of lateral ankle ligaments and their relationship to bony landmarks. Surg Radiol Anat. 2006;28:391–7.
21. Buzzi R, Todescan G, Brenner E, et al. Reconstruction of the lateral ligaments of the ankle: an anatomic study with evaluation of isometry. J Sports Traumatol Relat Res. 1993;15:55–74.
22. Laidlaw PP. The varieties of the Os Calcis. J Anat Physiol. 1904;38:133–43.
23. Jeys L, Korrosis S, Stewart T, et al. Bone anchors or interference screws? A biomechanical evaluation for autograft ankle stabilization. Am J Sports Med. 2004;32(7):1651–9.
24. Ozeki S, Yasuda K, Kaneda K, et al. Analysis of the isometry for reconstruction of the lateral ankle ligaments. J Jpn Soc Surg Foot. 1990;11:98–102.
25. Youn H, Kim YS, Lee J, et al. Percutaneous lateral ligament reconstruction with allograft for chronic lateral ankle instability. Foot Ankle Int. 2012;33(2):99–104.
26. Michels F, Matricali G, Guillo S, et al. An oblique fibular tunnel is recommended when reconstructing the ATFL and CFL. Knee Surg Sports Traumatol Arthrosc. 2020;28(1):124–31.
27. Kelian A. Sarafian's anatomy of the foot and ankle: descriptive topographical, functional. 3rd ed. Philadelphia: Lippincott Williams & Wilkins; 2011. p. 163–222.
28. Michels F, Matricali G, Wastyn H, et al. A calcaneal tunnel for CFL reconstruction should be directed to the posterior inferior medial edge of the calcaneal tuberosity. Knee Surg Sports Traumatol Arthrosc. 2020. https://doi.org/10.1007/s00167-020-06134-x.
29. Morimoto M, Utsumi M, Tohno Y, et al. Age-related changes of bone mineral density in human calcaneus, talus, and scaphoid bone. Biol Trace Elem Res. 2001;82(1–3):53–60.
30. Michels F, Cordier G, Guillo S, et al. Endoscopic ankle lateral ligament graft anatomic reconstruction. Foot Ankle Clin. 2016;21(3):665–80.

ATFL Anatomical Reconstruction

29

Youichi Yasui, Wataru Miyamoto, Kentaro Matsui, Shinya Miki, Maya Kubo, Hélder Pereira, and Masato Takao

29.1 Introduction

Arthroscopic anterior talofibular ligament (ATFL) anatomical reconstruction described in this chapter is a similar technique to Arthroscopic AntiRoLL (A-AntiRoLL) (see Chap. 31). The main difference between them is a graft shape.

In this chapter, we describe a surgical technique for arthroscopic ATFL anatomical reconstruction briefly and do discuss when and how isolated ATFL reconstruction alone or combined ATFL plus calcaneal fibular ligament (CFL) reconstruction would be chosen.

Y. Yasui (✉) · W. Miyamoto · K. Matsui · S. Miki · M. Kubo
Department of Orthopaedic Surgery, Teikyo University School of Medicine, Tokyo, Japan
e-mail: miyamoto@med.teikyo-u.ac.jp; kenor@nifty.com

H. Pereira
Knee and Ankle Orthopaedic Department, Centro Hospitalar Póvoa de Varzim, Vila do Conde, Portugal

Ripoll y De Prado Sports Clinic: FIFA Medical Centre of Excellence, Murcia-Madrid, Spain

ICVS/3B's – PT Government Associate Laboratory, University of Minho, Braga/Guimarães, Portugal

M. Takao
Clinical and Research Institute for Foot and Ankle Surgery, Jujo Hospital, Chiba, Japan
e-mail: m.takao@carifas.com

29.2 Surgical Technique

29.2.1 Position

The patient lays supine on the operative table with the hip ipsilateral to the injured flexed (Fig. 29.1). A thigh tourniquet is applied, but not typically used.

29.2.2 Step 1: Making Portals

Medial midline (MML) portal, accessory anterolateral (AAL) portal and subtalar portal (ST) are used (Fig. 29.2). Prior to any incisions, superficial peroneal nerve is marked to decrease the iatrogenic injury's risk for this nerve.

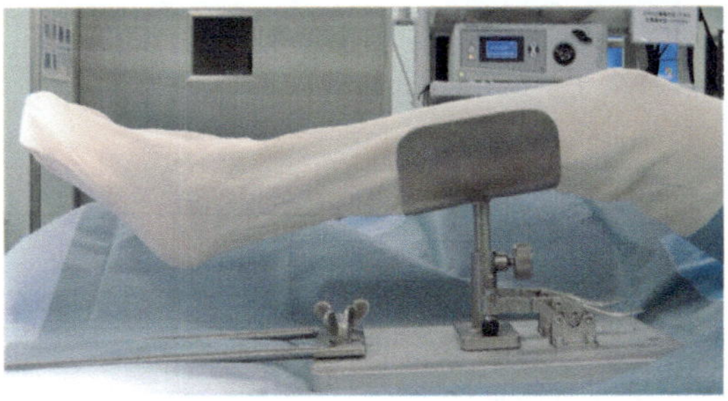

Fig. 29.1 Intraoperative position of operative foot

H. Pereira et al. (eds.), *Lateral Ankle Instability*, https://doi.org/10.1007/978-3-662-62763-1_29

29.2.3 Step 2: Systematic Diagnostic Examination for Intra-articular Disorder [1]

ATFL injury frequently accompanies concomitant ankle pathologies (e.g. synovitis, bony spur, ligament injuries). These lesions should be treated prior to ATFL reconstruction. It is a good idea to add more portals in treatment for those pathologies.

29.2.4 Step 3: Making a Graft from an Autologous Gracilis Tendon

An autologous gracilis tendon is harvested from the ipsilateral knee. For arthroscopic ATFL reconstruction, the length of the graft is 90 mm.

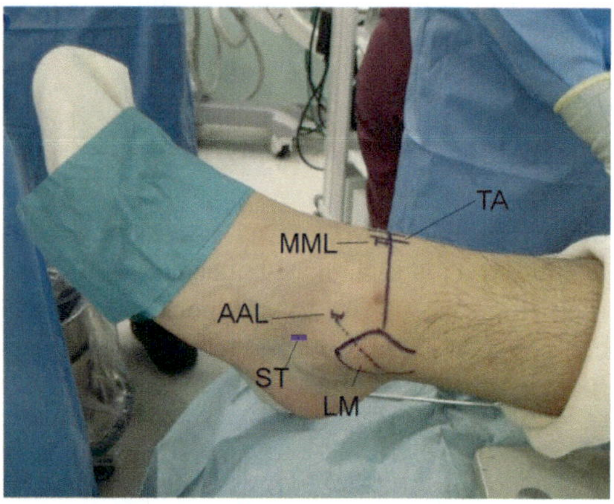

Fig. 29.2 Portals (same figure in Chap. 31)

The harvested tendon is folded at 45 mm from the end to become a twofold graft (Fig. 29.3).

29.2.5 Step 4: Making the Bone Tunnels at Each Attachment to Fibula and Talus (Fig. 29.4a, b)

Fibular and talar bone tunnels are made similarly to AntiRoLL. In arthroscopic ATFL reconstruction, a calcaneal bone tunnel is not made.

29.2.6 Step 5: Introducing the Graft into the Bone Tunnels and Fixing with the Interference Screw (Fig. 29.4c, d)

This step is also the same manner as AntiRoLL. After the graft is introduced through the portals, the fibular side is fixed using an interference screw. Then, the talar side is fixed with a neutral position of ankle and foot.

29.3 Post-operative Management

The elastic bandage is used approximately 2 days following surgery. A full weight-bearing is allowed according to pain from 1 day after surgery. Patients are allowed to return to sport and more physical activities 6–8 weeks after surgery.

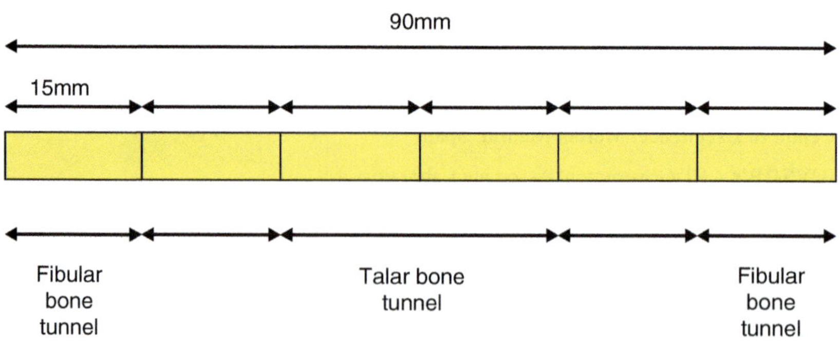

Fig. 29.3 The autologous gracilis tendon is folded at the site of 45 mm from the end to become a twofold graft. The ends are inserted into fibular bone tunnel

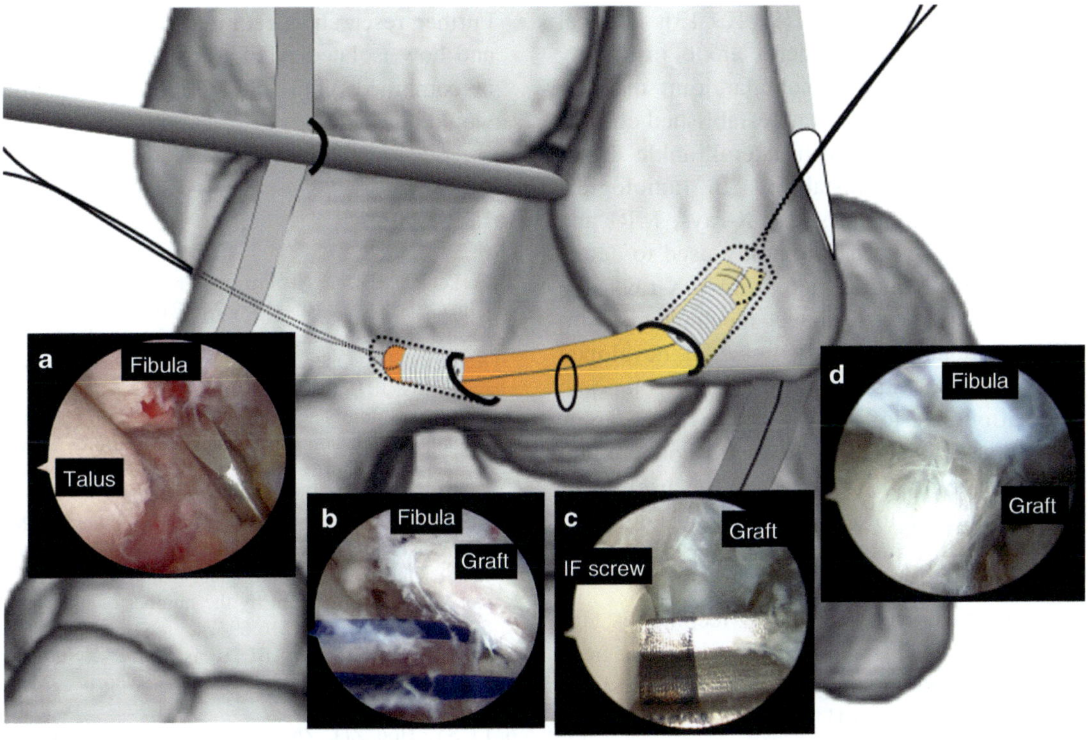

Fig. 29.4 (**a**, **b**) The ATFL is reconstructed as a similar manner to arthroscopic AntiRoLL technique. (**a**) The guide-wire is inserted into fibular through the portal. (**b**) The graft is introduced into the capsule using inside-out technique. (**c**) The ends of graft are fixed using interference screw. (**d**) Final appearance of ATFL

29.3.1 When and How Do You Prefer Isolated ATFL Reconstruction and Not the Full Combined ATFL Plus CFL Reconstruction

Most patients with chronic lateral ankle instability have ATFL injury alone, while 20% have combined ATFL and CFL injuries [2]. A variety of surgical techniques are currently in use for these pathologies. However, there is a lack of universal consensus in the treatment for concomitant ATFL and CFL injuries and how isolated ATFL reconstruction alone or combined ATFL plus CFL reconstruction would be chosen even in not only arthroscopic procedures but also open procedures [3]. In previous literature, the anatomy of CFL has been still unclear. A recent anatomical study by Edema et al. investigated the relationship between the ATFL and CRL in 81 legs from 43 cadavers, and found that a variety of attachments and these relationships were present [4]. The authors propose that the control function of the ankle may differ within each type and among types.

The function of CFL for ankle and subtalar joint has remained controversial. In the previous literature, CFL has been proposed as a primary stabilizer of the subtalar joint, while some researchers recently describe that interosseous talocalcaneal ligament (ITCL) or cervical ligament (CL) is the most important stabilizer [5–9]. Wang et al. found that the subtalar joint had no instability after sectioning of the CFL in 42 patients receiving open reduction and internal fixation for calcaneal fractures [10]. A recent study by Kim et al. proposes that anterior capsular ligament (ACL) may have the most critical role for subtalar joint stabilization [11].

In the clinical situation, both clinical and radiological diagnostic accuracy of CFL injuries are still challenging [9, 12, 13]. Clinical symptoms of chronic lateral ankle instability are similar to those of subtalar joint instability [11]. To date, there is no established clinical evaluation to distinguish lateral ankle instability or subtalar instability. In radiological diagnostic modalities, stress X-rays, MRI and ultrasound have been commonly used to detect CFL injuries. Among them, stress X-rays is a more dynamic test to detect mechanical instability of subtalar. Recently, Lee et al. developed a new manual stress radiographic technique: Supination-anterior drawer stress radiography, detecting subtalar instability with concomitant ankle instability [9]. However, the usefulness of stress X-rays to detect CFL insufficiency is still due to the uncertain function of CFL, as described above.

Anatomical reconstruction techniques for treating both ATFL and CFL injuries have been broadly divided into three categories: reconstruction of ATFL alone [14], reconstruction of ATFL with reinforcement of local tissue [15] and reconstruction of both ATFL and CFL [16]. Although abundant clinical evidence advocates the excellent clinical outcomes following each surgical technique, there is still a controversy on which surgical strategy is better than the other.

In summary, based on available evidence, operative treatment for accompanying CFL injury may not be required in all cases. Further research is required to clarify when and how isolated ATFL reconstruction alone or combined ATFL plus calcaneal fibular ligament reconstruction would be chosen.

Take-Home Messages

- Surgical technique of arthroscopic ATFL anatomical reconstruction is similar to the A-AntiRoLL. The main difference between them is a graft shape.
- Arthroscopic ATFL anatomical reconstruction is a potentially less invasive procedure for surgical treatment for ATFL injury alone.
- Further research is required to clarify when and how isolated ATFL reconstruction alone or combined ATFL plus CFL reconstruction would be chosen.

References

1. Ferkel RD, Fischer SP. Progress in ankle arthroscopy. Clin Orthop Relat Res. 1989;240:210–20.
2. Yasui Y, Murawski CD, Wollstein A, Takao M, Kennedy JG. Operative treatment of lateral ankle instability. JBJS Rev. 2016;4(5).
3. Yasui Y, Shimozono Y, Kennedy JG. Surgical procedures for chronic lateral ankle instability. J Am Acad Orthop Surg. 2018;26(7):223–30. https://doi.org/10.5435/JAAOS-D-16-00623. Review.
4. Edama M, Kageyama I, Kikumoto T, Nakamura M, Ito W, Nakamura E, Hirabayashi R, Takabayashi T, Inai T, Onishi H. Morphological features of the anterior talofibular ligament by the number of fiber bundles. Ann Anat. 2017;216:69–74.
5. Karlsson J, Eriksson BI, Renstrom PA. Subtalar ankle instability. A review. Sports Med. 1997;24(5):337–46.
6. Li SY, Hou ZD, Zhang P, Li HL, Ding ZH, Liu YJ. Ligament structures in the tarsal sinus and canal. Foot Ankle Int. 2013;34(12):1729–36.
7. Martin LP, Wayne JS, Monahan TJ, Adelaar RS. Elongation behavior of calcaneofibular and cervical ligaments during inversion loads applied in an open kinetic chain. Foot Ankle Int. 1998;19(4):232–9.
8. Kjaersgaard-Andersen P, Wethelund JO, Nielsen S. Lateral talocalcaneal instability following section of the calcaneofibular ligament: a kinesiologic study. Foot Ankle. 1987;7(6):355–61.
9. Lee BH, Choi KH, Seo DY, Choi SM, Kim GL. Diagnostic validity of alternative manual stress radiographic technique detecting subtalar instability with concomitant ankle instability. Knee Surg Sports Traumatol Arthrosc. 2016;24(4):1029–39.
10. Wang CS, Tzeng YH, Lin CC, Huang CK, Chang MC, Chiang CC. Radiographic evaluation of ankle joint stability after calcaneofibular ligament elevation during open reduction and internal fixation of calcaneus fracture. Foot Ankle Int. 2016;37(9):944–9.
11. Kim TH, Moon SG, Jung HG, Kim NR. Subtalar instability: imaging features of subtalar ligaments on 3D isotropic ankle MRI. BMC Musculoskelet Disord. 2017;18(1):475. https://doi.org/10.1186/s12891-017-1841-5.
12. Mittlmeier T, Wichelhaus A. Subtalar joint instability. Eur J Trauma Emerg Surg. 2015;41(6):623–9.

13. Park HJ, Lee SY, Park NH, Kim E, Chung EC, Kook SH, Lee JW. Usefulness of the oblique coronal plane in ankle MRI of the calcaneofibular ligament. Clin Radiol. 2015;70(4):416–23.
14. Maffulli N, Del Buono A, Maffulli GD, Oliva F, Testa V, Capasso G, Denaro V. Isolated anterior talofibular ligament Broström repair for chronic lateral ankle instability: 9-year follow-up. Am J Sports Med. 2013;41(4):858–64.
15. Matsui K, Takao M, Miyamoto W, Matsushita T. Early recovery after arthroscopic repair compared to open repair of the anterior talofibular ligament for lateral instability of the ankle. Arch Orthop Trauma Surg. 2016;136(1):93–100.
16. Takao M, Glazebrook M, Stone J, Guillo S. Ankle arthroscopic reconstruction of lateral ligaments (ankle anti-ROLL). Arthrosc Tech. 2015;4(5):e595–600.

Arthroscopic Anatomical Reconstruction of the Lateral Ankle Ligaments

30

Joao Teixeira, Haruki Odagiri, Ronny Lopes, Thomas Bauer, and Stéphane Guillo

30.1 Introduction

Ankle sprain is the most common sport trauma. Conservative functional management most often gives good results [1]. Nevertheless, 10–20% of these sprains will progress to chronic instability with variable clinical signs (simple chronic discomfort obliging to reduce or stop sports activities, anterolateral conflict, repeated sprains), responsible for rapid chondral lesions and leading to early tibio-talar osteoarthritis [2]. Surgical treatment of chronic ankle instability (CAI) is therefore justified to stabilize the ankle, to restore physiological joint kinematics and to prevent the occurrence of osteoarthritic degradation. Many procedures have been described to treat CAI, and globally it is possible to summarize them in either ligament repairs or ligament reconstructions. Ligament repairs (ligament retensionning with or without reinforcement) give good results in the medium and long term and remain indicated in first intention. However, they are insufficient in patients with poor-quality residual ligament and in obese or high-performance athletes [3–5]. In these situations, it is necessary to perform a ligament reconstruction interesting the anterior talofibular ligament (ATFL) and the calcaneo-fibular ligament (CFL). Non-anatomical reconstructions were the most popular and the most studied; they give excellent early results but can cause stiffness and osteoarthritic degradation of the subtalar joint [6–11]. This is why anatomical reconstructions have been developed and tend to impose in restoration of the articular physiology [12]. Gradually arthroscopic techniques of anatomic reconstruction have developed and confirmed their reliability in terms of reconstruction quality and safety [13, 14]. Therefore, arthroscopy become an indispensable tool in the treatment of CAI: in terms of diagnosis, it allows a precise lesion assessment guiding the choice of the most appropriate stabilization technique; on the therapeutic level, it offers the possibility to treat the associated lesions and perform ligament repairs

J. Teixeira
Department of Orthopaedic and Traumatology, Centro Hospitalar de Entre o Douro Vouga, Santa Maria da Feira, Portugal

Department of Foot and Ankle Surgery, Hospital da luz Arrábida, Vila Nova de Gaia, Portugal

H. Odagiri
Kumamoto Foot and Ankle Center, Hotakubo Orthopedic Hospital, Kumamoto, Japan

R. Lopes
Pied Cheville Nantes Atlantique, Atlantic Health, Saint Herblain, France

Breteche Clinic, Nantes, France

T. Bauer
Hopital Ambroise Paré, Boulogne-Billancourt, France
e-mail: thomas.bauer@aphp.fr

S. Guillo (✉)
SOS Pied Cheville Bordeaux, Bordeaux-Mérignac, France

H. Pereira et al. (eds.), *Lateral Ankle Instability*, https://doi.org/10.1007/978-3-662-62763-1_30

or anatomical reconstructions. This technical note reviews the arthroscopic anatomical reconstruction of ATFL and CFL.

30.2 Indications

Interventions for chronic lateral ankle instability should always be proposed after failure of well-conducted medical treatment (proprioceptive rehabilitation, plantar orthotics). Overall, in case of surgical indication always try to repair the ATFL first. However, there are certain situations where ligament reconstruction can be proposed from the outset as follows:

- The failures to repair the ATFL
- Morbid obesity
- Constitutional hyperlaxity
- Advanced degeneration of ATFL and retinaculum
- Professional high-demand sports patients

30.3 Surgical Technique

30.3.1 Instrumentation

The technique is performed using a standard 30° arthroscope of 4 mm. The complete exploration of the tibio-talar joint and the talofibular gutter is facilitated by laxity. Irrigation is provided by simple gravity, so an irrigation system is not essential. A 4.5-mm shaver (soft tissue cutter) is used for the preparation.

30.3.2 Positioning

The patient is placed ¾ supine to have a medial rotation of the lower limb and clear the lateral aspect of the ankle for reconstruction. This position allows the lateral rotation of the lower limb with flexion of the knee for gracilis harvest. Lateral decubitus installation is possible. The ankle protrudes from the end of the table and is free to allow dorsal flexion and plantar flexion (Fig. 30.1).

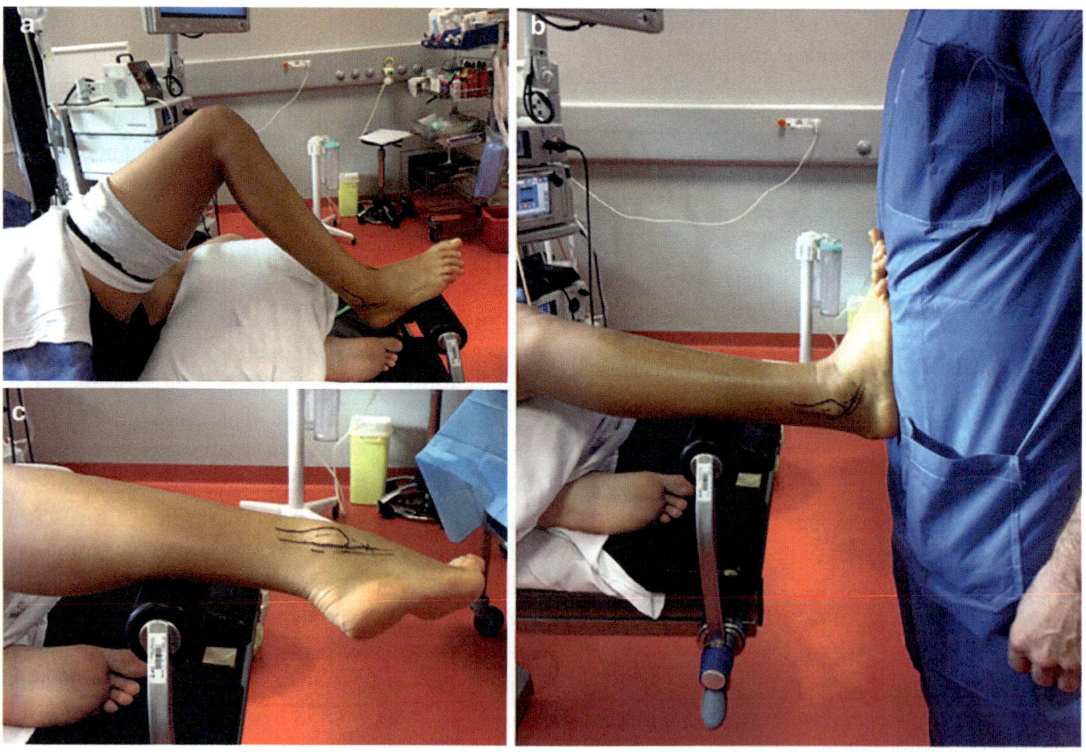

Fig. 30.1 (**a**) Position 1: Harvesting the graft. (**b**) Position 2: Anterior arthroscopy. (**c**) Position 3 Lateral endoscopy

30.3.3 Gracilis Harvest

Gracilis is collected and stored in physiological serum. The length of the graft should be approximately 12 cm (4 cm for LTFA transplant, 5 cm for LCF transplant, and 2–3 cm for fibular joint insertion). It is left free and a thread is snuck at each end.

30.3.4 Landmark Identification

Three portals are normally required to perform this procedure. The anteromedial approach is the first performed (Portal n° 1). The ankle should be placed in maximum dorsal flexion in order to have the most lateral route possible on the medial part of the anterior tibialis whose position is more medial in dorsiflexion than in plantar flexion. This way enables a larger working area and protects the cartilage when the ankle is dorsiflexed. The second approach is the equivalent of an accessory anterolateral approach, more lateral and more distal than the conventional anterolateral approach (Portal n° 2). This portal is not marked on the skin because it is performed by transillumination from portal 1 when the arthroscope is perfectly well positioned on the lateral gutter. This portal can be done using a needle to position it in the axis of the future talar tunnel (Fig. 30.2).

The portal n° 3, or tarsal sinus portal, is performed at the intersection of two lines. The first line corresponds to the upper edge of the peroneus brevis. The second line corresponds to the axis of the malleolar tunnel, oriented approximately 10° in relation to the long axis of the fibula (Fig. 30.3). This lateral approach makes it possible to leave the joint and to have a complete endoscopic vision of the lateral ligament complex.

30.3.5 Step 1: Arthroscopic Exploration of the Ankle and Ligament Balance

The arthroscope is placed in the anteromedial portal (P1). It is important to do it in dorsiflexion and on the medial edge of the tibialis anterior. The correct positioning of this portal allows a perfect view of the lateral gutter. Transillumination makes it possible to perform the anterolateral portal (P2). Using a needle, the anterolateral approach is placed in the axis of the future talar tunnel, so it is more distal than the anterolateral anteroposterior ankle arthroscopy. The dissection begins with the shaver and always follows the same plan. We begin by resecting the nearly constant anterolateral conflict tissue to visualize the lower part of the anterior tibio-fibular ligament (AITFL or Basset ligament). The most distal fibers are then followed until their malleolar insertion. The malleolar insertion zone of the ATFL is located just below the malleolar insertion of the AITFL and is easily visualized. The talus insertion zone of the ATFL can then be easily visualized. Residual ATFL resection and insertion zone preparation is done with the shaver.

30.3.6 Step 2: Calcaneal and Malleolar Tunnel

The patient is placed in lateral decubitus. The arthroscope is positioned in portal 2 for better vision of the lateral gutter. The arthroscopic dissection of the lateral side of the hind foot is carried out from de lateral gutter to the footprint of the CFL. An Halstead forceps is introduced through portal 3 toward the malleolus to prepare the working area. A shaver is then introduced by this route to continue the dissection. The arthroscope, introduced by portal 2, is positioned in the lateral groove to visualize the malleolus and the lateral surface of the talus (Fig. 30.4). The dissection should continue to the lower side of the lateral side of the slope from top to bottom. The anatomical landmarks are the subtalar line spacing and the fibular tendons outside and distally. The residual CFL is then easily visualized because it crosses the fibular tendons. The CFL fibers must be followed until it is calcaneal (Fig. 30.5). A guidewire is then placed through portal 3 at the calcaneal footprint insertion of the CFL. This pin is directed medially, back and distal so as to emerge at the posteromedial side of the heel. A cannulated drill of 5 or 6 mm is then

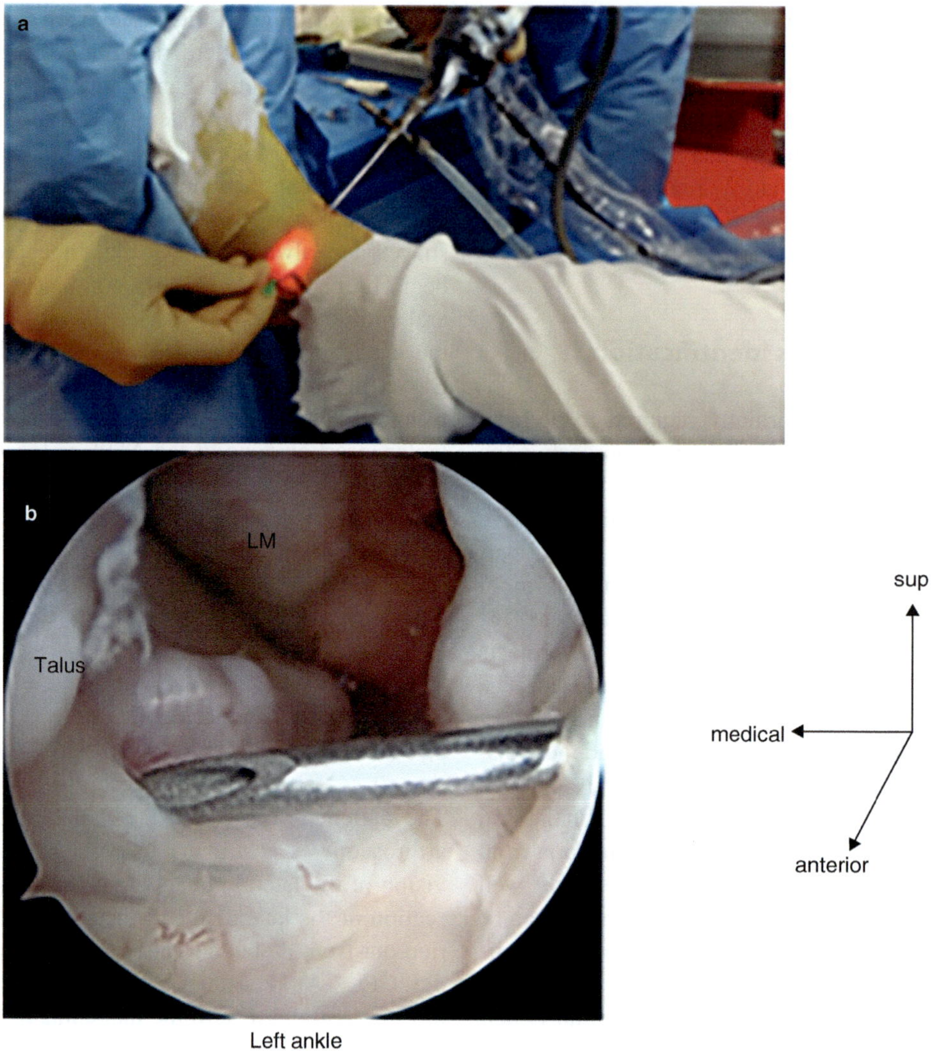

Fig. 30.2 (**a**) External view of **b**. (**b**) positioning of the first portal n° 2. It must be directed to the future tallar tunnel. *LM* lateral malleolus

passed over this pin to achieve a complete calcaneal tunnel. A lead suture is then introduced into the tunnel.

The dissection is then carried on the tip of the malleolus. The tunnel at this level must be positioned between the insertion of ATFL and that CFL. This spot is marked by a small ridge called the obscure tubercle [15], which marks the slight change in orientation of the anterior cortex of the malleolus (Fig. 30.6). This zone is quite distal and is visible only if the arthroscope is in portal 2; it is not well visualized if the arthroscope is in portal 1 and the risk is to do the malleolar tunnel too proximal. A guidewire is then introduced at this level through portal 3 and directed up and back with respect to the axis of the fibula and slightly outside. To ensure the correct positioning of this pin, it may be necessary to make a small concave mark using a cutter. Moreover, if the passage of the pin in the malleolus is done without arthroscopic control, it is useful to draw the cutaneous contour of the malleolus and the direction of the tunnel because it facilitates this step. A 4.5 mm cannulated drill is then passed from one cortex to the other by performing a posterior counter-pressure to protect the fibular tendons. A

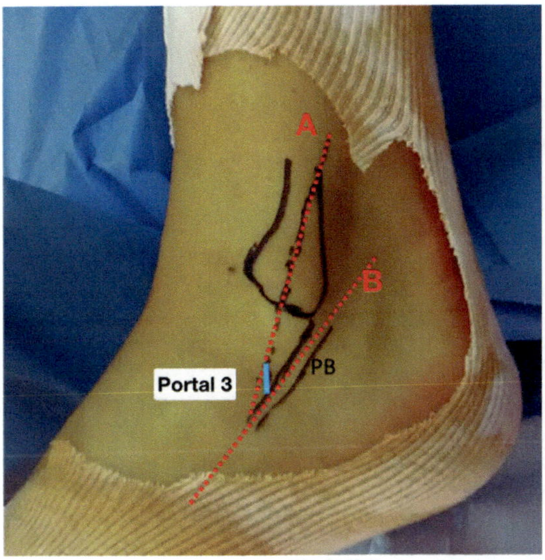

Fig. 30.3 Portal n° 3: One line passes through the upper edge of the peroneus brevis (line A) and another through the axis of the malleolar tunnel (line B)

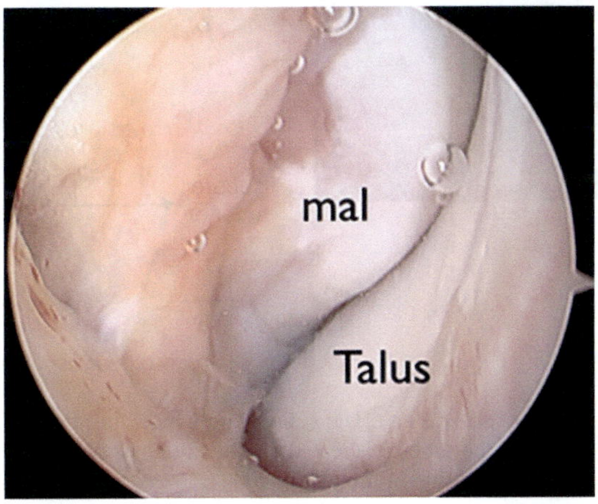

Fig. 30.4 View of the lateral gutter. The beginning of the arthroscopic dissection of the lateral side is clearing the anterior aspect of the malleolus bone from superior to inferior

6-mm drill then is passed in the first 15 mm of the tunnel in order to enable to adjust the tension of the transplants at the end of the procedure.

30.3.7 Step 3: Talar Tunnel

The talar tunnel is made through portal 2 with the arthroscope placed in either portal 1 or portal 3 according to the surgeon's preference and the quality of the visualization. The talus insertion zone of the ATFL is located on the supero-lateral rim of the talar neck just below a triangular zone without cartilage on the lateral edge of the anterior portion of the dome of the talus (Fig. 30.7). A pin is placed through portal 2 directed toward the center of the body of the talus to avoid any break either in the upper cortex of the neck of the talus or in the sinus of the tarsus [16]. A 5- or 6-mm cannulated drill is positioned to make a blind 2 cm tunnel.

30.3.8 Step 4: Fixing the Graft

All fixation will be made via portal 2. For that, it is needed to bring the two shuttle relay sutures from the calcaneal and the malleolar tunnel through portal 2. The graft is introduced into the talar tunnel via portal 2 (Fig. 30.8) using the bio tenodesis screw® (Arthrex, Munich). Its fixation is ensured by an interference screw of 5.5 mm, controlled by arthroscopy.

The preparation of the graft is then finished. Three marks are made: one at 1.5 cm from de talar tunnel, another one at 2 cm from the other mark, and a last one at 4.5 cm of the previous one. The tendon is sutured to itself at the end of the graft with a pulling suture.

An endobutton is then passed through the malleolar tunnel via portal 2 using the shuttle relay suture and is placed on the posterior cortical of the malleolus under direct visual control. The graft is then passed into the loop of the endobutton, and by pulling to close the loop, the endobutton is positioned between the two marks. The arthroscope is now placed in portal 3 to confirm the absence of tissue interposition. The loop of the endobutton is gradually closed to position the graft at the entrance of the malleolar tunnel (Fig. 30.9). During this maneuver, the graft is tensioned at its exit from the calcaneal tunnel, and the ankle is held in a neutral position at 90° dorsiflexion angle. The position of the graft at the entrance of the malleolar tunnel must be well controlled since tensioning may have removed it from the malleolar tunnel; it is therefore essen-

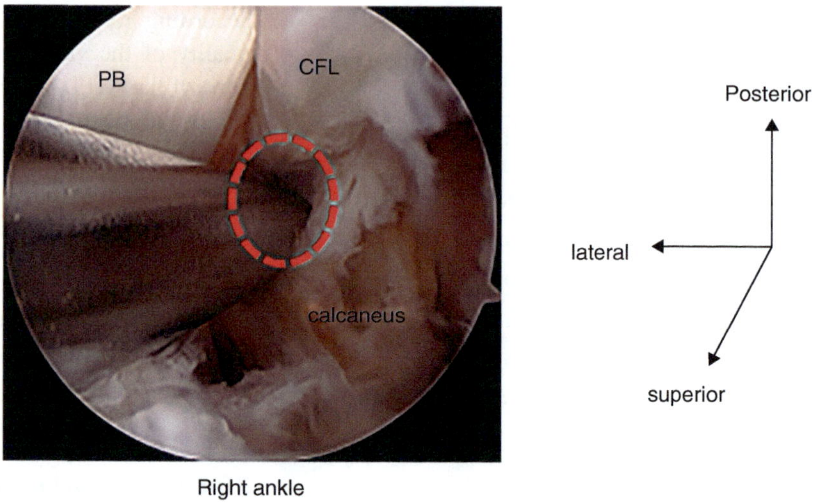

Fig. 30.5 Arthroscopic view of calcaneal CFL footprint materialized by a red circle. The arthroscope introduced by portal n° 2 looking down and down showing the space between the peroneus brevis (PB) on the left and the calcaneus on the right

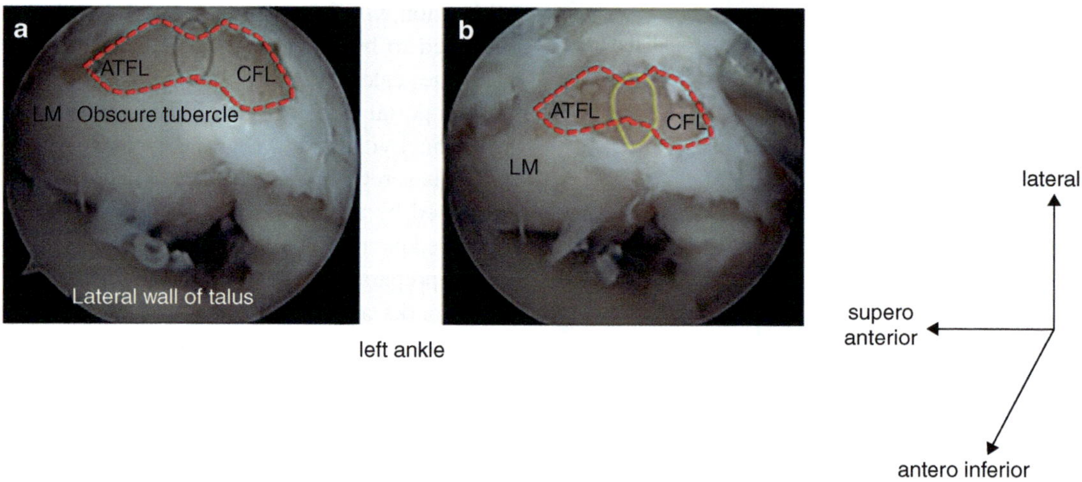

Fig. 30.6 Vision of malleolar footprint. Arthroscopic view from portal n° 2. Red lines indicate insertion of ATFL and CFL. The grey circle indicates the location of the dark tubercle (A). The yellow circle indicates the concavity at the tubercle created by the cutter to secure the insertion location of the guided pin (B)

tial, before perform the calcaneal fixation, to reposition the graft well at the entrance of the malleolar tunnel.

30.3.9 Step 5: Calcaneal Fixation and Tensioning of the Graft

The calcaneal fixation is provided by an interference screw (often oversized with respect to the tunnel diameter due to the porosity of the calcaneus bone). The screw is put in place by the portal 3 while keeping the graft in tension. The arthroscope is positioned in portal 2 and controls both the correct insertion of the screw (to avoid any conflict with the fibular) and the maintenance of the good position of the transplant at the entrance of the malleolar tunnel (Fig. 30.10).

After calcaneal fixation, the graft can be tensioned by pulling on the endobutton wire. The transplant thus enters the malleolar tunnel and carries out the tensioning of the ATFL and the CFL graft limbs. The tensioning must be carried out with the ankle in neutral position. The adjustment of the graft tension is the final step. Therefore, it is important to avoid complete

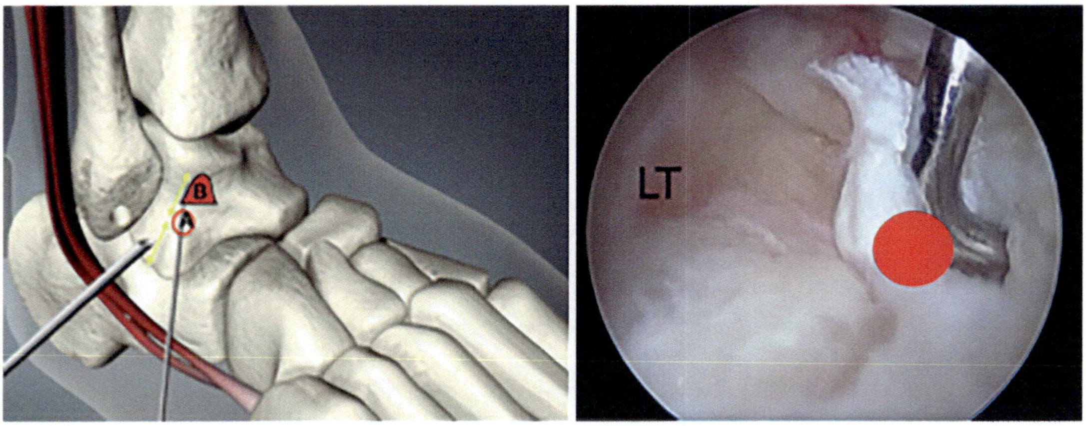

Fig. 30.7 Placement of the talar tunnel (B). Just below the area without cartilage (A) and mid distance from the height of the lateral articular surface. The red spot indicates the placement of the tunnel. *LT* lateral side of the talus

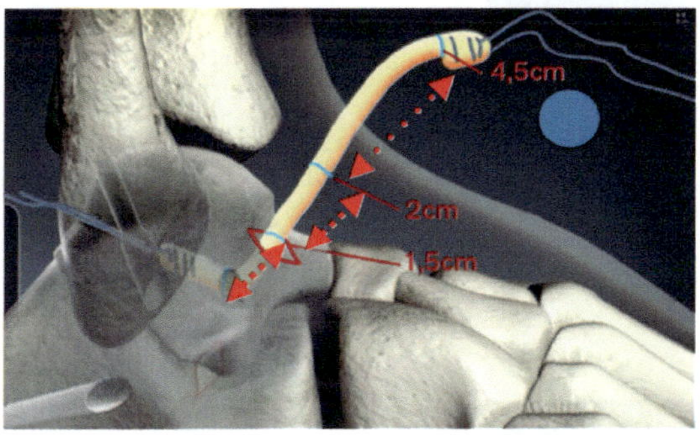

Fig. 30.8 The graft is prepared after being fixed at the level of the talar tunnel. It is marked at the level of its different zones: 1.5 cm for the ATFL, 2 cm for the malleolus, and 4.5 cm for the CFL

insertion of the graft into the malleolar tunnel before the calcaneal fixation in order to prevent lack of space available for final tensioning that can compromise the functional result (Fig. 30.11).

30.4 Technical Option for Making the Calcaneal Tunnel with a Percutaneous Technique

R Lopes (Ref Lopes R, Decante C, Geffroy L, Brulefert K, Noailles T. Arthroscopic anatomical reconstruction of the lateral ankle ligaments: A technical simplification. Orthop Traumatol Surg Res 2016;102:S317–S22.) has described a simplified variant involving percutaneous creation of the calcaneal tunnel for the distal attachment of the calcaneo-fibular ligament. The rationale for this technical stratagem was provided by a preliminary cadaver study that demonstrated a correlation between the lateral malleolus and the distal footprint of the calcaneo-fibular ligament. The Skin incision is made 1 cm inferiorly and posteriorly to the malleolus (Fig. 30.12). After a nick and spread technique to reach the contact with the bone, a key wire is positioned, and the calcaneal tunnel is made (Fig. 30.13).

30.5 Accessory Portal: Tendinoscopy

Some patients with CAI also have fibular tendons tendinopathy with or without rupture. Tendinoscopy allows visualization and can be useful in these cases. It is then necessary to do a fourth portal. This approach is performed after step # 2. The incision is located opposite the fibular tendons 1–2 cm more proximal than the tip of the malleolus. After the skin incision, it is important to expose the upper retinaculum. A longitudinal incision is then performed, and the access to the peroneal tendon is done with the aid of a Halstead clamp. The arthroscope is then introduced from proximal to distal. The two tendons are visualized as well as a small septum which marks the beginning of the proper tunnels of the

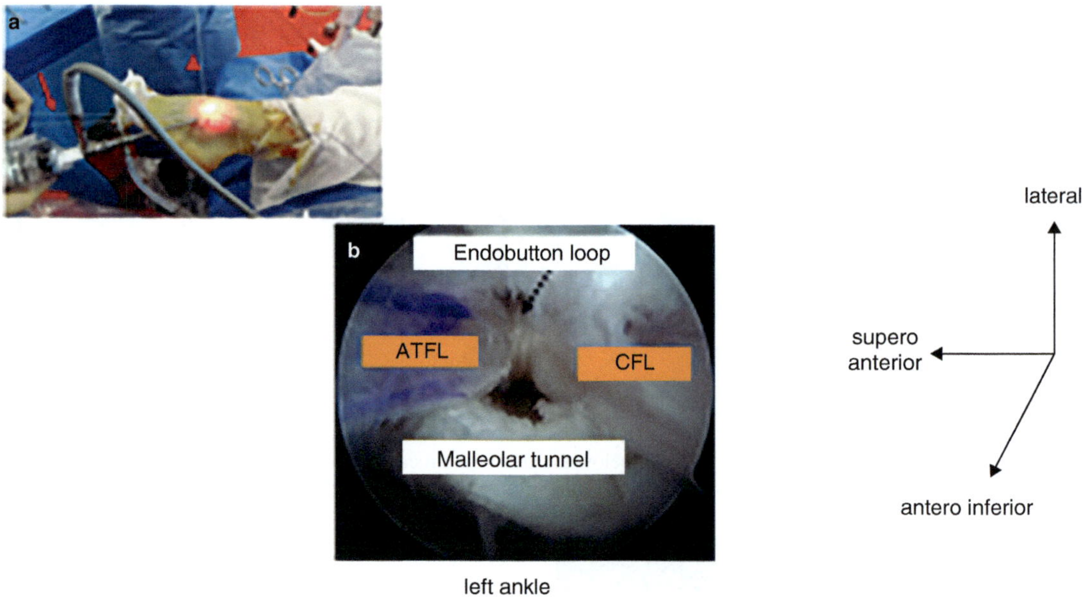

Fig. 30.9 The large arrow indicates the endobutton wires that will be used to push the graft into the malleolar tunnel. The triangle indicates the thread that has temporarily passed around the talar limb graft. Traction on this wire will increase the length of the ATFL graft. Before placing the calcaneal screw, it is important to check under arthroscopy the tension of the ATFL limb graft and the good malleolar introduction of the graft

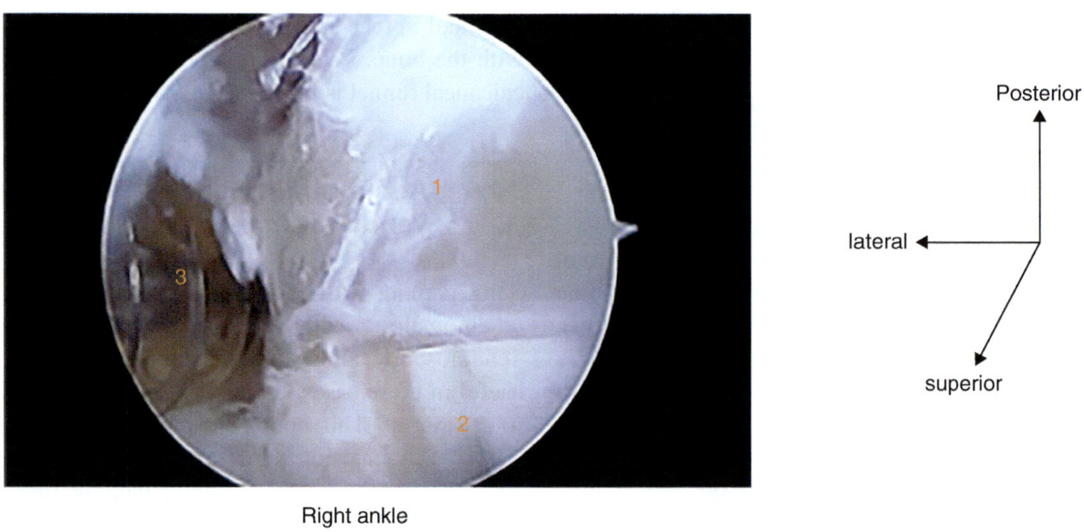

Fig. 30.10 Screw in the calcaneal tunnel; 1, CFL; 2, Sub Talar Joint; 3, Screw

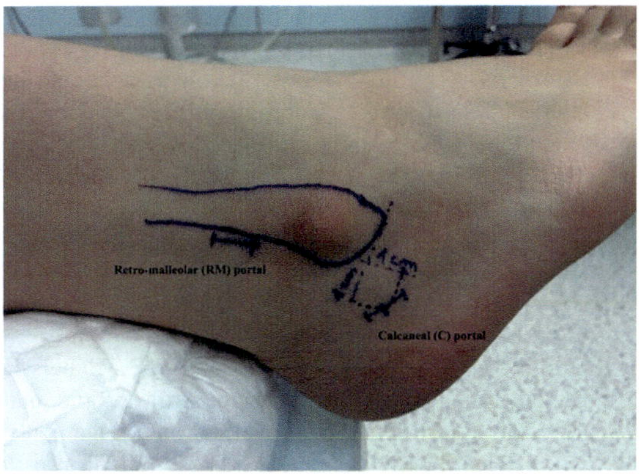

Fig. 30.11 Final aspect

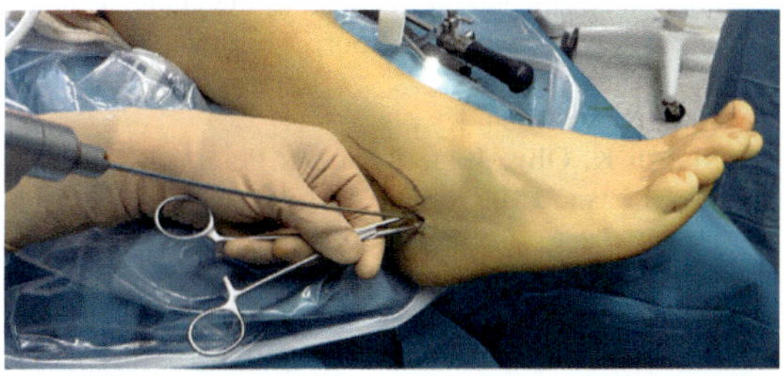

Fig. 30.12 Preparation of the landmark for the percutaneous calcaneal tunnel

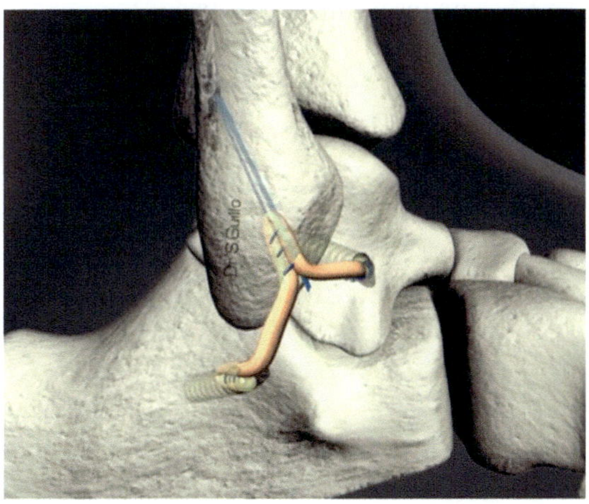

Fig. 30.13 Direction of the eyelet and the drill for making the calcaneal tunnel

short and the long fibular. Just before this septum, above the short fibular, we find the entrance of the tarsal sinus and more proximal the CFL footprint. The dissection can begin in the tarsal sinus and thus expose the CFL, the subtalar joint, as well as a possible fibular tendinopathy.

30.6 Post-operative Care

The intervention can be performed on an outpatient basis. Patients are immobilized in a removable ankle splint for 4–6 weeks. During the first 15 days, partial weight bearing, elevation, and icing of the ankle are recommended to fight edema and inflammatory phenomena. Rehabilitation is gradually started from the second week. The resumption of the sport can be considered at the 12th week and the competition at the 6th month.

30.7 Conclusion

Arthroscopic anatomical reconstruction of the lateral collateral ligament of the ankle using a gracilis tendon is a reliable technique [14]. This technique is indicated in cases of ligament deficiency prohibiting repair by Bröstöm Gould. Lateral endoscopy of the ankle allows for complete and reliable dissection of ATFL as well as CFL. It is then possible to perform an anatomical reconstruction of these two ligaments with probably more precise anatomical positioning than in the open techniques. The description of this five-step technique makes it reproducible. However, this arthroscopic technique has a learning curve (essentially related to the recognition of anatomical landmarks) quite short, but justifying learning about anatomical landmarks before taking care of patients. The development of auxiliary and specific implants will simplify and secure the technique. Multicentric clinical studies shows reproducibility and absence of morbidity of this technique and thus better define the place of arthroscopic anatomic ligamentoplasty of the ankle.

References

1. Garrick JG. The frequency of injury, mechanism of injury, and epidemiology of ankle sprains. Am J Sports Med. 1977;5(6):241–2.
2. Guillo S, Bauer T, Lee JW, Takao M, Kong SW, Stone JW, Mangone PG, Molloy A, Perera A, Pearce CJ, Michels F, Tourne Y, Ghorbani A, Calder J. Consensus in chronic ankle instability: aetiology, assessment, sur-

gical indications and place for arthroscopy. Orthopaed Traumatol Surg Res. 2013;99(8 Suppl):S411–9. https://doi.org/10.1016/j.otsr.2013.10.009.
3. Girard P, Anderson RB, Davis WH, Isear JA, Kiebzak GM. Clinical evaluation of the modified Brostrom-Evans procedure to restore ankle stability. Foot Ankle Int. 1999;20(4):246–52.
4. Karlsson J, Bergsten T, Lansinger O, Peterson L. Reconstruction of the lateral ligaments of the ankle for chronic lateral instability. J Bone Joint Surg Am. 1988;70(4):581–8.
5. Karlsson J, Lansinger O. Chronic lateral instability of the ankle in athletes. Sports Med. 1993;16(5):355–65.
6. Bahr R, Pena F, Shine J, Lew WD, Tyrdal S, Engebretsen L. Biomechanics of ankle ligament reconstruction. An in vitro comparison of the Brostrom repair, Watson-Jones reconstruction, and a new anatomic reconstruction technique. Am J Sports Med. 1997;25(4):424–32.
7. Becker HP, Ebner S, Ebner D, Benesch S, Frossler H, Hayes A, Gritze G, Rosenbaum D. 12-year outcome after modified Watson-Jones tenodesis for ankle instability. Clin Orthop Relat Res. 1999;358:194–204.
8. Colville MR, Marder RA, Zarins B. Reconstruction of the lateral ankle ligaments. A biomechanical analysis. Am J Sports Med. 1992;20(5):594–600.
9. Rosenbaum D, Becker HP, Sterk J, Gerngross H, Claes L. Functional evaluation of the 10-year outcome after modified Evans repair for chronic ankle instability. Foot Ankle Int. 1997;18(12):765–71.
10. Rosenbaum D, Becker HP, Wilke HJ, Claes LE. Tenodeses destroy the kinematic coupling of the ankle joint complex. A three-dimensional in vitro analysis of joint movement. J Bone Joint Surg. 1998;80(1):162–8.
11. Sammarco GJ, Idusuyi OB. Reconstruction of the lateral ankle ligaments using a split peroneus brevis tendon graft. Foot Ankle Int. 1999;20(2):97–103.
12. Takao M, Oae K, Uchio Y, Ochi M, Yamamoto H. Anatomical reconstruction of the lateral ligaments of the ankle with a gracilis autograft: a new technique using an interference fit anchoring system. Am J Sports Med. 2005;33(6):814–23. https://doi.org/10.1177/0363546504272688.
13. Guillo S, Takao M, Calder J, Karlson J, Michels F, Bauer T, Ankle Instability Group. Arthroscopic anatomical reconstruction of the lateral ankle ligaments. Knee Surg Sports Traumatol Arthrosc. 2015; https://doi.org/10.1007/s00167-015-3789-z.
14. Thes A, Klouche S, Ferrand M, Hardy P, Bauer T. Assessment of the feasibility of arthroscopic visualization of the lateral ligament of the ankle: a cadaveric study. Knee Surg Sports Traumatol Arthrosc. 2016;24(4):985–90. https://doi.org/10.1007/s00167-015-3804-4.
15. Matsui K, Oliva XM, Takao M, Pereira BS, Gomes TM, Lozano JM, Group EAAI, Glazebrook M. Bony landmarks available for minimally invasive lateral ankle stabilization surgery: a cadaveric anatomical study. Knee Surg Sports Traumatol Arthrosc. 2016; https://doi.org/10.1007/s00167-016-4218-7.
16. Michels F, Guillo S, Vanrietvelde F, Brugman E, Ankle Instability Group, Stockmans F. How to drill the talar tunnel in ATFL reconstruction? Knee Surg Sports Traumatol Arthrosc. 2016;24(4):991–7. https://doi.org/10.1007/s00167-016-4018-0.

31 Arthroscopic AntiRoLL Technique

Masato Takao and Mark Glazebrook

AntiRoLL is the word made by Dr. Glazebrook, aligning underlined parts of the phrase "Anatomical Reconstruction of the Lateral Ligament of the ankle" [1]. There are two types of AntiRoLL, arthroscopic (A-AntiRoLL) [1] and percutaneous [2] (P-AntiRoLL, see Chap. 17). In this chapter, we would like to describe A-AntiRoLL.

31.1 Indication

Choice of a surgical procedure is performed by evaluating the quality of the residual ligament with stress ultrasonography before surgery, and determined with arthroscopic evaluation during surgery (see Chap. 26). A-AntiRoLL is selected if there is no ligament fiber, and intra-articular co-morbid lesions including osteochondral lesions and/or anterior ankle impingement were clarified preoperatively. If there were no intra-articular lesions, it may be better to perform P-AntiRoLL which is a simpler technique than A-AntiRoLL (see Chap. 17).

M. Takao (✉)
Clinical and Research Institute for Foot and Ankle Surgery, Jujo Hospital, Chiba, Japan
e-mail: m.takao@carifas.com

M. Glazebrook
Department of Orthopaedic Surgery, Dalhousie University, Halifax, NS, Canada

There are four steps for AntiRoLL: step 1 as make the portals; step 2 as make a Y-shaped graft; step 3 as make the bone tunnels at each attachment to fibula, talus, and calcaneus; step 4 as introduce a Y-shaped graft into the bone tunnels and fix with the interference screw.

31.2 Surgical Procedure

31.2.1 Position

The position is supine, and the lower leg is held with a leg holder (see Chap. 26). The tourniquet is not normally used, but it should be worn on the thigh for use when the field of vision is hindered by bleeding.

31.2.2 Step 1: Make Portals

Medial midline (MML) portal, accessary anterolateral (AAL) portal, and subtalar portal (ST) are used (Fig. 31.1). If it is needed to treat the intra-articular lesions, we add anterolateral (AL) portal.

31.2.3 Step 2: Make a Y-shaped Graft

An autologous gracilis tendon is harvested from ipsilateral knee (Fig. 31.2a). Marking is done nine times every 15 mm, resulting 135 mm length

H. Pereira et al. (eds.), *Lateral Ankle Instability*, https://doi.org/10.1007/978-3-662-62763-1_31

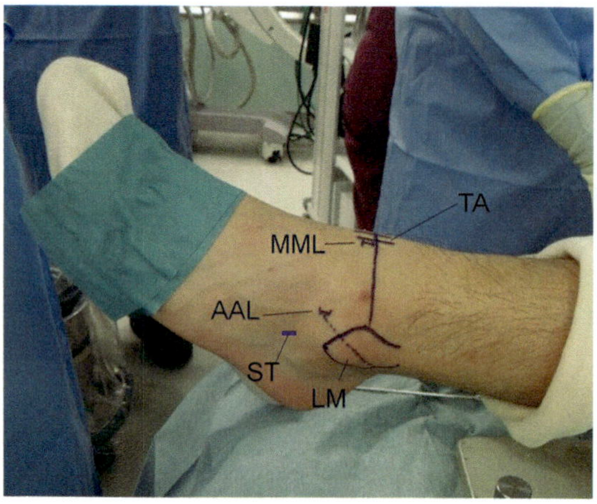

Fig. 31.1 Portals. *MML* medial midline portal, *AAL* accessary anterolateral portal, *ST* subtalar portal

tendon should be needed as a tendon graft (Fig. 31.2b). Next fold back at the site 60 mm from the end, pass the guide thread through this fold, and then suture the tendons with the 3-0 bio-absorbable thread at the position 15 mm from the turning point (Fig. 31.2c). Finally fold back at 15 mm from both ends, pass guide thread through folded back, and then suture the tendons with 3-0 bio-absorbable thread (Fig. 31.2d). The short leg of the Y-shaped tendon graft is ATFL and the long leg is CFL (Fig. 31.2e).

31.2.4 Step 3: Make the Bone Tunnels at Each Attachment to Fibula, Talus, and Calcaneus

Positioning of each fibular, talar, and calcaneal bone tunnels is made by using the landmarks existing on the bone surface as shown in Fig. 31.3a [3].

In making a fibular bone tunnel, a viewing portal is MML and a working portal is ST (Fig. 31.3b). A landmark for fibular bone tunnel is fibular obscure tubercle (FOT) which exists at the border of the foot prints of the ATFL and the CFL (Fig. 31.3c). After to show an FOT to remove a part of remnant of ATFL using motorized shaver, a guide wire for cannulated drill is inserted via ST portal and penetrates the center of the fibula at FOT toward the direction of proximal-posterior fibular cortex as 30° to the axis of fibula, and finally penetrates the posterior leg skin (Fig. 31.3b). Next an overdrilling of 6 mm in diameter and 20 mm in depth is done using cannulated drill. Finally, a guide wire is replaced to guide thread (Fig. 31.3d).

In making a talar bone tunnel, a viewing portal is MML and a working portal is AAL (Fig. 31.3e). A landmark for talar bone tunnel is anterolateral and posterolateral corners of the talar body (Fig. 31.3a). On the line to connect the anterolateral and posterolateral corners of the talar body, about 40% inferior point from anterolateral corner of the talar body is the center of the footprint of the ATFL. But in actual cases, there remains a ligament fiber at the attachment of the ATFL to the talus in most cases, and it is a good landmark to make a talar bone tunnel. A guide wire for cannulated drill is inserted via AAL portal and penetrates the center of the footprint at talus (Fig. 31.3f) toward the direction to tip of the medial malleolus, and finally penetrates the skin. Next an overdrilling of 6 mm in diameter and 20 mm in depth is done using cannulated drill (Fig. 31.3e). Finally, a guide wire is replaced to guide thread.

In making a calcaneal bone tunnel, a viewing portal is ST and a working portal is AAL (Fig. 31.3g). A landmark for calcaneal bone tunnel is posterior facet of the talocalcaneal joint (Fig. 31.3h). On the line perpendicular bisector of the posterior facet, 17 mm inferior point from posterior facet is the center of the footprint of the CFL. But in actual cases, peroneal tendons run just over the insertion of the CFL. To avoid the damage to the peroneal tendons, the authors make a calcaneal bone tunnel proximal to the peroneal tendon sheath, about 10 mm inferior point from posterior facet (Fig. 31.3a). A guide wire for cannulated drill is inserted via AAL portal and penetrates the calcaneus as the direction of center of the posterior corner of the calcaneus, and finally penetrates the posterior heel skin (Fig. 31.3g). Next an overdrilling of 6 mm in diameter and 20 mm in depth is done using cannulated drill. Finally, a guide wire is replaced to guide thread.

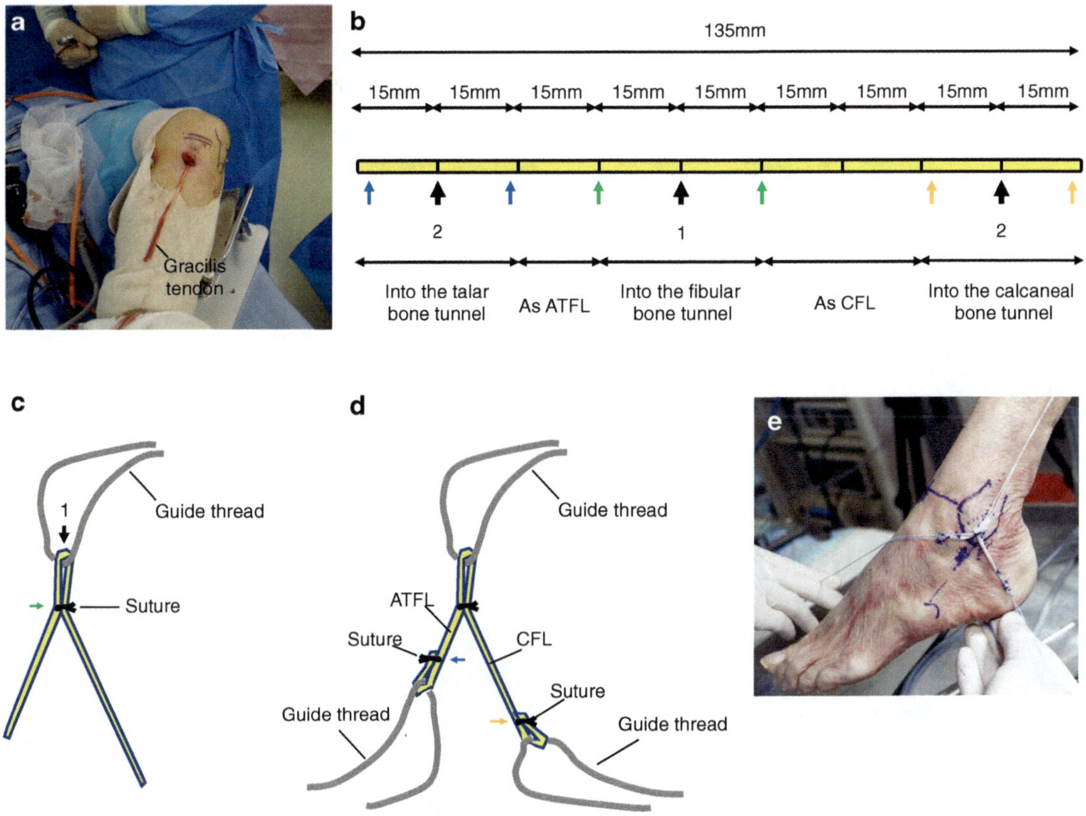

Fig. 31.2 Make a Y-shaped graft. (**a**) An autologous gracilis tendon is harvested from ipsilateral knee. (**b**) Marking on the harvested graft. Marking is done nine times every 15 mm, resulting 135 mm length tendon should be needed as a tendon graft. Black arrow: point to fold back, green arrow: marking suture for fibular bone tunnel, blue arrow: marking suture for talar bone tunnel, yellow arrow: marking suture for calcaneal bone tunnel. (**c**) At the site 60 mm from the end, pass the guide thread through this fold, and then suture the tendons with the 3-0 bio-absorbable thread at the position 15 mm from the turning point. (**d**) Fold back at 15 mm from both ends, pass guide thread through folded back, and then suture the tendons with 3-0 bio-absorbable thread. (**e**) The short leg of the Y-shaped tendon graft is ATFL and the long leg is CFL

In this time, a guide thread of the fibular bone tunnel is inserted via ST portal. This thread is grasped by forceps via AAL portal inside the joint, and introduced to the AAL portal. Accordingly, all guide threads are inserted via AAL portal.

31.2.5 Step 4: Introduce a Y-Shaped Graft into the Bone Tunnels and Fix with the Interference Screw

A Y-shaped graft is introduced and fixed into the bone tunnels firstly fibula, next talus, and finally calcaneus. It is important to insert a guide wire for interference screw before introducing a graft into the bone tunnels to prevent to penetrate the graft by a guide wire following graft damage by an interference screw.

Viewing a fibular bone tunnel via MML portal, a fibular end of a Y-shaped graft is introduced into the fibular bone tunnel using guide thread with inside-out technique at the level of the suture which ties the graft at the position 15 mm from the turning point (Fig. 31.4a, b). A graft is fixed into the bone tunnel with an interference screw 6 mm in diameter and 15 or 20 mm in length (Fig. 31.4c, d).

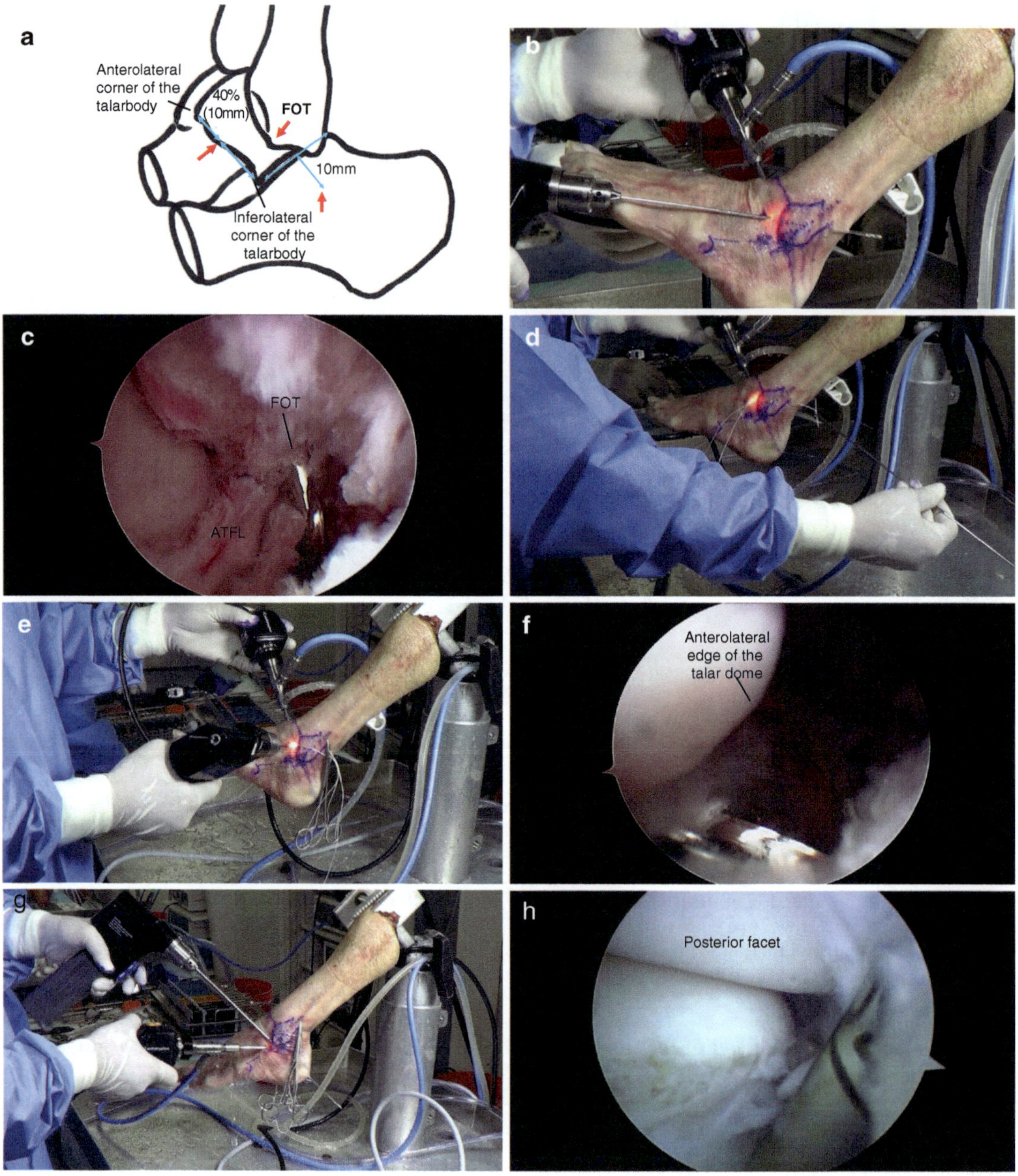

Fig. 31.3 Make the bone tunnels at each attachment to fibula, talus, and calcaneus. (**a**) Landmarks for each bone tunnels. A landmark for fibular bone tunnel is fibular obscure tubercle (FOT) which exists at the border of the foot prints of the ATFL and the CFL. For talar bone tunnel, on the line to connect the anterolateral and posterolateral corners of the talar body, about 40% inferior point from anterolateral corner of the talar body is the center of the footprint of the ATFL. For calcaneal bone tunnel, on the line perpendicular bisector of the posterior facet, 10 mm inferior point from posterior facet should be a landmark for calcaneal bone tunnel to avoid the damage to the peroneal tendons. (**b**) In making a fibular bone tunnel, a viewing portal is MML and a working portal is ST. (**c**) Arthroscopic view of the fibular obscure tubercle (FOT). (**d**) After an overdrilling of 6 mm in diameter and 20 mm in depth is done using cannulated drill, a guide wire is replaced to guide thread. (**e**) In making a talar bone tunnel, a viewing portal is MML and a working portal is AAL. (**f**) Arthroscopic view of the remaining ligament fiber at the attachment of the ATFL to the talus. (**g**) In making a calcaneal bone tunnel, a viewing portal is ST and a working portal is AAL. (**h**) For calcaneal bone tunnel, on the line perpendicular bisector of the posterior facet, 10 mm inferior point from posterior facet is the point to make a bone tunnel

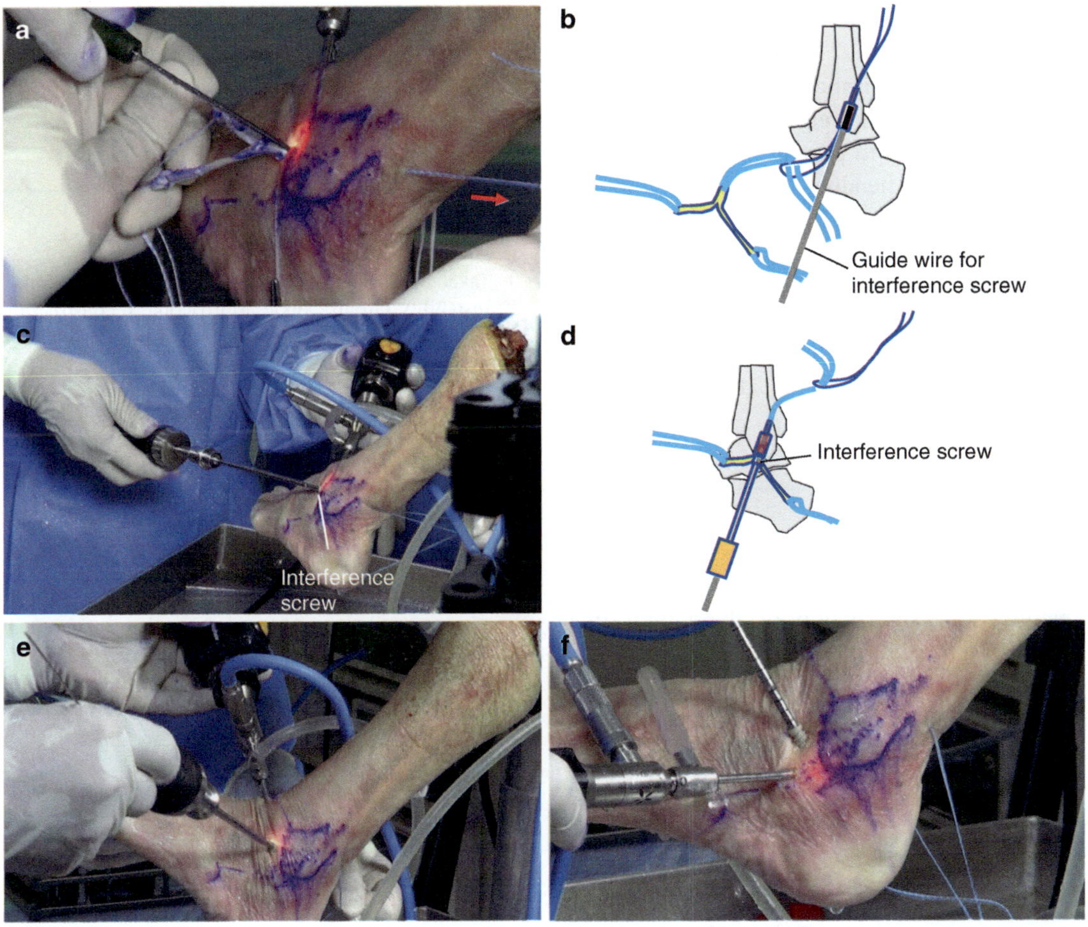

Fig. 31.4 Introduction of a Y-shaped graft into the bone tunnels and fixation with the interference screw. (**a**, **b**) Viewing a fibular bone tunnel via MML portal, a fibular end of a Y-shaped graft is introduced into the fibular bone tunnel using guide thread with inside-out technique at the level of the suture which ties the graft at the position 15 mm from the turning point. (**c**, **d**) Fixation of a graft into the bone tunnel with an interference screw of 6 mm in diameter and 15 or 20 mm in length. (**e**, **f**) Fixation of a graft into talar (**e**) and calcaneal (**f**) bone tunnel. As ankle is positioned in 0° neutral position and to tension the tendon graft by manually pulling a guide thread, a graft is fixed into the bone tunnel with an interference screw of 6 mm in diameter and 15 or 20 mm in length

Viewing a talar bone tunnel via MML portal, a talar end of a Y-shaped graft is introduced into the talar bone tunnel using guide thread with inside-out technique at the level of the suture which ties the graft at the position 15 mm from the turning point. As ankle positioned in 0° neutral position and to tensile the tendon graft pulling a guide thread manually, a graft is fixed into the bone tunnel with an interference screw 6 mm in diameter and 15 or 20 mm in length (Fig. 31.4e).

Viewing a calcaneal bone tunnel via ST portal, a calcaneal end of a Y-shaped graft is introduced into the calcaneal bone tunnel using guide thread with inside-out technique at the level of the suture which ties the graft at the position 15 mm from the turning point. As ankle positioned in 0° neutral position and to tensile the tendon graft pulling a guide thread manually, a graft is fixed into the bone tunnel with an interference screw 6 mm in diameter and 15 or 20 mm in length (Fig. 31.4f).

All guide thread can be removed easily to cut the one end near the skin and pull the other end manually.

31.3 Postoperative Management

After surgery, the elastic bandage is applied for 2 days, and the full weight-bearing walking is allowed according to pain from a day after surgery. The bone tendon attachment gradually increases the strength of biological bonding and becomes nearly normal strength at 4 weeks postoperatively [4]. Accordingly, jogging and proprioceptive training will be from 4 weeks postoperatively and return to sports without external fixation shall be after 6–8 weeks postoperative.

31.4 Summary

Arthroscopic AntiRoLL (A-AntiRoLL) is an anatomical reconstruction of the lateral ligaments of the ankle performing all arthroscopically with minor invasion. The author recommends it for surgical treatment of lateral instability of the ankle if there is no ligament fiber and if there are intra-articular co-morbid lesions including osteochondral lesions and/or anterior ankle impingement.

References

1. Takao M, Glazebrook MA, Stone JW, Guillo S, Ankle Instability Group. Ankle arthroscopic reconstruction of lateral ligaments (Ankle Anti-ROLL). Arthrosc Tech. 2015;4:e595–600.
2. Glazebrook M, Stone J, Matsui K, Guillo S, Takao M, ESSKA-AFAS Ankle Instability Group. Percutaneous ankle reconstruction of lateral ligaments (Perc-Anti RoLL). Foot Ankle Int. 2016;37:659–64.
3. Matsui K, Oliva XM, Takao M, Pereira BS, Gomes TM, Lozano JM, ESSKA AFAS Ankle Instability Group, Glazebrook M. Bony landmarks available for minimally invasive lateral ankle stabilization surgery: a cadaveric anatomical study. Knee Surg Sports Traumatol Arthrosc. 2017;25:1916–24.
4. Rodeo SA, Arnoczky SP, Torzilli PA, Hidaka C, Warren RF. Tendon-healing in a bone tunnel. A biomechanical and histological study in the dog. J Bone Joint Surg Am. 1993;75:1795–803.

The Plantaris Tendon Option for Anatomical Reconstruction

32

Pedro Diniz, Diego Quintero, Lautaro Ezpeleta, Nasef Abdelatif, Jorge Batista, and Hélder Pereira

Fact Box

- In an anatomical study by van Sterkenburg et al., a plantaris tendon was identified in all specimens [1].
- Biomechanical strength of a quadrupled plantaris tendon is higher than a native anterior talofibular ligament or Broström repair [2–4].
- The location and integrity of the plantaris tendon can be checked with magnetic resonance imaging, or ultrasound [5].

32.1 Introduction

Anatomical reconstructions are the preferred option when ligament remnants are absent or of low quality [6, 7]. These reconstructive procedures require the use of a graft, with several options being described in the literature [8–10]. As with all grafting procedures, donor site morbidity should be considered [11], such as when a peroneal tendon is used, which may itself impair ankle function [12]. This has prompted a search for graft alternatives, including allografts, and autografts in locations other than the ankle.

The plantaris tendon is a viable option for lateral ligament reconstruction. It is locally accessible and has also been used for reconstruction of

P. Diniz (✉)
Department of Orthopaedic Surgery, Hospital de Sant'Ana, Parede, Portugal

Institute for Bioengineering and Biosciences, Instituto Superior Técnico, Universidade de Lisboa, Lisbon, Portugal

Fisiogaspar, Lisbon, Portugal

D. Quintero · L. Ezpeleta
Department of Applied Anatomy in Orthopedic Physiatry and Traumatology of the Museum of Morphological Sciences of the Chair of Normal Anatomy of the Faculty of Medical Sciences, Rosario University, Rosário, Argentina

N. Abdelatif
Orthopedic Reconstructive Foot & Ankle Surgery Unit, Cairo, Egypt

J. Batista
Clinical Department Club Atletico Boca Juniores, CAJB – Centro Artroscopico, Buenos Aires, Argentina

H. Pereira
Knee and Ankle Orthopaedic Department, Centro Hospitalar Póvoa de Varzim, Vila do Conde, Portugal

Ripoll y De Prado Sports Clinic: FIFA Medical Centre of Excellence, Murcia-Madrid, Spain

ICVS/3B's – PT Government Associate Laboratory, University of Minho, Braga/Guimarães, Portugal

H. Pereira et al. (eds.), *Lateral Ankle Instability*, https://doi.org/10.1007/978-3-662-62763-1_32

other anatomical structures, including the Achilles tendon [13, 14], peroneal tendon retinaculum [15], and long flexor tendons of the hand [16].

32.2 Anatomy

The plantaris muscle has a mean size of 1.5 × 10 cm and is located deep and medial to the lateral head of the gastrocnemius, and lateral to the popliteal vessels and tibial nerve [5]. The plantaris muscle is mainly a weak plantar flexor of the ankle, but also contributes to ankle inversion [17, 18].

The plantaris tendon runs between the gastrocnemius and soleus muscles (Fig. 32.1), in an distal and medial direction, running parallel to the Achilles tendon (Fig. 32.2) before inserting on the calcaneus or on the Achilles tendon itself [5]. Its mean length varies between 24.7 and 35 cm, and its width varies between 1.9 and 4.1 mm [5].

Some authors refer to the plantaris tendon as being absent in 7.7% [19] to 19.2% [20] of the population, but an anatomical study by van Sterkenburg et al. found that a plantaris tendon could be identified in all of the 107 lower extremities dissected, albeit subject to several anatomical variations [1]. In their study, 11 of the specimens had a plantaris tendon firmly attached to the Achilles tendon, but which when dissected proximally could always be individualized and traced back to the plantaris muscle. Overall, nine different insertion sites for the plantaris tendon could be identified.

In a classic study from Daseler and Anson, which involved the dissection of 750 limbs, the plantaris tendon insertion was categorized into four types: Type 1, a fan-shaped insertion into the medial aspect of the superior calcaneal tuberosity, next to the Achilles tendon; Type 2, a fan-shaped insertion, possibly extending to the retinaculum, 0.5–2.5 cm anterior to the adjacent margin of the Achilles tendon; Type 3, a large and wide insertion medial to the terminal portion of the Achilles tendon; and Type 4, in which the plantaris tendon inserts into directly into the medial edge of the Achilles tendon, clearly proximal to its distal insertion [21].

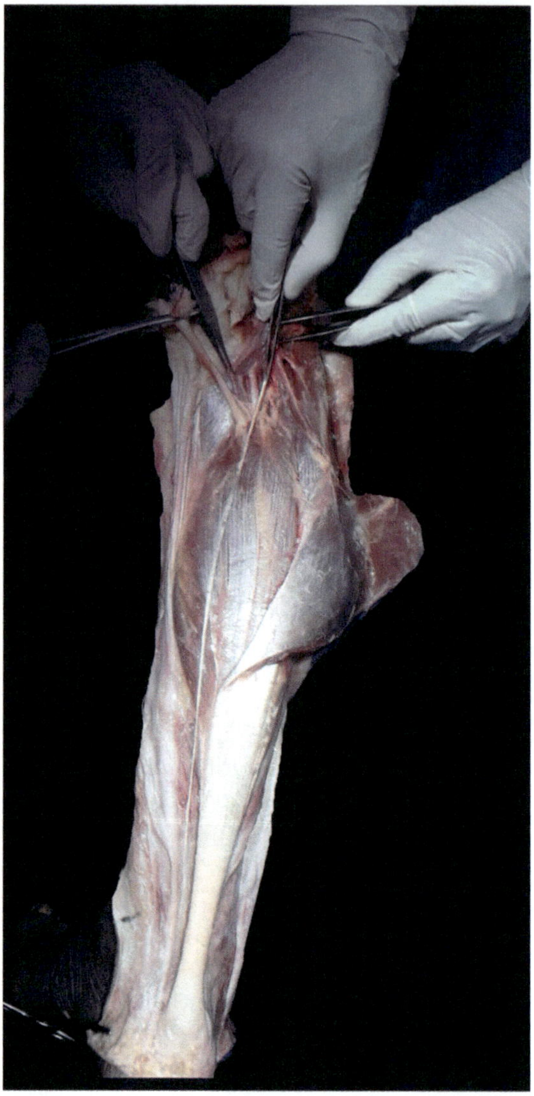

Fig. 32.1 Anatomical dissection of the entire length of the *plantaris tendon* (pointed by pincet)

32.3 Biomechanical Properties

The biomechanical properties of a double or quadrupled plantaris tendon construct were examined by Jackson et al. [2]. Thirty-five fresh-frozen human cadaver specimens, with a mean age of 66 (range: 43–89) years old, were used. All constructs had a minimum of 20 mm of functional length. Quadrupled constructs had a tensile strength of 205.8 ± 68.2 N and a stiffness of 133.1 ± 46.3 N/mm. Single strands had a tensile strength of 66.9 ± 26.3 N and a stiffness of 43.8 ± 14.7 N/mm.

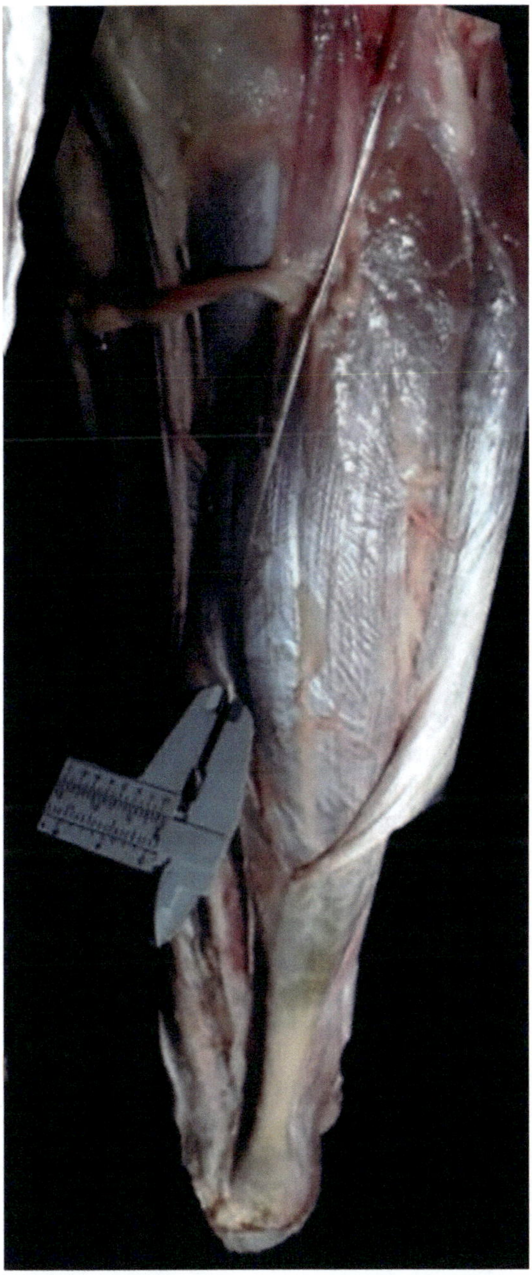

Fig. 32.2 Anatomical dissection and measurements of the *plantaris tendon*

The native anterior talofibular ligament (ATFL) tensile strength has a reported maximum load to failure of 138.9 ± 23.5 N [4, 22] to 160.9 ± 72.2 N [3]. The Broström repair has its time zero tensile strength rated at 68–79 N [3]. This supports the assumption that the plantaris tendon is well suited for anatomical reconstruction of the lateral ankle ligaments.

32.4 Surgical Technique

32.4.1 Indications

Lateral ligament reconstruction is indicated in patients in whom conservative treatment for chronic ankle instability has failed, and that have been deemed to have insufficient soft tissue quality to perform an anatomical repair technique.

32.4.2 Preoperative Planning

A thorough history collection and physical exam is required, with special attention to the presence of hyperlaxity, concurrent pathology, or limb alignment issues.

Surgeons should be cognizant of possible involvement of the plantaris tendon in patients with previous Achilles tendinopathy [18]. Magnetic resonance imaging, or ultrasound, can be used to assess location and status of the plantaris tendon preoperatively (Fig. 32.3) [5].

Patients should always be counseled before an ATFL repair that ligament remnants may be insufficient or unsuitable for repair, and that a reconstructive procedure may be required.

32.4.3 Harvest

Two approaches for harvesting are here presented. Plantaris tendon harvesting can also be performed with arthroscopic assistance (Figs. 32.4 and 32.5).

32.4.3.1 Proximal Harvest

A proximal harvest technique was described by Pangenstert et al. [9]. In this technique, a 2-cm longitudinal skin incision is made, 25–30 cm from the tip of the medial malleolus, in the medial side of the triceps surae muscle. Blunt dissection of the subcutaneous tissue is performed until the fascia is apparent, taking care not to injure the

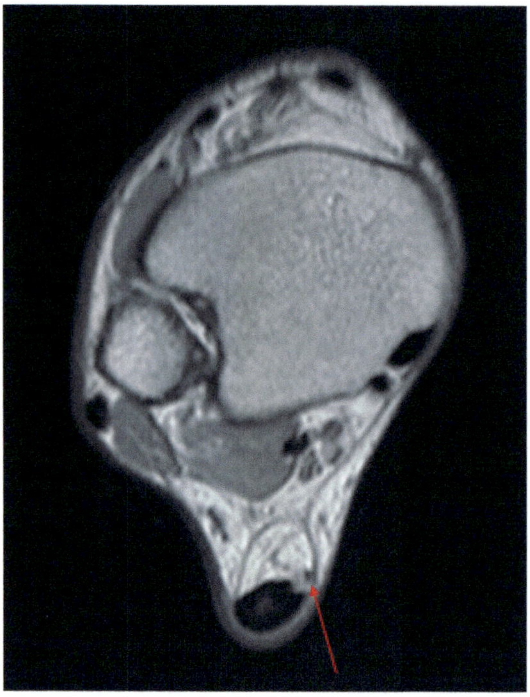

Fig. 32.3 MRI axial view of the *plantaris tendon* (red arrow)

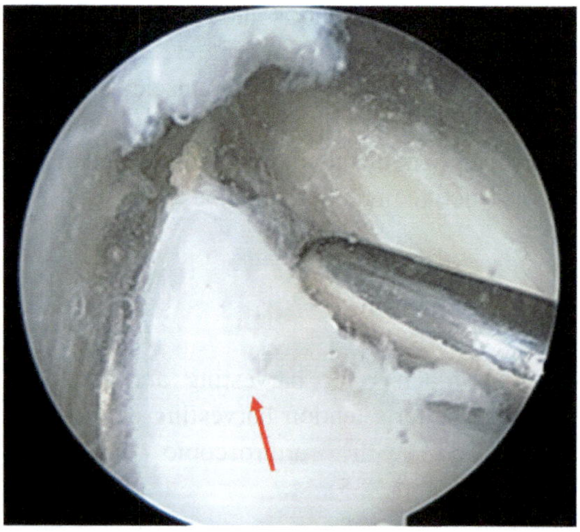

Fig. 32.4 Endoscopic view of the *plantaris tendon* separated from the *Achilles tendon* at its medial side

saphenous nerve and vein. The fascia is then incised longitudinally, and blunt dissection, with the finger, between the gastrocnemius and soleus muscles is performed. The plantaris tendon can then be palpated. The tendon is further individualized with the help of a finger or a nerve retractor. The tendon is fixed with a clamp, then cut and secured with a running locking stitch technique. A 4-mm blunt tendon stripper is then introduced and advanced while keeping the plantaris tendon under tension. At the level of the ankle joint, the stripper is rotated in a medial direction and the plantaris tendon is retrieved.

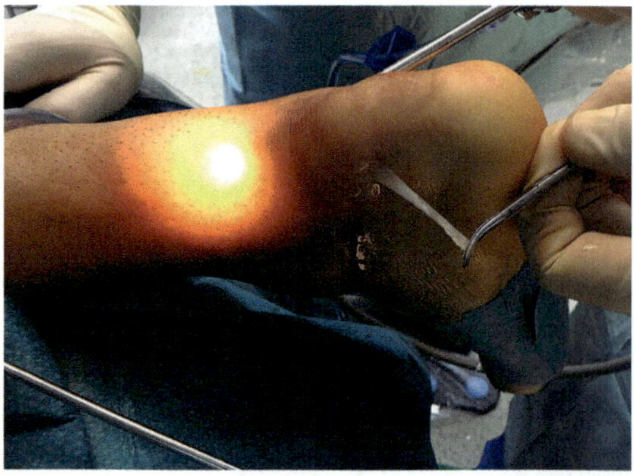

Fig. 32.5 Endoscopic harvesting of the *plantaris tendon*

32.4.3.2 Distal Harvest

A distal harvest technique was described by Jackson et al. [2]. Using this technique, the authors were able to harvest seven of nine tendon through a distal minimally invasive approach. The average length of the incision was 2.9 (2.5–3.5) cm. The plantaris tendon could be found in the two remaining specimens by extending the incision proximally.

In this technique, an incision is made on the posteromedial aspect of the calcaneus; the plantaris tendon is identified, and released from the insertion site. The tendon is secured with a running locking stitch, and then harvested using a 4.0-mm tendon stripper. In this series, the authors report a case of a graft that was significantly shorter due to the presence of unreleased attaching bands to the Achilles tendon, but which length was still adequate for a quadruple construct creation.

32.4.4 Anatomical Lateral Ligament Reconstruction

Several techniques of anatomical lateral ankle ligaments reconstruction using tendon grafts have been described and can be found elsewhere in this book. Herein we describe the technique of Hua et al. (Fig. 32.6) [8].

After arthroscopic ankle assessment, a straight skin incision is made from the tip of the distal fibula to the talar insertion of the ATFL. The tip of the fibula is exposed to show the fibular insertion of the ATFL and calcaneofibular (CFL) ligaments. At this level, a second straight longitudinal incision is made at the posterior aspect of the lateral malleolus.

Two tunnels are then drilled in an oblique direction, parallel to each other in a distal-anterior to proximal-posterior direction, using 3.5 mm drill, with anterior starting points at 7 and 13 mm from the tip of the fibula. Two more 3.5 mm tunnels are drilled, in a convergent direction, at the edge of the cartilage and 18 mm proximal do the subtalar joint, in the talus, near the ATFL attachment.

A third incision is made, below and parallel to the first incision, exposing the calcaneal tubercle, and a guide wire is introduced, exiting medially. A 6 mm reamer is used, for a 25 mm depth. One end of the graft is then introduced in the calcaneal tunnel and fixed with a 7-mm interference screw. The graft is then passed under the peroneal tendons, through the inferior tunnel in a posterior direction, through the superior tunnel in an anterior direction, and then through both tunnels in the talus.

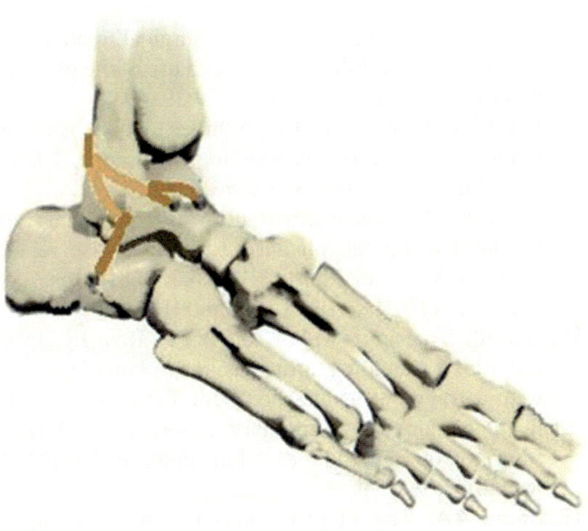

Fig. 32.6 ATFL and CFL reconstruction using the *plantaris tendon* graft as described by Hua et al. [8]

Full range of motion in the ankle is confirmed for 20 cycles, and tension in the graft is adjusted. The free end of the graft is then sutured to itself, with the ankle in neutral position. The capsule and skin incision are closed. The anterior drawer and talar tilt tests are performed for final confirmation. Sterile dressings and a posterior splint in the neutral position are applied.

32.5 Postoperative Care

Patients can be discharged on the same day, except if other procedures, such as osteotomies, have been performed on the same surgery and there are concerns about pain management.

First postoperative visit at 7–10 days for removal of sutures. These can be removed after 14–20 days if concerns about wound healing exist. The splint is removed, and the patient is placed on a short leg cast. Isometric exercises for muscles around the ankle are permitted since the day of surgery.

The cast is kept for the first 6 weeks, before being replaced by an ankle stirrup brace and passive range of motion exercises started. Weight bearing is allowed at 8 weeks after surgery. Sports activities with high strain are permitted after 3 months.

32.6 Outcomes

Hintermann and Rengli published a case series of 48 patients (52 ankles), with an average age of 28.6 (range: 16–46) years old. There were 30 ankles in men and 22 ankles in women. Fifty ankles were available for a final follow-up at an average of 3.5 (range: 1–10 years) years. Average

AOFAS was 97.9 (range: 90–100). The functional result was deemed excellent in 39 ankles (78%), good in 9 ankles (18%), fair in 2 ankles (4%), and poor in 0 ankles. There were no cases of restricted dorsiflexion or plantarflexion. Two ankles presented minor restriction of supination range of motion. Forty-seven of the 48 patients were highly satisfied with the surgery in regard to ankle stability. No worsening over time was evident [23].

Take-Home Messages

- The plantaris tendon can be considered as an option for lateral ligament reconstruction. Magnetic resonance imaging or ultrasound can be used to determine the location and integrity of the tendon. It can be harvested using a proximal or distal approach with minimally invasive techniques.
- Proximal and distal approaches for harvesting are here in presented. Harvesting can also be performed with arthroscopic assistance. Several techniques of anatomical lateral ankle ligaments reconstruction using tendon grafts have been described and can be used with a plantaris tendon graft.

References

1. van Sterkenburg MN, Kerkhoffs GMMJ, Kleipool RP, Niek van Dijk C. The plantaris tendon and a potential role in mid-portion Achilles tendinopathy: an observational anatomical study. J Anat. 2011;218:336–41. https://doi.org/10.1111/j.1469-7580.2011.01335.x.
2. Jackson JB, Philippi MT, Kolz CW, Suter T, Henninger HB. Characterization of Plantaris tendon constructs for ankle ligament reconstruction. Foot Ankle Int. 2014;35:922–8. https://doi.org/10.1177/1071100714539663.
3. Waldrop NE III, Wijdicks CA, Jansson KS, LaPrade RF, Clanton TO. Anatomic suture anchor versus the Brostrom technique for anterior talofibular ligament repair: a biomechanical comparison. Am J Sports Med. 2012;40:2590–6. https://doi.org/10.1177/0363546512458420.
4. Attarian DE, McCrackin HJ, DeVito DP, McElhaney JH, Garrett WE. Biomechanical characteristics of human ankle ligaments. Foot Ankle. 1985;6:54–8. https://doi.org/10.1177/107110078500600202.
5. Spang C, Alfredson H, Docking SI, Masci L, Andersson G. The plantaris tendon: a narrative review focusing on anatomical features and clinical importance. Bone Joint J. 2016;98-B:1312–9. https://doi.org/10.1302/0301-620X.98B10.37939.
6. Pereira H, Vuurberg G, Spennacchio P, Batista J, D'Hooghe P, Hunt K, Van Dijk N. Surgical treatment paradigms of ankle lateral instability, osteochondral defects and impingement. Adv Exp Med Biol. 2018;1059:85–108. https://doi.org/10.1007/978-3-319-76735-2_4.
7. Vuurberg G, Pereira H, Blankevoort L, van Dijk CN. Anatomic stabilization techniques provide superior results in terms of functional outcome in patients suffering from chronic ankle instability compared to non-anatomic techniques. Knee Surg Sports Traumatol Arthrosc. 2018;26:2183–95. https://doi.org/10.1007/s00167-017-4730-4.
8. Hua Y, Chen S, Jin Y, Zhang B, Li Y, Li H. Anatomical reconstruction of the lateral ligaments of the ankle with semitendinosus allograft. Int Orthop. 2012;36:2027–31. https://doi.org/10.1007/s00264-012-1577-7.
9. Pagenstert GI, Valderrabano V, Hintermann B. Lateral ankle ligament reconstruction with free plantaris tendon graft. Tech Foot Ankle Surg. 2005;4:104–12. https://doi.org/10.1097/01.btf.0000152574.09654.80.
10. Guillo S, Archbold P, Perera A, Bauer T, Sonnery-Cottet B. Arthroscopic anatomic reconstruction of the lateral ligaments of the ankle with gracilis autograft. Arthrosc Tech. 2014;3:e593–8. https://doi.org/10.1016/j.eats.2014.06.018.
11. Diniz P, Pacheco J, Flora M, Quintero D, Stufkens S, Kerkhoffs G, Batista J, Karlsson J, Pereira H. Clinical applications of allografts in foot and ankle surgery. Knee Surg Sports Traumatol Arthrosc. 2019;27:1847–72. https://doi.org/10.1007/s00167-019-05362-0.
12. Tourné Y, Mabit C. Lateral ligament reconstruction procedures for the ankle. Orthop Traumatol Surg Res. 2017;103:S171–81. https://doi.org/10.1016/j.otsr.2016.06.026.
13. Dekker M, Bender J. Results of surgical treatment of rupture of the Achilles tendon with use of the plantaris tendon. Arch Chir Neerl. 1977;29:39–46.
14. Lynn TA. Repair of the torn Achilles tendon, using the plantaris tendon as a reinforcing membrane. J Bone Joint Surg Am. 1966;48:268–72.
15. Hansen BH. Reconstruction of the peroneal retinaculum using the plantaris tendon: a case report. Scand J Med Sci Sports. 1996;6:355–8. https://doi.org/10.1111/j.1600-0838.1996.tb00107.x.
16. Bertelli JA, Santos MA, Kechele PR, Rost JR, Tacca CP. Flexor tendon grafting using a plantaris tendon with a fragment of attached bone for fixation to the distal phalanx: a preliminary cohort study. J Hand Surg. 2007;32:1543–8. https://doi.org/10.1016/j.jhsa.2007.08.022.
17. Spina AA. The plantaris muscle: anatomy, injury, imaging, and treatment. J Can Chiropr Assoc. 2007;51:158–65.

18. van Sterkenburg MN, van Dijk CN. Mid-portion Achilles tendinopathy: why painful? An evidence-based philosophy. Knee Surg Sports Traumatol Arthrosc. 2011;19:1367–75. https://doi.org/10.1007/s00167-011-1535-8.
19. Nayak SR, Krishnamurthy A, Prabhu LV, Madhyastha S. Additional tendinous origin and entrapment of the plantaris muscle. Clinics (Sao Paulo, Brazil). 2009;64:67–8. https://doi.org/10.1590/s1807-59322009000100012.
20. Wehbé MA. Tendon graft donor sites. J Hand Surg. 1992;17:1130–2. https://doi.org/10.1016/s0363-5023(09)91079-6.
21. Daseler E, Anson B. The plantaris muscle an anatomical study of 750 specimens. J Bone Joint Surg. 1943;25:822.
22. Attarian DE, McCrackin HJ, Devito DP, McElhaney JH, Garrett WE. A biomechanical study of human lateral ankle ligaments and autogenous reconstructive grafts. Am J Sports Med. 1985;13:377–81. https://doi.org/10.1177/036354658501300602.
23. Hintermann B, Renggli P. [Anatomic reconstruction of the lateral ligaments of the ankle using a plantaris tendon graft in the treatment of chronic ankle joint instability]. Orthopade. 1999;28:778–84.

33 Rehabilitation After Acute Lateral Ankle Ligament Injury and After Surgery

Christopher Pearce and Anthony Perera

33.1 Introduction

Ankle sprains are the most common injuries sustained during sporting activity. In the UK, there are approximately 5600 incidences per day, accounting for between 3% and 5% of all Emergency Department attendances [1]. In the USA, the figures are 30,000 per day or 2 million per year [2, 3]. The actual incidence of ankle sprain is, of course, much higher than this as it is estimated that as many as 55% of patients do not seek evaluation or treatment from a healthcare professional [4]. In a Systematic Review and Meta-Analysis of Prospective Epidemiological Studies, Doherty et al. [5] found that female sex, lower age and athletes competing in indoor and court sports are the subgroups most at risk of ankle sprain. The majority of ankle sprains will recover without surgery, but around 20% of patients will go on to develop chronic ankle instability [6] and up to 34% will sprain their ankle again within 3 years of the initial injury [7]. There is no correlation between the initial severity of the sprain and the subsequent development of chronic instability [8]; therefore, other factors are responsible for the outcome of these injuries. Without adequate diagnosis and treatment, ankle injuries may lead to chronic instability, osteoarthritis and other permanent sequelae [9–11].

There are two main issues to consider when choosing a rehabilitation programme after an initial ankle sprain or after surgery for chronic ankle instability, namely how the ligamentous tissues heal and how the neuromuscular control mechanisms (strength and static/dynamic targeted ankle proprioception) are regained after injury or surgery and how these are affected by activity [9, 12].

33.2 Functional Rehabilitation

Traditionally, significant ankle ligament injuries were treated with prolonged periods (4 weeks) in a cast with restricted weight-bearing. Recently it has become apparent that active rehabilitation programmes yield superior results in many areas of orthopaedic and sports injuries [13–15]. There is a need for athletes, especially professionals, to return to play as quickly as is safely possible but more generally, as awareness of the complications of immobilsation such as thromboembolic events, neuromuscular deconditioning and chronic regional pain syndrome increases, the balance has swung towards earlier mobilisation and early weight-bearing [16]. Moreover, even

C. Pearce (✉)
Jurong Health, NTFGH, Singapore, Singapore
e-mail: chris.pearce@doctors.org.uk

A. Perera
Spire Cardiff Hospital, Cardiff, Wales, UK
e-mail: anthony@footandankleuk.com

H. Pereira et al. (eds.), *Lateral Ankle Instability*, https://doi.org/10.1007/978-3-662-62763-1_33

short periods of joint immobilisation, even in healthy subjects, can lead to functional deconditioning [17].

There have been several studies [10, 18–26] concerning neuromuscular rehabilitation in acute injuries and for non-operatively treated chronic ankle instability. One of the goals of an active rehabilitation programme is to strengthen the active stabilisers of the ankle to control potentially traumatic ankle inversion movements. Weakness of the ankle evertor muscles has been shown to be one of the major factors in chronic instability [21]. The other major goal is the restoration of proprioceptive acuity [22]; proprioceptive training has been a major part of ankle instability rehabilitation since Freeman's original publications in 1965 [10, 20]. Restoring proprioceptive acuity aims to reduce functional deficits, symptoms of giving way, as well as reduce the risk of re-injury and improve postural control [23]. Thonnard [27] demonstrated that a pre-activation (activation before foot contact with the floor) of 80–100 ms of the ankle evertor muscles is observed in healthy subjects when walking on uneven ground, running and on landing from a jump. This pre-activation pre-empts the 75 ms of electromechanical delay (i.e. delay between the electrical muscle activation and the beginning of force production) of the evertor muscle [28], and thus ensures an effective eversion force when the foot hits the ground. This pre-activation is lost after an ankle ligament injury and those patients who are unable to regain this ability and wish to continue sporting activities usually require surgical intervention.

There is high-level evidence for functional rehabilitation. Kerkhoffs et al. in 2002 [13] conducted a Cochrane review and meta-analysis of the results of immobilisation or functional treatment for acute lateral ankle ligament injuries in adults that included 2184 patients from 21 trials. Statistically significant differences in favour of functional treatment when compared with immobilisation were found for seven outcome measures. Most notably more patients returned to sport in the long term; return to work and sports was faster in the patients who underwent functional rehabilitation. There were also fewer patients with objective instability as tested by stress X-ray, and patients were more satisfied with their treatment after a functional treatment programme. Similar advantages of an active rehabilitation over immobilisation were observed in another more recent systematic review [29].

Kerkhoffs et al. in another Cochrane review showed that the use of an elastic bandage has fewer complications than taping, but it is associated with a slower return to work and sport and more reported instability than a semi-rigid ankle support [30]. A lace-up ankle support is effective in reducing swelling in the short term compared with a semi-rigid ankle support, elastic bandage, or tape [30].

33.3 Rehabilitation After Surgery

The factors that must be considered when designing a rehabilitation protocol after ankle ligament surgery are the strength of the initial repair, or fixation strength of the ligament to the bone if performing a reconstruction, compared to the stress that the ligament will be under during weight-bearing or ankle movements, the mechanism by which ligaments or tendon grafts heal to bone and later the prevention of re-injury by safely returning the patient to activities based on an objective assessment of strength and neuromuscular control [16].

Loading of both bony and ligamentous structures is vital for normal homeostasis, and it is well established in animal models that stress deprivation leads to a decrease in the mechanical properties of both the ligaments themselves and their insertions [31, 32]. The absence of load has also been shown to be detrimental to tendon-to-bone healing [33–35].

The normal histological anatomy of the bone–tendon or bone–ligament interface is a four-zone gradient from bone to mineralised fibrocartilage, to unmineralised fibrocartilage to tendon or ligament [36]. The mechanical properties of each zone are different, and thus this transitional arrangement limits stress concentration in any one region of the insertion by having a graduated evolution from the stiff bone to the elastic ligament [37–40]. Re-establishment of this transitional insertion site is vital as without it the strength of the insertion is an order of magnitude weaker [40]. Whether the surgery for ankle ligaments involves a direct repair of the ligament to the bone (as in a modified Brostrom-Gould procedure) or reconstruction using tendon graft; the strength of the repair to the bone is affected by the rehabilitation protocol that is adopted. A balance needs to be achieved between excessive load, which will damage the repairing insertion site, and insufficient load, which will lead to a catabolic environment [35, 41, 42].

Animal studies have been conducted on the rotator cuff insertion into the humerus (which is a similar situation to the anterior talo-fibular ligament (ATFL) and calcaneofibular ligament (CFL) repairing to the fibula after a modified Broström type procedure), and in Anterior Cruciate Ligament (ACL) reconstruction (which is a similar situation to the tendon graft procedures in the ankle) comparing the strength of the repair with different post-operative mobilisation regimes. The evidence from these studies [33–35, 40–48] clearly shows that, in order to establish the best quality repair, some mechanical stimulus is required. Without the correct mechano-biological environment, the four-zone gradient from tendon to bone is not established, and fibrovascular (scar) tissue forms in the gap instead [42, 45] and the repair is an order of magnitude weaker [40].

It would appear from these studies that the strongest repair at the bone tendon/ligament interface is achieved with a short period of immobilisation (to allow resolution of acute post-operative inflammation) followed by controlled mechanical loads [43]. This is convenient as many foot and ankle surgeons like to employ a short (10–14 days) period of immobilisation and elevation of the limb until the best chance of wound healing is given without complication. The fear being that excessive swelling and oedema in the immediate post-operative period may lead to tension on the sutures and subsequent ischaemia of the skin as well as wound leakage which may result in infection. Having said that, the studies on ankle ligament surgery where immediate weight-bearing was employed did not report any increased wound complication rates [49, 50].

References

1. Cooke MW, Lamb SE, Marsh J, Dale J. A survey of current consultant practice of treatment of severe ankle sprains in emergency departments in the United Kingdom. Emerg Med J. 2003;20(6):505–7.
2. DiGiovanni CW, Brodsky A. Current concepts: lateral ankle instability. Foot Ankle Int. 2006;27(10):854–66. https://doi.org/10.1177/107110070602701019.
3. Waterman BR, Owens BD, Davey S, Zacchilli MA, Belmont PJ Jr. The epidemiology of ankle sprains in the United States. J Bone Joint Surg Am. 2010;92(13):2279–84. https://doi.org/10.2106/JBJS.I.01537.
4. McKay GD, Goldie PA, Payne WR, Oakes BW. Ankle injuries in basketball: injury rate and risk factors. Br J Sports Med. 2001;35(2):103–8.
5. Doherty C, Delahunt E, Caulfield B, Hertel J, Ryan J, Bleakley C. The incidence and prevalence of ankle sprain injury: a systematic review and meta-analysis of prospective epidemiological studies. Sports Med. 2014;44(1):123–40. https://doi.org/10.1007/s40279-013-0102-5.
6. Corte-Real NM, Moreira RM. Arthroscopic repair of chronic lateral ankle instability. Foot Ankle Int. 2009;30(3):213–7. https://doi.org/10.3113/FAI.2009.0213.
7. van Rijn RM, van Os AG, Bernsen RM, Luijsterburg PA, Koes BW, Bierma-Zeinstra SM. What is the clinical course of acute ankle sprains? A systematic literature review. Am J Med. 2008;121(4):324–331.e326. https://doi.org/10.1016/j.amjmed.2007.11.018.
8. Konradsen L, Bech L, Ehrenbjerg M, Nickelsen T. Seven years follow-up after ankle inversion trauma. Scand J Med Sci Sports. 2002;12(3):129–35.
9. Bosien WR, Staples OS, Russell SW. Residual disability following acute ankle sprains. J Bone Joint Surg Am. 1955;37-A(6):1237–43.
10. Freeman MA. Instability of the foot after injuries to the lateral ligament of the ankle. J Bone Joint Surg. 1965;47(4):669–77.
11. van den Bekerom MP, Kerkhoffs GM, McCollum GA, Calder JD, van Dijk CN. Management of acute lateral ankle ligament injury in the athlete. Knee Surg Sports Traumatol Arthrosc. 2013;21(6):1390–5. https://doi.org/10.1007/s00167-012-2252-7.
12. Hiller CE, Kilbreath SL, Refshauge KM. Chronic ankle instability: evolution of the model. J Athl Train. 2011;46(2):133–41. https://doi.org/10.4085/1062-6050-46.2.133.
13. Kerkhoffs GM, Rowe BH, Assendelft WJ, Kelly K, Struijs PA, van Dijk CN. Immobilisation and functional treatment for acute lateral ankle ligament injuries in adults. Cochrane Database

Syst Rev. 2002;(3):CD003762. https://doi.org/10.1002/14651858.CD003762.
14. Petersen OF, Nielsen MB, Jensen KH, Solgaard S. [Randomized comparison of CAM walker and light-weight plaster cast in the treatment of first-time Achilles tendon rupture]. Ugeskr Laeger. 2002;164(33):3852–5.
15. Saleh M, Marshall PD, Senior R, MacFarlane A. The Sheffield splint for controlled early mobilisation after rupture of the calcaneal tendon. A prospective, randomised comparison with plaster treatment. J Bone Joint Surg Br. 1992;74(2):206–9.
16. Pearce CJ, Tourne Y, Zellers J, Terrier R, Toschi P, Silbernagel KG, Group E-AAI. Rehabilitation after anatomical ankle ligament repair or reconstruction. Knee Surg Sports Traumatol Arthrosc. 2016;24(4):1130–9. https://doi.org/10.1007/s00167-016-4051-z.
17. Fortuna M, Teixeira S, Machado S, Velasques B, Bittencourt J, Peressutti C, Budde H, Cagy M, Nardi AE, Piedade R, Ribeiro P, Arias-Carrion O. Cortical reorganization after hand immobilization: the beta qEEG spectral coherence evidences. PLoS One. 2013;8(11):e79912. https://doi.org/10.1371/journal.pone.0079912.
18. Collado H, Coudreuse JM, Graziani F, Bensoussan L, Viton JM, Delarque A. Eccentric reinforcement of the ankle evertor muscles after lateral ankle sprain. Scand J Med Sci Sports. 2010;20(2):241–6. https://doi.org/10.1111/j.1600-0838.2009.00882.x.
19. David P, Halimi M, Mora I, Doutrellot PL, Petitjean M. Isokinetic testing of evertor and invertor muscles in patients with chronic ankle instability. J Appl Biomech. 2013;29(6):696–704.
20. Freeman MA, Dean MR, Hanham IW. The etiology and prevention of functional instability of the foot. J Bone Joint Surg. 1965;47(4):678–85.
21. Hartsell HD, Spaulding SJ. Eccentric/concentric ratios at selected velocities for the invertor and evertor muscles of the chronically unstable ankle. Br J Sports Med. 1999;33(4):255–8.
22. Postle K, Pak D, Smith TO. Effectiveness of proprioceptive exercises for ankle ligament injury in adults: a systematic literature and meta-analysis. Man Ther. 2012;17(4):285–91. https://doi.org/10.1016/j.math.2012.02.016.
23. Rozzi SL, Lephart SM, Sterner R, Kuligowski L. Balance training for persons with functionally unstable ankles. J Orthop Sports Phys Ther. 1999;29(8):478–86. https://doi.org/10.2519/jospt.1999.29.8.478.
24. Sale DG. Neural adaptation to resistance training. Med Sci Sports Exerc. 1988;20(5 Suppl):S135–45.
25. Thepaut-Mathieu C, Van Hoecke J, Maton B. Myoelectrical and mechanical changes linked to length specificity during isometric training. J Appl Physiol. 1988;64(4):1500–5.
26. Thorstensson A. Observations on strength training and detraining. Acta Physiol Scand. 1977;100(4):491–3. https://doi.org/10.1111/j.1748-1716.1977.tb05975.x.
27. Thonnard JL. La pathogénie de l'entorse du ligament latéral externe de la cheville. Evaluation d'une hypothèse. Thèse en vue de l'obtention du grade de Docteur en réadaptation. Université Catholique de Louvain, Faculté de médecine, Institut d'Éducation physique et de réadaptation; 1988.
28. Konradsen L. Sensori-motor control of the uninjured and injured human ankle. J Electromyogr Kinesiol. 2002;12(3):199–203.
29. Petersen W, Rembitzki IV, Koppenburg AG, Ellermann A, Liebau C, Bruggemann GP, Best R. Treatment of acute ankle ligament injuries: a systematic review. Arch Orthop Trauma Surg. 2013;133(8):1129–41. https://doi.org/10.1007/s00402-013-1742-5.
30. Kerkhoffs GM, Struijs PA, Marti RK, Assendelft WJ, Blankevoort L, van Dijk CN. Different functional treatment strategies for acute lateral ankle ligament injuries in adults. Cochrane Database Syst Rev. 2002;3:CD002938. https://doi.org/10.1002/14651858.CD002938.
31. Gomez MA, Woo SL, Amiel D, Harwood F, Kitabayashi L, Matyas JR. The effects of increased tension on healing medical collateral ligaments. Am J Sports Med. 1991;19(4):347–54.
32. Woo SL, Gomez MA, Sites TJ, Newton PO, Orlando CA, Akeson WH. The biomechanical and morphological changes in the medial collateral ligament of the rabbit after immobilization and remobilization. J Bone Joint Surg Am. 1987;69(8):1200–11.
33. Thomopoulos S, Kim HM, Rothermich SY, Biederstadt C, Das R, Galatz LM. Decreased muscle loading delays maturation of the tendon enthesis during postnatal development. J Orthop Res. 2007;25(9):1154–63. https://doi.org/10.1002/jor.20418.
34. Thomopoulos S, Marquez JP, Weinberger B, Birman V, Genin GM. Collagen fiber orientation at the tendon to bone insertion and its influence on stress concentrations. J Biomech. 2006;39(10):1842–51. https://doi.org/10.1016/j.jbiomech.2005.05.021.
35. Thomopoulos S, Zampiakis E, Das R, Silva MJ, Gelberman RH. The effect of muscle loading on flexor tendon-to-bone healing in a canine model. J Orthop Res. 2008;26(12):1611–7. https://doi.org/10.1002/jor.20689.
36. Benjamin M, Evans EJ, Copp L. The histology of tendon attachments to bone in man. J Anat. 1986;149:89–100.
37. Lu HH, Thomopoulos S. Functional attachment of soft tissues to bone: development, healing, and tissue engineering. Annu Rev Biomed Eng. 2013;15:201–26. https://doi.org/10.1146/annurev-bioeng-071910-124656.
38. Thomopoulos S, Genin GM, Galatz LM. The development and morphogenesis of the tendon-to-bone insertion - what development can teach us about healing. J Musculoskelet Neuronal Interact. 2010;10(1):35–45.
39. Thomopoulos S, Williams GR, Gimbel JA, Favata M, Soslowsky LJ. Variation of biomechanical, structural, and compositional properties along the tendon to

bone insertion site. J Orthop Res. 2003;21(3):413–9. https://doi.org/10.1016/S0736-0266(03)00057-3.
40. Thomopoulos S, Williams GR, Soslowsky LJ. Tendon to bone healing: differences in biomechanical, structural, and compositional properties due to a range of activity levels. J Biomech Eng. 2003;125(1):106–13.
41. Dagher E, Hays PL, Kawamura S, Godin J, Deng XH, Rodeo SA. Immobilization modulates macrophage accumulation in tendon-bone healing. Clin Orthop Relat Res. 2009;467(1):281–7. https://doi.org/10.1007/s11999-008-0512-0.
42. Galatz LM, Charlton N, Das R, Kim HM, Havlioglu N, Thomopoulos S. Complete removal of load is detrimental to rotator cuff healing. J Shoulder Elbow Surg. 2009;18(5):669–75. https://doi.org/10.1016/j.jse.2009.02.016.
43. Bedi A, Kovacevic D, Fox AJ, Imhauser CW, Stasiak M, Packer J, Brophy RH, Deng XH, Rodeo SA. Effect of early and delayed mechanical loading on tendon-to-bone healing after anterior cruciate ligament reconstruction. J Bone Joint Surg Am. 2010;92(14):2387–401. https://doi.org/10.2106/JBJS.I.01270.
44. Galatz LM, Rothermich SY, Zaegel M, Silva MJ, Havlioglu N, Thomopoulos S. Delayed repair of tendon to bone injuries leads to decreased biomechanical properties and bone loss. J Orthop Res. 2005;23(6):1441–7. https://doi.org/10.1016/j.orthres.2005.05.005.1100230629.
45. Galatz LM, Sandell LJ, Rothermich SY, Das R, Mastny A, Havlioglu N, Silva MJ, Thomopoulos S. Characteristics of the rat supraspinatus tendon during tendon-to-bone healing after acute injury. J Orthop Res. 2006;24(3):541–50. https://doi.org/10.1002/jor.20067.
46. Gimbel JA, Van Kleunen JP, Williams GR, Thomopoulos S, Soslowsky LJ. Long durations of immobilization in the rat result in enhanced mechanical properties of the healing supraspinatus tendon insertion site. J Biomech Eng. 2007;129(3):400–4. https://doi.org/10.1115/1.2721075.
47. Peltz CD, Dourte LM, Kuntz AF, Sarver JJ, Kim SY, Williams GR, Soslowsky LJ. The effect of postoperative passive motion on rotator cuff healing in a rat model. J Bone Joint Surg Am. 2009;91(10):2421–9.
48. Thomopoulos S, Hattersley G, Rosen V, Mertens M, Galatz L, Williams GR, Soslowsky LJ. The localized expression of extracellular matrix components in healing tendon insertion sites: an in situ hybridization study. J Orthop Res. 2002;20(3):454–63.
49. Miyamoto W, Takao M, Yamada K, Matsushita T. Accelerated versus traditional rehabilitation after anterior talofibular ligament reconstruction for chronic lateral instability of the ankle in athletes. Am J Sports Med. 2014;42(6):1441–7. https://doi.org/10.1177/0363546514527418.
50. Petrera M, Dwyer T, Theodoropoulos JS, Ogilvie-Harris DJ. Short- to medium-term outcomes after a modified Brostrom repair for lateral ankle instability with immediate postoperative weightbearing. Am J Sports Med. 2014;42(7):1542–8. https://doi.org/10.1177/0363546514530668.

34 Goal-Based Protocol for Rehabilitation

Noelene G. Davey

34.1 Introduction

This chapter provides both a pre- and post-operative rehabilitation guide for patients with chronic ankle instability undergoing anatomical ankle ligament repair or reconstruction stabilisation surgery. The concept of pre-operative rehabilitation, also known as 'prehabilitation', is discussed as it has the potential to improve surgical outcomes, but it is not currently considered routinely for this ankle surgery. The ESSKA-AFAS Ankle Instability Group post-operative protocol [1] is then presented in an easily accessible format, alongside examples of strategies that can be employed to address deficits.

34.2 Pre-operative Rehabilitation

The current state of the evidence regarding potential predictors of poor outcome in ankle instability surgery has been summarised by Guillo et al. [2], but at the time of writing there have been no studies exploring the effect that a pre-operative rehabilitation protocol, also known as prehabilitation or 'prehab,' might have on outcomes.

N. G. Davey (✉)
Imperial College Healthcare NHS Trust, St Mary's Hospital, London, UK
e-mail: noelene@kineticphysio.org, Noelene.Davey@nhs.net

In the knee, a systematic review of anterior cruciate ligament reconstruction surgery found that, whilst reduced knee extension range or reduced quadriceps strength predicted poorer surgical outcomes, prehabilitation improved them [3]. Ankle stabilisation surgery has good outcomes with 80% reporting a good to excellent result over a 15-year follow-up [4] and 94% return to sport [5], but research into the effect of a prehabilitation would be of interest as it has the potential to improve these outcomes even further.

Most CAI patients will have undertaken a period of conservative rehabilitation prior to being offered surgery, but prehabilitation is different in that it prepares the patient both physically and mentally for not only the surgery but also the commitment required for post-operative rehabilitation.

A prehabilitation programme should include the following:

- An easily manageable exercise routine to maintain any gains made during conservative rehabilitation.
- Include proximal strengthening exercises because ipsilateral hip strength is reduced after an ankle sprain [6], and risk of re-injury is reduced if hip strength is improved [7].
- A preview of the post-operative protocol, explaining the timeline in relation to the phases of tissue healing and remodelling and the length of time it takes to retrain normal

H. Pereira et al. (eds.), *Lateral Ankle Instability*, https://doi.org/10.1007/978-3-662-62763-1_34

neuromuscular function. Short- and long-term goals can also be set with reference to these timeframes.

- Review of the immediate post-operative phase instructions as physiotherapy may not start until after the plaster has been removed. Ensure they understand that early rehabilitation is important in order to minimise muscle atrophy caused by immobilisation and arthrogenic muscle inhibition.
- Management of patient expectations because negative pre-surgical expectations can predict a poorer outcome [8].
- Mental preparation for the post-operative rehabilitation period:
  - Encourage a positive and resilient attitude. For example, 'focus on what you can do, not what you can't do';
  - Forewarn and prepare them for setbacks and reassure them that this is normal. For example, there is often a flare-up of pain and swelling with transition out of the boot, or after the first attempt at jogging;
  - Try to see this as a period of potential opportunity. For example, use this time to increase general muscle mass, improve swimming technique, learn a new skill or take up a new hobby.

Prehabilitation also allows time to:

- Collect baseline measures and outcome measures;
- Screen for factors that may have a negative effect on outcome, such as poor health literacy [9], mood disorders and psychosocial factors [10];
- Develop good rehabilitation habits and build rapport with their physiotherapist;
- Consider undergoing a course of formal sports psychology as this improves the likelihood of a successful return to sport and can reduce the risk of re-injury [11];

34.3 Post-operative Rehabilitation

The ESSKA-AFAS Ankle Instability Group ankle stabilisation surgery post-operative protocol serves to protect the surgical repair, regain normal musculoskeletal function and facilitate appropriate loading of the healing tissues in order to maximise the tissue remodelling process. However, regaining normal ankle musculoskeletal function involves more than just rehabilitating joint range of motion and strength; some functions such as balance and proprioception are 'sensorimotor' meaning that they rely on both motor *and* sensory functions [12]. Therefore, sensory deficits must also be addressed in order to maximise recovery after ankle stabilisation surgery. For example, chronic ankle instability patients often have reduced plantar sensitivity [13, 14] that impairs balance [15], so in order to make a full recovery of balance sensory deficits must also be addressed.

The protocol is presented in an easily accessible format, and examples of strategies that can be employed to address deficits are displayed alongside. Progression onto the next phase of rehabilitation is permitted only if the current phase goals have been achieved and the markers for progression met.

34.3.1 Immediate Post-operative Phase

0 to 10–14 Days

- NWB in plaster

Goals of this Phase

- Minimise sensory deficits
- Minimise muscle atrophy both locally and proximally

34.3.1.1 Sensory Rehabilitation

- Massage and touch exposed areas of skin in order to minimise shrinkage of the foot and ankle region in the somato*sensory* cortex. Include the plantar surface as this area often has reduced sensation in the CAI group [13, 14].

34.3.1.2 Motor Rehabilitation

- Maintain proximal hip strength to reduce the risk of recurrent sprains [7] and improve lower limb motor control.
- Minimise loss of somato*motor* cortical representation by performing mental practice of movements and moving the contralateral ankle. If available, apply vibration to the tendons through windows in the cast [16].
- Isometric contractions (press/push against the inside of the cast) in all directions, particularly eversion. 'Foot shortening' intrinsic muscle exercises can also be performed.
- Strengthen the contralateral leg as the non-exercised immobilised side will also benefit from a 7–8% increase in voluntary strength [17].
- Reduce pain and swelling (elevate the foot above the hip) in order to minimise weakness caused by arthrogenic muscle inhibition [18].

Arthrogenic muscle inhibition (AMI) is the excessive discharge of afferent flow (ascending neural signals) from the sensory receptors of the joint [18]. AMI can be caused by pain, swelling, laxity, stiffness or structural damage to joint afferents and leads to inhibition of efferent (descending) neural signal, leading to myogenic inhibition which will be reflected as weakness. AMI can be modulated by:

- Deep cooling of the joint (20 min) [18]
- Reduction of pain (analgesics, NSAIDs, TENS machine, relaxation breathing techniques)
- Reduction of swelling—elevate the foot above the hip, or even above the heart
- Normalising joint range of motion

34.3.2 Post-operative Phase

Week 2–6

- FWB in below knee walking boot. Walking without protection is contraindicated until week 6.
- Patients are allowed to remove the boot to perform active dorsiflexion (DF) and plantarflexion (PF), and a small amount of inversion/eversion is allowed to a maximum of 10–15°

Goals of this Phase

- Regain range of movement within allowed limits*
- Minimise sensory deficits
- Minimise muscle atrophy locally and proximally

**If there have been concurrent procedures, there may be contraindications to certain movements.*

34.3.2.1 Sensory Rehabilitation

Boot off, sitting in a chair:

- Massage the plantar surface of the foot [19] or brush the sole of the foot along a textured surface on carpet to give sensory input.
- Lightly tap the foot up and down; make sure the foot is landing flat with no inversion.
- Apply pressure to a bathroom scale. Do not exceed 50% body weight, and the thigh must stay in contact with the chair (see Fig. 34.1).

34.3.2.2 Motor Rehabilitation

- Once plaster removed, apply ice for 20 min twice per day in order to deep cool the joint. This reduces afferent outflow from the joint thereby reducing arthrogenic muscle inhibition [20], which along with disuse atrophy contributes to weakness.
- Isometrics in varying degrees of DF and PF range. Use a towel to keep the foot in a neutral (or midline) position (see Fig. 34.2).

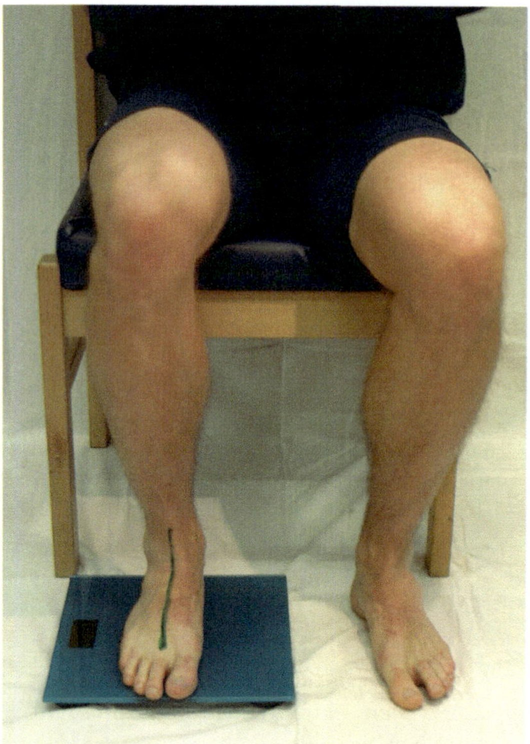

Fig. 34.1 Apply mechanical pressure through the plantar surface of the foot using bathroom scales for visual feedback. Do not exceed 50% of bodyweight, and the thigh must not lift off the chair

- Seated heel raises, see Fig. 34.3a. Ensure good quality of movement—do not allow the ankle to roll out into inversion (Fig. 34.3b), which could be a sign of poor joint position sense or functional peroneal weakness.
- Plantarflexion against resistance over the edge of a book or step, maintaining neutral rearfoot alignment (Fig. 34.4). Progressively increase both the resistance and the number of repetitions and make sure that the eccentric phase of the contraction is also well controlled. Then increase speed. Make sure to also control the up phase, returning to dorsiflexion.

34.3.3 Early Rehabilitation Phase

From Week 6
- FWB no boot, no brace
- Stationary exercise bicycle can start

Goals of this Phase
- Restore normal gait
- MECHANICAL—regain range of motion

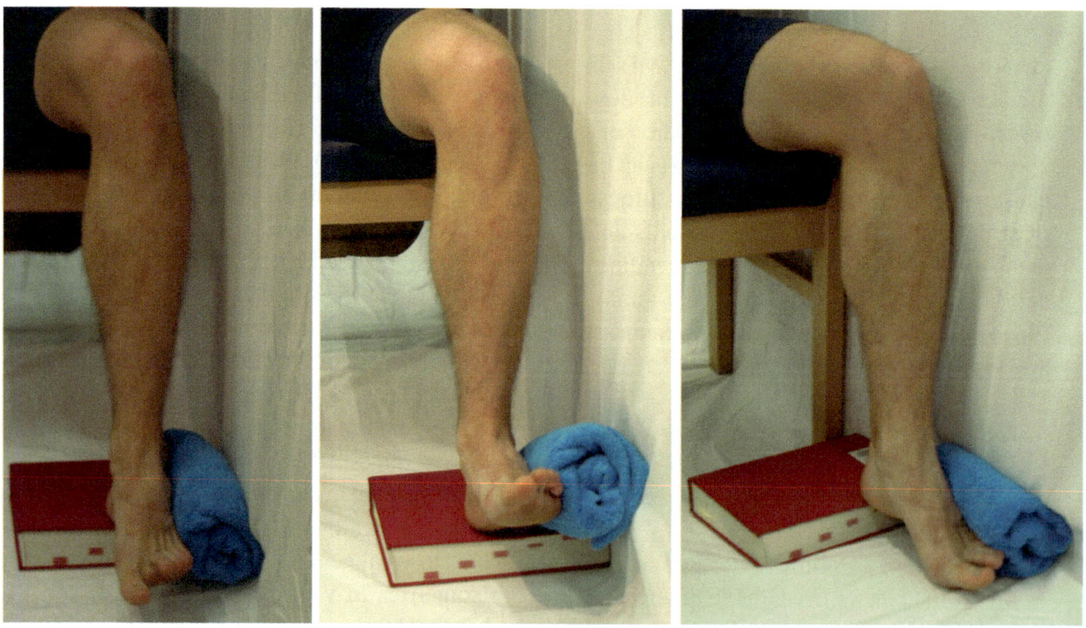

Fig. 34.2 Isometric eversion in varying degrees of dorsiflexion and plantarflexion

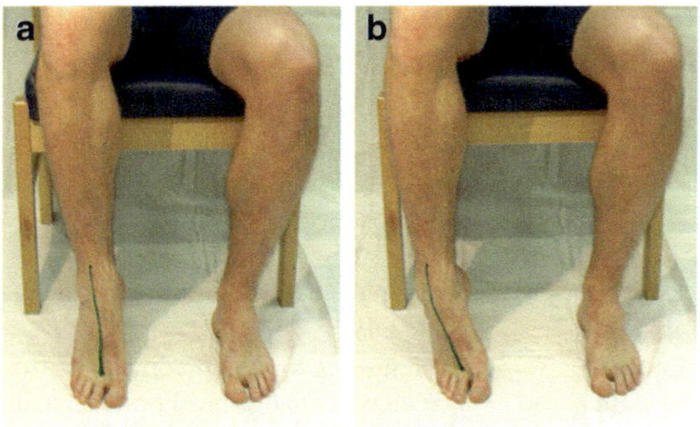

Fig. 34.3 (**a**) Seated heel raise with good alignment (weight-bearing through the second metatarsal head). (**b**) Seated heel raise demonstrating poor alignment; rolling out into inversion with weight-bearing over the third/fourth metatarsal heads

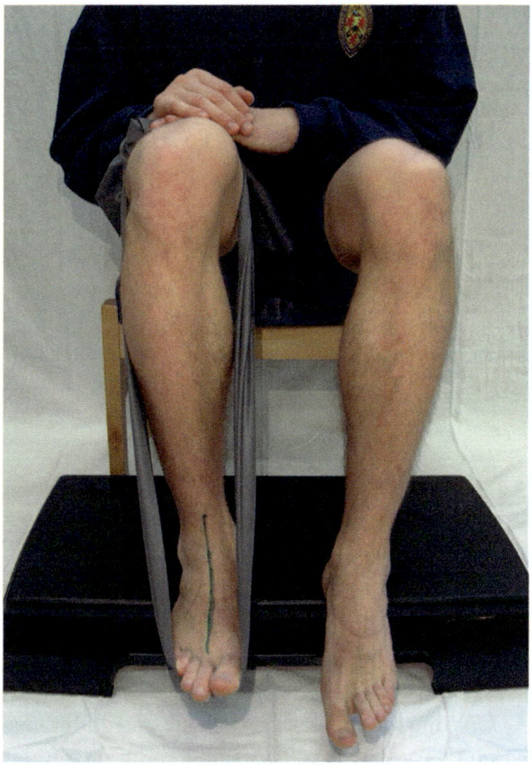

Fig. 34.4 DF against resistance whilst controlling the rearfoot position

- SENSORY—improve proprioception (balance and joint position sense)
- MOTOR—increase strength, particularly of the evertors
- Improve dynamic postural control (DPC)

34.3.3.1 Sensory Rehabilitation

- Use bathroom scales to give feedback on whether an equal amount of pressure is being applied through each foot. Weight-bearing is often reduced on the operated side due to reduced plantar mechanoreception. The scales can also be used to practice weight transfer (Fig. 34.5).

34.3.3.2 Proprioceptive Rehabilitation

- Balance
  - Patients with CAI have reduced plantar sensitivity to light touch and pressure [13, 14], and wearing socks further reduces plantar sensitivity [21]. Therefore, perform balance exercises in bare feet as much as possible for the first few months in order to help increase the amount of sensory information received from the periphery.
  - Adding cognitive demands reduces postural stability in CAI patients [22], so use this to increase difficulty. For example, counting backwards from 100 by 7's or spelling difficult words whilst performing balancing tasks.
  - Balance exercises on an unstable surface do reduce frequency of giving way [23], but they do not target ankle proprioception [24]. Rearfoot-specific ankle destabilisation devices that target the subtalar joint Henke axis, around which inversion sprains occur [25–27], do improve ankle proprio-

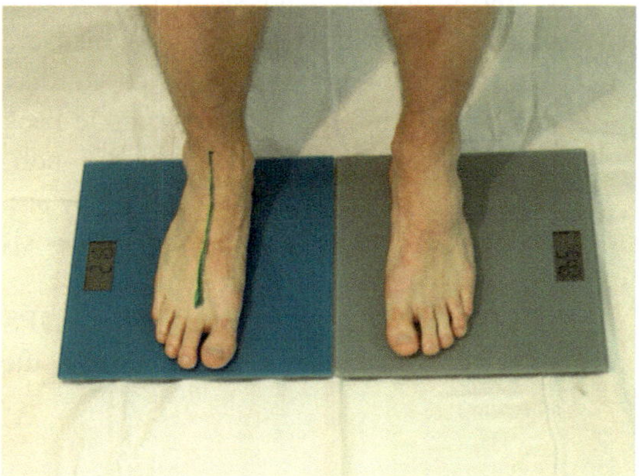

Fig. 34.5 Practicing weight transfer using bathroom scales to give feedback

ception, increase peroneal muscle amplitudes and reaction times [28].

Ankle inversion sprains occur around the subtalar joint Henke axis [25–27]. In response to research that showed traditional rehabilitation exercises performed on an unstable surfaces, do not target the rearfoot axis and do not increase ankle proprioception activity [24], but rearfoot-specific ankle destabilisation devices do increase proprioception at the ankle and also evertor muscle activation [28, 29]. These boot or sandal-type devices can be worn whilst performing rehabilitation tasks such as the Star Excursion Balance Test (SEBT), balance drills and hopping tasks.

- Progress difficulty of the balance exercises—see Table 34.1.

- Joint Position Sense (JPS)

  Patients with CAI have reduced JPS [30, 31]. Extrapolating from proprioception research in cervical whiplash and ACL-deficient knees, you can try these novel ideas to improve JPS:

  - With a laser pointer taped onto the foot, move the ankle to trace around pictures of shapes and random squiggles that attached to a wall [32]. Try to block visual input so they cannot see their foot, for example, by laying a place of cardboard over their knees.
  - Using an inclinometer smart phone App, position the patient's ankle and measure the joint angle [33]. Ask the patient to relax and then try to reposition their ankle back into the same position, then use the inclinometer to measure how accurate they are. Did they overshoot or under shoot the position? Give feedback and repeat.
  - Use these principles to create your own JPS practice drills. For example, stand the patient on a mark on the floor. With their eyes closed, ask them to step away then step straight back onto the spot—did they over- or undershoot the target? Give feedback and repeat until performance improves. Practice all directions.

Table 34.1 Progressing the difficulty of balance exercises

Easiest	More difficult
Flat stable surface	On an uneven, unstable or moving surface
	Rearfoot-specific destabilisation device
Knee straight, ankle at 0°	Varying degrees of knee flexion and ankle DF/PF
Looking straight ahead	Head turning to look up/down/ sideways to change head position and challenge vestibular system
Eyes open	Eyes close, 2–3 s, or H-pattern tracking eye movement
Quiet environment	Noisy environment
Good lighting	Dark or poor lighting, strobe lighting
No concurrent task	Concurrent tasks such as catching a ball
No cognitive demands	Add cognitive demands
No external perturbation	Unpredictable external perturbation
	Combine various combinations of the above

34.3.3.3 Motor Rehabilitation

- Strengthen all muscle groups, particularly the evertors that are weak in CAI patients [29].
- Strengthening is very functional and specific: strengthen through the full joint range and progress to faster speeds [34] and in upright WB postures [35].
- Continue to increase resistance and endurance and vary between power and endurance training sessions.
- Progress double heel raise to single leg heel raise (range 0° DF–full PF) and then off a step in order to strengthen the full range 15°–20° DF–30°–40° PF (Fig. 34.6). Ensure good rear-

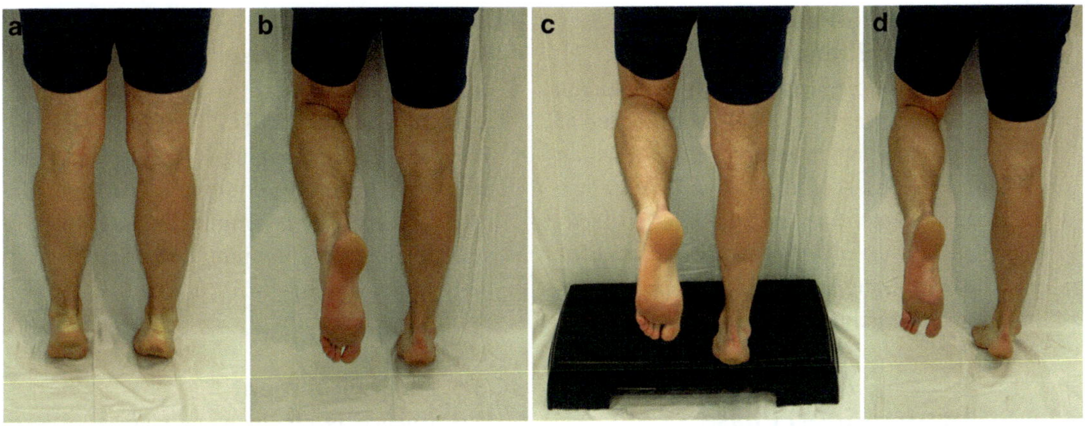

Fig. 34.6 Heel raise progressions. (**a**) Double heel raise. (**b**) Single heel raise off floor, demonstrating good alignment (WB through the second metatarsal). (**c**) Progression to single leg heel raises over edge of a step or book to strengthen through whole range. (**d**) Single heel raise demonstrating poor alignment (rolling out into inversion and WB through the third and fourth metatarsals)

foot alignment is maintained; i.e. do not allow the ankle to roll out into inversion (Fig. 34.6d).

- Regain good quality of movement (minimise compensatory trunk and arm movements).
- Using a rearfoot ankle destabilisation device can increase peroneal activation [36].
- Regain full hip strength and proximal control.

Strengthening the ipsilateral hip muscles reduces the risk of re-injury [7].

34.3.3.4 Dynamic Postural Control Rehabilitation

Dynamic Postural Control (DPC) drills include the following:

- The star excursion balance test (SEBT) and simplified Y excursion balance test (YEBT) [37] can be used for both assessment of DPC deficit and as a training exercise.
- Throwing, hitting or catching tasks.

34.3.4 Late Rehabilitation Phase

Week 8–12

Markers for progression onto this phase (only progress when markers achieved)

- *Strength at least 90% compared to the contralateral side*
- *Good static balance*
- *Normal gait with no pain when changing direction/turning*

Goals of this Phase

- Straight line jogging—refer to jogging progressions and soreness rules guides [1]
- Plyometrics can start once ×25 single leg heel raises achieved. Start with double leg jumping and progress onto single leg hopping drills.
- Progress DPC drills

34.3.4.1 Dynamic Postural Control Rehabilitation

- Jumping and hopping (*landing*) drills. Patients with CAI often land on the lateral border of the foot/in excessive inversion [38, 39], which increases their risk of re-injury. To retrain a different movement pattern, give verbal feedback to '*land on a flat foot*'. Progress difficulty by combining jumping and hopping with throwing and catching drills.

34.3.5 Return to Sport Phase

Week 12–16
Marker for progression onto this phase

- *Functional DPC tests (SEBT or YEBT and hop tests* [1]) *are ≥90%*

Goals of this Phase

- Slow jogging → faster jogging → changes of direction → straight line running → fast changes of direction
- Agility drills
- Towards week 16 independent sports-specific drills → one-on-one → team practice. Prophylactic bracing or taping is advised during team practice in order to reduce the risk of re-injury [40]

Dynamic Systems Theory [41] is a useful tool to help you identify variables specific to each patient's rehabilitation needs. By the return to sport phase of rehabilitation, the patient deficits should be minimal and the focus now shifts towards addressing task-related and environmental demands. Individual's progress at their own rate based on their ability to perform movements and drills error-free.

34.3.5.1 Task

- Agility drills. Progress to multidirectional, complex patterns and fast, e.g. cone running and carioca ladder drills.
- Progress DPC hopping (*landing*) drills—increasing difficulty, complexity and specificity to sports. For example for basketball or volleyball players, hopping down from a gradually increasing height.
- Sports-specific drills.

34.3.5.2 Environment

- Performance is challenged in noisy or very busy environments due to the increased attentional demands on the central processing system—have them transfer some of their practice sessions into these real-life situations.
- Practice drills in other difficult environments such as challenging surfaces (cobblestones or a rough or muddy field) or in low lighting conditions.
- Train when fatigued to mimic the negative effects this might have on performance (e.g. in the last quarter of game play).
- Unpredictable perturbation to mimic contact with other players.
- Confront as many conditions and situations as possible as it is better to first meet challenges within the rehabilitation environment rather than in game play.

34.3.6 Return to Competitive Play

After 16 Weeks
Markers for return to competitive play:

- *No DPC deficits*
- *Full strength distally and proximally with good quality of movements*
- *Able to fully participate in practice without any increase in symptoms*
- *The player feels ready*

Prophylactic bracing or taping is advised when returning to competitive play in order to reduce the risk of re-injury or reduce the severity of injury if an inversion sprain occurs again [40].

Take-Home Messages

- Due to the multi-factorial nature of CAI, a multi-faceted approach is needed when rehabilitating patients after ankle stabilisation surgery; mechanical, motor *and* sensory deficits all need to be addressed in a comprehensive post-operative rehabilitation programme in order to maximise outcomes and safely return patients to activities and sports.
- It will be interesting to see whether prehabilitation does further improve surgical outcomes. In the present day however, this protocol helps highlight the importance of early intervention in the immediate post-operative period, and following the guidance of markers for progression, it allows for faster rehabilitation. In conclusion, the return to sport phase must provide sufficiently challenging tasks and environments in order to achieve maximal results from rehabilitation and to reduce the risk of future injury.

References

1. Pearce CJ, Tourné Y, Zellers J, Terrier R, Toschi P, Silbernagel KG. Rehabilitation after anatomical ankle ligament repair or reconstruction. Knee Surg Sports Traumatol Arthrosc. 2016;24(4):1130–9. https://doi.org/10.1007/s00167-016-4051-z.
2. Guillo S, Bauer T, Lee JW, Takao M, Kong SW, Stone JW, Mangone PG, Molloy A, Perera A, Pearce CJ, Michels F, Tourné Y, Ghorbani A, Calder J. Consensus in chronic ankle instability: aetiology, assessment, surgical indications and place for arthroscopy. Orthop Traumatol Surg Res. 2013;99(8):S411–9. https://doi.org/10.1016/j.otsr.2013.10.009.
3. van Melick N, van Cingel REH, Brooijmans F, Neeter C, van Tienan T, Hullegie W, Nijhuis-van der Sanden MW. Evidence-based clinical practice update: practice guidelines for anterior cruciate ligament rehabilitation based on a systematic review and multidisciplinary consensus. Br J Sports Med. 2016;50(24):1506–15. https://doi.org/10.1136/bjsports-2015-095898.
4. Krips R, Brandsson S, Swensson C, van Dijk CN, Karlsson J. Anatomical reconstruction and Evans tenodesis of the lateral ligaments of the ankle. Clinical and radiological findings after follow-up for 15 to 30 years. J Bone Joint Surg Br. 2002;84(2):232–6. https://doi.org/10.1302/0301-620X.84B2.12143.
5. Li X, Killie H, Guerrero P, Busconi BD. Anatomical reconstruction for chronic lateral ankle instability in the high-demand athlete. Am J Sports Med. 2009;37(3):488–94. https://doi.org/10.1177/0363546508327541.
6. Friel K, McLean N, Myers C, Caceres M. Ipsilateral hip abductor weakness after inversion ankle sprain. J Athl Train. 2006;41(1):74–8.
7. Smith BI, Docherty CL, Curtis D. Effects of hip strengthening on neuromuscular control, hip strength, and self-reported functional deficits in individuals with chronic ankle instability. J Sport Rehabil. 2017;12:1–23. https://doi.org/10.1123/jsr.2016-0143.
8. Waljee J, McGlinn EP, Sears ED, Chung KC. Patient expectation and patient-reported outcomes in surgery: a systematic review. Surgery. 2014;155(5):799–808. https://doi.org/10.1016/j.surg.2013.12.015.
9. Berkman ND, Sheridan SL, Donahue KE, Halpern DJ, Crotty K. Low health literacy and health outcomes: an updated systematic review. Ann Intern Med. 2011;155(2):97–107. https://doi.org/10.7326/0003-4819-155-2-201107190-00005.
10. Rosenberger P, Jokl P, Ickovics J. Psychosocial factors and surgical outcomes: an evidence-based literature review. J Am Acad Orthop Surg. 2006;14(7):397–405.
11. Ardern CL, Taylor NF, Feller JA, Webster KE. A systematic review of the psychological factors associated with returning to sport following injury. Br J Sports Med. 2013;47(17):1120–6. https://doi.org/10.1136/bjsports-2012-091203.
12. Riemann BL, Lephart SM. The sensorimotor system, part II: the role of proprioception in motor control and functional joint stability. J Athl Train. 2002;37(1):80–4.
13. Hoch MC, McKeon PO, Andreatta RD. Plantar vibrotactile detection deficits in adults with chronic ankle instability. Med Sci Sports Exerc. 2012;44:666–72. https://doi.org/10.1249/MSS.0b013e3182390212.
14. Powell MR, Powden CJ, Houston MN, Hoch MC. Plantar cutaneous sensitivity and balance in individuals with and without chronic ankle instability. Clin J Sport Med. 2014;24:490–6. https://doi.org/10.1097/JSM.0000000000000074.
15. Wang T, Lin S. Sensitivity of plantar cutaneous sensation and postural stability. Clin Biomech. 2008;23(4):493–9. https://doi.org/10.1016/j.clinbiomech.2007.11.014.
16. Roll R, Kavounoudias A, Albert F, Legre R, Gay A, Fabre B, Roll JP. Illusory movements prevent cortical disruption caused by immobilization. NeuroImage. 2012;62(1):510–9. https://doi.org/10.1016/j.neuroimage.2012.05.016.

17. Carroll TJ, Herbert RD, Munn J, Lee M, Gandevia SC. Contralateral effect of unilateral strength training: evidence and possible mechanisms. J Appl Physiol. 2006;101(5):1514–22. https://doi.org/10.1152/japplphysiol.00531.2006.
18. Rice DA, McNair JP. Quadriceps arthrogenic muscle inhibition: neural mechanisms and treatment perspectives. Semin Arthritis Rheum. 2010;40(3):250–66. https://doi.org/10.1016/j.semarthrit.2009.10.001.
19. McKeon PO, Wikstrom EA. Sensory-targeted ankle rehabilitation strategies for chronic ankle instability. Med Sci Sports Exerc. 2016;48(5):776–84. https://doi.org/10.1249/MSS.0000000000000859.
20. Rice D, McNair PJ, Dalbeth N. Effects of cryotherapy on arthrogenic muscle inhibition using an experimental model of knee swelling. Arthritis Rheum. 2009;61(1):78–83. https://doi.org/10.1002/art.24168.
21. Burcal CJ, Hoch MC, Wikstrom EA. Effects of a stocking on plantar sensation in individuals with and without ankle instability. Muscle Nerve. 2017;55(4):513–9. https://doi.org/10.1002/mus.25362.
22. Rahnama L, Salvati M, Akhbari B, Mazaheri M. Attentional demands and postural control in athletes with and without functional ankle instability. J Orthop Sports Phys Ther. 2010;40(3):180–7. https://doi.org/10.2519/jospt.2010.3188.
23. Webster KA, Gribble PA. Functional rehabilitation interventions for chronic ankle instability: a systematic review. J Sport Rehabil. 2017;19(1):98–114.
24. Kiers H, Brumagne S, van Dieën J, van der Wees P, Vanhees L. Ankle proprioception is not targeted by exercises on an unstable surface. Eur J Appl Physiol. 2012;112(4):1577–85. https://doi.org/10.1007/s00421-011-2124-8.
25. Fong DT, Hong Y, Shima Y, Krosshaug T, Yung PS, Chan KM. Biomechanics of supination ankle sprain: a case report of an accidental injury event in the laboratory. Am J Sports Med. 2009;37(4):822–7. https://doi.org/10.1177/0363546508328102.
26. Fong DT, Ha SC, Mok KM, Chan CW, Chan KM. Kinematics analysis of ankle inversion ligamentous sprain injuries in sports: five cases from televised tennis competitions. Am J Sports Med. 2012;40(11):2627–32. https://doi.org/10.1177/0363546512458259.
27. Hertel J. Functional anatomy, pathomechanics, and pathophysiology of lateral ankle instability. J Athl Train. 2002;37(4):364–75.
28. Donovan L, Hart JM, Saliba SA, Park J, Feger MA, Herb CC, Hertel J. Rehabilitation for chronic ankle instability with or without destabilization devices: a randomized controlled trial. J Athl Train. 2016;51(3):233–51. https://doi.org/10.4085/1062-6050-51.3.09.
29. Terrier R, Degache F, Fourchet F, Gojanovic B, Forestier N. Assessment of evertor weakness in patients with chronic ankle instability: functional versus isokinetic testing. Clin Biomech. 2017;41:54–9. https://doi.org/10.1016/j.clinbiomech.2016.12.002.
30. Konradsen L. Factors contributing to chronic ankle instability: kinesthesia and joint position sense. J Athl Train. 2002;37(4):381–5.
31. Konradsen L. Sensori-motor control of the uninjured and injured human ankle. J Electromyogr Kinesiol. 2002;12(3):199–203.
32. Kristjansson E, Treleaven J. Sensorimotor function and dizziness in neck pain: implications for assessment and management. J Orthop Sports Phys Ther. 2009;3(5):364–77. https://doi.org/10.2519/jospt.2009.2834.
33. Mourcou Q, Fleury A, Diot B, Franco C, Vuillerme N. Mobile phone-based joint angle measurement for functional assessment and rehabilitation of proprioception. Biomed Res Int. 2015;2015:328142. https://doi.org/10.1155/2015/328142.
34. Jones DA, Rutherford OM, Parker DF. Physiological changes in skeletal muscle as a result of strength training. Exp Physiol. 1989;74(3):233–56. https://doi.org/10.1113/expphysiol.1989.sp003268.
35. Wilson GJ, Murphy AJ, Walshe A. The specificity of strength training: the effect of posture. Euro J Appl Physiol. 1996;73(3–4):346–52. https://doi.org/10.1007/BF02425497.
36. Forestier N, Toschi P. The effects of an ankle destabilization device on muscular activity while walking. Int J Sports Med. 2014;26(6):464–70. https://doi.org/10.1055/s-2004-830336.
37. Hertel J, Braham RA, Hale SA, Olmsted-Kramer LC. Simplifying the star excursion balance test: analyses of subjects with and without chronic ankle instability. J Orthop Sports Phys Ther. 2006;36(3):131–7. https://doi.org/10.2519/jospt.2006.36.3.131.
38. Docherty CL, Arnold BL, Gansneder BM, Hurwitz S, Gieck J. Functional-performance deficits in volunteers with functional ankle instability. J Athl Train. 2005;40(1):30–4.
39. Eechaute C, Roel De Ridder R, Maes T, David Beckwée D, Swinnen E, Buyl R, Vaes P. Evidence of a different landing strategy in subjects with chronic ankle instability. Gait Posture. 2017;52:62–7. https://doi.org/10.1016/j.gaitpost.2016.11.002.
40. Doherty C, Bleakley C, Delahunt E, Holden S. Treatment and prevention of acute and recurrent ankle sprain: an overview of systematic reviews with meta-analysis. Br J Sports Med. 2017;51:113–25. https://doi.org/10.1136/bjsports-2016-097339.
41. Wikstrom EA, Hubbard-Turner T, McKeon PO. Understanding and treating ankle sprains and their consequences: a constraints based approach. Sports Med. 2013;43(6):385–93. https://doi.org/10.1007/s40279-013-0043-z.

35 Rehabilitation Options for Chronic Ankle Instability: What Is New?

Romain Terrier, Yves Tourné, Brice Picot, and Nicolas Forestier

35.1 Background: Current Methods of Rehabilitation of the Chronically Unstable Ankle

35.1.1 Current Management of Functional Ankle Instability

Simultaneously with the management of pain and oedema, and the restoration of joint range of motion, there is an international consensus to recommend an early neuromuscular reprogramming. Muscle and proprioceptive deficits induced by trauma and deteriorated by immobilization must be functionally re-educated through a sensorimotor reprogramming to restore the active joint protection system. Specifically, it means strengthening the ankle stabilizing muscles (eversors) associated with proprioceptive work.

Although management protocols clearly lack standardization, the vast majority of physiotherapists use methods and tools which are similar in their characteristics. Strengthening the fibular muscles is conventionally done in non-weight-bearing stance with the physiotherapist applying manual resistance or by using an electrostimulation device. Some therapists use a rubber band to offer resistance to the eversors. As regards proprioceptive restoration work, the tools that are used by the patients with instructions to keep their balance generate multidirectional destabilization. This family of tools, based on the concept of optimization of the reflex loop described over 45 years ago by Freeman and colleagues [1], includes the wobble board, the trampoline, foam supports, or else the Dotte swing. Only rarely do some therapists use unidirectional destabilization tools (Vaast table, propriofoot). These methods and tools briefly presented here are a good illustration of the neuromuscular rehabilitation path now followed by most patients suffering from an acute ankle sprain episode or from a chronic ankle instability condition. It is therefore appropriate to question the effectiveness of this management, in terms of recurrence rate.

R. Terrier (✉) · N. Forestier
Inter-University Laboratory of Human Movement Science (EA 7424), Département STAPS, University Savoie Mont-Blanc, Mont-Blanc, France
e-mail: Nicolas.Forestier@univ-savoie.fr

Y. Tourné
Foot & Ankle Surgery, Osteo-Articular Center of Cèdres - Parc Galaxie Sud, Echirolles, France

B. Picot
Physiotherapy Practice, Aix-les-Bains, France

H. Pereira et al. (eds.), *Lateral Ankle Instability*, https://doi.org/10.1007/978-3-662-62763-1_35

35.1.2 How Effective Is this Conventional Approach?

Functional treatment has been recognized as the most suitable therapy for over two decades [2, 3]; however, the study of its effectiveness, when the management is done with the most commonly used techniques, proves to be much more complex and nuanced as regard the traumatic recurrence rate.

The analysis on the subject is rather disappointing: Hertel [4] concluded that current techniques do nothing to prevent re-injury as recurrence rates are generally higher than 30% and may reach 73%. The same author stated that the first factor that exposes us to the risk of lateral ankle sprain is having had a previous ankle sprain, which implies that the level of initial joint protection has not been restored following rehabilitation. Among sports people, various studies have reported, for over two decades, recurrence rates of 70–80% in patients who had neuromuscular rehabilitation [5, 6]. In the same vein, questionnaires have been available to STAPS students at the University of Savoy for 3 years [7]. Every year, the results of more than 200 young athletes show comparable recurrence rates (over 50%) in groups (1) having not had any physiotherapy management or (2) having had physiotherapy management.

Finally, the meta-analysis of Postle et al. [8] concludes that proprioceptive rehabilitation on unstable surfaces has not proved its effectiveness with respect to traumatic recurrence. To sum up, although neuromuscular rehabilitation is necessary, it seems essential to seriously consider improvement areas. In this chapter, we will try to develop detailed specifications for optimizing the functional rehabilitation of unstable ankles, based on current scientific knowledge in terms of proprioceptive acuity development, muscle strengthening, and neuromuscular reprogramming. This is a particularly appropriate time for this work since, as we have previously stated, the commonly used techniques with their limited effectiveness are based on old concepts [1] and have not yet been updated.

35.2 Toward an Optimization of Rehabilitation Methods

35.2.1 Optimizing Ankle Proprioceptive Work

35.2.1.1 Why Include Proprioceptive Rehabilitation in the Management of Unstable Ankles?

When anatomical lesions have occurred, for instance when one or more bundles of the lateral collateral ligament of the ankle are affected, the proprioception sense can be altered [9]. Indeed, the injury mechanism leads to a stretching of the capsular ligament system which deteriorates mechanoreceptors. Besides, post-trauma immobilization (strict or partial) which facilitates the ligament healing process also increases the proprioceptive deficit through deconditioning effects. Finally, nociceptive information and the presence of a periarticular edema in the early post-traumatic days result in impaired proprioceptive signals. Thus, since the work of Freeman et al. [1], the restoration of satisfactory proprioceptive acuity has been part of standard ankle sprain rehabilitation. It should be remembered though the reasons why quality proprioceptive work is essential to ankle rehabilitation.

Satisfactory proprioceptive acuity enables a person to know her ankle position with accuracy in all circumstances and without using her sight. This allows for a well-adapted positioning of the joint, and especially during critical phases such as jump landing or heel striking when running. The fact that the central nervous system (CNS) integrates ankle movements rapidly and accurately allows the detection of potentially lesional movements (quick inversion) and so makes it possible to develop the required joint protection strategies such as weight unloading associated with fibular activation.

Quality proprioceptive information allows proactively (feedforward) the integration into the initial motor program of motor commands protective of the ankle. For instance, the detection of an inversion ankle when jumping will allow the integration into the initial motor program of fibular activation before the foot touches the ground, so as to replace the ankle in neutral position and lock it. Activation of this protective motor control is based on the integration of reliable and accurate proprioceptive data.

It is now clear that proprioceptive work following an ankle sprain is an essential element of rehabilitation. So we will now examine the limitations of the tools typically used in this context by therapists.

35.2.1.2 Lack of Specificity of the Commonly Used Tools

Traditionally, physical therapists use various tools mentioned previously that mostly result in multidirectional destabilization. Proprioceptive training is grounded in the concept of destabilization, but the tools that are used have important limitations. Their main limitations are due to the fact that they generate multidirectional destabilizations that are quite removed from the injury mechanism. Indeed, the inversion/eversion axis of the rearfoot as well as the dissociation between forefoot and rearfoot are seldom reproduced. Now, the patient's foot never completely gives away when the sprain occurs. There is therefore in any potentially lesional ankle movement a differential couple at midfoot level. This couple represents a significant source of proprioceptive signal not to be overlooked. So what it really means is that the tools used do not seem specific enough to work on ankle proprioceptive acuity. This was corroborated by the results of the recent study by Kiers et al. [10]. The authors used the proprioceptive disruption caused by tendon vibration (artificial discharge of spindles) as a probe to investigate the recourse to different sources of proprioceptive data. Thanks to this experiment, and in the same line as previous work [11], Kiers et al. [10] demonstrated that equilibration work on unstable multidirectional surfaces does not target proprioceptive work of the ankle. Indeed, with this type of tool, the patients chiefly resort to proprioceptive information from the lumbar area (and most certainly to vestibular information as well). Such data suggest that a patient whose postural performance improves on unstable platforms is not in fact a patient whose ankle proprioceptive acuity has been optimized. In other words, you can become an expert on unstable surfaces without necessarily having restored your ankle proprioceptive acuity. This is also confirmed by the results of Bernier and Perrin [12] who observed, following rehabilitation on unstable platforms, postural performance improvement which was not associated with better proprioceptive acuity assessed through a repositioning test. In conclusion, the conventionally used tools seem to lack specificity to effectively optimize and target ankle proprioceptive acuity. Moreover, the impossibility to work in locomotion (walking, running, changing direction, stairs), whereas ankle sprains always occur in locomotion, represents major limitations for these tools. And last, early proprioceptive work is recommended, but the absence of destabilization amplitude adjustment allowing for progression in rehabilitation makes it impossible for the patients to use these tools from the early days of functional rehabilitation. It is indeed an additional limitation.

35.2.1.3 How to Give Proprioceptive Work the Specificity It Clearly Needs?

Proprioceptive work must ideally be performed in conditions that are as close as possible to the injury mechanism, while ensuring a secured environment. This means that a very specific work is essential to proprioception optimization and efficient detection of potentially lesional joint movements. As Vanbiervliet indicated [9], the natural location of mechanoreceptors involves optimal detection of physiological movements. Regarding the ankle, this concept is supported by shorter reaction time values of the fibular when sudden ankle destabilization occurs along the physiological axis of the subtalar joint (Henke's axis) compared to destabilization along a sagittal axis [13]. This result strongly suggests that solicitation along the physiological axis optimizes the sensorimotor loop by promoting detection of the ankle movements through peripheral proprioceptors. Besides, data have proved that equilibration in unipodal stance loads the fibular muscles, all the more so as destabilization is generated specifically around Henke's axis [14]. That also represents a strong argument for the need of specifically geared destabilization to optimize proprioceptive rehabilitation of the ankle. Finally, in line with the work of Kiers et al. [10], our team (in collaboration with the Research Group of Movement Analysis and Ergonomics—GRAME—Laval University, Quebec, Canada) recently demonstrated that equilibration work on a specific destabilization tool whose characteristics are inspired by the functional anatomy of the rearfoot and which allows a metatarsal anchoring makes it possible to specifically solicit the ankle peripheral proprioceptive information and targets the recruiting of the fibular muscles [15].

35.2.2 Optimizing Ankle Evertors Strengthening

Like proprioceptive work, muscle building is a process-specific training. This fact is well known by physical trainers, and it is supported by various publications, most of which are decades old. The specificity of the muscle building process implies that its effects are limited to working conditions, or in this case to the conditions adopted during rehabilitation. These conditions relate to different factors.

The gain obtained from muscle strengthening is superior in the angular sector of work, compared to the other joint angles [16]. If we want the fibular muscles to be able to initiate a protective eversion moment on the whole joint amplitude, then we should work on the largest physiological joint amplitude possible.

The objective of fibular muscles strengthening should be to enable these muscles to initiate a moment of evertor force capable of effectively protecting and stabilizing the ankle in potential trauma situations. The load to be supported corresponds to the patient's bodyweight plus the kinetic energy developed on jump landing or heel striking when running. Low-load muscular work does not effectively increase maximum strength [17]. So during fibular muscles strengthening exercises a load equal to the patient's bodyweight at least should be imposed by the end of rehabilitation management.

Muscle strengthening work is specific to the contraction mode in which the muscle group is solicited [18]. The fibular muscles protect the ankle in eccentric (control action of the inversion movement) and in concentric (generates eversion movement). Moreover, Stauber [19] showed that work in eccentric mode allows for the optimization of strength gains compared to concentric work in similar angular sectors of work. Collado et al. [20] recently demonstrated the application of this principle to fibular muscles strengthening in patients suffering their first lateral ankle sprain. Thus, all these data show that it is necessary to add to concentric strengthening exercises, protocols of fibular eccentric strengthening in the management of unstable ankles, especially as patients with chronic instability show a control deficit (eccentric) of ankle inversion in weight-bearing support [21].

Muscle strengthening work in a given position, performing a specific movement, is particularly transferable to the reproduction of the same movement in tasks performed in the same position [22]. As regards fibular muscles strengthening, this conclusion strongly suggests the importance of weight-bearing work in inversion/eversion. Such weight-bearing work also offers the advantage of opposing body weight resistance if the patient is in unipodal support.

To summarize, in order to optimize fibular muscles strengthening as part of ankle sprain or chronic ankle instability functional rehabilitation, the physiotherapist must make sure to:

- Target fibular muscles training by performing inversions/eversion
- Work on the largest physiological joint amplitude possible
- Impose a sufficient load for the fibular muscles to be able to produce a real stabilizing evertor moment in a potentially traumatic context
- Integrate modes of concentric and eccentric contractions of the fibular muscles

- Work in conditions as close to injury mechanisms as possible, namely in weight-bearing stance and possibly in locomotion or jump landing.

35.2.3 Integrating a Neuromuscular Reprogramming Component

The previous paragraphs have enabled us to define the major characteristics that determine the efficiency of ankle proprioceptive acuity optimization, on the one hand, and fibular strengthening optimization, on the other hand. These two aspects are the pillars of functional rehabilitation of the ankle. They should however not be considered as an end in itself. They are in fact essential and complementary prerequisites for neuromuscular reprogramming of joint protection strategies. Neuromuscular reprogramming consists in putting to music quality afferent proprioceptive information and efferent motor information which activate a powerful muscular system in order to develop and integrate neuromuscular strategies of effective joint protection. To do so, the patient should be placed in conditions that are close to the injury mechanism but in a secured context. Those conditions must include various motor situations whose difficulty gradually evolves, and which eventually gets closer to the patient's usual solicitation, i.e., to their sporting activity(es), when applicable. The two effective joint protection strategies are fibular proactivation to prevent destabilization in inversion and body weight unloading to avoid trauma in case of sudden destabilization.

35.2.3.1 Proactivation of the Fibular Muscles

Patients with chronic ankle instability show activation deficits of the eversor muscles. As a matter of fact, during the gait cycle in the case of the unstable ankle, the fibulars are activated to a lesser extent as compared to the healthy ankle [23]. Besides, the proactivation level (activation, 100 ms before foot comes into contact with the ground) of these same muscles when jump landing is inferior among subjects with chronic instability, compared to healthy subjects [24]. This proactivation deficit of the fibular muscles particularly puts the subject at risk of chronic instability, even if proprioceptive and strength production qualities have been satisfactorily restored. Indeed, fibular proactivation (activation before foot hits the ground) is the main neuromuscular strategy of ankle protection. So why develop an efficient production capacity of evertors moment if the central nervous system (CNS) cannot activate the fibular muscles in time to protect the joint?

Thonnard demonstrated in 1988 [25] that an ankle sprain could occur in just 30 ms, while the implementation of the feedback loop which activates the fibular muscles requires 60–70 ms [13, 26]. This feedback loop refers to the latency between the beginning of ankle destabilization and electromyographic activation of the fibular: it is peroneal reaction time (PRT). Konradsen [26] reported that an evertors moment occurs about 150 ms after destabilization. This means that about 80 ms are required after fibular activation to initiate a force moment protective of the ankle. This additional delay refers to the electromechanical delay (EMD) of the fibular. This is the necessary time between muscle activation and force production. The sequence of these inescapable events is shown in Fig. 35.1. Faced with these findings, it appears that activation of the fibular via a sensorimotor feedback loop does not represent the optimal joint protection mechanism.

Moreover, Thonnard's studies show that when performing tasks that particularly constrain the ankle such as walking downstairs or jumping below, the fibular muscles are always activated before heel strikes the ground. So it seems that the feedback loop deficit is counterbalanced by ankle stabilization before the foot impacts the ground. This locking is the result of proactivation of the fibular muscles. Functional rehabilitation should consequently focus on restoring the integrity of motor programs that incorporate this early activation of the fibular muscles in the various at-risk activities for ankle sprains.

As illustrated in Fig. 35.2, Forestier and Toschi [15] reported fibular activation 77 ms, on average, before heel striking in subjects who were

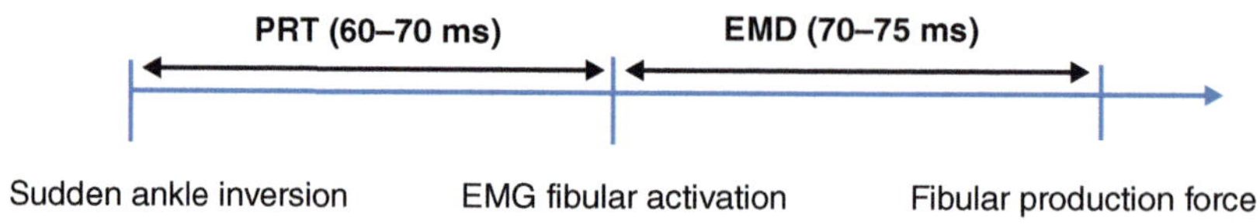

Fig. 35.1 Diagram of the chronology of events occurring between sudden ankle destabilization and ankle evertor muscles force production

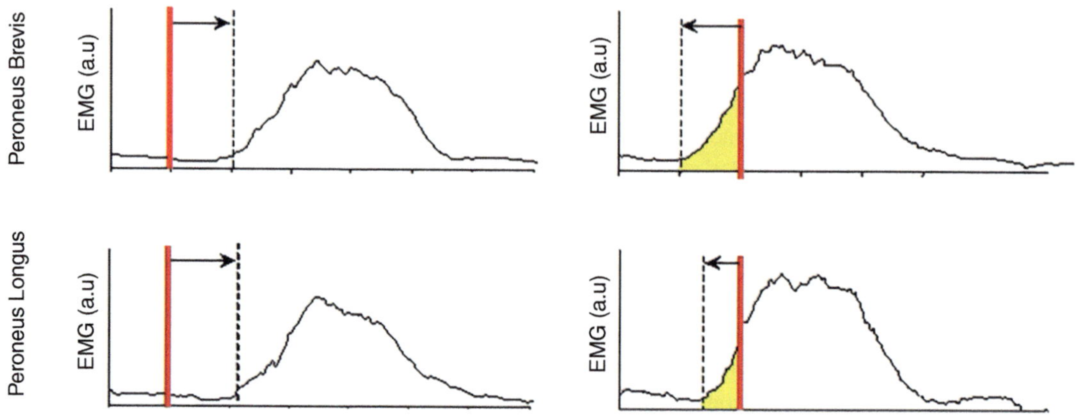

Fig. 35.2 Illustration of fibular proactivation when walking with destabilizing rearfoot articulator boots. Left: normal walking; right: destabilized walking. Top: fibularis brevis activity, below fibularis longus activity. The vertical red line indicates when heel strikes the ground; the black dotted line indicates muscle activation. From Forestier and Toschi [15]

walking with destabilizing rearfoot articulators boots which destabilized their ankles in inversion. This proactivation allowed subjects to walk naturally by blocking destabilization before heel striking. In fact, in order to do this, proactivation of the fibular muscles should be initiated at a time value which corresponds to their electromechanical delay, that is 75–80 ms. Such proactivation allows rearfoot stabilization before heel hits the ground without altering the walking pattern since the fibular force production coincides with the loading. It therefore appears that destabilization close to the injury mechanism and in a secured context encourages fibular proactivation strategies. It is interesting to note that the results of Forestier and Toschi [15] have recently been reproduced by the team of Pr Hertel [27, 28] at the University of Virginia (USA).

It is also useful to note that in case of significant destabilization (such as setting foot on a sidewalk kerb), 80 ms proactivation allowing to set foot on the ground simultaneously with the genesis of the evertors moment is not sufficient to prevent destabilization. However, such proactivation allows, by increasing muscle stiffness, a reduction of peroneal reaction time on the one hand, and electromechanical delay on the other hand [29].

In light of the findings mentioned above, it is legitimate to raise a major question: how is it possible for the CNS to integrate into the initial motor program a fibular activation order 80 ms before setting foot on the ground whatever the nature and speed of the locomotion movements (running, lateral leaps, jump landing, etc.). The answer to this question lies in the predictive ability of the central nervous system. Through the efference copy (i.e., copy of motor command generated by the primary motor cortex and conveyed to other cortical areas and the cerebellum), the central nervous system is able to predict the sensory consequences of future actions and to refine them pro-actively (feedforward). The efference copy concept was widely described by Schmidt [30] and is a major neurophysiological pillar of internal models theory [31].

Specifically, the motor command generated to perform a stride allows the CNS to predict the moment when the foot hits the ground and integrate proactively (i.e., before any sensory feedback from potential ankle destabilization) a fibular activation command about 80 ms before foot/ground impact. In addition, the CNS relies on the integration of sensory information to determine whether such proactivation is necessary for joint protection. These data useful to determine the potential danger to the ankle can be visual (e.g., unstable ground, roots, scree) or proprioceptive (e.g., inversion ankle during the lifting phase). This is particularly in that sense that proprioceptive restoration, as discussed above, represents a major challenge for functional rehabilitation.

In summary, functional rehabilitation of the ankle must focus on the restoration of a satisfactory capacity of fibular force production. Restoration of proprioceptive acuity is also essential for sensory integration which allows the detection of at-risk situations such as an ankle positioned in inversion before the foot hits the ground. These sensory inputs condition the feedforward motor programming of joint protection strategies such as proactivation of the fibular muscles. To restore the capacity to have recourse to these proactivation strategies requires neuromuscular reprogramming training built on the specific characteristics described in the following.

- A rearfoot destabilization as close as possible to the injury mechanism (inversion).
- A dynamic work capacity in locomotion, performing several steps, and consecutive leaps. Indeed, behavioral neurosciences have demonstrated repeatedly that motor programming of individual tasks (discrete, such as an isolated jump) is widely different from that of continuous tasks (such as a jump followed by running). But ankle sprains occur during continuous tasks such as running (sequence of strides) or changes of direction while walking. Reprogramming the ability to resort to pro-fibular activation strategies should ideally be based on continuous and destabilizing dynamic exercises such as walking, running, or performing lateral leaps. It thus seems important that thc destabilizing element should be placed under the patient's rearfoot.
- Capacity to solicit proactivation at an early stage during rehabilitation. In other words, the patient should work on a dynamic and little constraining mode such as walking at first (while ensuring that it generates proactivation, which means destabilizing the ankle).
- Capacity to resort to proactivation fibular strategies in the most varied dynamic tasks adapted to the progressive process of rehabilitation. In other words, rehabilitation must cover a whole range of situations the patient is commonly faced with, so the exercises will start with early walking to the most demanding activities (according to their sporting activities).

35.2.3.2 Body Weight Unloading Strategies

It must be recalled that ankle inversion is a physiological movement and thus not systematically traumatic even with large amplitudes. It is the combination of large amplitudes in inversion and body weight loading which generates trauma [26, 32]. With this in mind, Schmitt et al. [33] suggested that in case of sudden destabilization in inversion, the critical moment for traumatic risk corresponded to maximum loading after destabilization. These authors also suggested that the delay (though they did not actually calculate it) between EMG activation of the fibular muscles and that critical moment could be of great interest to evaluate the eversors capacity to actively protect the ankle in case of sudden destabilization. In other words, if this delay is superior to the EMG fibular activation (delay between muscle activation and force production, see Fig. 35.1), the fibular muscles would be able to actively stabilize the destabilized ankle at the critical moment.

To address this critical question, our team has developed a study to measure the delay between fibular activation and maximum loading following an ankle sudden inversion. The essential prerequisite for such a study is to replicate sudden destabilization as closely as possible to the traumatic mechanism. To do so, the subjects were in unipodal stance on a device generating sudden inversion by means of an articulator inspired by the subtalar mechanics and controlled by an electromagnet. It was also necessary to ensure that the inversion speeds generated approached the real traumatic mechanism. To do so, we can refer to recent data from Fong et al. [34] and Kristianslund et al. [35] who reported peak values of inversion speed during real ankle sprains of around 623°/s and 559°/s, respectively.

For the tests associated with inversion velocity peaks superior to 550°/s, we calculated the time between fibular activation and maximum loading on the destabilized support (critical moment). It is clear from this analysis that the delay was consistently higher than the 75 ms fibular electromechanical delay with an average of 90 ms. Finally, this result strongly suggests that the fibular muscles have the capacity to actively protect the ankle in case of sudden inversion, which enables us to understand that sprain can be avoided in the event of sudden destabilization. However, we have to understand what strategies are developed to ensure adequate delay between muscle activation and maximum loading.

Analysis of the vertical force profiles in the study previously presented highlights the systematic use of an unloading strategy. Such organization reflects temporary relief which can delay the critical moment, i.e., the loading peak. Konradsen [26] was the first author to declare that such a relief mechanism might play a crucial role in ankle joint protection in the event of sudden inversion. He even suggested that unloading may be the result of a deliberate action, a global pattern in response to ankle destabilization. Along the same lines, Santos and Liu [36] analyzed the postural reactions of subjects with no previous ankle injury to which they applied nociceptive stimuli to their leg lateral compartment. It is interesting to note that unloading strategies were found only when the patients' ankle was in inversion at the time of the painful stimuli. These unloading strategies were the result of a triple hip–knee–ankle flexion. The same stimuli applied to the same subjects, ankle in neutral position, did not lead to any postural reaction. This differential result, although obtained using an experimental protocol that did not integrate the reproduction of ankle sprain mechanism, is a strong argument in favor of voluntary use of unloading strategies as a means of ankle joint protection.

The knowledge developed here becomes especially interesting for the therapist if it turns out that the use of unloading strategies can be optimized by rehabilitation. That is precisely what Konradsen [26] suggested who considered unloading strategies as an "active muscular defense mechanism to sudden ankle destabilization of cortical origin and therefore likely to react positively to training." Moreover, Santos et al. [36] reported that the unloading strategies observed when nociceptive stimuli were applied on subjects' leg lateral compartment, ankle in inversion, have larger amplitude and are implemented faster in subjects with chronic ankle instability than in healthy subjects. The authors interpreted this result as the expression of a learning phenomenon that results from frequent real-life situations from subjects suffering chronic ankle instability in their recurring destabilizing episodes.

Finally, the currently available scientific data allow us to consider unloading strategies as an effective mechanism for ankle joint protection. This is the last defense when joint stabilization is found deficient. Besides, it also appears that the use of these active joint protection strategies can be optimized by training, which gives the therapists a practical perspective on their rehabilitation programs. The kind of action that appears most relevant in this regard is to place the patient—toward the end of their rehabilitation and when all the other objectives have been achieved—in situations close to the injury mechanism while ensuring a secured environment. Specifically, what should be done is generate sudden inversion, at speeds comparable to the injury mechanism, while providing a mechanical lock that prevents injury in case of inadequate response from the patient (secured context).

35.2.4 Presentation of the Myolux™ Concept

The optimization axes of unstable ankles' neuromuscular rehabilitation that have previously been developed represented real specifications for our team whose aim is to offer a more effective alternative. Our reflection on the basis of those specifications resulted in the development of the Myolux™ concept. Figure 35.3 shows the device currently available to professionals in charge of functional rehabilitation.

On the one hand, Myolux Medik e-volution is equipped with a rearfoot articulator inspired by the rearfoot functional anatomy (Henke's axis): destabilization is generated in inversion/eversion and metatarsal anchoring is allowed. An Inertial Measurement Unit has been integrated, and a specific Software has been developed allowing proprioceptive impairment assessment (position sense) as well as specific stimulation and evolution under unweight and weight-bearing (Fig. 35.4) conditions.

Different destabilization amplitude settings of the rearfoot and stabilization or destabilization of the forefoot (optional anchoring of the metatarsal support) allow progression in the difficulty of the exercises proposed during the management of the injury. Such a device allows rehabilitation professionals to optimize proprioceptive work [37]. This is due to a specific and targeted work on the ankle which is the only structure whose muscular system is able to control generated destabilization. In line with the work of Kiers et al. [10], our team (in collaboration with the Research Group in Movement Analysis and Ergonomics—GRAME—Laval University, Quebec, Canada) recently demonstrated that equilibration work on this destabilization device specifically solicits ankle peripheral proprioceptive information and targets the recruiting of the fibular muscles [38].

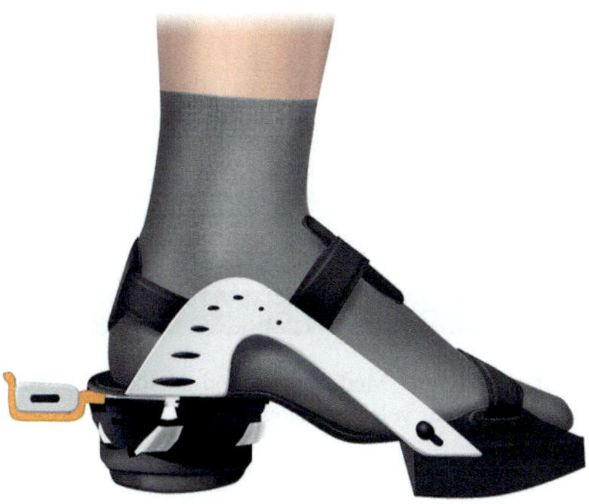

Fig. 35.3 Illustration of the Myolux Medik e-volution orthosis

Myolux Medik e-volution also optimizes evertor weakness assessment and strengthening since, by the end of the progressive rehabilitation, it allows a targeted weight-bearing work, with maximal physiological amplitude, and in concentric and eccentric modes. The superiority of such a protocol over strengthening against manual resistance or by electrostimulation was demonstrated [39]. Moreover, our works allowed to identify an accessible and functional parameter for evertor weakness assessment [21, 40]. Patients just have to control ankle inversion movements in weight-bearing conditions without exceeding a threshold of 60°/s (Fig. 35.5).

The Myolux Medik e-volution software allows proprioceptive and evertor performance assessment and follow-up by means of an intuitive interface presented in Fig. 35.6.

Finally, the possibility of working in locomotion offers the opportunity to generate and automate fibular proactivation strategies [15, 27, 28]. Moreover, sudden destabilization, caused by muscle fatigue during body weight eversors strengthening or by the therapist manual destabilization, allows us to generate inversions associated with angular velocity peaks comparable to those observed during a real sprain injury [13]. This capacity to simulate the real trauma kinematic characteristics (trajectory, speed) in a secured environment enables the patients to resort to unloading strategies [41].

All these features allow the Myolux™ device and its associated rehabilitation protocols to optimize the management of unstable ankles. A preliminary clinical study [41] reported a 12%

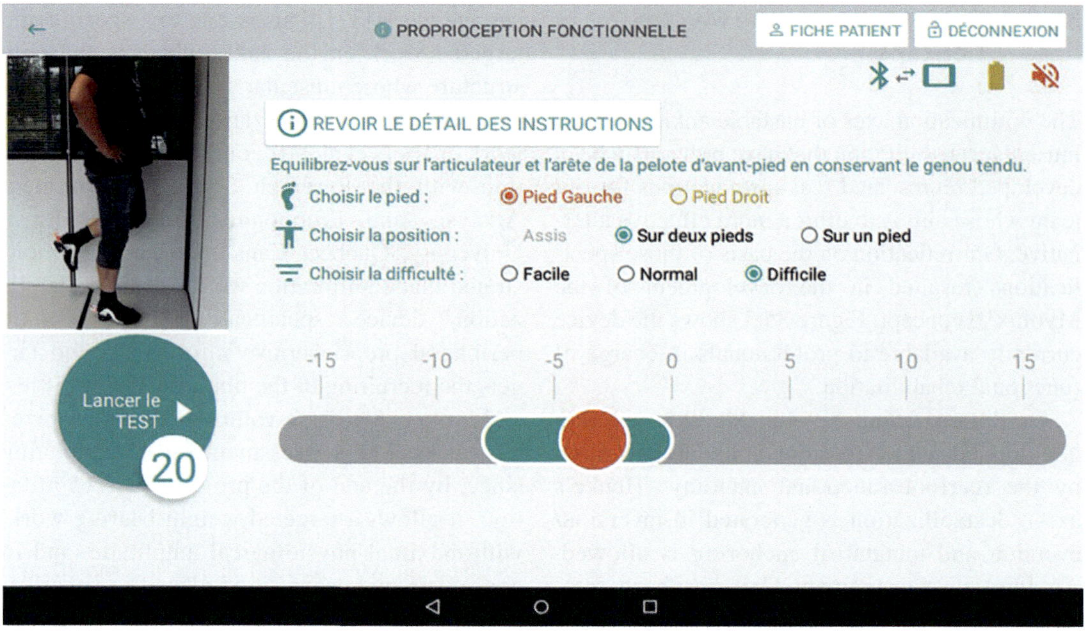

Fig. 35.4 Ankle proprioception assessment and stimulation with the Myolux Medik e-volution device. The patient has to keep the orange ball representing rearfoot position into the green area

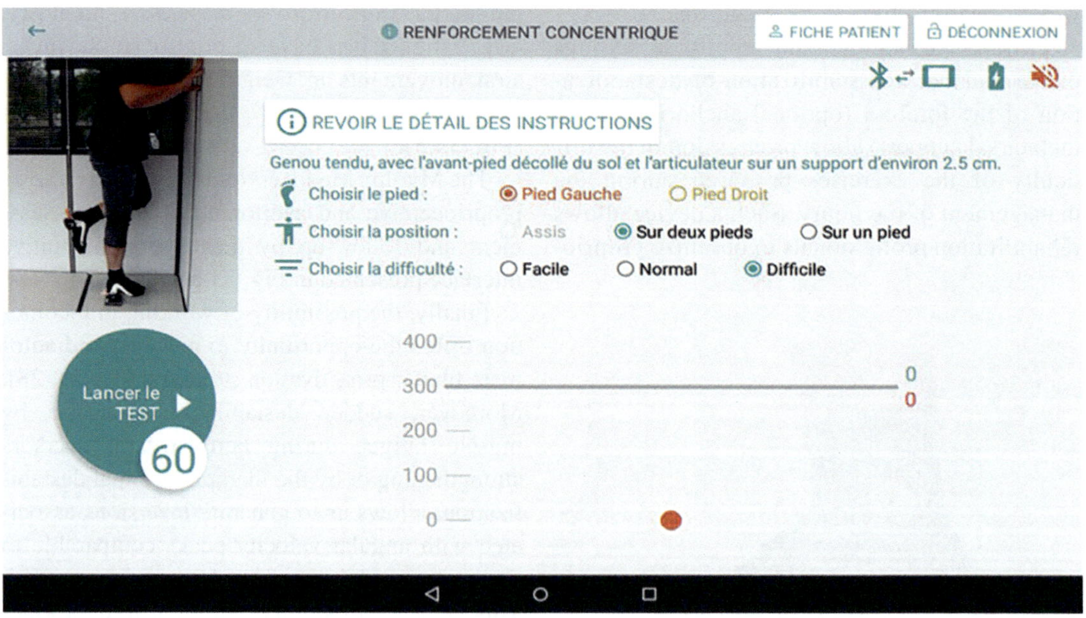

Fig. 35.5 Ankle evertor eccentric assessment and stimulation with the Myolux Medik e-volution device. The patient has to control ankle inversion in weight-bearing condition keeping the angular velocity below 60°/s

recurrence rate after 18 months in a population having had a ten-session rehabilitation. This recurrence rate falls to 3% for patients who have had a monthly booster session. These results are well below the recurrence rate commonly reported in scientific literature and mentioned in

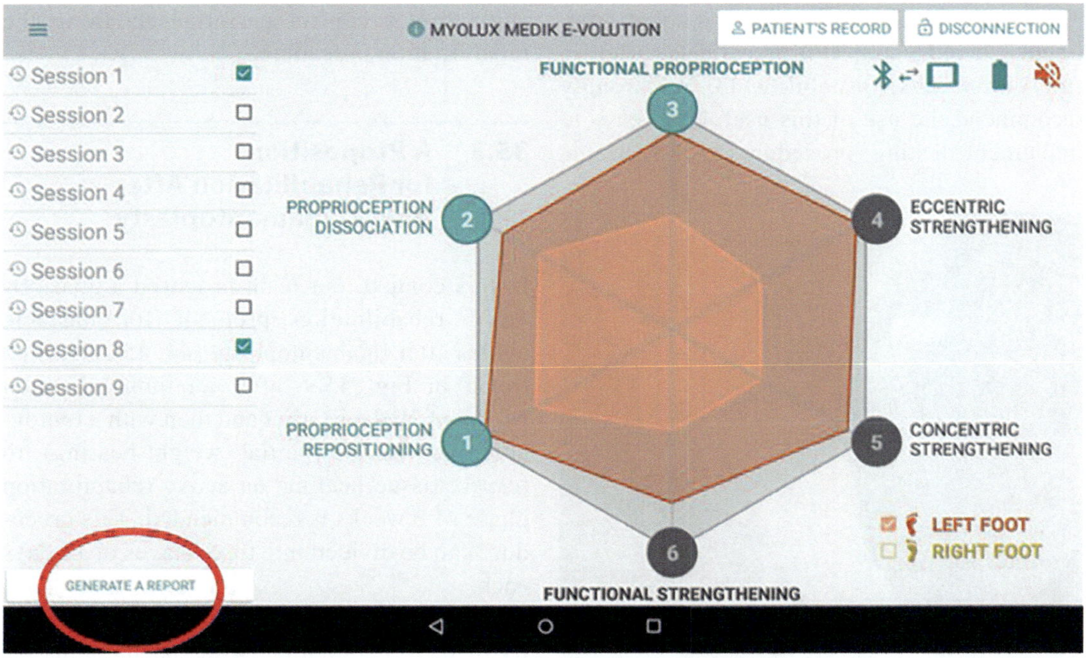

Fig. 35.6 Example of the assessment screen of the Myolux Medik e-volution. This patient had strong evertor strength deficit (4-5-6) during the first session, and this weakness was clearly reduced during session 8

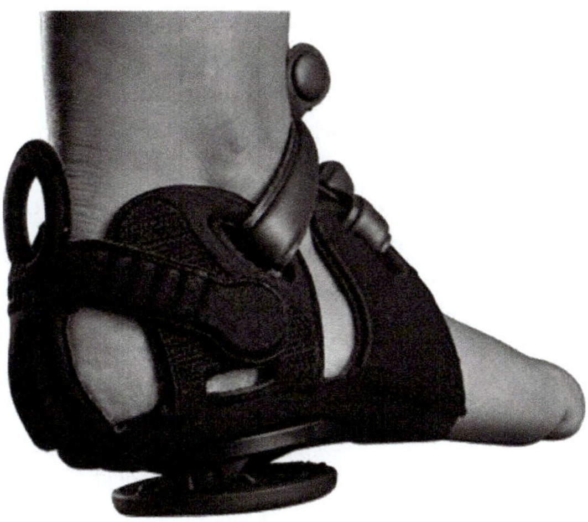

Fig. 35.7 Illustration of the Myolux Soft™ device

the introduction to this chapter. The interest of a regular maintenance work of active joint protection must be seen in light of these results. It is in this spirit that a maintenance device Myolux Soft has been developed for patients to use independently (Fig. 35.7).

A comparative, multicenter, and randomized study of clinical validation is currently underway. This work is coordinated by the team of Prof. Hertel (Virginia University—USA).

35.2.5 Ankle Motor Control Assessment

There is a growing evidence of the interest of dynamic postural control tests (Star Excursion Balance Test or Y Balance Test) to assess lower limb motor control and recovery [42]. This test is particularly easy to implement on the field, and data collection (reached distance expressed as a percentage of the lower limb length) can be made without any specific material. However, as highlighted by the authors, this testing procedure is not specific to a joint. In this context, our team showed that Y Balance Test performance could reveal specific ankle motor control deficit is patients are placed under a modified configuration. This configuration consists in a specific and physiological rearfoot destabilization (Fig. 35.8), and we have evidenced that a threshold performance of

82% of the lower limb length was able to distinguish healthy subject from patients suffering from chronic ankle instability [43]. We strongly recommend the use of this useful and easy to implement testing procedure to assess the ankle motor control performance along the rehabilitation procedure.

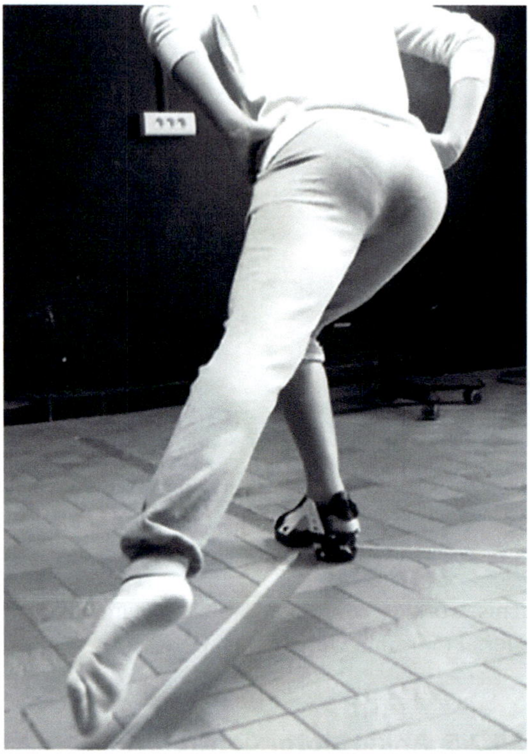

Fig. 35.8 Configuration of the modified Y Balance Test. The right (tested) ankle is placed on a specific and physiological rearfoot destabilization (a Myolux™ device here)

35.3 A Proposition for Rehabilitation After Ankle Ligamentoplasty

In this context, our team proposed a goal oriented rehabilitation protocol for unstable ankles after ligamentoplasty [44, 45]. As illustrated in Fig. 35.9, after an immobilization period of 30 days (strict and then with a removable cast and a partial weight-bearing) to respect tissue healing, an active rehabilitation phase of 6 weeks is recommended. This procedure can be divided into three stages of 15 days each.

It is very important to respect the progressivity of the rehabilitation, with specific aims for each stage, as mentioned in Fig. 35.9. During the first stage, cutaneous and antalgic works are the main objectives, but the triceps sural stretching and "passive" motor (electrostimulation) and proprioceptive stimulation by means of illusions associated with tendinous vibrations can be implemented. During the second stage, proprioception acuity recovery represents the main goal. The purpose of the third stage is to restore proximal and distal muscular performance. It is important to at least assess proprioception acuity at the end of the second stage and ankle ever-

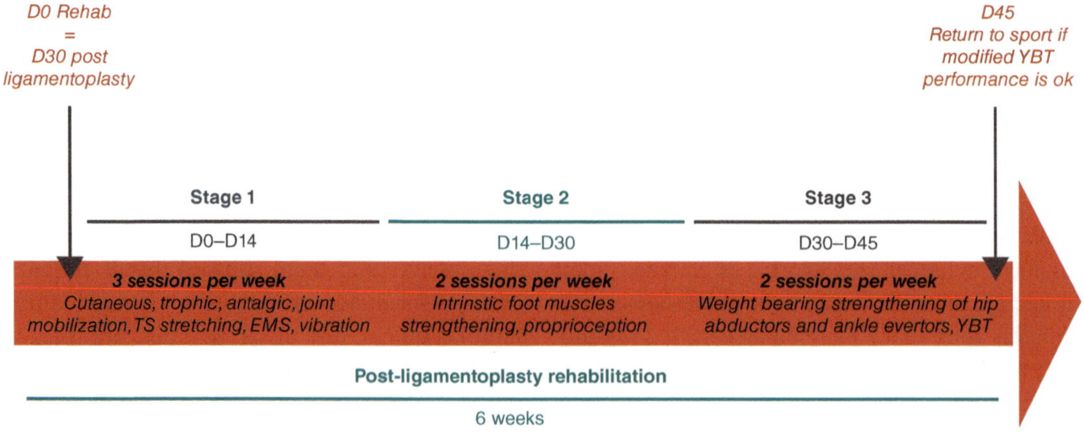

Fig. 35.9 Illustration of the main stages of ankle rehabilitation after a ligamentoplasty

tor muscles performance at the end of the third stage. Easy to reach and functional assessing procedures have been mentioned above in this chapter. Moreover, we strongly recommend a "return to sport" decision validated by a dynamic postural control performance assessed by means of the modified (unstable) Y Balance Test procedure.

References

1. Freeman MAR, Dean MRE, Haman IWF. The etiology and prevention of functional instability of the foot. J Bone Joint Surg. 1965;47:678–85.
2. Kannus P, Renstrom P. Treatment for acute tears of the lateral ligaments of the ankle: operation, cast, or early controlled mobilization. J Bone Joint Surg Am. 1991;73:305–12.
3. Kerkhoffs GM, Struijs PA, Marti RK, Blankevoort L, Assendelft WJ, van Dijk CN. Functional treatments for acute ruptures of the lateral ankle ligament: a systematic review. Acta Orthop Scand. 2003;74(1):69–77.
4. Hertel J. Functional anatomy, pathomechanics, and pathophysiology of lateral ankle instability. J Athl Train. 2002;37(4):364–75.
5. Webster KA, Gribble PA. Functional rehabilitation interventions for chronic ankle instability: a systematic review. J Sport Rehabil. 2010;19:e98–114.
6. Yeung MS, Chan KM, So CH, Yuan WY. An epidemiological survey on ankle sprain. Br J Sports Med. 1994;28:112–6.
7. Picot B, Terrier R, Forestier N. Le contrôle moteur et la protection articulaire de la cheville: concepts de base. Kinésithérapie Scientifique. 2012;530:57–8.
8. Postle K, Pak D, Smith TO. Effectiveness of proprioceptive exercises for ankle ligament injury in adults: a systematic literature and meta-analysis. Man Ther. 2012;17:285–91.
9. Vanbiervliet W. Circonstances et mécanismes d'altération de la proprioception au cours de lésions anatomiques. In: Julia M, et al., editors. La proprioception. Montpellier: Sauramps Medical; 2012. p. 66–77.
10. Kiers H, Brumagne S, van Dieën J, van der Wees P, Vanhees L. Ankle proprioception is not targeted by exercises on an unstable surface. Eur J Appl Physiol. 2012;112(4):1577–85.
11. Brumagne S, Janssens L, Knapen S, Claeys K, Suuden-Johansson ES. Persons with recurrent low back pain exhibit a rigid postal control strategy. Eur Spine J. 2008;17(9):1177–84.
12. Bernier JN, Perrin DH. Effect of coordination training on proprioception of the functionally instable ankle. J Orthop Sports Phys Ther. 1998;27(4):264–75.
13. Forestier N, Terrier R. Peroneal reaction time measurement in unipodal stance for two different destabilization axes. Clin Biomech. 2011;26:766–71.
14. Coutagne X, Monnet S, Lempereur J-J. Activité des muscles fibulaires sur différents appareils de rééducation proprioceptive. Mesure par électromyographie de surface sur plateau de Freeman, table de Vaast et Myolux. Kinésithérapie la Revue. 2008;83(8):34–8.
15. Forestier N, Toschi P. The effects of an ankle destabilization device on muscular activity while walking. Int J Sport Med. 2005;26(6):464–70.
16. Thépaut-Mathieu C, Van Hoecke J, Maton B. Myoelectrical and mechanical changes linked to length specificity during isometric training. J Appl Physiol. 1988;64(4):1500–5.
17. Sale DG. Neural adaptation to resistance training. Med Sci Sports Exerc. 1988;20(5):135–45.
18. Tomberlin JP, Basford JR, Schwen EE, Orte PA, Scott SC, Laughman RK, Ilstrup DM. Comparative study of isokinetic eccentric and concentric quadriceps training. J Orthop Sports Phys Ther. 1991;14(1):31–6.
19. Stauber WT. Eccentric action of muscles. Physiology, injury, adaptation. Exerc Sport Sci Revue. 1989;19:157.
20. Collado H, Coudreuse JM, Graziani F, Bensoussan L, Viton JM, Delarque A. Eccentric reinforcement of the ankle evertor muscles after lateral ankle sprain. Scand J Med Sci Sports. 2010;20:241–6.
21. Terrier R, Rose-Dulcina K, Toschi B, Forestier N. Impaired control of weight bearing ankle inversion in subjects with chronic ankle instability. Clin Biomech. 2014;29:439–43.
22. Thorstensson A. Observations on strength training and detraining. Acta Physiol Scand. 1977;100(4):491–3.
23. Santilli V, Frascarelli MA, Paoloni M, Frascarelli F, Camerota F, De Natale L, De Santis F. Peroneus longus muscle activation pattern during gait cycle in athletes affected by functional ankle instability: a surface electromyographic study. Am J Sports Med. 2005;33(8):1183–7.
24. Suda EY, Amorim CF, Sacco Ide C. Influence of ankle functional instability on the ankle electromyography during landing after volleyball blocking. J Electromyogr Kinesiol. 2009;19(2):e84–93.
25. Thonnard JL. La pathogénie de l'entorse du ligament latéral externe de la cheville. Evaluation d'une hypothèse. Thèse en vue de l'obtention du grade de Docteur en réadaptation. Université Catholique de Louvain, Faculté de médecine, Institut d'Éducation physique et de réadaptation; 1988.
26. Konradsen L. Sensori-motor control of the uninjured and injured human ankle. J Electromyogr Kinesiol. 2002;12:199–203.
27. Donovan L, Hart JM, Hertel J. Lower-extremity electromyography measures during walking with ankle-destabilization devices. J Sport Rehabil. 2014;23(2):134–44.
28. Donovan L, Hart JM, Hertel J. Effects of 2 ankle destabilization devices on electromyography mea-

sures during functional exercises in individuals with chronic ankle instability. J Orthop Sports Phys Ther. 2015;45(3):219–31.
29. Gasq D, Montoya R, Dupui P. Bases théoriques de l'évaluation du système proprioceptif. In: Julia M, et al., editors. La proprioception. Montpellier: Sauramps Medical; 2012. p. 9–18.
30. Schmidt RA, Lee T. Motor control and learning: a behavioral emphasis. 4th ed. Champaign, IL: Human Kinetics; 2005.
31. Kawato M. Internal models for motor control and trajectory planning. Curr Opin Neurobiol. 1999;9:718–27.
32. Ashton-Miller JA, Ottaviani RA, Hutchinson C, Wojtys EM. What best protects the inverted weight-bearing ankle against further inversion? Evertor muscle strength compares favorably with shoe height, athletic tape, and three orthoses. Am J Sports Med. 1996;24:800–9.
33. Schmitt S, Melnyk M, Alt W, Gollhofer A. Novel approach for a precise determination of short-time intervals in ankle sprain experiments. J Biomech. 2009;42:2823–5.
34. Fong DTP, Hong Y, Shima Y, Krosshaug T, Yung PSH, Chan KM. Biomechanics of supination ankle sprain: a case report of an accidental injury invent in the laboratory. Am J Sport Med. 2009; 37:822–7.
35. Kristianslund E, Bahr R, Krosshaug T. Kinematics and kinetics of an accidental lateral ankle sprain. J Biomech. 2011;44(14):2576–8.
36. Santos MJ, Liu H, Liu W. Unloading reactions in functional ankle instability. Gait Posture. 2008;27:589–94.
37. Pitrat R. Evolution du sens de position en inversion de cheville chez les basketteurs: comparaison du travail avec Myolux et plateau de Freeman. Travail de fin d'études pour l'obtention du grade académique de Master en kinésithérapie. Haute Ecole Louvain en Hainaut; 2011. p. 31.
38. Forestier N, Terrier R, Teasdale N. Ankle muscular proprioceptive signals relevance for balance control on various support surfaces. An exploratory study. Am J Phys Med Rehabil. 2014;94(1):20–7.
39. Marechal S. Évaluation de trois méthodes d'entrainement différentes sur la force des éverseurs. Travail de fin d'études pour l'obtention du grade académique de Master en kinésithérapie. Haute Ecole Robert Schuman; 2008. p. 15.
40. Terrier R, Degache F, Fourchet F, Gojanovic B, Forestier N. Assessment of evertor weakness in patients with chronic ankle instability: functional versus isokinetic testing. Clin Biomech. 2017;41:54–9.
41. Terrier R, Picot B, Forestier N. Le contrôle moteur et la protection articulaire de la cheville. Optimization de la reprogrammation neuromusculaire: les stratégies de délestage. Kinésithérapie Scientifique. 2012;537:71–4.
42. Gribble PA, Hertel J, Plisky P. Using the star excursion balance test to assess dynamic postural-control deficits and outcomes in lower limb extremity injury: a literature and systematic review. J Athl Train. 2012;47(3):339–47.
43. Terrier R, Forestier N. Quels tests en pratique clinique quotidienne pour diagnostiquer les déficits fonctionnels associés à l'instabilité chronique de cheville? Intérêts du dispositif Myolux™. Mains Libres. 2015;7:275–9.
44. Pearce CJ., Tourné Y., Zellers J., Terrier R., Toschi P., Grävare Silbernagel K., , ESKKA-AFAS Ankle Instability Group. Rehabilitation after anatomical ankle ligament repair or reconstruction. Knee Surg Sports Traumatol Arthrosc 2016. DOI https://doi.org/10.1007/s00167-016-4051-z, 24, 1130.
45. Tourné Y, Peruzzi M. Lateral collateral ligament repair anatomical ligament reinsertion with augmentation using inferior extensor retinaculum flap. Oper Orthop Traumatol. 2019;31:169. https://doi.org/10.1007/s00064-019-0599-3.

Part IV

Further Implications of Ankle Instability

Lower Extremity Alignment and Ankle Instability

36

Jorge Pablo Batista and Hélder Pereira

Lesions of the lateral ligament complex of the ankle is one of the most frequent sports-related injuries. Generally, the lateral ligament injury progresses favorably with rehabilitation protocols and medical treatment; however, the chronic lateral instability develops as a sequel in almost 30% of these patients [1–4].

The use of arthroscopy in ankle ligament repair was first described by Hawkins in 1987 [5].

During the last 15 years, a lot of techniques had been published for surgical repair or reconstruction of the lateral ligaments of the ankle in patients with complaints of chronic lateral ankle instability [6–19].

Open, endoscopic, or percutaneous procedures has gained popularity in different parts of the world; however, direct repair or reconstruction of the ligaments was often not an option in combination with inframalleolar or supramalleolar osteotomies [6, 17, 18, 20–27].

The surgical treatment of symptomatic ankle instability can be approached through different techniques: anatomical repairs, non-anatomical procedures, and anatomical reconstructions [6–13, 16, 19–21]. The Broström procedure is the classic repair of the lateral ligaments and in several occasions it is associated with the Gould procedure, which is an augmentation with a proximal advancement of the inferior extensor retinaculum [7, 8, 12]. These techniques (Anatomical repairs) are still considered the gold standard for treatment of symptomatic chronic instability [6, 9, 10, 13, 20, 21]. Although the modified Broström procedure is widely used for the surgical treatment of chronic lateral ankle instability, contraindications have now been suggested after further experience with this direct ligament repair, including failed previous reconstructive surgery, the presence of long-standing ankle instability, generalized ligamentous laxity, or increased size or weight [28–30]. Lateral ankle ligament reconstruction using an allograft or autograft tendon is used for a lot of surgeons, and it is recommended for patients with chronic lateral ankle instability with severely attenuated or deficient lateral ankle ligaments, which are expected to have a poor outcome with direct ligament repair alone [28–30].

Recently, several authors have reported good results using an arthroscopy-assisted lateral liga-

J. P. Batista (✉)
Centro Artroscópico Jorge Batista SA, AV. Pueyrredon 2446 First Floor, Buenos Aires, Argentina

Professional Soccer Department Club Atlético Boca Juniors, CABA, Buenos Aires, Argentina
e-mail: http://www.cajb.com.ar

H. Pereira
Ripoll y De Prado Sports Clinic: FIFA Medical Centre of Excellence, Murcia-Madrid, Spain

Orthopaedic Department, Centro Hospitalar Póvoa de Varzim, Vila do Conde, Portugal

ICVS/3B's – PT Government Associate Laboratory, University of Minho, Braga/Guimarães, Portugal

H. Pereira et al. (eds.), *Lateral Ankle Instability*, https://doi.org/10.1007/978-3-662-62763-1_36

ment repair [6, 10, 18, 20, 21, 26, 31, 32] Most of them also attempted to reinforce the repair by using the inferior external retinaculum (IER) but found that this was both technically difficult and added significant surgery time to the procedure [33, 34].

There is also a concern that when using the IER, this is not strictly an anatomical repair since its calcaneal attachment is 10 mm anterior to that of the calcaneofibular ligament (CFL), and this may thus restrict full plantar flexion of the ankle. The need to reinforce lateral ligament repair with the IER is therefore debatable [34, 35].

Complications related to the superficial peroneal nerve have been reported with arthroscopic and percutaneous techniques in the ankle [36–40].

Neuritis of the superficial peroneal or sural nerve, and pain or discomfort due to a prominent anchor or suture knot are the most frequent complications reported in percutaneous reconstructions [6, 10, 18].

The good and excellent results of these techniques in patients with mild, moderate, or severe ankle instability are well known, but many patients present severe chronic ankle instability associated with post-traumatic and idiopathic cavovarus deformity on whom conservative and orthopedic treatment failed to show acceptable results.

In these cases even if the ligament is repaired, the patients will develop an ankle osteoarthritis (OA) if the malalignment is not corrected. The problem is that these patients with post-traumatic osteoarthritis and idiopathic cavovarus deformity of the ankle are usually active and young if we compare with patients with end-stage degenerative OA of the hip or knee. An optimal treatment option in this group of patients with lower extremities deformities associated with chronic lateral ankle instability is to perform an endoscopic procedure to treat the ligament injury associated with joint preserving surgeries [20, 21]. These procedures include joint debridement [41, 42], osteochondral resurfacing [43], and corrective osteotomies (supramalleolar or inframalleolar osteotomies) in order to avoid joint-sacrificing procedures such as ankle arthrodesis and total ankle replacement in the future [44, 45].

Valderrabano et al. [46] performed an etiological, clinical, and radiographic review of 33 ankles with ligamentous post-traumatic ankle OA. The majority of the patients (85%) had injuries of the lateral ankle ligaments, and 15% had injury of the medial and medial–lateral ligaments. The mean latency time between injury and end-stage ankle OA was 34.3 years. In this study, lateral ankle sprains in sports were the main cause of ligamentous post-traumatic ankle OA with significant concomitant varus malalignment of the hindfoot [44].

Supramalleolar or inframalleolar osteotomies are being used to correct lower extremity, ankle and foot deformities in adults to prolong ankle function and avoid the need for an ankle arthrodesis. The goal of these procedures is to realign the limb in the setting of these deformities and to redistribute the loads on the ankle joint, thereby improving the biomechanics of the lower extremity [47].

Although the current literature is lacking data on sports activity after realignment surgery for varus or valgus ankle OA, the restoration of pain-free sporting activity may be possible [48, 49].

The goal of supramalleolar or inframalleolar osteotomies is to realign the low extremity deformity and to redistribute the loads on the ankle joint, improving the biomechanics of the lower limb.

36.1 Supramalleolar Osteotomies

This procedure is indicated to correct the deformity above or below the ankle joint, and in ankle arthrosis associated with intra-articular varus or valgus deformity (Fig. 36.1). When the patient is standing, the center of force transmission is medialized in a varus ankle and lateralized in a valgus ankle. The forces within the joint are amplified by activation of the triceps surae. The posterior tibial tendon and the Achilles tendon may become an invertor in patients with varus deformities, and specifically the Achilles tendon may be an evertor in patients with valgus deformities, thereby exerting an additional deforming force on the hindfoot [50].

In patients with tibia or hindfoot varus deformity, an osteotomy can be used to correct

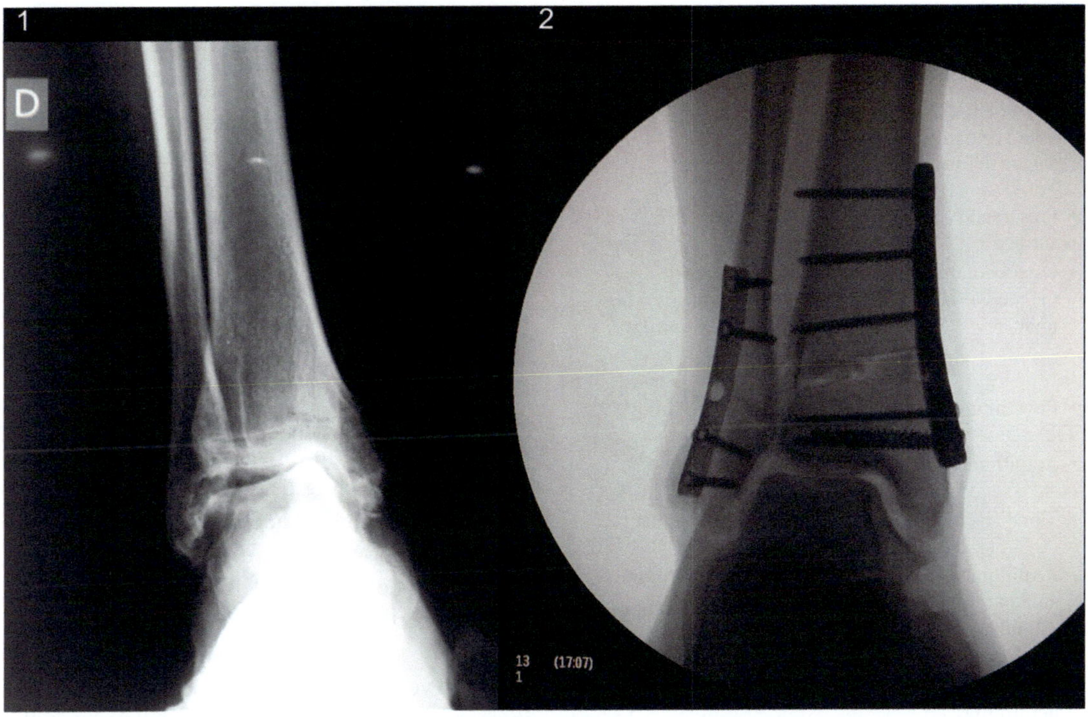

Fig. 36.1 Anteroposterior X ray of a patient with supramalleolar tibial and fibular osteotomy

the malalignment and to prevent the development of degenerative changes, or in cases with ankle osteoarthritis, to modify joint mechanics and shift loads onto intact articular cartilage [47].

The goal of supramalleolar osteotomy is to maintain the weight-bearing axis of the lower extremity centered over the tibiotalar and subtalar joints in both the coronal and sagittal planes in order to realign the hindfoot, and to improve the direction of the force vector of the triceps surae. Supramalleolar osteotomy is also a very useful adjunct to the correction of an intra-articular varus deformity associated either with recurrent ankle instability or congenital distal tibia vara (Table 36.1).

36.1.1 Indications

The main indication for supramalleolar osteotomy in patients with chronic ankle instability is: symptomatic instability combined with asymmetric varus ankle, without osteoarthritis or with degenerative changes while preserving at least 50% of the tibiotalar joint surface.

Supramalleolar osteotomies can also be used to optimize alignment of total ankle arthroplasty or ankle arthrodesis in the treatment of end-stage ankle OA.

36.1.2 Contraindications

Patients with hindfoot instability that a ligament repair or reconstruction is not performed is an absolute contraindication. If we plan to perform a supramalleolar osteotomy, we must repair or reconstruct the lateral ligaments.

Severe vascular and neurologic deficiency in the affected extremity, inflammatory disease, neuroarthropathy, osteoporosis, and acute or chronic infection of the ankle are absolute contraindications.

Patient age >65 years and smokers are relative contraindications for supramalleolar osteotomy.

Table 36.1 Indications and contraindications of supramalleolar osteotomies

Indications	Contraindications
• Asymmetric ankle osteoarthritis with varus/valgus deformity and ≥50% • Preserved tibiotalar joint surface	*Absolute*
• Osteochondral lesion of the medial/lateral tibiotalar joint	• Severe ankle osteoarthritis with >50% of cartilage damage of joint surface
• Physeal growth arrest	• Severe hindfoot instability
• Autoimmune arthropaties	• Acute/chronic infection
• Tibial fracture malunion	• Severe vascular deficiency
• Realignment before total ankle arthroplasty	• Severe neurologic deficiency
• Tibiotalar arthrodesis malunion	• Neuropathic disorders
• Residual paralytic deformities	*Relative*
• Congenital talipes equinovarus sequelae	• Patient noncompliance
• Hemophilic arthropathy	• Elderly patients
	• Moderate or severe osteoporosis
	• Smokers
	• DBT
	• Chronic skin abnormalities or soft tissue defects

36.2 Inframalleolar Osteotomies

In patients with symptomatic foot and ankle malalignment, the osteotomy of the calcaneus plays an important role in restoring hindfoot biomechanics (Fig. 36.2). Osteotomies through the calcaneus body not only realign the tuberosity but also redirect the pull of the Achilles tendon making it a corrective rather than a deforming force [51].

Different types of posterior calcaneal osteotomy are used for calcaneal realignment. Calcaneal osteotomy is an extra-articular procedure that is used in the correction of cavovarus and planovalgus foot deformity, and it is usually performed through a lateral approach.

Complications are rare with this procedure, but wound dehiscence, delayed union, and soft tissue or peroneal tendon fibrosis along the osteotomy site can occur and have been presented [52]. Dwyer popularized calcaneal osteotomy for the correction of cavovarus foot alignment in the 1950s. The original description was that of a removal of a laterally based wedge to produce a neutral or valgus position of the heel. The wedge is taken proximally to the posterior articular facet [51, 53, 54].

Patients with symptomatic foot and ankle malalignment can have relief of their symptoms with a calcaneus osteotomy which improves/aims to restore, the hindfoot biomechanics.

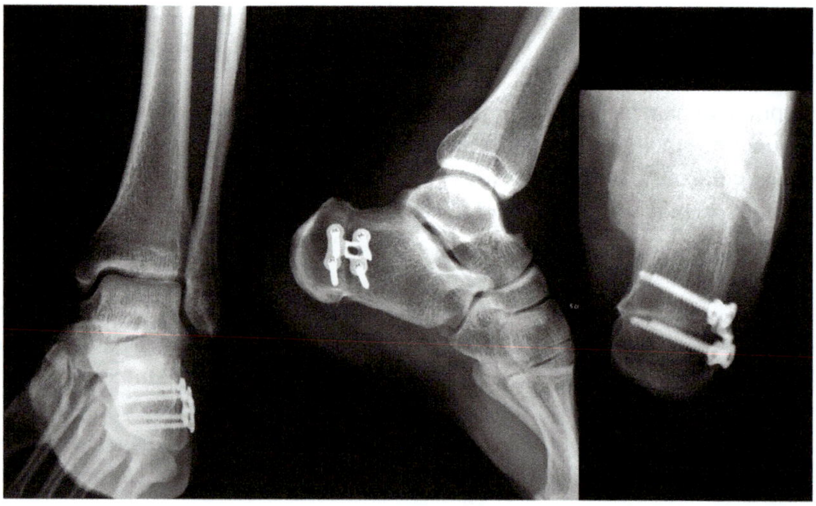

Fig. 36.2 Anteroposterior, lateral and axial view of an ankle with an inframalleolar (calcaneal) osteotomy using a step plate

Table 36.2 Indications and contraindications of inframalleolar osteotomies (Dwyer/Lateral sliding calcaneal Osteotomies)

Indications	Contraindications
• Cavovarus foot	*Absolute*
• Planovalgus foot	• Severe ankle osteoarthritis with >50% of cartilage damage of joint surface • Osteoarthritis of the subtalar joint • Irreducible hindfoot instability
• Osteochondral lesion of the medial/lateral tibiotalar joint	• Idiopatic or posttraumatic varus of the distal tibia
• Severe ankle osteoarthritis with <50% of cartilage damage of joint surface	• Acute/chronic infection
• Severe chronic ankle instability	• Severe vascular deficiency
• Failure of previous ankle instability surgeries	• Severe neurologic deficiency
	• Neuropathic disorders
• Residual paralytic deformities	*Relative*
	• Patient noncompliance
	• Elderly patients (>65–70 years)
	• Moderate or severe osteoporosis
	• Smokers
	• DBT
	• Chronic skin abnormalities or soft tissue defects

Closing wedge osteotomies (Dwyer) or single plane translational osteotomies (Sliding osteotomies) are performed through open or endoscopic techniques associated with an anterior ankle arthroscopy procedure in the majority of the times to treat the intra-articular-associated lesions but without repairing or reconstructing the ligaments injured [53–57] (Table 36.2).

36.2.1 Indications

The main indication for a corrective osteotomy of the calcaneus is a cavovarus or planovalgus foot deformity due to a malaligned calcaneus with a flexible subtalar joint.

In patients with chronic ankle instability, an endoscopic or open repair of the injured ligaments is indicated.

36.2.2 Contraindications

The main contraindication to calcaneal osteotomy includes pre-existing subtalar arthritis. In the presence of subtalar arthritis, subtalar arthrodesis alleviates pain and an extra-articular osteotomy is required.

Relative contraindications include smoking, diabetes, peripheral vascular disease obesity, and poor skin conditions.

36.3 Endoscopic ATFL Repair Combined with Supramalleolar/Inframalleolar Osteotomies

Chronic lateral ankle instability has been suggested to be an etiologic factor in the development of ankle arthritis [58, 59]. Long-term ankle incongruency or instability presumably increases ankle contact stress that exceeds the capacity of the ankle joint to repair itself or adapt [60]. Excessive varus or valgus alignment of the calcaneus or distal tibia has been shown to alter contact characteristics and ligament strain at the level of the ankle joint and therefore has the potential to contribute to ankle arthritis [61, 62] (Fig. 36.1).

Morscher in 1986 presented one of the few articles in which he suggests a combination of fibulotalar syndesmoplasty with osteotomy of the calcaneus according to Dwyer in cases of patients with chronic ankle instability after a supination trauma with a pathological calcaneus varus as opposed to physiological calcaneus valgus [63].

A combination of endoscopic lateral ligament repair of the ankle combined with supramalleolar or inframalleolar osteotomies according with the deformity of the lower extremity provides a very good, patient-reported, satisfaction rate [20, 21].

Table 36.3 Indications and contraindications of combined Endoscopic ATFL repair associated with inframalleolar osteotomies (Dwyer/Lateral sliding calcaneal Osteotomies)

Indications	Contraindications
• Cavovarus foot (Hindfoot deformity)	*Absolute*
• Moderate or severe chronic ankle instability	• Severe ankle osteoarthritis with >50% of cartilage damage of joint surface • Osteoarthritis of subtalar joint • Irreducible hindfoot instability
• Osteochondral lesion of the medial/lateral tibiotalar joint	• Idiopatic or posttraumatic varus of the distal tibia
• Faillure of previous conservative or orthopedic treatments	• Acute/chronic infection
• Severe ankle osteoarthritis with <50% of cartilage damage of joint surface	• Severe vascular deficiency
• Failure in previous ankle instability surgeries	• Severe neurologic deficiency
	• Neuropathic disorders
	Relative
	• Patient noncompliance
	• Elderly patients (>65–70 years)
	• Moderate or severe osteoporosis
	• Smokers
	• DBT
	• Chronic skin abnormalities or soft tissue defects

Positive outcome includes complete resumption to previous activities of daily living and, in several cases, return to sports activities. This combined procedures aims to restore adequate stability and correct the cavovarus deformities in cases with severe lateral ankle ligaments injuries and malalignement/deformities. Such previously described cases are expected to have a poor outcome with direct ligament repair alone (Table 36.3).

36.3.1 Indication

The indications for this combined procedure are patients with severe chronic ankle instability associated with post-traumatic and/or idiopathic cavovarus deformity in whom conservative or orthopedic treatment failed to provide positive results.

36.3.2 Contraindication

The absolute contraindication was osteoarthritis of the subtalar joint; however, there were relative contraindications too: irreducible hindfoot instability, deep or superficial infections, neurovascular impairment of the lower extremity, Charcot arthropathy, severe osteoporosis, elderly patients, diabetes mellitus, and smokers.

36.4 Preoperative Assessment

36.4.1 Clinical Evaluation

Surgical planning begins with physical examination of the patient.

Clinical and radiologic examinations were performed before surgery to assess the presence of mechanical instability and associated pathologies.

It is essential to make the clinical evaluation of the alignment of the lower limbs with the patient standing/weightbearing (Fig. 36.3). Furthermore, in some cases, the deformity is exacerbated with the patient in the tiptoe position, and this is important to recognize in order to evaluate if the deformity is affected by the contraction of the posterior tibial tendon or the eccentric pull of Achilles tendon. Tenderness and pain on palpation of the lateral gutter and lateral ligament region are common in this pathology.

Pain is exacerbated during the weight-bearing and when the patient intents to walk, run, or jump. Medial and lateral ankle stability is assessed when the patient is sitting. Clinical talar tilt test and anterior drawer test and overall limb alignment were assessed with attention to any concomitant knee or tibia deformity that may have contributed to the hindfoot malalignment.

It is important to measure both passive and active joint range of motion, aiming to assess and

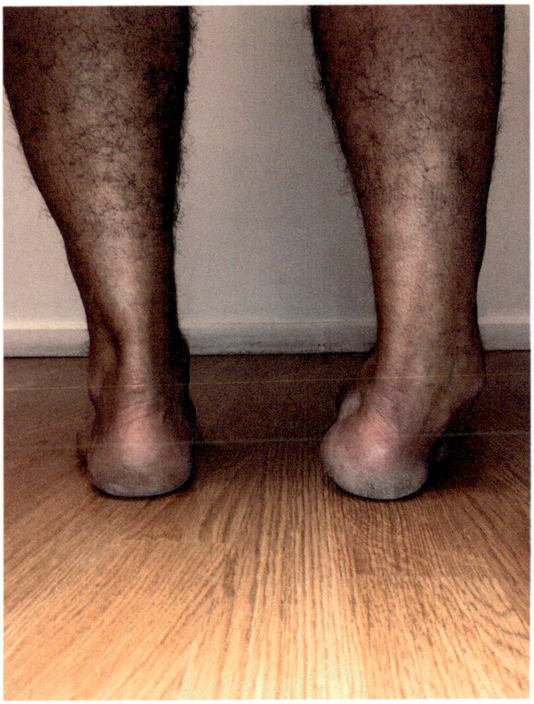

Fig. 36.3 Patient with a severe malalignment of his right hindfoot

determine any limitation degree of dorsiflexion or plantarflexion.

36.4.2 Radiologic Evaluation

Planning of the extremity correction starts with full-length radiographs of the bilateral lower extremities. Anteroposterior and lateral radiographs of the feet and ankles were taken to exclude ossicles, malleolar or talar old fractures that can result from ankle sprains. Saltzman's view in 20° and 45° were performed to evaluate the alignment of the limbs of all the patients pre- and postoperatively.

The most important aspect of preoperative planning is the assessment of the origin of the deformity [64]. A complete clinical and radiographic evaluation of the lower extremity from the hip through the foot is imperative for identifying the deformity. For preoperative planning the calculation of the degree of surgical correction is recommended using weight-bearing anteroposterior and lateral radiographs of the ankle. One of the most important radiographic parameters for quantification of the supramalleolar varus or valgus deformity is the medial distal tibial angle or distal tibial surface angle (TAS). The tibial plafond on the anteroposterior (AP) radiographic view forms an angle of 90° (R = 86°–93°) with the mechanical axis of the tibia called the distal tibial ankle surface angle (TAS). On the lateral radiograph, this angle is referred to as the tibial lateral surface angle (TLS), normal averaging 80° (R = 78°–82°) (Fig. 36.4). When performing a distal osteotomy, the surgeon should be to restore the TAS and TLS back to within normal values when compared with the contralateral limb [44, 47, 65, 66].

Multiplanar deformities are not the topic of this chapter but often involve coronal and sagittal components. Such complex cases can result in a combination of deformities such as ankle varus, valgus, recurvatum, procurvatum, translation, and rotation, and in these cases the types of deformities are measured and described by the center of rotation and angulation (CORA).

Another radiographic parameter which should be considered for the preoperative planning is the talar tilt. The talar tilt is defined as the difference between the distal tibial ankle surface angle (TAS) and the tibiotalar angle (normal value 91.5 ± 1.2°). In neutrally aligned ankles, the talar tilt should be less than 4° [67, 68].

The angle of the lateral calcaneal wall can be used as a measure of calcaneal malalignment (e.g., inframalleolar deformity). Hintermann suggests obtaining a Saltzman view in 20° and 45° for the assessment of hindfoot alignment [50, 69] (Fig. 36.5).

The use of CT scan or magnetic resonance imaging (MRI) is not essential. However, it might be used in order to identify associated intra-articular pathology, identify required additional surgical procedures such as treatment of intra-articular loose bodies, ligament's insufficiency, or tendinous pathology. In cases of hindfoot arthrosis with or without instrumentation, the use of SPECT-CT has simplified the study of these complex cases since the examination is capable to suggest the origin of the pain [69–71] (Fig. 36.6).

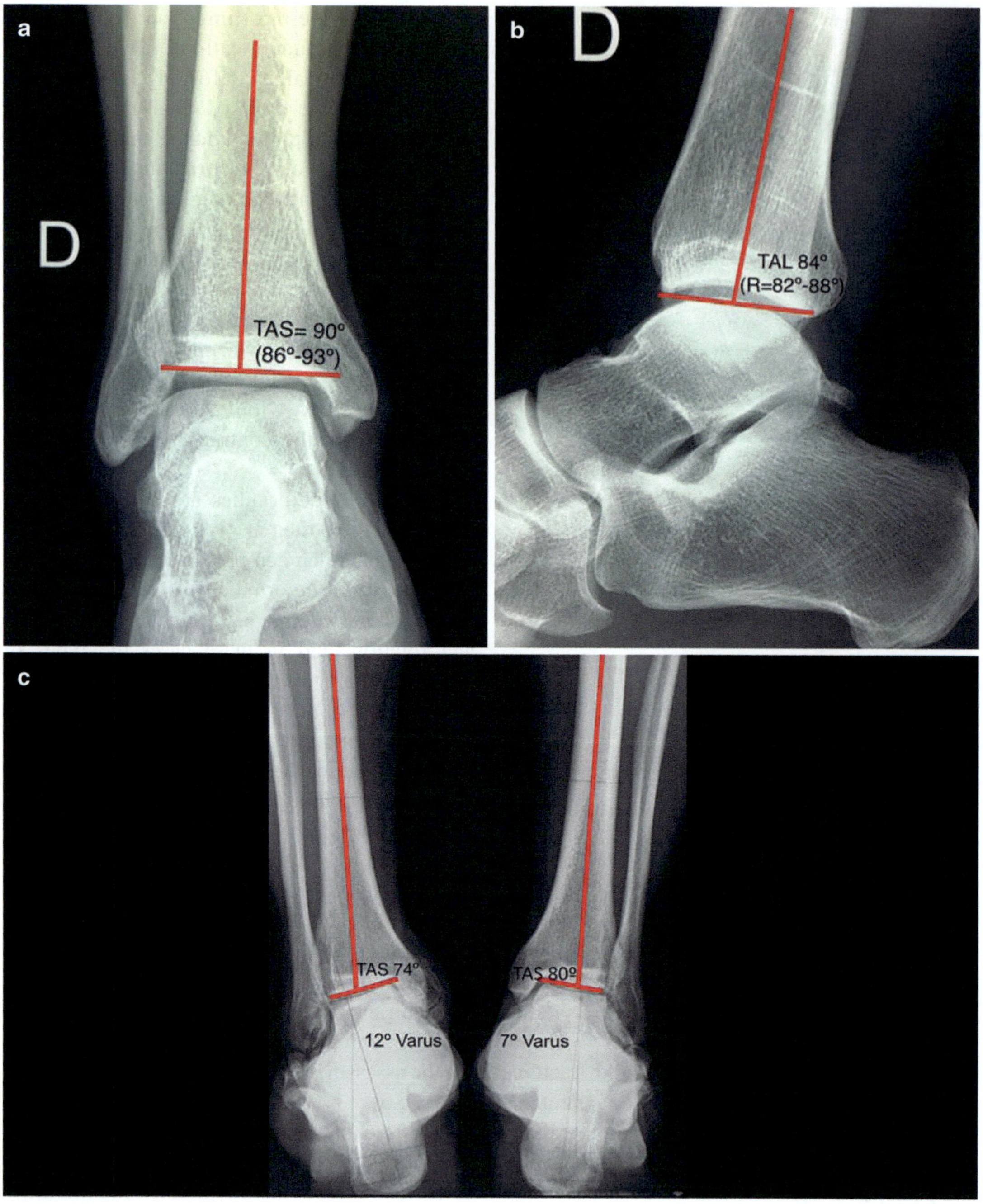

Fig. 36.4 (**a**) The tibial plafond on the antero-posterior (AP) radiographic view forms an angle of 90° (*R* = 86°–93°) with the mechanical axis of the tibia called the distal tibial ankle surface angle (TAS). (**b**) On the lateral radiograph, this angle is referred to as the tibial lateral surface angle (TLS), normal averaging 80° (*R* = 78°–82°). (**c**) Pathologic AP X-rays with abnormal distal tibial ankle surface angle (TAS)

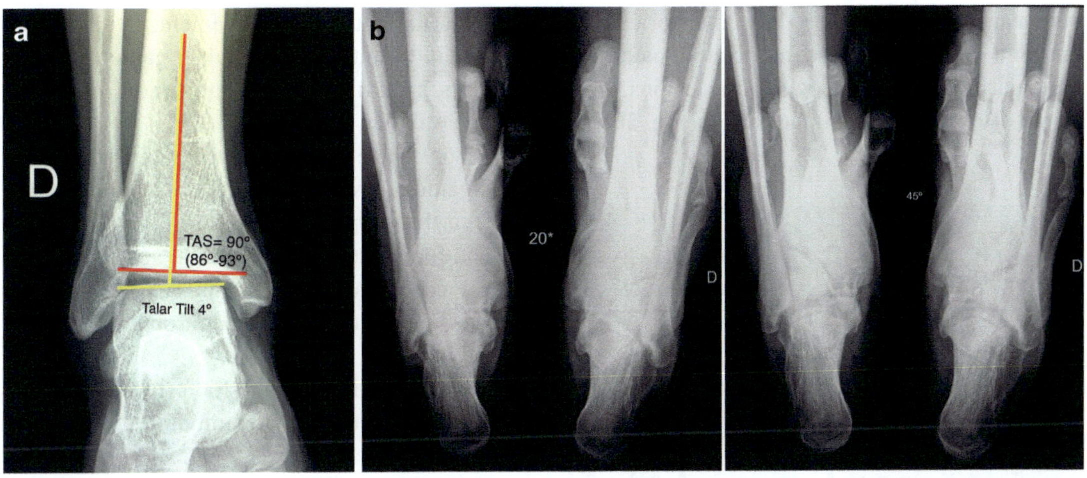

Fig. 36.5 (**a**) Anteroposterior X ray of a right ankle with the talar tilt measured. (Normal value 91.5 ± 1.2°). In neutrally aligned ankles the talar tilt should be less than 4°. (**b**) Saltzman view in 20° and 45° for assessment of hindfoot alignment

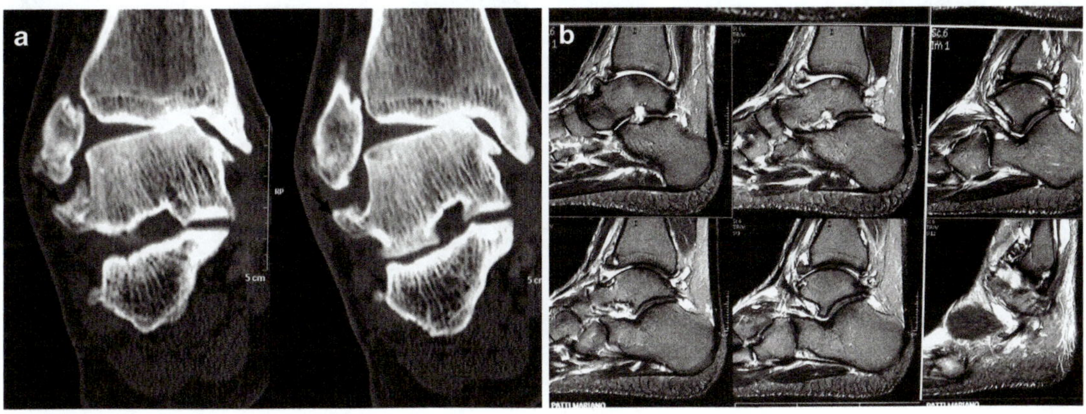

Fig. 36.6 (**a**) Ankle CT scan showing a prominent lateral talar osteophyte and talar tilt. (**b**) Magnetic Resonance Imaging (MRI) shows tibial and talar osteophytes, loose bodies, and subchondral geodes

36.5 Surgical Technique

36.5.1 Anterior Ankle Arthroscopy (Endoscopic Anterior Talofibular Ligament Repair Through Two Portals)

The patients were placed in supine position, both the hip and the knee were extended with the ankle on the tip of the table to allow flexo-extension movement during the surgery. A pneumatic tourniquet located on the ipsilateral tight is inflated to 300 mmHg in order to exsanguinate the lower extremity. General or subarachnoid anesthesia is often used. Anterior ankle arthroscopy was performed using only the two classic anteromedial and anterolateral portals described by Prof. van Dijk [72, 73] (Fig. 36.7).

Distraction of the ankle was not used during this arthroscopic procedure routinely. A 4-mm 30° arthroscope is introduced through anteromedial portal. The ankle is positioned in maximum dorsiflexion to relax the capsular joint and to obtain the optimal view of the lateral gutter.

In this position, anterolateral portal is made by transillumination taking care of the superficial peroneal nerve. We explored the anterior talocrural joint and treated the associated pathology (sinovial processes, osteochondral lesions, tibial spurs, osteophytes, and talar beaks) (Fig. 36.8).

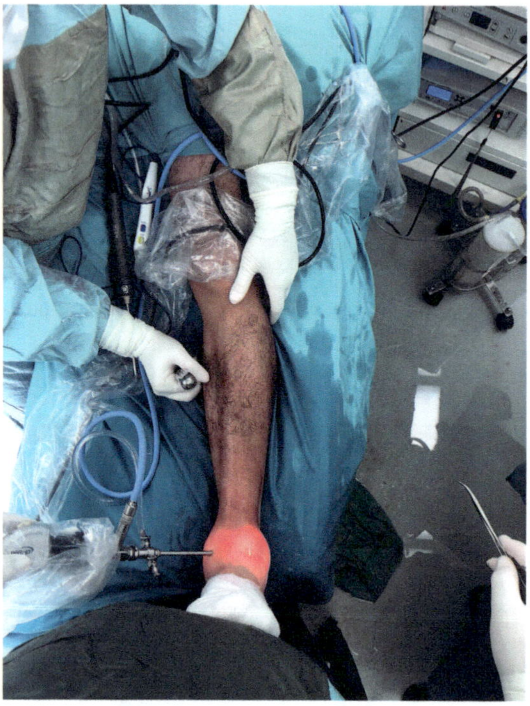

Fig. 36.7 Patient placed in supine position, both the hip and the knee extended with the ankle on the tip of the table to allow flexo-extension movement during the surgery

Prior to reattach the ligament, it should be defined if the anterior talofibular ligament (ATFL) presents a partial or complete lesion and if the calcaneofibular ligament (CFL) is broken (Fig. 36.9). The remnant of the anterior talofibular ligament (ATFL) should be repaired under direct arthroscopic visualization.

The footprint for the fibular attachment of the lateral collateral ligaments is debrided with a shaver or a curette introduced through the anterolateral portal.

Perform the hole on the footprint in the distal tip of the fibula through the initiator of the anchor by drilling. The drill was directed from anterior

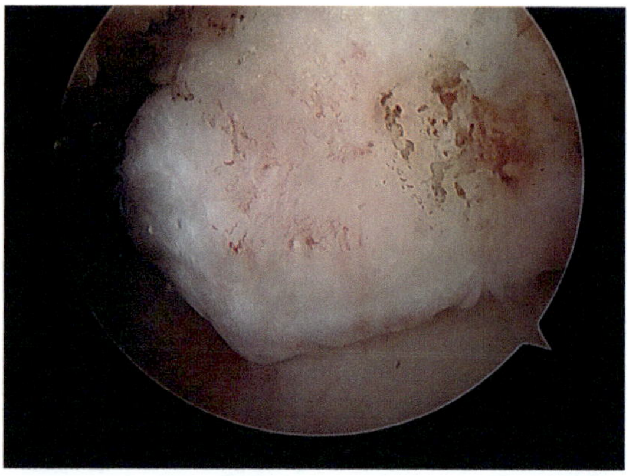

Fig. 36.8 Arthroswcopic view of a prominent talar osteophyte

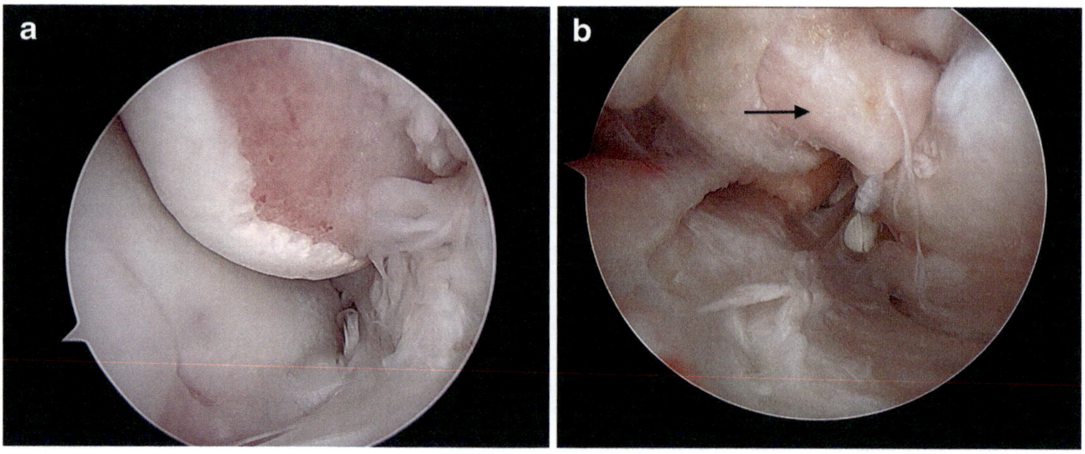

Fig. 36.9 (**a**) Arthroscopic view of the lateral gutter with a chronic rupture of the anterior talo fibular ligament (ATFL). (**b**) Arthroscopic view of the lateral gutter with a fibular osteophyte (black arrow) and a chronic rupture of the calcaneal fibular ligament (CFL). The peroneal tendons can be identificated in the depth

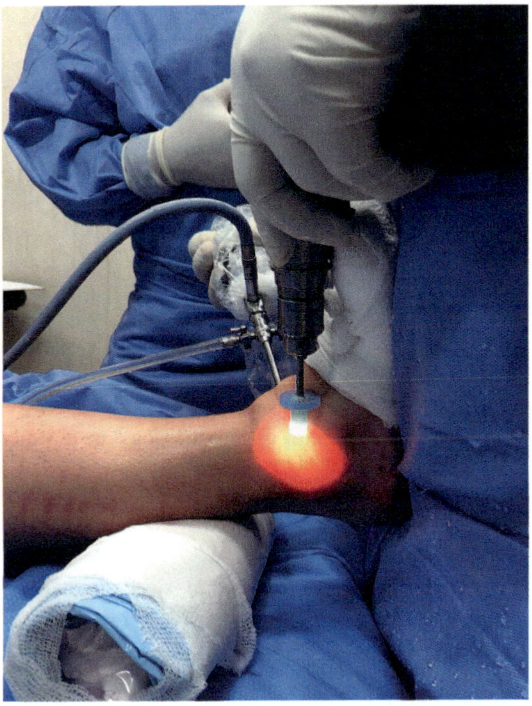

Fig. 36.10 The drill was directed from anterior to posterior, and parallel to the plantar plane as well as the plane of the lateral gutter in order to perform the fibular hole

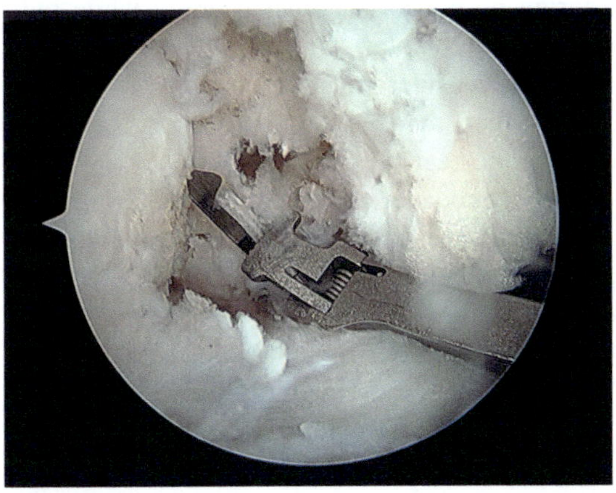

Fig. 36.11 A suture passer Mini Scorpion (Arthrex Inc., Naples, FL, USA), a 2:0 or 0 nonabsorbable suture, and a 4.5 mm knotless anchor (Foot Print Ultra 4.5 mm, Smith & Nephew Plc) is used for catch the remnant tissue of the ATFL

to posterior, and parallel to the plantar plane as well as the plane of the lateral gutter (Fig. 36.10). A suture passer Mini Scorpion (Arthrex Inc., Naples, FL, USA), a 2:0 or 0 nonabsorbable suture, and a 4.5 mm knotless anchor (Foot Print Ultra 4.5 mm, Smith & Nephew Plc) were used for ligament repair (Fig. 36.11).

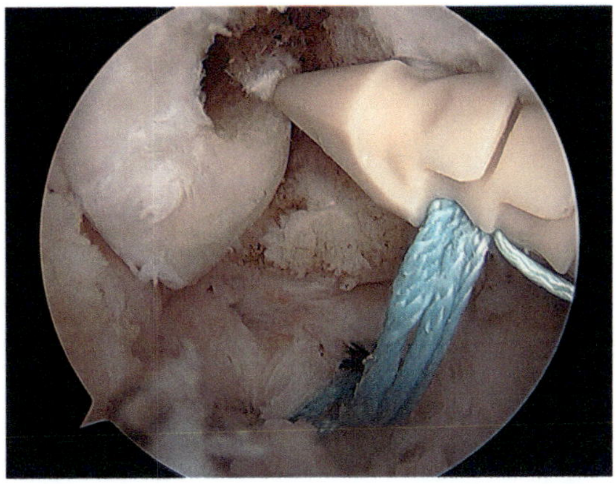

Fig. 36.12 A 4.5 mm knotless anchor (Smith & Nephew Plc) is introduced by impactation under direct visualization

The Mini Scorpion suture passer is introduced through the anterolateral portal, and under direct arthroscopic visualization, the remnant ATFL is penetrated from lateral to medial with a double suture. The suture is pulled back with the Mini Scorpion gripper through the anterolateral portal. Pull back the suture to be sure if there is a firm and acceptable capture of the remnant tissue. The limbs of the suture are passed through the hole in the upper side of the knotless anchor. Be careful that the tension of the suture can be modified only before introducing the anchor. Once the anchor is introduced by impaction, the tension of suture cannot be modified. Cut the remnant suture with a specific endoscopic scissor (Fig. 36.12).

36.5.2 Calcaneal Osteotomy

In patients with inframalleolar deformities, we suggest add this procedure to the endoscopic ATFL repair. The objective of the translational osteotomies of the calcaneus is to realign the posterior part of the foot tripod through a simple transverse osteotomy at the body of the calcaneus. The tuberosity can then be translated laterally in order to correct the varus of the hindfoot. We suggest translate the calcaneal tuberosity

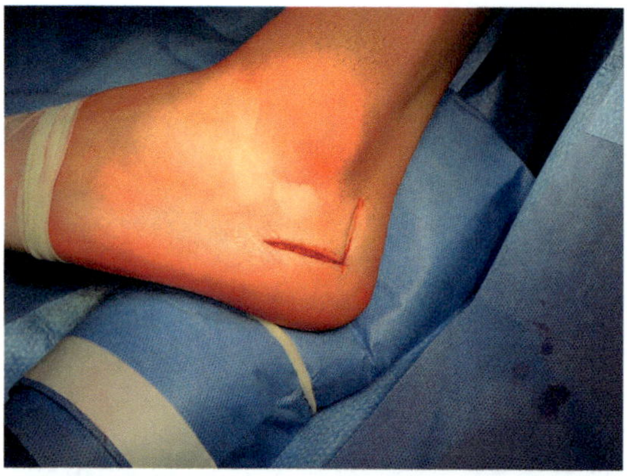

Fig. 36.13 An "L shaped" mini extensile lateral incision to elevate a full thickness skin flap is performed in order to expose the lateral calcaneous cortex

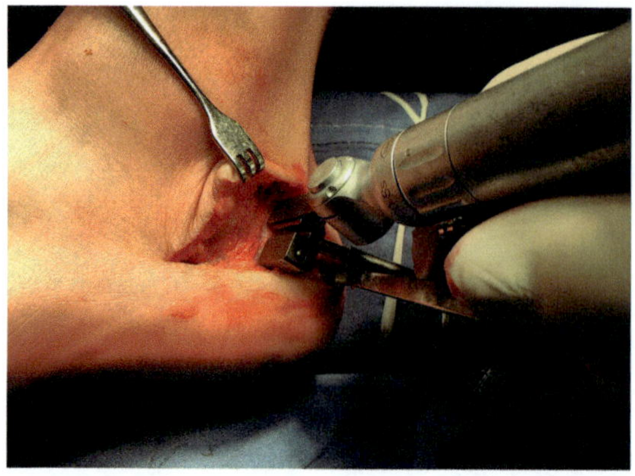

Fig. 36.14 The calcaneal osteotomy should be made in the safe zone established by projecting anteriorly 11 mm from a line drawn between the posterosuperior apex of the calcaneus and the plantar fascia origin

while the ankle is in full plantarflexion to relax the Achilles tendon.

After endoscopic ATFL repair, the patient may be repositioned in either the lateral position and a removable bump under the ipsilateral hip allows the leg to be internally rotated. Two types of approach can be used for osteotomies: an "L-shaped" mini extensile lateral incision or an oblique incision. With oblique incisions in lateral surgical approaches to the calcaneus, nerve injuries have been well studied in the anatomy and trauma literature, and can result in transitory or permanent irritation along the course of the sural nerve at the heel with neuroma formation and distal dysesthesia [74, 75].

We prefer an "L-shaped" mini extensile lateral incision to elevate a full thickness skin flap in order to expose the lateral calcaneous cortex (Fig. 36.13). This preserves the integrity of the lateral calcaneal artery reducing the risk of edge ischemia, infection, and wound breakdown. There is a "safe zone" defined by Talusan and colleagues that is established by projecting anteriorly 11 mm from a line drawn between the posterosuperior apex of the calcaneus and the plantar fascia origin. The incision should be made directly in the middle of the tuberosity at the anterior edge of the safe zone (Fig. 36.14). Several variations of the calcaneal osteotomy exist for the correction of hindfoot varus. Dwyer [53] originally described the removal of a wedge from the lateral wall of the bone while leaving the medial side intact as a periosteal hinge. This osteotomy is intrinsically stable and could be performed with minimal fixation. The use of a lateral shift allows the surgeon for greater correction and adequate stability. A 5–10 mm lateral-based wedge of bone is removed prior to the osseous stabilization (Depending of the hindfoot deformity). It displaces the weight-bearing portion of the heel laterally while redirecting the plantar surface into more valgus. Carmont consider that this technique is advantageous when there is overloading on the lateral edge of the heel [51, 76].

Other procedure that can be used is a lateral sliding calcaneal osteotomy. A single plane translational osteotomy was made initially with an oscillating saw and finished with a bone chisel. Be careful in order to avoid over-penetration of the saw blade toward medial neurovascular structures. The osteotomy is then gently distracted with a laminar spreader. The osteotomy was stabilized with a blocked staple plate or two cannulated screw followed by wound closure (Arthrex Inc., Naples, FL, USA) (Fig. 36.15).

A compressive bandage and a walking boot keeping the ankle in 90° is indicated in all patients and maintained for 6 weeks. Crutches are used for 3 weeks. No weight-bearing was indicated for 2 weeks. Fourteen days after surgery the patients showed partial weight-bearing, and after this time gradually full weight-bearing was allowed.

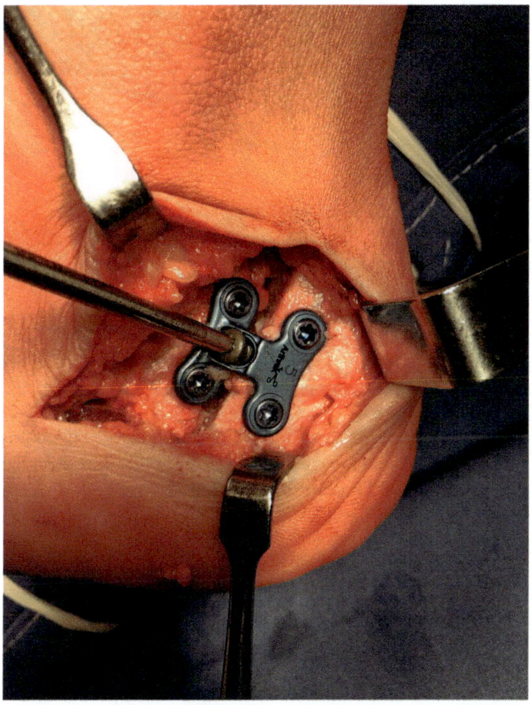

Fig. 36.15 The osteotomy is stabilized with a blocked staple plate. (Arthrex Inc., Naples, FL, USA)

Thromboprophylaxis was used in patients who were over 30 years old.

Balance training and proprioceptive exercises were encouraged. Before starting sports activities, when patients experienced ankle instability and a giving way sensation, they were advised to delay their sports activities and were encouraged to concentrate more on balance training and peroneal strengthening exercises.

Clinical research studies show good results of calcaneal osteotomies, most of which include the procedure associated with other techniques. Kraus described a modification of lateral closing wedge technique combined with lateral translation to minimize the amount of shortening from wedge resection and presented a very good result with this combined technique [76].

Our group presented 11 patients treated with combined inframalleolar osteotomies and endoscopic ATFL repair in cases with severe chronic ankle instability and varus extremity deformities with very good results and a very low complications rate [20, 21].

Barg and Valderrabano presented very good results with Dwyer osteotomies in 31 patients. All of them had a substantial inframalleolar cavovarus deformity with preoperative moment arm of the calcaneus of -17.9 ± 3.3 mm, which improved significantly to 1.6 ± 5.9 mm and a significantly improved of The American Orthopaedic Foot and Ankle Society score and pain relief [55].

The most important complications with calcaneal osteotomies include under-correction, nonunion and local complications to the sural nerve and skin [77]. Tarsal tunnel syndrome has been associated too with lateralizing calcaneal osteotomy in patients with greater translation of the osteotomy and osteotomies performed more anteriorly on the tuberosity [51, 78].

Some surgeons suggest plantar fascia release after these procedures to avoid plantar fascia pain during the postoperative period.

Overcorrection is an uncommon complication and has been reported only in one case for a planovalgus foot overcorrected into varus by medial slide osteotomy [77]. Screw heads can cause pain if placed in the posteroinferior tuberosity and are potential sources of hardware-related pain [79].

36.5.3 Supramalleolar Osteotomy

The patient was placed in supine position with a pneumatic tourniquet located on the ipsilateral tight inflated to 300 mmHg in order to exsanguinate the lower extremity. Both the hip and the knee were extended with the ankle on the tip of the table to allow flexo-extension movement during the surgery. We identify and perform landmarks on the anterior joint line, which is easily palpated by moving the joint through plantar and dorsiflexion. A perfect lateral fluoroscopic image should be obtained.

Ankle varus deformity may be associated with chronic ankle instability, and the deformity can be tibial, calcaneal, or intra-articular.

In patients with supramalleolar varus deformities, the surgeon can choose from two surgical options: medial opening wedge osteotomy or lateral closing wedge osteotomy (anti-varus osteotomy) [46].

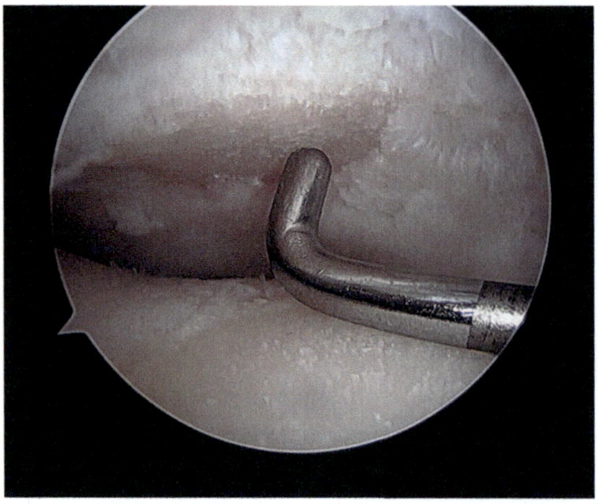

Fig. 36.16 Arthroscopic image of a patient with lateral chronic ankle instability with hindfoot varus deformity. We can see the lack of cartilage in medial talar and tibial bone

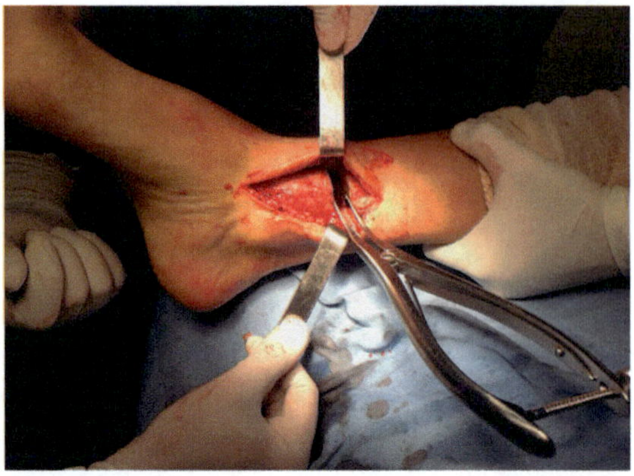

Fig. 36.17 A wide saw blade is used to perform the osteotomy under water irrigation to reduce thermal damage during the cut. The osteotomy may be refined using a chisel or osteotome

Osteotomy selection requires careful evaluation of multiple conditions and factors. The surgeon should know the advantages and disadvantages to help choose the best procedure in each patient.

Lateral osteotomies are difficult to perform because of the proximity of the fibula and the risk of postoperative peroneal weakness, and therefore are often avoided. However, when greater than 10°–12° of varus exists, a lateral closing wedge osteotomy is recommended. We prefer medial opening wedge osteotomy in most of the cases.

Prior to perform the tibial osteotomy, anterior ankle arthroscopy is performed in all patients in order to assess if the cartilage degeneration of the joint is > or <50% (Fig. 36.16). If necessary, loose bodies are removed and anterior ankle impingement is debrided. Endoscopic ATFL repair or arthroscopic ligament reconstruction with gracilis tendon can be performed in some patients.

The medial opening wedge osteotomy is indicated in cases with a varus deformity less than 10°.

An 8- to 10-cm longitudinal incision is centered along the medial malleolus and carried proximally in line with the tibial crest. The saphenous nerve and vein are typically anterior to the incision, but branches may need to be addressed. A full-thickness flap is most reliable in avoiding injury to the anterior neurovascular structures. The sheath of the posterior tibial tendon is incised to allow posterior retraction of the tendon and visualization of the distal tibia. Once adequate exposure of the tibia is achieved, soft tissue structures must be protected to avoid iatrogenic injury. Using fluoroscopy, only one Kirschner wire is necessary for orientation and saw blade guidance, and it is positioned parallel to the joint surface to act as a reference during correction.

Using a wide saw blade, the osteotomy is performed under water irrigation to reduce thermal damage during the cut. The osteotomy may be refined using a chisel or osteotome (Fig. 36.17). It should be clearly exposed that 1 mm of opening corresponds to 1.3° of correction of the deformity.

The lateral cortex is typically preserved to enhance the intrinsic stability of the osteotomy, and so the intact fibula does not hinder the desired tibial correction.

The gap can be filled with allograft or autograft harvested from the ipsilateral iliac crest bone. The fixation of the osteotomy is performed using a T-shaped 3.5-mm LCP plate with angular stabilizing screws. Fixation stability is vital to outcomes (Fig. 36.18).

As a general rule, if identical deformities are located in the fibula and the tibia, an osteotomy should be performed at the same level in both bones.

We recommend to evaluate the tibial deformity and decide if a tibial and fibular opening wedge or tibial opening wedge and fibular closing wedge is better to perform.

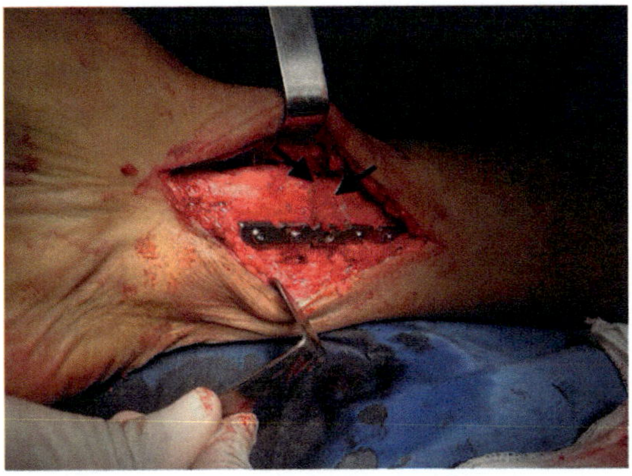

Fig. 36.18 The gap was filled with autograft harvested from the ipsilateral iliac crest bone (black arrows). The fixation of the osteotomy is performed using a T-shaped 3.5-mm LCP plate with angular stabilizing screws

When using a translation/angulation osteotomy, the fibula should be osteotomized slightly distal to the tibia. If there is no fibular deformity and the tibial deformity angulates the plafond toward the fibula, the fibula does not require an osteotomy, because it will not be affected during reduction [80, 81].

Patients are immobilized for 4–6 weeks and strictly non-weight-bearing is indicated after the surgery. Deep drain is not routinely used. Sutures are removed between 2 and 3 weeks, based on the degree of soft tissue swelling. Complications with supramalleolar osteotomies are rare. The most common is decreased range of motion and stiffness of the ankle. Nonunion, delayed union, persistent pain, wound complications, superficial or deep late infections, nerve damage, fracture, deep venous thrombosis, and compartment syndrome are some of the complications with these procedures. Wound healing problems and infections may be resolved by i.v. antibiotics and/or surgical debridement and irrigation. Intraoperative complications may include injuries of neurovascular structures and tendons. Anatomical knowledge of surgical approaches is required.

References

1. Bosien WR, Staples OS, Russell SW. Residual disability following acute ankle sprains. J Bone Joint Surg Am. 1955;37-A(6):1237–43. https://doi.org/10.2106/00004623-195537060-00011.
2. Ekstrand J, Tropp H. The incidence of ankle sprains in soccer. Foot Ankle. 1990;11(1):41–4. https://doi.org/10.1177/107110079001100108.
3. Freeman MA. Instability of the foot after injuries to the lateral ligament of the ankle. J Bone Joint Surg Br. 1965;47(4):669–77.
4. Garrick JG. The frequency of injury, mechanism of injury, and epidemiology of ankle sprains. Am J Sports Med. 1977;5(6):241–2. https://doi.org/10.1177/036354657700500606.
5. Hawkins RB. Arthroscopic stapling repair for chronic lateral instability. Clin Podiatr Med Surg. 1987;4:875–83.
6. Acevedo JI, Mangone PG. Arthroscopic lateral ligament reconstruction. Tech Foot Ankle Surg. 2011;10:111–6.
7. Broström L. Sprained ankles. V. Treatment and prognosis in recent ligament ruptures. Acta Chir Scand. 1966;132:537–50.
8. Broström L. Sprained ankles. VI Surgical treatment of "chronic" ligament ruptures. Acta Chir Scand. 1966;132:551–65.
9. Clanton TO, Viens NA, Campbell KJ, LaPrade RF, Wijdicks CA. Anterior talofibular ligament ruptures, Part 2. Am J Sports Med. 2013;42:412–41.
10. Corte-Real NM, Moreira RM. Arthroscopic repair of chronic lateral ankle instability. Foot Ankle Int. 2009;30:213–7.
11. Evans DL. Recurrent instability of the ankle. A method of surgical treatment. Proc R Soc Med. 1953;46(5):343–4.
12. Gould N, Seligson D, Gassman J. Early and late repair of lateral ligament of the ankle. Foot Ankle. 1980;1:94–9.
13. Guillo S, Bauer T, Lee JW, Takao M, Kong SW, Stone JW, Mangone PG, Molloy A, Perera A, Pearce CJ, Michels F, Tourné Y, Ghorbani A, Calder J. Consensus in chronic ankle instability: aetiology, assessment, surgical indications and place for arhthroscopy. Orthop Traumatol Surg Res. 2013;99:411–9.
14. Matsui K, Burgesson B, Takao M, Stone J, Guillo S, Glazebrook M, ESSKA AFAS Ankle Instability Group. Minimally invasive surgical treatment for chronic ankle instability: a systematic review. Knee Surg Sports Traumatol Arthrosc. 2016;24:1040–8. https://doi.org/10.1007/s00167-016-4041-1.
15. Michels F, Pereira H, Calder J, Matricali G, Glazebrook M, Guillo S, Karlsson J, The ESSKA-AFAS Ankle Instability Group. Searching for consensus in the approach to patients with chronic lateral ankle instability: ask the expert. Knee Surg Sports Traumatol Arthrosc. 2017; https://doi.org/10.1007/s00167-017-4556-0.
16. Snook GA, Chrisman OD, Wilson TC. Long-term results of the Chrisman-Snook operation for reconstruction of the lateral ligaments of the ankle. J Bone Joint Surg Am. 1985;67(1):1–7.
17. Takao M, Glazebrook M, Stone J, et al. Ankle arthroscopic reconstruction of lateral ligaments (Ankle Anti-ROLL). Arthrosc Tech. 2015;4:595–600.
18. Vega J, Golano P, Pellegrino A, Rabat E, Pena F. Allinside arthroscopic lateral collateral ligament

repair for ankle instability with a knotless suture anchor technique. Foot Ankle Int. 2013;34:1701–9.
19. Watson-Jones R. Recurrent forward dislocation of the ankle joint. J Bone Joint Surg. 1952;34B:519–22.
20. Batista JP, Del Vecchio Jorge J, Patthauer L, Ocampo M. Arthroscopic lateral ligament repair through two portals in chronic ankle instability. Open Orthop J. 2017;11:3–00.
21. Batista JP, Arrondo G, Joannas G, Del Vecchio J, Patthauer L, Pereira DH, Vega J. Endoscopic lateral ligament repair associated with calcaneous osteotomy. New insights in the treatment of chronic ankle instability. Free paper. AIG Congress Bordeaux. 21–22 Sept 2017.
22. Guillo S, Archbold P, Perera A, Bauer T, Sonnery-Cottet B. Arthroscopic anatomic reconstruction of the lateral ligaments of the ankle with gracilis autograft. Arthrosc Tech. 2014;3:e593–8.
23. Guillo S, Cordier G, Sonnery-Cottet B, Bauer T. Anatomical reconstruction of the anterior talofibular and calcaneofibular ligaments with an all-arthroscopic surgical technique. Orthop Traumatol Surg Res. 2014;100:S413–7.
24. Michels F, Cordier G, Burssens A, et al. Endoscopic reconstruction of CFL and the ATFL with a gracilis graft: a cadaveric study. Knee Surg Sports Traumatol Arthrosc. 2016;24:1007–14.
25. Michels F, Cordier G, Guillo S, et al. Endoscopic ankle lateral ligament graft anatomic reconstruction. Foot Ankle Clin. 2016;21:665–80.
26. Nery C, Raduan F, Buono AD, Asaumi ID, Cohen M, Maffulli N. Arthroscopic-assisted Broström–Gould for chronic ankle instability: a long-term follow-up. Am J Sports Med. 2011;39:2381–8.
27. Takao M, Matsui K, Stone James W, Glazebrook Mark A, Kennedy John G, Guillo S, Calder James D, Karlsson J, Ankle Instability Group. Arthroscopic anterior talofibular ligament repair for lateral instability of the ankle. Knee Surg Sports Traumatol Arthrosc. 2016;24:1003–6. https://doi.org/10.1007/s00167-015-3638-0.
28. Ahn JH, Choy W, Kim H. Reconstruction of the lateral ankle ligament with a long extensor tendon graft of the fourth toe. Am J Sports Med. 2011;39(3):637–44.
29. Coughlin MJ, Schenck RC, Grebing BR, Treme G. Comprehensive reconstruction of the lateral ankle for chronic instability using a free gracilis graft. Foot Ankle Int. 2004;25(4):231–41.
30. Jung HG, Kim TH, Park JY, Bae EJ. Reconstruction of the anterior talofibular and calcaneofibular ligaments using a semitendinosus tendon allograft and interference screws. Knee Surg Sports Traumatol Arthrosc. 2012;20(8):1432–7.
31. Kim ES, Lee KT, Park JS, Lee YK. Arthroscopic anterior talofibular ligament repair for chronic ankle instability with a suture anchor technique. Orthopedics. 2011;34:1–5.
32. Matsui K, Takao M, Miyamoto W, Innami K, Matsushita T. Arthroscopic Broström repair with Gould argumentation via an accessory anterolateral port for lateral instability of the ankle. Arch Orthop Trauma Surg. 2014;134:1461–7.
33. Aydogan U, Glisson RR, Nunley JA. Extensor retinaculum augmentation reinforces anterior talofibular ligament repair. Clin Orthop Relat Res. 2006;442:210–5.
34. Dalmau-Pastor M, Yasui Y, Calder JD, Karlsson J, Kerkhoffs GMMJ, Kennedy JG. Anatomy of the inferior extensor retinaculum and its role in lateral ankle ligament reconstruction: a pictorial essay. Knee Surg Sports Traumatol Arthrosc. 2016;24:957–62. https://doi.org/10.1007/s00167-016-4082-5.
35. Behrens SB, Drakos M, Lee BJ, Paller D, Hoffman E, Koruprolu S, DiGiovanni CW. Biomechanical analysis of Brostrom versus Brostrom–Gould lateral ankle instability repair. Foot Ankle Int. 2013;34:587–92.
36. Barber FA, Click J, Britt BT. Complications of ankle arthroscopy. Foot Ankle. 1990;10:263–6.
37. De Leeuw PAJ, Golanó P, Sierevelt IN, et al. The course of the superficial peroneal nerve in relation to the ankle position: anatomical study with ankle arthroscopic implications. Knee Surg Sports Traumatol Arthrosc. 2010;18:612–7.
38. Ferkel RD, Heath DD, Guhl JF. Neurological complications of ankle arthroscopy. Arthroscopy. 1996;12:200–8.
39. Ferkel RD, Small HN, Gittins JE. Complications in foot and ankle arthroscopy. Clin Orthop Relat Res. 2001;391:89–104.
40. Zengerink M, van Dijk CN. Complications in ankle arthroscopy. Knee Surg Sports Traumatol Arthrosc. 2012;20:1420–31.
41. Ogilvie-Harris DJ, Gilbart M. Treatment modalities for soft tissue injuries of the ankle: a critical review. Clin J Sport Med. 1995;5(3):175–86. https://doi.org/10.1097/00042752-199507000-00008.
42. Ogilvie-Harris DJ, Sekyi-Otu A. Arthroscopic debridement for the osteoarthritic ankle. Arthroscopy. 1995;11(4):433–6. https://doi.org/10.1016/0749-8063(95)90197-3.
43. Wiewiorski M, Barg A, Valderrabano V. Cartilage reconstruction in osteochondral lesions of the talus (OCLT). Foot Ankle Clin. 2013. (Accepted for publication).
44. Barg A, Pagenstert GI, Horisberger M, Jochen P, Gloyer M, Henninger HB, Valderrabano V. Supramalleolar osteotomies for degenerative joint disease of the ankle joint: indication, technique and results. Orthopaedics (SICOT). 2013;37:1683–95. https://doi.org/10.1007/s00264-013-2030-2.
45. Tanaka Y. The concept of ankle joint preserving surgery: why does supramalleolar osteotomy work and how to decide when to do an osteotomy or joint replacement. Foot Ankle Clin. 2012;17(4):545–53.
46. Valderrabano V, Hintermann B, Horisberger M, Fung TS. Ligamentous posttraumatic ankle osteoarthritis. Am J Sports Med. 2006;34(4):612–20.
47. Becker AS, Myerson MS. The indications and technique of supramalleolar osteotomy. Foot Ankle Clin

N Am. 2009;14:549–61. https://doi.org/10.1016/j.fcl.2009.06.002.
48. Takakura Y, Takaoka T, Tanaka Y, Yajima H, Tamai S. Results of opening-wedge osteotomy for the treatment of a post-traumatic varus deformity of the ankle. J Bone Joint Surg Am. 1998;80(2):213–8.
49. Takakura Y, Tanaka Y, Kumai T, Tamai S. Low tibial osteotomy for osteoarthritis of the ankle. Results of a new operation in 18 patients. J Bone Joint Surg Br. 1995;77(1):50–4.
50. Hintermann B, Knupp M, Barg A. Supramalleolar osteotomies for the treatment of ankle arthritis. J Am Acad Orthop Surg. 2016;24:424–32.
51. Tennant JN, Carmont M, Phisitkul P. Calcaneus osteotomy. Curr Rev Musculoskelet Med. 2014;7:271–6. https://doi.org/10.1007/s12178-014-9237-8.
52. Mendicino RW, Catanzariti AR, Reeves CL. Posterior calcaneal displacement osteotomy: a new percutaneous technique. J Foot Ankle Surg. 2004;43:332–5.
53. Dwyer FC. Osteotomy of the calcaneum for pes cavus. J Bone Joint Surg Br. 1959;41:80–6.
54. Dwyer FC. The present status of the problem of pes cavus. Clin Orthop Relat Res. 1975;106:254–75.
55. Barg A, Hörterer H, Jacxsens M, Wiewiorski M, Paul J, Valderrabano V. Dwyer osteotomy: lateral sliding osteotomy of calcaneus. [Article in German]. Oper Orthop Traumatol. 2015;27(4):283–97. https://doi.org/10.1007/s00064-015-0409-5. Epub 2015 Jul 22.
56. Hintermann B, Knupp M, Barg A. Osteotomies of the distal tibia and hindfoot for ankle realignment. Orthopade. 2008;37:212–3.
57. Lui TH. Percutaneous posterior calcaneal osteotomy. J Foot Ankle Surg. 2015;54(6):1188–92. https://doi.org/10.1053/j.jfas.2015.04.027. Epub 2015 Jul 16.
58. Harrington KD. Degenerative arthritis of the ankle secondary to long-standing lateral ligament instability. J Bone Joint Surg. 1979;61A:354–61.
59. Rieck B, Reiser M, Bernet P. Posttraumatic arthrosis of the upper ankle joint in chronic insufficiency of the fibular ligament. Orthopade. 1986;6:466–71.
60. Buckwalter JA, Saltzman CL. Ankle osteoarthritis: distinctive characteristics. AAOS Instruct Course Lect. 1999;48:233–42.
61. Resnick RB, Jahss MH, Choueka J, Kummer F, Hersch JC, Okereke E. Deltoid ligament forces after tibialis posterior tendon rupture: effects of triple arthrodesis and calcaneal displacement osteotomies. Foot Ankle Int. 1995;16:14–20.
62. Steffensmeier SJ, Saltzman CL, Berbaum KS, Brown TD. Effects of medial and lateral displacement calcaneal osteotomies on tibiotalar joint contact stresses. J Orthop Res. 1996;14:980–5.
63. Morscher E, Hefti F, Baumann JU. Combined lateral ligament-plasty and calcaneus osteotomy in recurrent foot dislocation. [Article in German]. Orthopade. 1986;15(6):461–5.
64. Knupp M, Barg A, Bolliger L, et al. Reconstructive surgery for overcorrected club-foot in adults. J Bone Joint Surg Am. 2012;94:e1101–7.
65. Egol KA, Kubiak EN, Fulkerson FJ, et al. Biomechanics of locked plates and screws. J Orthop Trauma. 2004;18(8):488–93.
66. Mangone PG. Distal tibial osteotomies for the treatment of foot and ankle disorders. Foot Ankle Clin. 2001;6(3):583–97.
67. Cox JS, Hewes TF. "Normal" talar tilt angle. Clin Orthop Relat Res. 1979;140:37–41.
68. Tanaka Y, Takakura Y, Fujii T, Kumai T, Sugimoto K. Hindfoot alignment of hallux valgus evaluated by a weightbearing subtalar x-ray view. Foot Ankle Int. 1999;20(10):640–5.
69. Saltzman CL, el-Khoury GY. The hindfoot alignment view. Foot Ankle Int. 1995;16(9):572–6.
70. Reilingh ML, Beimers L, Tuijthof Gabriëlle JM, Stufkens Sjoerd AS, Maas M, van Dijk CN. Measuring hindfoot alignment radiographically: the long axial view is more reliable than the hindfoot alignment view. Skelet Radiol. 2010;39:1103–8. https://doi.org/10.1007/s00256-009-0857-9.
71. Dann K, Wahler G, Neubauer N, Steiner R, Titze W, Wagner M. Sportverletz Sportschaden. 1996;10(3):67–9. https://doi.org/10.1055/s-2007-993402.
72. van Dijk CN, Scholte D. Arthroscopy of the ankle joint. Arthroscopy. 1997;13:90–6.
73. van Dijk CN, Van Bergen CJ. Advancements in ankle arthroscopy. J Am Acad Orthop Surg. 2008;16:635–46.
74. Eastwood DM, Irgau I, Atkins RM. The distal course of the sural nerve and its significance for incisions around the lateral hindfoot. Foot Ankle. 1992;13(4):199–202.
75. Haugsdal J, Dawson J, Phisitkul P. Nerve injury and pain after operative repair of calcaneal fractures: a literature review. Iowa Orthop J. 2013;33:202–7.
76. Kraus JC, Fischer MT, McCormick JJ, et al. Geometry of the lateral sliding, closing wedge calcaneal osteotomy: review of the two methods and technical tip to minimize shortening. Foot Ankle Int. 2014;35(3):238–42. Recent review of technique for performing a valgus-producing (closing wedge or lateral sliding) calcaneal osteotomy.
77. Koman LA, Mooney JF III, Goodman A. Management of valgus hindfoot deformity in pediatric cerebral palsy patients by medial displacement osteotomy. J Pediatr Orthop. 1993;13(2):180–3.
78. Den Hartog BD, DiGiovanni CW, VanValkenburg SM, et al. Nerve injury associated with lateral calcaneal osteotomy, in American orthopaedic foot and ankle specialty day, American academy of orthopaedic surgeons annual meeting. New Orleans, LA; 2014.
79. Maskill MP, Maskill JD, Pomeroy GC. Surgical management and treatment algorithm for the subtle cavovarus foot. Foot Ankle Int. 2010;31(12):1057–63.
80. Mulhern JL, Protzman NM, Brigido SA, Deol Premjit PS. Supramalleolar osteotomy indications and surgical techniques. Clin Podiatr Med Surg. 2015;32:445–61. https://doi.org/10.1016/j.cpm.2015.03.006.
81. Siddiqui NA, Herzenberg JE, Lamm BM. Supramalleolar osteotomy for realignment of the ankle joint. Clin Podiatr Med Surg. 2012;29:465–82.

Ankle Instability and Gastrocnemius Tightness

37

Pierre Barouk

37.1 Introduction

Gastrocnemius tightness has been recognized to be involved in many foot pathologies [1]. Those who are secondary to a forefoot overload: hallux valgus, hammer toes, metatarsalgia, Morton's neuroma, Lisfranc arthritis [1]. And those who are secondary to a tension in the tendino-muscular structures: plantar aponeurosis [2], Achillis tendinopathy [3], tennis leg [4], and calf cramps and tensions [5]. Also, those who are secondary to a hyperlordosis given by the equinus [6].

We also showed in our monography [7] that there is a relation between ankle instability and gastrocnemius tightness.

37.2 Clinical Examination

Assessment of GC tightness is made by the Silfverskiold test [8].

The rear foot must be in neutral position and must keep the tibialis anterior relaxed. The pressure below the second and third metatarsal heads must be light, around 2 kg (Fig. 37.1). Appreciation must be done by the lateral aspect of the foot. A negative passive dorsal flexion signs a gastrocnemius tightness [9].

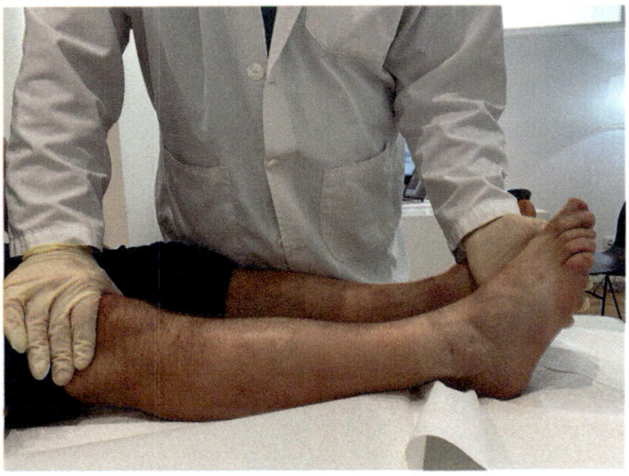

Fig. 37.1 Examination, rear foot reduced, smooth force applied under the second and third metatarsals, with tibialis anterior relaxed

37.3 What Kind of Instability Are We Talking About?

We note a difference between a sensation of instability, what we call a subjective instability, and a real instability with recurrent ankle sprains, what we call an objective instability.

P. Barouk (✉)
Centre de Chirurgie Orthopédique et Sportive, Clinique du Sport de Bordeaux Mérignac, Mérignac, France

H. Pereira et al. (eds.), *Lateral Ankle Instability*, https://doi.org/10.1007/978-3-662-62763-1_37

37.3.1 Subjective Instability

This is a sensation of instability. This impression of instability reveals itself by an apprehension, an impression of losing one's balance, and even falls. These phenomena are not followed by sprains. It is a rare motivation for a foot surgeon consultation. Interrogation is of major importance. By questioning the patient, we will b able to find these "signs" which are often neglected or progress faintly without any explanation.

In our series of 354 proximal gastrocnemius lengthening [7] (mostly combined with forefoot surgery), we asked preoperatively the question to the patient: "do you feel instable on your legs?." Of them, 52.5% answered "yes." This instability disappeared in 79% of the cases, and had been improved in 19% after the proximal gastrocnemius lengthening. So there has been a positive effect of the gastrocnemius lengthening on the subjective instability in 98% of the cases.

37.3.2 Objective Instability

This is the recurrence of real lateral ankle sprains with lesion of the lateral ligaments. The line between objective and subjective instability is often small. The fact of suffering repetitive sprains can be the consequence of a more important gastrocnemius tightness or ligament laxity, or of a more "at-risk" sport practice, comparing to the patients suffering subjective instability.

In the same series, 27% patients had recurrent ankle sprains. It was not the subject of the consultation except in five cases.

After the gastrocnemius lengthening, only 3% had ankle instability. And those five patients who initially seeked assistance due to ankle instability, did not experience further ankle sprains after being treated by gastrocnemius lengthening.

These results encouraged us to search and treat the gastrocnemius tightness in every patient that comes for ankle instability.

37.4 Biomechanics Elements

We try to explain this relation by several explanations.

37.4.1 The Talus

The position of the talus when the ankle is in equinus is a key point in the instability.

During the gait, at the toe off phase, when the knee is in extension, the gastrocnemius is maximally contracted. This is the zone C or point x of Cazaux [10] (Fig. 37.2).

If the gastrocnemius is short, this dorsiflexion cannot be reached totally. The talus stays in plantar flexion and is not locked between the malleolus because it is narrower posteriorly [11] (Figs. 37.3 and 37.4).

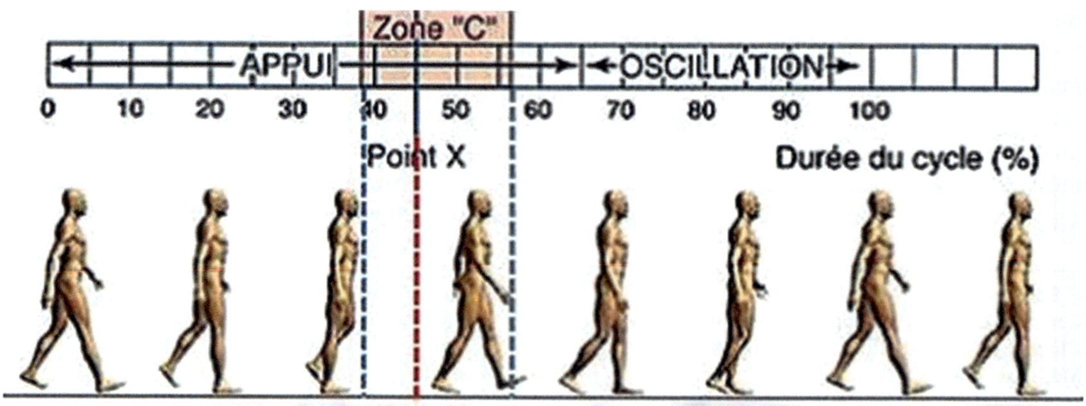

Fig. 37.2 Zone C: maximum of contraction of the gastrocnemius (when the ankle is in plantar flexion)

37.4.2 The Valgus

Several authors observe more valgus rear foot than varus when there is gastrocnemius tightness [11–13].

The lack of dorsiflexion when the knee is extended forces the calcaneum to slide laterally to gain some dorsal flexion. And, as the "neutral" position is in valgus, this valgus increases.

According to Kowalski [13], this valgus induces a hypotony, a weakness of the peroneal brevis that could not act as a stabilizator of the varus stress.

We are here in a paradoxal situation of a valgus rear foot (characterized by a flat foot) with a varus instability. This is typical of the gastrocnemius tightness. Figure 37.5 shows a valgus rear foot with a varus deformity of the shoe, in a patient that suffers of recurrent sprains and has gastrocnemius tightness.

In the series of LS Barouk [11], the valgus was increased after GC lengthening, when it was severe preoperatively. It did not change when it was mild. The rare cases of varus rear foot did not change and were associated to poorer results on the instability.

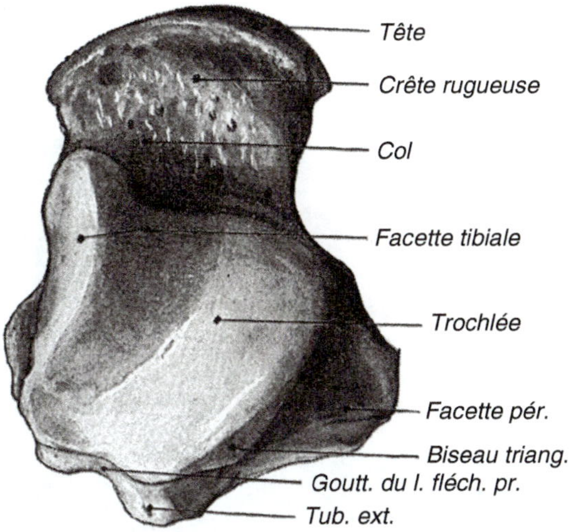

Fig. 37.3 The talus is larger at the front

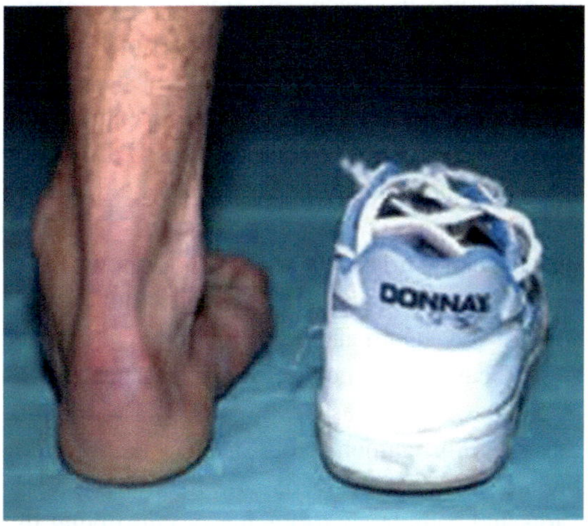

Fig. 37.5 Valgus rear foot but shoe deformed in varus

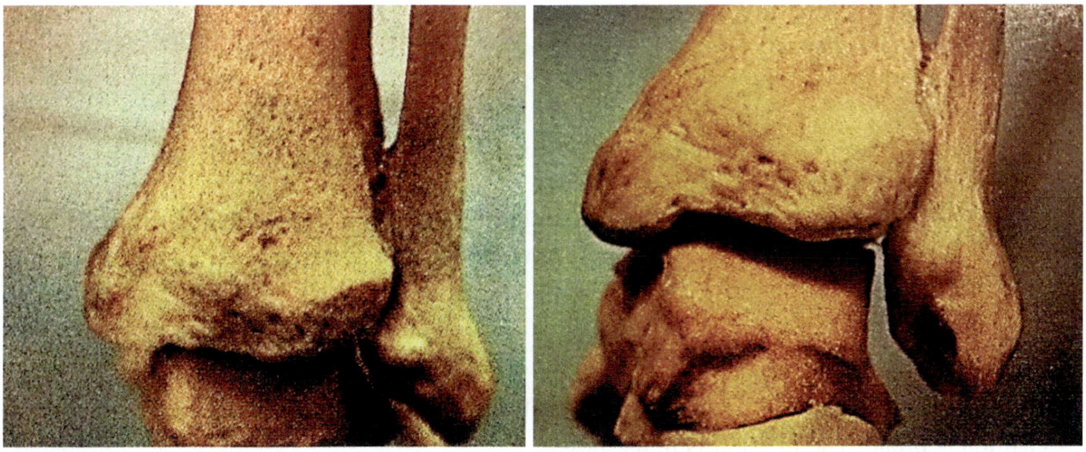

Fig. 37.4 Decoaptation of the lateral gutter when the ankle is in plantar flexion

37.4.3 Plantar Contact Area

The equinus decreased the contact area of the sole of the foot. This may lead to instability.

37.5 Discussion

We observed in our practice an association of ankle instability and gastrocnemius tightness. Patients visited us mainly for forefoot problems, and it is the interrogatory that reveal a present or a past history of recurrent ankle instability.

We think that it starts with a subjective instability, and once the ligaments (mainly the anterior talo-fibular) are elongated than ruptured, the instability increases and it becomes an objective instability. For us there is a lot of ankle instability that are due to gastrocnemius tightness. Particularly those who have a valgus rear foot. The treatment of this tightness is crucial because it is logical to treat the cause first. We succeed in five cases in our series by doing a proximal gastrocnemius release without any ligament reconstruction. Since then, several cases have been done with success. It is also possible to associate the gastrocnemius release with ligament reconstruction if there is a big instability with decoaptation of the talus in varus and completely torn anterior talo-fibular ligament. It seems logical to treat the cause and the consequences. As the proximal GC lengthening can be considered harmless [14, 15], it is possible to start with the lengthening procedure before proposing a ligament reconstruction, in case of concomitant GC tightness and ankle instability (with injured ligaments).

We do not know the rate of GC tightness in the population of ankle instability. This is a research way for the future. Once we have a reproductible device for equinus measurement.

The physiotherapy can also be done to lengthen the gastrocnemius, but we believe more in the harmless surgical lengthening and have the experience by over 2000 procedures done.

Our technique is simple:

Position is prone. The incision is in the flexion crease, 1 cm lateral to the medial fovea. It is approximately 3 cm in length (Fig. 37.6). At this level there are no vascular or nervous structures that can be damaged, as well described by the anatomic study of Hamilton and Solan [9]. The sub-cutaneous fat is retracted, and we find the posterior fascia of the leg. This is opened in the axis of the leg. We find, just underneath, the medial gastrocnemius covered by a thin aponeurosis and marked by a fat layer of variable thickness. The tendon is on the medial side, extending anteriorly (Fig. 37.7). All the white fibers are cut with scissors (Fig. 37.8). We check that there is no more tension in the muscle, using a finger, while we move the ankle into dorsiflexion.

There is no need for postoperative immobilization.

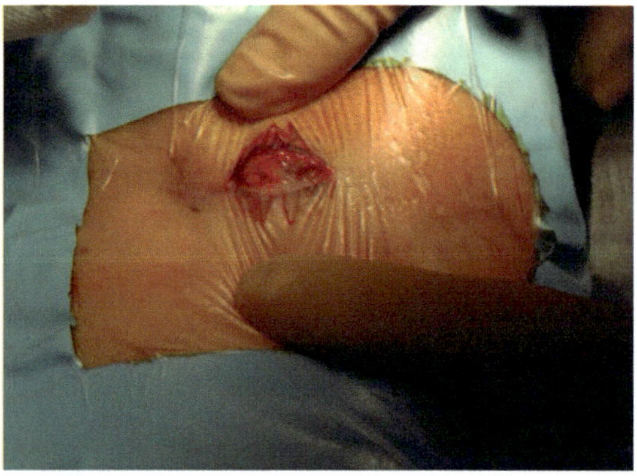

Fig. 37.6 Incision in the flexion crease of the knee

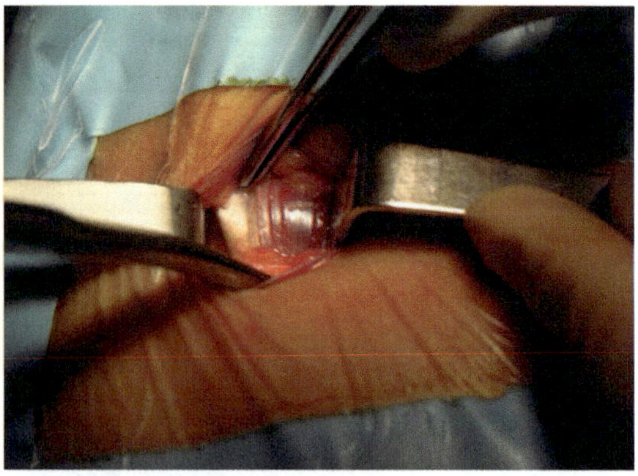

Fig. 37.7 The tendinous structure of the medial gastrocnemius becomes thicker medially and at the anterior aspect of the muscle

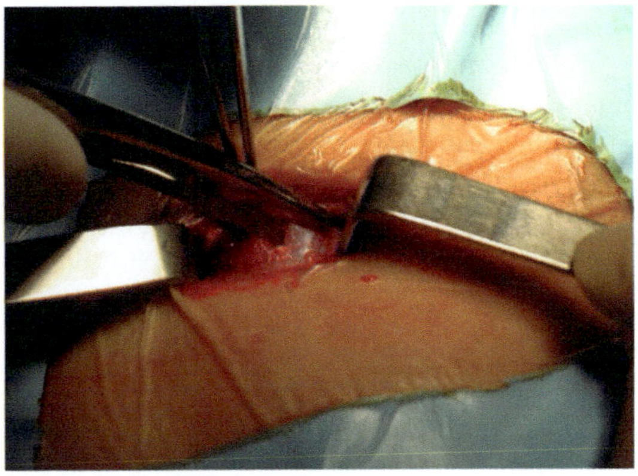

Fig. 37.8 Section of the white fibers of the medial gastrocnemius

37.6 Conclusion

We find often instability symptoms when there is a gastrocnemius tightness. This association is underestimated by the physicians who deal with patients who suffers from instability. We propose a simple and effective surgical solution (proximal medial gastrocnemius release), alone or associated with ligament reconstruction when it is needed. The assessment should be systematic. Further studies should be run to evaluate the rate of GC tightness and the effect of gastrocnemius lengthening in a population of instable patients.

References

1. DiGiovanni CW, Kuo R, Tejwani N, Price R, Hansen ST Jr, Cziernecki J, et al. Isolated gastrocnemius tightness. J Bone Joint Surg Am. 2002;84-A(6):962–70.
2. Bolívar YA, Munuera PV, Padillo JP. Relationship between tightness of the posterior muscles of the lower limb and plantar fasciitis. Foot Ankle Int. 2013;34(1):42–8.
3. Molund M, Lapinskas SR, Nilsen FA, Hvaal KH. Clinical and functional outcomes of gastrocnemius recession for chronic Achilles tendinopathy. Foot Ankle Int. 2016;37(10):1091–7.
4. Baudet B. Tennis leg. In: Brièveté des gastrocnémiens. Montpellier: Sauramps; 2012. p. 270–6.
5. Barouk P. Signes directs. In: Brièveté des gastrocnémiens. Montpellier: Sauramps; 2012. p. 175–81.
6. Barouk P. Lombalgies. In: Brièveté des gastrocnémiens. Montpellier: Sauramps; 2012. p. 180–2.
7. Barouk P. Instabilité des membres inférieurs. In: Brièveté des gastrocnémiens. Montpellier: Sauramps; 2012. p. 183–6.
8. Silfverskiold N. Reduction of the uncrossed two joints muscles of the leg to one joint muscles in spastic conditions. Acta Chir Scand. 1924;56:315–104.
9. Barouk P, Barouk LS. Clinical diagnosis of gastrocnemius tightness. Foot Ankle Clin. 2014;19(4):659–67.
10. Cazeau C. Biomechanics of the gastrocnemius tightness on the foot. The gastrocnemius. Foot Ankle Clin. 2014;19(4):649–58.
11. Barouk LS, Barouk P. Instabilité de cheville et brièveté tricipitale. In: Yourné Y, Mabit C, editors. La cheville instable. France: Elsevier Masson; 2014.
12. Colombier JA. Libération Proximale Pure dans la prise en charge thérapeutique des Gastrocnemiens. Courts Symposium « Brieveté desGastrocnemiens », Journées de Printemps SFMCP-AFCP, Toulouse, 2006. Med Chir Pied. 2006;22:156–7.
13. Kowalski C, Diebold P, Pennecot GF. Le tendon calcanéen court. In: Encyclopédie Medico-Chirurgicale 27-060. Amsterdam: Elsevier; 1999.
14. Barouk P. Technique for proximal medial gastrocnemius lengthening. The gastrocnemius. Foot Ankle Clin. 2014;19(4):659–67.
15. Hamilton PD, Brown M, Ferguson N, Adebibe M, Maggs J, Solan M. Surgical anatomy of the proximal release of the gastrocnemius: a cadaveric study. Foot Ankle Int. 2009;30(12):1202–6.

38 Concurrent Pathology and Ankle Instability

Hélder Pereira, Pieter D'Hooghe, Kenneth J. Hunt, Akos Kynsburg, A. Pereira de Castro, and Henrique Jones

38.1 Introduction

Ankle sprain is a very frequent lesion which can cause functional limitations. It has been described as one of the most frequent injuries during sports activity (either in athletes or general population). Nevertheless, guidelines or evidence-based criteria for return to activity are scarce [1]. Some gestures such as rapid changes in direction, inadequate footwear, walk in uneven ground or landings from jumps or falls might exceed the mechanical resistance of the ankle joint leading to injury [2, 3].

An inversion mechanism is the most frequently implicated in an acute ankle sprain [4]. This characteristically happens after a jump or twist, when landing on the lateral border of the foot, but might also occur if the foot gets locked on the ground, while the body continues to rotate.

This will cause an abrupt increase in both inversion and internal rotation forces, which combines either dorsi- or plantarflexion, producing enough loads which might lead to rupture of the lateral ligaments, cause loose bodies, osteochondral lesions, anterior or posterior joint impingement, or even further ligaments and tendons lesions (Fig. 38.1) [5, 6]. The anterior talofibular ligament (ATFL) is always injured first (Fig. 38.2), but with increased inversion and rotation the calcaneofibular ligament (CFL) might also be torn [7]. An isolated rupture of the ATFL occurs in around 65% of cases, while

H. Pereira (✉)
Orthopedic Department of Póvoa de Varzim, Vila do Conde Hospital Centre, Vila do Conde, Portugal

Ripoll y De Prado Sports Clinic: Murcia-Madrid FIFA Medical Centre of Excellence, Murcia-Madrid, Spain

International Centre of Sports Traumatology of the Ave, Vila do Conde, Portugal

ICVS/3B's - PT Government Associated Laboratory, University of Minho, Braga-Guimarães, Portugal

P. D'Hooghe
Department of Orthopaedic Surgery, Aspire Zone, Aspetar Orthopaedic and Sportsmedicine Hospital, Doha, Qatar
e-mail: pieter.dhooghe@aspetar.com

K. J. Hunt
Department of Orthopaedic Surgery, University of Colorado School of Medicine, Aurora, CO, USA
e-mail: KENNETH.J.HUNT@cuanschutz.edu

A. Kynsburg
Sports Medicine, Podiatry, Landesklinikum Scheibbs – Traumatology, Scheibbs, Austria
e-mail: kynsburg@tmo.at

A. P. de Castro
DESPORSANO, Sports Clinic, Lisbon, Portugal

H. Jones
Montijo Orthopaedic and Sports Medicine Clinica, Montijo, Portugal

Hospital da Luz, Setúbal, Portugal

Lusófona University, Lisbon, Portugal

H. Pereira et al. (eds.), *Lateral Ankle Instability*, https://doi.org/10.1007/978-3-662-62763-1_38

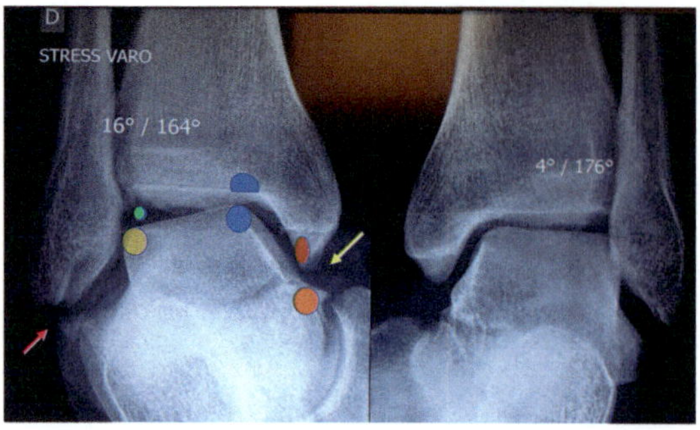

Fig. 38.1 On the right ankle it is visible the asymmetric; varus stress X-ray, representing lateral ankle instability. Possible consequences are shown such as medial impingement (orange colors—"kissing lesions"), anteromedial impingement (blue colors—"kissing lesions"), lateral talar impingement (light color). All these can lead to spur formation, osteochondral lesions, or loose bodies (green color)

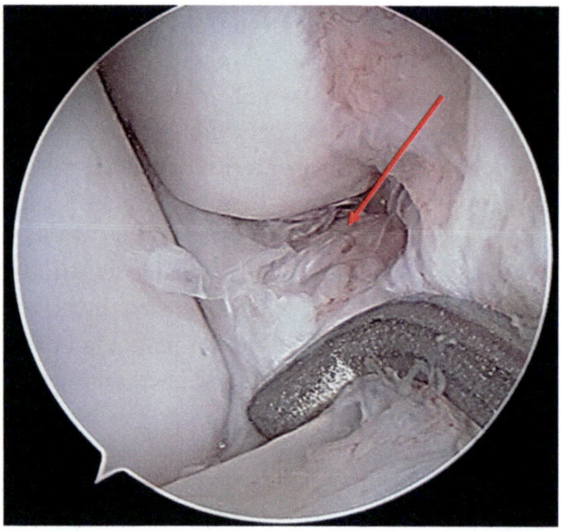

Fig. 38.2 Arthroscopic view of the anterior tibiofibular ligament (ATFL) remnant detached from the fibula (red arrow)

combined ruptures of the ATFL and CFL happens in about 20% [8, 9]. The posterior talofibular ligament (PTFL) is rarely injured in inversion mechanism sprains (Fig. 38.1) [10, 11]. A complete rupture of lateral ankle ligaments happens in approximately 10–15% of all inversion injuries [12]. However, 50% of these cases will have concomitant injuries (Fig. 38.1) in the joint (medial ligaments injuries, syndesmotic injuries, loose bodies, osteochondral defects (OCD)) [13].

The progression to chronic lateral ankle instability (CLAI) can aggravate such consequences with progression of osteochondral defects, ankle impingement, synovitis, and post-traumatic ankle arthritis [14–17]. Moreover, patients with CAI have changed joint kinematics which leads to higher risk for further recurrence of ankle sprains [18].

Repeated "micro-traumatisms" will increase the possibility for cartilage and osteochondral degeneration as well as anterior and/or posterior impingement. In case of failure of conservative treatment, patients who suffer from recurrent ankle sprains can be effectively treated by means of surgical stabilization [19–21]. Surgical treatment aims to restore joint kinematics and improve clinical outcome [22]. With the objective to minimize surgical aggression and enable immediate treatment of comorbidities, arthroscopic techniques have been developed and optimized, providing at least similar outcome as open techniques while also enabling dealing with most of the concomitant pathologies [19]. For this reason, this approach is growing in popularity [23].

38.2 From Ankle Sprain to Chronic Lateral Ankle Instability

Though the natural history of ankle sprains is not completely comprehended, the intrinsic stability of the ankle mortice and its congruency plays a role in the fact that complete but isolated ATFL ruptures have good prognosis, but also dictates possible damage when this congruency is put at risk. Despite most cases are effectively treated with conservative treatment [24], some argue that, in selected cases (e.g., elite athletes), early surgery can be considered as a first-line treatment. The goal would be to achieve a faster return to play and identify all possible concomitant lesions which are not easily identified in early imaging [25, 26].

Despite adequate conservative treatment, around 20–30% of patients will develop CLAI with persistent symptoms (persistent pain, fear of reinjury limiting activity, sense of giving away, and recurrent sprains) [25, 27, 28]. Definitive criteria guiding return to play for athletes or active people are insufficient in literature and there are no objective guidelines to aid in making this decision [1] .

CAI derives from numerous functional and mechanical factors [7, 29, 30]. These include proprioceptive deficits, disturbance of normal reflexes, or (peroneal) muscle weakness [29]. Consequently, a careful rehabilitation program emphasizing proprioceptive, neuromuscular control, and balance training is required, based on success rates up to 80% for functional rehabilitation programs [10, 25].

Surgery is required upon failure of conservative treatment [24, 28]. The surgical options to treat CAI include "anatomical" and nonanatomical repair/reconstructions (with the latest being connected to worst outcome and higher complications) [31, 32].

Presently, there is no evidence to support any specific superior surgical intervention over any other in the treatment of chronic ankle instability [27, 33].

However, there is a growing movement on the development of arthroscopic techniques, based on the positive outcome of repairs/reconstruction based on such approaches [23, 34–38]. This might lower the surgical morbidity, and shorten the time of recovery [39, 40]. Arthroscopy enables the treatment of concomitant intra-articular lesions in addition to ankle stabilization [14, 41]. However, we must emphasize that arthroscopy is a tool but not an obsession and the goal is to treat effectively the patient by whatever means required or depending on the surgeon's experience [19, 39, 40].

38.3 Loose Bodies, Ankle Osteochondral Defects, and CLAI

By definition, an osteochondral defect (OCD) is a lesion involving the articular hyaline cartilage and its subchondral bone (Fig. 38.3). The first classifications was proposed by Berndt and Harty in the late 1950s, but several others subsided [42]. OCDs are usually caused by traumatic

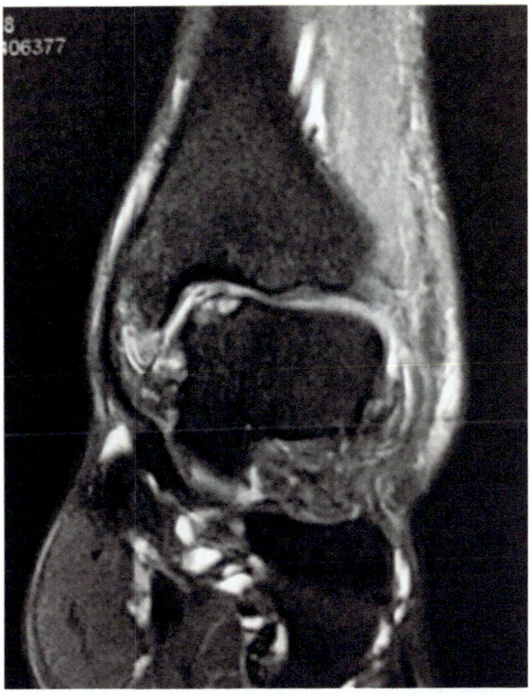

Fig. 38.3 MRI with visible talar osteochondral lesion with cartilage detachment (red arrow) as well as lateral bony edema secondary to lateral impingement

events (single or multiple), but nontraumatic, idiopathic OCD of the ankle is also admitted [43–46]. The anatomical grid proposed by Raikin and Elias has proven to be useful both in the talus and in the tibial plafond [47, 48]. The defect initially can comprise only superficial cartilage damage produced by shearing stress forces, but after a high-impact force, an OCD or even a bony defect can be created [49]. The formation of subchondral bone cysts is often linked to the development of the lesion (Fig. 38.4). Such cysts are related with recurrent deep ankle pain leading to further functional limitation. Most OCDs of the talus are found on the anterolateral or posteromedial talar dome [50]. Lateral OCDs are usually shallow oval shaped, and a shear mechanism has been proposed as the most frequent cause. Opposingly, medial lesions are usually deeper, and cup-shaped, advocating a torsional impaction and axial loading mechanism [44, 45]. The complete etiology and pathogenesis are still not fully comprehended of ankle OCDs and remain to be clarified.

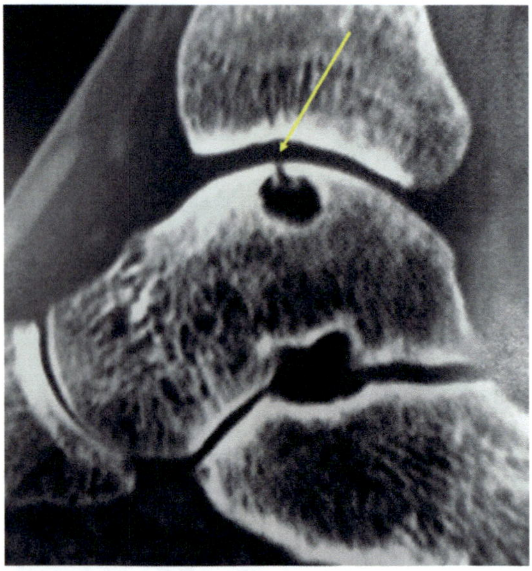

Fig. 38.4 Talar osteochondral lesion. It is visible the interruption of the talar dome which is conceivably connected to hydrostatic pressure involved in cystic formation

A traumatic event is generally accepted as the most significant cause of an OCD of the talus. For lateral talar defects, trauma has been implicated in 93–98% and for medial defects in 61–70% [51]. OCDs etiology can be divided into nontraumatic and traumatic defects [45]. Genetics as well as vascular causes with ischemia and consequent necrosis have been proposed as possible etiologies [44]. OCDs are bilateral in 10% of patients [52]. Moreover, OCDs have been found in identical twins and siblings [53]. Traumatic injuries of the cartilage comprises three groups: microdamage or blunt trauma, chondral fractures, and osteochondral fractures [54].

An OCD might have an acute onset or chronic onset. However the formation of subchondral cysts requires a slower development [55]. It is still unclear the reason why some OCDs remain asymptomatic, while others with apparently similar characteristics are painful (usually aggravated by effort), present bone edema on MRI and ultimately progress to subchondral cystic lesions. The comprehension of this pathophysiology would be of major relevance in order to prevent further joint degenerative changes [55].

Ankle sprains have a major role in the etiology of traumatic OCDs and most probably represent the most frequent traumatic events leading to these lesions [13]. Considering the anatomy and its inherent congruent morphology, during an ankle sprain, once the talus twists inside its "bony mortice," the cartilage overlying the talus can be damaged by direct impactions causing a real OCD, bone bruise, cartilage crack, or delamination. Shearing forces might cause split of the superficial cartilage cover [45]. Loose bodies can be produced, or OCDs might remain partially stable in its position (Fig. 38.5).

Formation of lateral ankle OCDs were reproduced under testing conditions by powerfully inverting a dorsiflexed ankle: as the foot was inverted: the lateral border of the talar dome was compressed against the fibula, and when the lateral ligament ruptured, it caused cartilage avulsion (Fig. 38.6). During application of excessive inverting force, the talus rotated laterally in the frontal plane within the mortise, thus impacting and compressing the lateral talar margin against the articular surface of the fibula. With this mechanism, a portion of the talar margin was delaminated causing a lateral OCD. A medial lesion could also be reproduced by forcing plantarflexion of the ankle in combination with anterior displacement of the talus under the tibia, while inverting and internally rotating the talus [42, 45].

For this reason, one can assume a close link between most ankle OCDs and CAI which is the topic for reflection in the herein presented paper.

Sometimes, OCDs are only asymptomatic incidental findings of the ankle, including in athletes [56].

Asymptomatic and/or low symptomatic OCDs can generally be treated conservatively, despite clinical and/or imaging follow-up is recommended. Conservative treatment includes orthobiologics (growth factors, hyaluronic acid, stem cells), physiotherapy, periods of rest, or immobilization (e.g., Walker Boot) [43, 50].

Upon failure of conservative treatment, symptomatic ankle OCDs can be surgically addressed (Fig. 38.7) by several approaches depending on the characteristics of the lesion and patient-

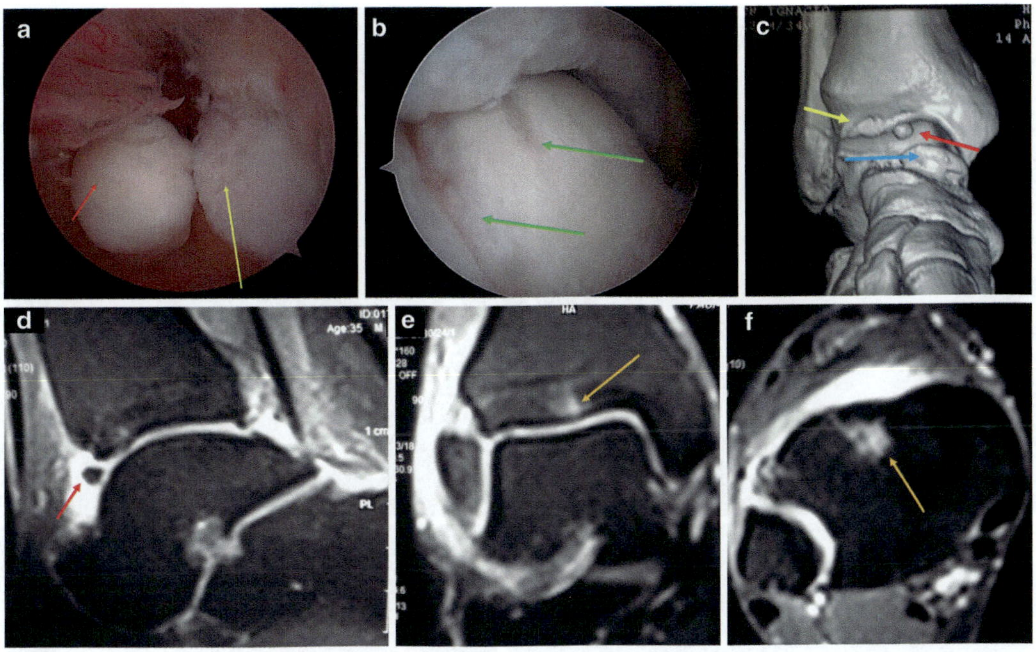

Fig. 38.5 (**a**) Loose body (red arrow) with cartilage conflict and damage (yellow arrow); (**b**) talar dome longitudinal defects caused by loose bodies (green arrows); (**c**) CT 3D image showing loose body (red arrow) as well as talar (light blue arrow) and tibial (yellow arrow) spurs related to ankle anterior impingement; (**d–f**) MRI view with loose body (red arrow) as well as tibial bony edema related to impingement (orange arrow)

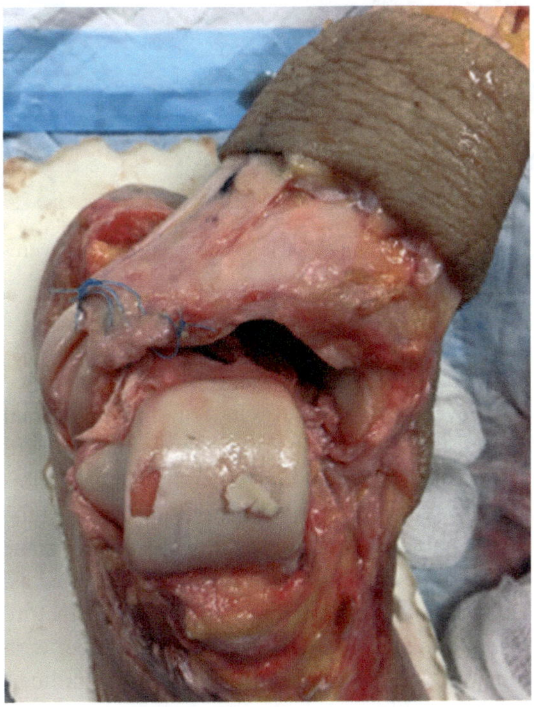

Fig. 38.6 Cadaveric Model representing lateral cartilage lesions secondary to ankle inversion mechanism

specific factors including expectations. There is currently no consensus in literature about a clear superiority of any surgical treatment over another in either primary or secondary ankle OCDs [50, 57, 58].

Preoperative planning is of paramount relevance and it always should include standing X-rays for assessment of alignment and global evaluation including the status of surrounding joints. The CT is very important and provides more feasible assessment of the dimensions of the bone defects under the lesion which can be overestimated by the edema visible in MRI (mostly in T2 sequences). However, edema in T2 MRI images insinuates activity around the injury. Moreover, CT lateral view in plantar flexion or dorsiflexion is helpful to determine if it is possibly an anterior or posterior arthroscopic approach. In some cases, an open approach by means of medial malleolar osteotomy is required for medial defects, or detachment of the lateral ligaments followed by its reinsertion in lateral defects.

An arthroscopic approach (Fig. 38.7) is presently the most frequent method for either

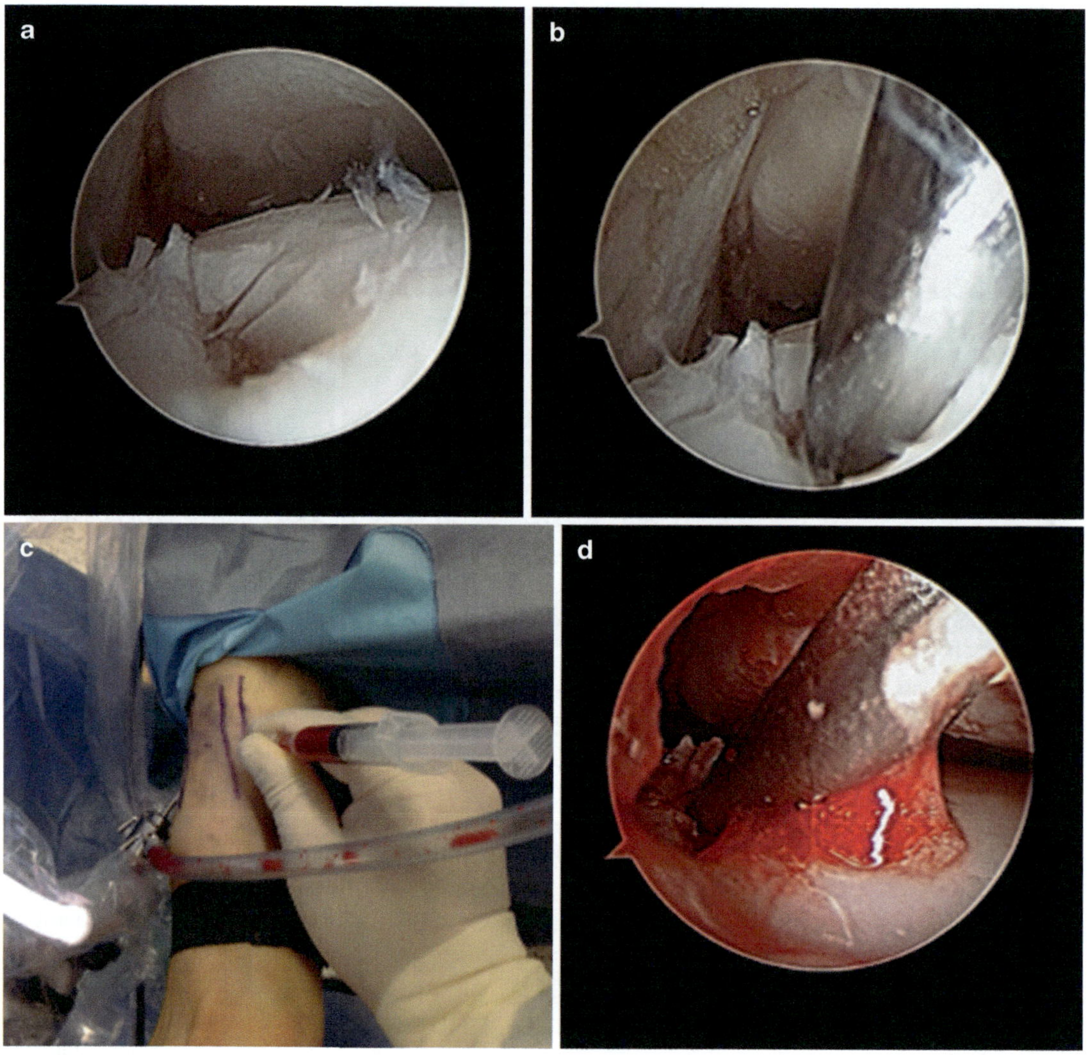

Fig. 38.7 (**a**) Talar osteochondral lesion; (**b**) microfractures; (**c** and **d**) demonstrate local injection with adhesive hydrogel imbedded with stem cells (experimental therapy)

anterior or posterior compartment's OCDs [59]. The percentage of complications is extremely low, particularly if no fixed distraction is used [60].

Considering the lack of evidence of any superior treatment, most authors favor the less aggressive procedures, usually less prone to complications and stating lower cost for either primary or secondary lesions. The final therapeutic option also considers the patient profile and injury characteristics.

Any ankle OCD should be fixed in place whenever possible (sufficient size and minimal layer of underlying bone). The so-called "Lift, Drill, Fill, Fix" technique should always be considered (either open or arthroscopic) and it is the one capable to preserve most of the native tissue and hyaline cartilage [61]. It can be described as, Lift: the defect, Drill: by making microfracture or bone marrow stimulation, Fill: the defect with bone graft; and Fix: the fragment with metallic or bioabsorbable screws or pins.

In OCDs up to 15 mm, bone marrow stimulation techniques, most frequently by means of microfractures, aims to stimulate the underlying mesenchymal stem cells (MSCs) and growth factors (GFs) from the subchondral bone. By creating/enhancing pathways to these bioactive agents, these techniques have the goal to promote fibrocartilage coverage of the defect and provide around 85% of successful outcome at 5 years follow-up [62]. Acknowledging the positive clinical outcome and its limited aggression, such approach may also be considered in bigger lesions (unsuitable for fixation or secondary injuries) [50, 57, 58].

Large cystic lesions (either in talus or tibia) can be treated by retrograde drilling. This technique aims to lower the pressure within the cyst and, if required and possible, the defect might be filled with bone graft or substitutes [57, 63].

The technique of osteochondral autologous transplantation surgery (OATS) for treatment of an ankle OCD comprises harvesting osteochondral plugs from the knee to fill an ankle injury. Even if some authors present a high rate of successful outcome, a recent systematic review has shown that it might be connected to a high rate of complications [64]. Many authors defend OATS as a procedure with specific indications such as larger OCDs or secondary injuries (following the failure of a previous operation).

Several cell-based therapies, scaffolds and augmentation with hydrogels and/or GFs, have been proposed isolated or as augmentation options for "classical" surgeries [65]. Even if such therapies are growing in popularity and seem to be the "road for future," until now they have not proven systematic clinical superiority concerning outcome when compared to the previously described techniques. Bearing this fact in mind, and considering their significant cost, they are seen as a possibility for augmentation of biological response and some cases of revision surgeries or large injuries not amenable by any of the previous, but are still considered as "experimental" and should be used under controlled research application aiming to improve our knowledge about their effect [66–83]. The particular case of use of platelet-rich plasma ("pool" of autologous GFs with different methodologies and characteristics) in orthopedics and cartilage treatment (Fig. 38.7), besides considered as safe, has been surrounded by some controversy [70, 84–89]. Nevertheless, advanced Tissue Engineering and Regenerative Medicine approaches promise new options for future and under intense research and development [65].

When biological healing fails, partial replacement of a medial talar dome defect by a recent metallic implant designed for secondary defects (Hemicap®) has enabled positive outcome on recent to mid-term follow-up [90].

Osteotomies, by providing biomechanical realignment (either calcaneal sliding or supramalleolar), remain powerful surgical options [91, 92]. By providing some more favorable biomechanical conditions for OCD healing they can be used, either isolated or combined, with either of the previously described options [91, 92].

Ankle arthrodesis or arthroplasty are considered the last resource, for very selected cases upon failure of all the above possibilities [91].

38.4 Ankle Impingement Syndromes and CLAI

Ankle impingement syndromes are based upon clinical diagnosis in which the key sentence is: "pain reproduced by local palpation during physical examination," usually described as superficial opposing to deep ankle pain (as referred for OCDs). Patients might refer persistent pain in walking, intensified by climbing stairs. Ankle dorsiflexion or local pressure might cause compression of bone, loose bodies, or soft tissue/synovitis between two bony surfaces (Fig. 38.8). Osteophytes might be visible in anterior or anteromedial impingement; however these are not enthesophytes [93]. They do not result from insertional traction, and they are within -"included in-, the limits of the capsule [93].

Repetitive microtrauma to the anterior aspect of the ankle joint might create bony spurs which leads to bony anterior impingement syndrome [63]. These microtrauma events might derive

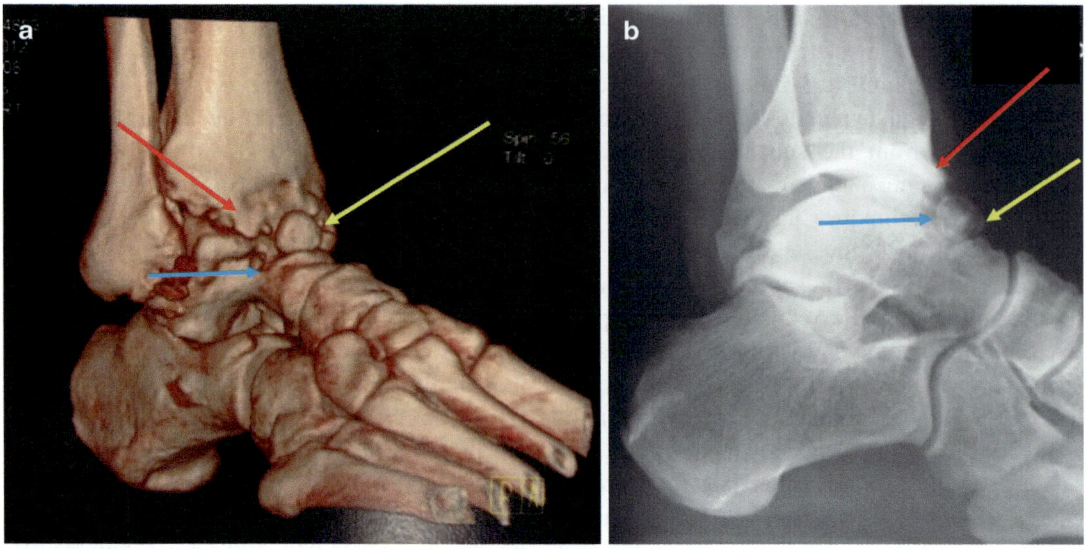

Fig. 38.8 (**a**) 3D CT demonstrating anterior impingement caused by tibial (red arrow) and talar spurs (light blue arrow) aggravated by loose body; (**b**) similar features visible on lateral X-ray

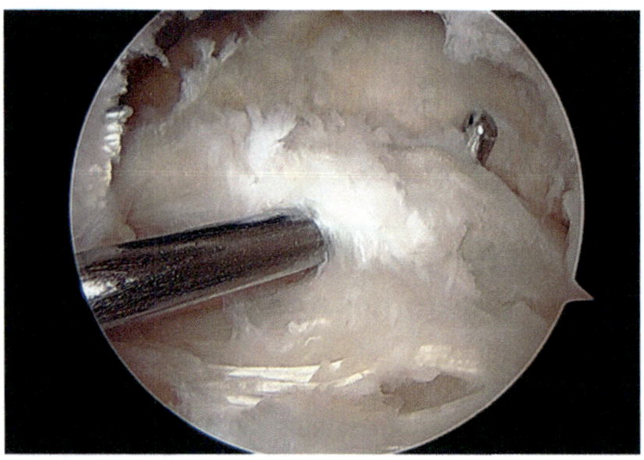

Fig. 38.9 Synovial hypertrophy causing soft tissue impingement

from CAI or repeated direct impact force (e.g., kicking a ball) [94]. Pain connected to ankle impingement has been described in about 30% of patients with CAI [63]. Injury of the anterior-inferior talofibular ligament can be associated to the "so-called" meniscoid lesion which might cause anterolateral soft tissue impingement, as well as synovial hypertrophy might lead to anterior or posterior impingement (Fig. 38.9) [63]. X-ray (including the AMIC view—anteromedial oblique view) [95] or CT can be useful for preoperative planning and identification of concomitant loose bodies or painful broken osteophytes. MRI is usually less required, and more useful in soft tissue conditions.

Repeated hyperplantarflexion might lead to the development of a mechanical conflict which is in the origin of posterior impingement [96]. It can be either acute (*os trigonum* or stieda process fracture or dislocation) after trauma [97] or chronic (repetitive microtrauma, in some cases also linked to CAI) (Fig. 38.10) [98, 99]. Chronic cases can be caused by hypertrophic *os trigonum* or posterior talar process as well as correlated to fractures or soft tissue mass effect (e.g., cysts). It is often observed in footballers, cyclists, swimmers, gymnasts, or ballet dancers [98, 99]. It is also a clinical syndrome. The posterior impingement test often confirms the diagnosis and imaging is used mostly for preoperative planning [100]. Surgical treatment is recommended upon failure of conservative management (physiotherapy, injections, change in shoe wear).

38.4.1 Anterior Impingement

The surgical treatment of anterior ankle impingement in any of its several presentations: anteromedial, anterolateral, bony or soft tissue ankle impingement is currently achieved

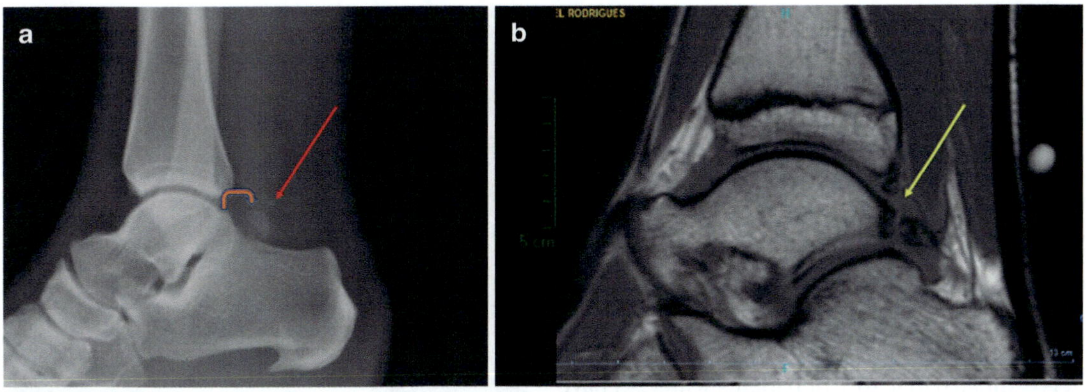

Fig. 38.10 (**a**) Lateral X-ray demonstrating dislocated *Os trigonum* (red arrow and line) and (**b**) dislocated *Os trigonum* in a children after inversion ankle sprain in patients with anterolateral ankle instability

arthroscopically. The medial portal is created in dorsiflexion, medial to the crossing line between the anterior tibialis tendon and the joint line [101]. This method ensures that the cartilage surface is protected under the tibial plafond, and the working space is "opened." Moreover, ankle arthroscopy performed without permanent traction is linked to a lower rate of complications [60, 102]. The lateral portal is performed under transillumination and once more in dorsiflexion to avoid nerve damage (the superficial peroneal never moves posteriorly) [102]. The tibial osteophyte shall be removed from superior to inferior and the talar osteophyte from distal to ensure control of the bony morphology during the procedure [93, 100]. It should be avoided to remove more bone than the really required to solve the conflict, in order to minimize aggression and avoid possibly derived secondary instability due to loss of bony contact when too much bone is removed [93, 100]. The less aggression is created during the procedure, the faster one can expect the full recover from it with return to normal activity [93, 100]. This intervention is performed as an outpatient procedure and the patient can weight bear from day 1 as long as tolerated. It is also essential to start active dorsiflexion-plantarflexion mobility from day 1 to avoid stiffness. Stiches are removed at 2 weeks and full return to activity is possible within 4–6 weeks. Satisfactory result has been published in about 85–90% of cases at 5 years' follow-up and around 80% remain asymptomatic at 8 years' follow-up [93, 100]. However, patients should be advised that the surgery is much more effective in treating pain than improving range of motion (ROM). However, they should also be informed that even if ROM remains unchanged, they should feel and perform better once they get free of the pain. Moreover, even if a relevant number might have recurrence of the osteophytes, most remain asymptomatic on the long term [63, 96, 100].

38.4.2 Posterior Impingement

The two-portals endoscopic approach for the hindfoot described by Van Dijk et al. enabled a significant improvement in the surgical treatment of these and other posterior pathologies around the ankle [103]. Such approach enabled to diminish the surgical aggressiveness, improve outcome, and lower complication rate of both bony and/or soft tissue impingement (including same cases with concomitant *Flexor Halluces Longus—FHL*—secondary tenosynovitis) [96, 100]. As described for anterior impingement, this is an outpatient procedure and the patient usually tolerates (and should be encouraged to) weight bear from day 1. Once more, it is "key to success" to start active dorsiflexion-plantarflexion exercises from the first day. Stiches are removed at 2 weeks and full return to activity is possible within 4–6 weeks for isolated procedures [96]. The FHL tendon is used as an important landmark to avoid the medial neurovascular bundle (just medial to it), thus defining a "safe" working area.

The step-by-step technique has been described elsewhere; however we emphasize that the knowledge of the arthroscopic anatomy is essential [104].

38.5 Tendons and Additional Ligaments Injuries After CLAI

It is estimated that 40% of patients with CAI have a combined partial deltoid injury [41, 105].

Rotational ankle instability occurs when the anterior fascicle of the deltoid ligament is injured in patients with chronic ankle instability [106]. In some cases of lateral ankle ligaments injury (either isolated ATFL or combined ATFL and CFL), a tear affecting the anterior area of the deltoid ligament might occur. This is referred as "open book" tear, once the ligament was separated from the medial malleolus when applying passive internal rotation of the tibio-talar joint [106]. Arthroscopic repair of these injuries has been demonstrated to be effective [106].

One might assume that CAI will lead to increased demand of the structures which function as "agonists" of the lateral ligaments complex. By acknowledging the previous, one can understand that there might be a link between CAI and peroneal tendon's pathology [107]. For such reason, peroneal tendon's pathology is an essential differential diagnosis of CAI and vice versa. With repetitive trauma or contraction of the peroneal muscles, the *peroneal brevis tendon* (Fig. 38.11) [108] as well as the *peroneal longus tendon* [109] may suffer degeneration or rupture.

Less frequently, tibialis posterior injuries have also been reported after ankle sprains [110].

Moreover, as previously referred, the anterior inferior tibiofibular (AITF) ligament as well as the anterior talofibular ligament [111] may be injured concomitantly to ankle sprain or CAI.

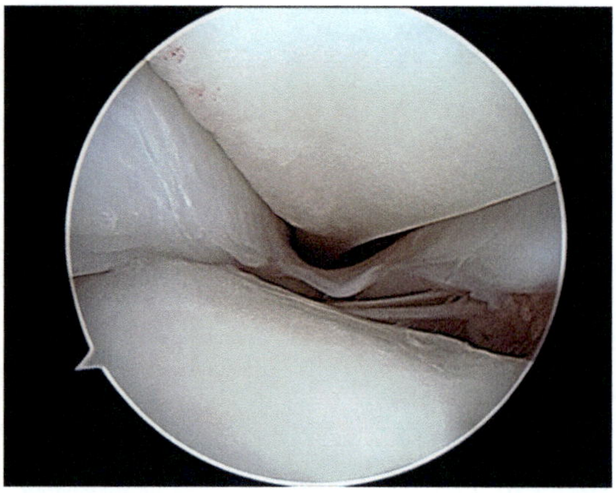

Fig. 38.11 *Peroneus brevis* split longitudinal tear. This can be either linked or differential diagnosis with chronic anterolateral ankle instability

Take-Home Messages

- Even in the case of ligament ruptures, the majority of inversion ankle sprains are effectively treated conservatively.
- There is increasing support on the effectiveness of arthroscopic approach (repair or reconstruction) for CAI treatment. So far, the reported outcomes are at least comparable to those of open techniques. However, further research is required.
- CAI is a major etiology of traumatic OCDs. However, osteochondral defects can have traumatic and nontraumatic etiology.
- The most frequent surgical treatment remains Bone Marrow Stimulation Techniques (e.g., debridement and microfractures). This is based on the high rate of positive clinical outcome, lower aggression, as well as the fact that no surgical procedure has, so far, demonstrated regular advantage over this. However, in order to preserve biology, the fixation of an OCD should be performed whenever possible.
- Orthobiologics and Tissue Engineering and Regenerative Medicine promises to provide further treatment options in a near future.

- Anterior and posterior impingement syndromes are based on clinical diagnosis while imaging is helpful in preoperative planning.
- Etiology anterior and posterior impingement syndromes can be traumatic such as a severe ankle sprain or the repeated microtrauma resulting from CAI.
- Arthroscopic/endoscopic approaches for both these entities enable high rate of good results, fast return to previous activity, and low percentage of complications.
- Combined lateral ankle ligaments injuries with lesions of other ligaments is not rare (e.g., deltoid ligament, AITFL, anterior talofibular ligament, or even posterior tibial tendon).
- Moreover, tendon's pathology, mainly affecting the peroneals can also be implicated and should always be considered a differential diagnosis.
- CAI, as herein explained, is a major entity which can cause further damage in other relevant structures around the ankle joint. Adequate treatment of CAI should also aim to avoid this secondary damage.
- When surgery is required, arthroscopy often enables the simultaneous treatment of concomitant pathology.

Fact Box 1: Ankle Lateral Instability

- Inversion ankle sprain is one of the most frequent sport-related injuries.
- Frequent mechanisms of injuries of lateral ligaments (ankle sprain): landing on the lateral border of the foot; foot blocked on the ground, while the body continues to turn.
- Lesion of the ATFL alone occurs in 65% of cases, while combined injuries of the ATFL and CFL occur in approximately 20%.
- Even after correct conservative treatment, around 20% of patients will develop chronic lateral ankle instability.
- After failure of conservative treatment, anatomic repair or reconstruction techniques have achieved high percentage of good results.
- Arthroscopy/endoscopy enables dealing concomitantly with lateral ligaments lesions as well as associated lesions (e.g., loose bodies, osteochondral lesions, medial ligaments, anterior-inferior tibiofibular ligament, tendon's injurues).

Fact Box 2: Osteochondral Defects (OCD) and Loose Bodies of the Ankle

- Traumatic and nontraumatic etiology have been proposed.
- OCD's etiology includes ankle fracture, sprain, or chronic ankle instability.
- Fixation of a large fragment shall be performed whenever possible.
- In most cases, OCDs can be treated arthroscopically.
- Loose bodies might be a consequence of ankle sprain or chronic ankle instability.
- Besides symptom of joint locking and pain, they can cause further cartilage damage.

Fact Box 3: Ankle Anterior and Posterior Impingement

- Despite imaging can be helpful (mainly for preoperative planning), the diagnosis of both anterior and posterior impingement is based on clinical findings.

- Arthroscopic treatment of bony or soft tissue impingement is the most frequent approach after failure of conservative treatment.
- Arthroscopic surgical treatment is commonly outpatient surgery with immediate range of motion and early weight-bearing. Full return to activity is usually achieved between 4 and 6 weeks.
- In order to avoid stiffness, it is very important to start active dorsiflexion-plantarflexion exercises from the first day after surgery.

Fact Box 4: Ankle Lateral Instability and Tendons and Other Ligaments Injuries

- In the presence of ankle instability complaints, peroneal tendons pathology must always be ruled out.
- On the other hand, in the presence of peroneal tendons complaints, ankle instability must also be ruled out.
- Injury of the anterior-inferior tibiofibular ligament can happen after ankle sprain or chronic ankle instability and lead to anterolateral soft tissue impingement syndrome.
- The deltoid ligament, particularly its deep portion, can be injured during ankle sprain or chronic ankle instability.
- Around 40% of patients with chronic ankle instability have a partial deltoid injury.
- Tendon's pathology, mainly affecting the peroneals, can also be implicated and should always be considered a differential diagnosis.

References

1. Hunt KJ, Fuld RS, Sutphin BS, Pereira H, D'Hooghe P. Return to sport following lateral ankle ligament repair is under-reported: a systematic review. J ISAKOS Joint Disord Orthopaed Sports Med. 2017;2:234. https://doi.org/10.1136/jisakos-2016-000064.
2. Lindner M, Kotschwar A, Zsoldos RR, Groesel M, Peham C. The jump shot - a biomechanical analysis focused on lateral ankle ligaments. J Biomech. 2012;45(1):202–6. https://doi.org/10.1016/j.jbiomech.2011.09.012.
3. Kristianslund E, Krosshaug T. Comparison of drop jumps and sport-specific sidestep cutting: implications for anterior cruciate ligament injury risk screening. Am J Sports Med. 2013;41(3):684–8. https://doi.org/10.1177/0363546512472043.
4. D'Hooge P, Giza E, Longo G. Torn ankle ligaments in elite handball: does a player require surgery? Aspetar Sports Med J.
5. Fong DT, Ha SC, Mok KM, Chan CW, Chan KM. Kinematics analysis of ankle inversion ligamentous sprain injuries in sports: five cases from televised tennis competitions. Am J Sports Med. 2012;40(11):2627–32. https://doi.org/10.1177/0363546512458259.
6. Kristianslund E, Bahr R, Krosshaug T. Kinematics and kinetics of an accidental lateral ankle sprain. J Biomech. 2011;44(14):2576–8. https://doi.org/10.1016/j.jbiomech.2011.07.014.
7. Brostroem L. Sprained ankles. I. Anatomic lesions in recent sprains. Acta Chir Scand. 1964;128:483–95.
8. Hunt K, D'Hooghe P, Kelley JZ, Anderson N, Fuld R, Baldini TH, Isakos Laf Committee, Pereira H. The role of calcaneofibular ligament (CFL) injury in ankle instability: implications for surgical management. Arthroscopy. 2017;33(10 Suppl):e51–2. https://doi.org/10.1016/j.arthro.2017.08.024.
9. Pereira H, D'Hooghe P, Anderson N, Fuld R, Kelley JZ, Baldini TH, Isakos Laf Committee, Hunt K. Ankle and subtalar joint kinematics following lateral ligament repair-implications for early surgical treatment. Arthroscopy. 2017;33(10):e101. https://doi.org/10.1016/j.arthro.2017.08.106.
10. Baumhauer JF, O'Brien T. Surgical considerations in the treatment of ankle instability. J Athl Train. 2002;37(4):458–62.
11. Lynch SA. Assessment of the injured ankle in the athlete. J Athl Train. 2002;37(4):406–12.
12. Brostroem L. Sprained ankles. V. Treatment and prognosis in recent ligament ruptures. Acta Chir Scand. 1966;132(5):537–50.

13. van Dijk CN, Bossuyt PM, Marti RK. Medial ankle pain after lateral ligament rupture. J Bone Joint Surg Br. 1996;78(4):562–7.
14. Ferkel RD, Chams RN. Chronic lateral instability: arthroscopic findings and long-term results. Foot Ankle Int. 2007;28(1):24–31. https://doi.org/10.3113/fai.2007.0005.
15. Harrington KD. Degenerative arthritis of the ankle secondary to long-standing lateral ligament instability. J Bone Joint Surg Am. 1979;61(3):354–61.
16. Lee J, Hamilton G, Ford L. Associated intra-articular ankle pathologies in patients with chronic lateral ankle instability: arthroscopic findings at the time of lateral ankle reconstruction. Foot Ankle Spec. 2011;4(5):284–9.
17. D'Hooge P, Giza E, Longo G. Torn ankle ligaments in elite handball: does a player require surgery? Aspetar Sports Med J. Volume 3 Targeted Topic-Sports Medicine in Handball. 186–194.
18. Kobayashi T, Gamada K. Lateral ankle sprain and chronic ankle instability: a critical review. Foot Ankle Spec. 2014;7(4):298–326. https://doi.org/10.1177/1938640014539813.
19. Drakos MC, Behrens SB, Paller D, Murphy C, DiGiovanni CW. Biomechanical comparison of an open vs arthroscopic approach for lateral ankle instability. Foot Ankle Int. 2014;35(8):809–15. https://doi.org/10.1177/1071100714535765.
20. Guillo S, Takao M, Calder J, Karlson J, Michels F, Bauer T. Arthroscopic anatomical reconstruction of the lateral ankle ligaments. Knee Surg Sports Traumatol Arthrosc. 2015;24:998. https://doi.org/10.1007/s00167-015-3789-z.
21. Struijs PA, Kerkhoffs GM. Ankle sprain. BMJ Clin Evid. 2010;2010:1115.
22. Ferran NA, Oliva F, Maffulli N. Ankle instability. Sports Med Arthrosc Rev. 2009;17(2):139–45. https://doi.org/10.1097/JSA.0b013e3181a3d790.
23. Pereira H, Vuurberg G, Gomes N, Oliveira JM, Ripoll PL, Reis RL, Espregueira-Mendes J, Niek van Dijk C. Arthroscopic repair of ankle instability with all-soft knotless anchors. Arthrosc Tech. 2016;5(1):e99–e107. https://doi.org/10.1016/j.eats.2015.10.010.
24. Michels F, Pereira H, Calder J, Matricali G, Glazebrook M, Guillo S, Karlsson J, Group E-AAI, Acevedo J, Batista J, Bauer T, Calder J, Carreira D, Choi W, Corte-Real N, Glazebrook M, Ghorbani A, Giza E, Guillo S, Hunt K, Karlsson J, Kong SW, Lee JW, Michels F, Molloy A, Mangone P, Matsui K, Nery C, Ozeki S, Pearce C, Pereira H, Perera A, Pijnenburg B, Raduan F, Stone J, Takao M, Tourne Y, Vega J. Searching for consensus in the approach to patients with chronic lateral ankle instability: ask the expert. Knee Surg Sports Traumatol Arthrosc. 2017;26:2095. https://doi.org/10.1007/s00167-017-4556-0.
25. Kerkhoffs GM, van den Bekerom M, Elders LA, van Beek PA, Hullegie WA, Bloemers GM, de Heus EM, Loogman MC, Rosenbrand KC, Kuipers T, Hoogstraten JW, Dekker R, Ten Duis HJ, van Dijk CN, van Tulder MW, van der Wees PJ, de Bie RA. Diagnosis, treatment and prevention of ankle sprains: an evidence-based clinical guideline. Br J Sports Med. 2012;46(12):854–60. https://doi.org/10.1136/bjsports-2011-090490.
26. White WJ, McCollum GA, Calder JD. Return to sport following acute lateral ligament repair of the ankle in professional athletes. Knee Surg Sports Traumatol Arthrosc. 2016;24(4):1124–9. https://doi.org/10.1007/s00167-015-3815-1.
27. de Vries JS, Krips R, Sierevelt IN, Blankevoort L. Interventions for treating chronic ankle instability. Cochrane Database Syst Rev. 2006;4:CD004124. https://doi.org/10.1002/14651858.CD004124.pub2.
28. Doherty C, Bleakley C, Delahunt E, Holden S. Treatment and prevention of acute and recurrent ankle sprain: an overview of systematic reviews with meta-analysis. Br J Sports Med. 2017;51(2):113–25. https://doi.org/10.1136/bjsports-2016-096178.
29. Hertel J. Functional anatomy, pathomechanics, and pathophysiology of lateral ankle instability. J Athl Train. 2002;37(4):364–75.
30. McKay GD, Goldie PA, Payne WR, Oakes BW. Ankle injuries in basketball: injury rate and risk factors. Br J Sports Med. 2001;35(2):103–8.
31. Vuurberg G, Pereira H, Blankevoort L, van Dijk CN. Anatomic stabilization techniques provide superior results in terms of functional outcome in patients suffering from chronic ankle instability compared to non-anatomic techniques. Knee Surg Sports Traumatol Arthrosc. 2017;26:2183. https://doi.org/10.1007/s00167-017-4730-4.
32. Vuurberg G, Veen OC, Pereira H, Blankevoort L, van Dijk CN. Tenodesis reconstruction in patients with chronic lateral ankle instability is associated with a high risk of complications compared with anatomic repair and reconstruction: a systematic review and meta-analysis. J ISAKOS Joint Disord Orthopaed Sports Med. 2017; https://doi.org/10.1136/jisakos-2016-000121.
33. de Vries JS, Krips R, Sierevelt IN, Blankevoort L, van Dijk CN. Interventions for treating chronic ankle instability. Cochrane Database Syst Rev. 2011;8:CD004124. https://doi.org/10.1002/14651858.CD004124.pub3.
34. Corte-Real NM, Moreira RM. Arthroscopic repair of chronic lateral ankle instability. Foot Ankle Int. 2009;30(3):213–7. https://doi.org/10.3113/FAI.2009.0213.
35. Guillo S, Takao M, Calder J, Karlson J, Michels F, Bauer T, Ankle Instability Group. Arthroscopic anatomical reconstruction of the lateral ankle ligaments. Knee Surg Sports Traumatol Arthrosc.

2016;24(4):998–1002. https://doi.org/10.1007/s00167-015-3789-z.
36. Matsui K, Burgesson B, Takao M, Stone J, Guillo S, Glazebrook M, Group EAAI. Minimally invasive surgical treatment for chronic ankle instability: a systematic review. Knee Surg Sports Traumatol Arthrosc. 2016;24(4):1040–8. https://doi.org/10.1007/s00167-016-4041-1.
37. Takao M, Matsui K, Stone JW, Glazebrook MA, Kennedy JG, Guillo S, Calder JD, Karlsson J, Ankle Instability Group. Arthroscopic anterior talofibular ligament repair for lateral instability of the ankle. Knee Surg Sports Traumatol Arthrosc. 2016;24(4):1003–6. https://doi.org/10.1007/s00167-015-3638-0.
38. Vega J, Golano P, Pellegrino A, Rabat E, Pena F. All-inside arthroscopic lateral collateral ligament repair for ankle instability with a knotless suture anchor technique. Foot Ankle Int. 2013;34(12):1701–9. https://doi.org/10.1177/1071100713502322.
39. Matsui K, Takao M, Miyamoto W, Matsushita T. Early recovery after arthroscopic repair compared to open repair of the anterior talofibular ligament for lateral instability of the ankle. Arch Orthop Trauma Surg. 2016;136(1):93–100. https://doi.org/10.1007/s00402-015-2342-3.
40. Yeo ED, Lee KT, Sung IH, Lee SG, Lee YK. Comparison of all-inside arthroscopic and open techniques for the modified Brostrom procedure for ankle instability. Foot Ankle Int. 2016;37(10):1037–45. https://doi.org/10.1177/1071100716666508.
41. Hintermann B, Boss A, Schafer D. Arthroscopic findings in patients with chronic ankle instability. Am J Sports Med. 2002;30(3):402–9. https://doi.org/10.1177/03635465020300031601.
42. Berndt AL, Harty M. Transchondral fractures (osteochondritis dissecans) of the talus. J Bone Joint Surg Am. 1959;41-A:988–1020.
43. O'Loughlin PF, Heyworth BE, Kennedy JG. Current concepts in the diagnosis and treatment of osteochondral lesions of the ankle. Am J Sports Med. 2010;38(2):392–404. https://doi.org/10.1177/0363546509336336.
44. Schachter AK, Chen AL, Reddy PD, Tejwani NC. Osteochondral lesions of the talus. J Am Acad Orthop Surg. 2005;13(3):152–8.
45. van Dijk CN, Reilingh ML, Zengerink M, van Bergen CJ. Osteochondral defects in the ankle: why painful? Knee Surg Sports Traumatol Arthrosc. 2010;18(5):570–80. https://doi.org/10.1007/s00167-010-1064-x.
46. Ventura A, Terzaghi C, Legnani C, Borgo E. Treatment of post-traumatic osteochondral lesions of the talus: a four-step approach. Knee Surg Sports Traumatol Arthrosc. 2013;21(6):1245–50. https://doi.org/10.1007/s00167-012-2028-0.
47. Elias I, Raikin SM, Schweitzer ME, Besser MP, Morrison WB, Zoga AC. Osteochondral lesions of the distal tibial plafond: localization and morphologic characteristics with an anatomical grid. Foot Ankle Int. 2009;30(6):524–9. https://doi.org/10.3113/FAI.2009.0524.
48. Elias I, Zoga AC, Morrison WB, Besser MP, Schweitzer ME, Raikin SM. Osteochondral lesions of the talus: localization and morphologic data from 424 patients using a novel anatomical grid scheme. Foot Ankle Int. 2007;28(2):154–61. https://doi.org/10.3113/FAI.2007.0154.
49. Vellet AD, Marks PH, Fowler PJ, Munro TG. Occult posttraumatic osteochondral lesions of the knee: prevalence, classification, and short-term sequelae evaluated with MR imaging. Radiology. 1991;178(1):271–6. https://doi.org/10.1148/radiology.178.1.1984319.
50. Zengerink M, Struijs PA, Tol JL, van Dijk CN. Treatment of osteochondral lesions of the talus: a systematic review. Knee Surg Sports Traumatol Arthrosc. 2010;18(2):238–46. https://doi.org/10.1007/s00167-009-0942-6.
51. Verhagen RA, Struijs PA, Bossuyt PM, van Dijk CN. Systematic review of treatment strategies for osteochondral defects of the talar dome. Foot Ankle Clin. 2003;8(2):233–42, viii–ix.
52. Hermanson E, Ferkel RD. Bilateral osteochondral lesions of the talus. Foot Ankle Int. 2009;30(8):723–7. https://doi.org/10.3113/FAI.2009.0723.
53. Woods K, Harris I. Osteochondritis dissecans of the talus in identical twins. J Bone Joint Surg. 1995;77(2):331.
54. Frenkel SR, Di Cesare PE. Degradation and repair of articular cartilage. Front Biosci. 1999;4:671–85.
55. Durr HD, Martin H, Pellengahr C, Schlemmer M, Maier M, Jansson V. The cause of subchondral bone cysts in osteoarthrosis: a finite element analysis. Acta Orthop Scand. 2004;75(5):554–8. https://doi.org/10.1080/00016470410001411.
56. Saxena A, Luhadiya A, Ewen B, Goumas C. Magnetic resonance imaging and incidental findings of lateral ankle pathologic features with asymptomatic ankles. J Foot Ankle Surg. 2011;50(4):413–5. https://doi.org/10.1053/j.jfas.2011.03.011.
57. Dahmen J, Lambers KTA, Reilingh ML, van Bergen CJA, Stufkens SAS, Kerkhoffs G. No superior treatment for primary osteochondral defects of the talus. Knee Surg Sports Traumatol Arthrosc. 2017;26:2142. https://doi.org/10.1007/s00167-017-4616-5.
58. Lambers KTA, Dahmen J, Reilingh ML, van Bergen CJA, Stufkens SAS, Kerkhoffs G. No superior surgical treatment for secondary osteochondral defects of the talus. Knee Surg Sports Traumatol Arthrosc. 2017;26:2158. https://doi.org/10.1007/s00167-017-4629-0.
59. van Dijk CN, van Bergen CJ. Advancements in ankle arthroscopy. J Am Acad Orthop Surg. 2008;16(11):635–46.
60. Zengerink M, van Dijk CN. Complications in ankle arthroscopy. Knee Surg Sports Traumatol Arthrosc. 2012;20(8):1420–31. https://doi.org/10.1007/s00167-012-2063-x.

61. Kerkhoffs GM, Reilingh ML, Gerards RM, de Leeuw PA. Lift, drill, fill and fix (LDFF): a new arthroscopic treatment for talar osteochondral defects. Knee Surg Sports Traumatol Arthrosc. 2016;24(4):1265–71. https://doi.org/10.1007/s00167-014-3057-7.
62. Doral MN, Bilge O, Batmaz G, Donmez G, Turhan E, Demirel M, Atay OA, Uzumcugil A, Atesok K, Kaya D. Treatment of osteochondral lesions of the talus with microfracture technique and post-operative hyaluronan injection. Knee Surg Sports Traumatol Arthrosc. 2012;20(7):1398–403. https://doi.org/10.1007/s00167-011-1856-7.
63. Ross KA, Murawski CD, Smyth NA, Zwiers R, Wiegerinck JI, van Bergen CJ, Dijk CN, Kennedy JG. Current concepts review: arthroscopic treatment of anterior ankle impingement. Foot Ankle Surg. 2017;23(1):1–8. https://doi.org/10.1016/j.fas.2016.01.005.
64. Ferreira C, Vuurberg G, Oliveira JM, Espregueira-Mendes J, Pereira H, Reis RL, Ripoll P. Assessment of clinical outcome after osteochondral autologous transplantation technique for the treatment of ankle lesions: a systematic review. J Isakos. 2016; https://doi.org/10.1136/jisakos-2015-000020.R2.
65. Correia SI, Pereira H, Silva-Correia J, Van Dijk CN, Espregueira-Mendes J, Oliveira JM, Reis RL. Current concepts: tissue engineering and regenerative medicine applications in the ankle joint. J R Soc Interface. 2014;11(92):20130784. https://doi.org/10.1098/rsif.2013.0784.
66. Bhattarai N, Gunn J, Zhang M. Chitosan-based hydrogels for controlled, localized drug delivery. Adv Drug Deliv Rev. 2010;62(1):83–99. https://doi.org/10.1016/j.addr.2009.07.019.
67. Brittberg M. Cell carriers as the next generation of cell therapy for cartilage repair: a review of the matrix-induced autologous chondrocyte implantation procedure. Am J Sports Med. 2010;38(6):1259–71. https://doi.org/10.1177/0363546509346395.
68. Candrian C, Miot S, Wolf F, Bonacina E, Dickinson S, Wirz D, Jakob M, Valderrabano V, Barbero A, Martin I. Are ankle chondrocytes from damaged fragments a suitable cell source for cartilage repair? Osteoarthrit Cartilage. 2010;18(8):1067–76. https://doi.org/10.1016/j.joca.2010.04.010.
69. Caron MMJ, Emans PJ, Coolsen MME, Voss L, Surtel DAM, Cremers A, van Rhijn LW, Welting TJM. Redifferentiation of dedifferentiated human articular chondrocytes: comparison of 2D and 3D cultures. Osteoarthr Cartil. 2012;20(10):1170–8. https://doi.org/10.1016/j.joca.2012.06.016.
70. Centeno CJ, Schultz JR, Cheever M, Robinson B, Freeman M, Marasco W. Safety and complications reporting on the re-implantation of culture-expanded mesenchymal stem cells using autologous platelet lysate technique. Curr Stem Cell Res Ther. 2010;5(1):81–93.
71. Che JH, Zhang ZR, Li GZ, Tan WH, Bai XD, Qu FJ. Application of tissue-engineered cartilage with BMP-7 gene to repair knee joint cartilage injury in rabbits. Knee Surg Sports Traumatol Arthrosc. 2010;18(4):496–503. https://doi.org/10.1007/s00167-009-0962-2.
72. Clar C, Cummins E, McIntyre L, Thomas S, Lamb J, Bain L, Jobanputra P, Waugh N. Clinical and cost-effectiveness of autologous chondrocyte implantation for cartilage defects in knee joints: systematic review and economic evaluation. Health Technol Assess. 2005;9(47):iii–iv, ix–x, 1–82.
73. Dhollander AA, De Neve F, Almqvist KF, Verdonk R, Lambrecht S, Elewaut D, Verbruggen G, Verdonk PC. Autologous matrix-induced chondrogenesis combined with platelet-rich plasma gel: technical description and a five pilot patients report. Knee Surg Sports Traumatol Arthrosc. 2011;19(4):536–42. https://doi.org/10.1007/s00167-010-1337-4.
74. DiGiovanni CW, Lin SS, Baumhauer JF, Daniels T, Younger A, Glazebrook M, Anderson J, Anderson R, Evangelista P, Lynch SE. Recombinant human platelet-derived growth factor-BB and beta-tricalcium phosphate (rhPDGF-BB/beta-TCP): an alternative to autogenous bone graft. J Bone Joint Surg Am. 2013;95(13):1184–92. https://doi.org/10.2106/JBJS.K.01422.
75. Enea D, Gwynne J, Kew S, Arumugam M, Shepherd J, Brooks R, Ghose S, Best S, Cameron R, Rushton N. Collagen fibre implant for tendon and ligament biological augmentation. In vivo study in an ovine model. Knee Surg Sports Traumatol Arthrosc. 2012; https://doi.org/10.1007/s00167-012-2102-7.
76. Gurkan UA, Tasoglu S, Kavaz D, Demirci U. Emerging technologies for assembly of microscale hydrogels. Adv Healthc Mater. 2012;1:149–58.
77. Harris JD, Siston RA, Pan X, Flanigan DC. Autologous chondrocyte implantation: a systematic review. J Bone Joint Surg Am. 2010;92(12):2220–33. https://doi.org/10.2106/JBJS.J.00049.
78. Jones HJ, Virgolino M. Biological approaches in ankle chondral defects. In: ECTES 2015 - 16th European Congress of Trauma & Emergency Surgery 10–12 May 2015, Amsterdam; 2015.
79. Nagura I, Fujioka H, Kokubu T, Makino T, Sumi Y, Kurosaka M. Repair of osteochondral defects with a new porous synthetic polymer scaffold. J Bone Joint Surg Br. 2007;89(2):258–64. https://doi.org/10.1302/0301-620X.89B2.17754.
80. Pereira D, Silva-Correia J, Pereira H, Espregueira-Mendes J, Oliveira JM, Reis RL. Gellan gum-based bilayered scaffolds for application in ostheochondral tissue engineering. J Tissue Eng Regen Med. 2013;7(1)
81. Shive MS, Stanish WD, McCormack R, Forriol F, Mohtadi N, Pelet S, Desnoyers J, Methot S, Vehik K, Restrepo A. BST-CarGel(R) treatment maintains cartilage repair superiority over microfracture at 5 years in a multicenter randomized controlled trial. Cartilage. 2015;6(2):62–72. https://doi.org/10.1177/1947603514562064.

82. Stanish WD, McCormack R, Forriol F, Mohtadi N, Pelet S, Desnoyers J, Restrepo A, Shive MS. Novel scaffold-based BST-CarGel treatment results in superior cartilage repair compared with microfracture in a randomized controlled trial. J Bone Joint Surg Am. 2013;95(18):1640–50. https://doi.org/10.2106/JBJS.L.01345.
83. Vinatier C, Mrugala D, Jorgensen C, Guicheux J, Noel D. Cartilage engineering: a crucial combination of cells, biomaterials and biofactors. Trends Biotechnol. 2009;27(5):307–14. https://doi.org/10.1016/j.tibtech.2009.02.005.
84. DeChellis DM, Cortazzo MH. Regenerative medicine in the field of pain medicine: prolotherapy, platelet-rich plasma therapy, and stem cell therapy—theory and evidence. Tech Region Anesth Pain Manag. 2011;15:74–80.
85. Engebretsen L, Steffen K, Alsousou J, Anitua E, Bachl N, Devilee R, Everts P, Hamilton B, Huard J, Jenoure P, Kelberine F, Kon E, Maffulli N, Matheson G, Mei-Dan O, Menetrey J, Philippon M, Randelli P, Schamasch P, Schwellnus M, Vernec A, Verrall G. IOC consensus paper on the use of platelet-rich plasma in sports medicine. Br J Sports Med. 2010;44(15):1072–81. https://doi.org/10.1136/bjsm.2010.079822.
86. Evans CH. Advances in regenerative orthopedics. Mayo Clin Proc. 2013;88(11):1323–39. https://doi.org/10.1016/j.mayocp.2013.04.027.
87. Lopez-Vidriero E, Goulding KA, Simon DA, Sanchez M, Johnson DH. The use of platelet-rich plasma in arthroscopy and sports medicine: optimizing the healing environment. Arthroscopy. 2010;26(2):269–78. https://doi.org/10.1016/j.arthro.2009.11.015.
88. Sheth U, Simunovic N, Klein G, Fu F, Einhorn TA, Schemitsch E, Ayeni OR, Bhandari M. Efficacy of autologous platelet-rich plasma use for orthopaedic indications: a meta-analysis. J Bone Joint Surg Am. 2012;94(4):298–307. https://doi.org/10.2106/JBJS.K.00154.
89. Soomekh DJ. Current concepts for the use of platelet-rich plasma in the foot and ankle. Clin Podiatric Med Surg. 2011;28(1):155–70. https://doi.org/10.1016/j.cpm.2010.09.001.
90. Ettinger S, Stukenborg-Colsman C, Waizy H, Becher C, Yao D, Claassen L, Noll Y, Plaass C. Results of HemiCAP(R) implantation as a salvage procedure for osteochondral lesions of the talus. J Foot Ankle Surg. 2017;56(4):788–92. https://doi.org/10.1053/j.jfas.2017.04.001.
91. Badekas T, Takvorian M, Souras N. Treatment principles for osteochondral lesions in foot and ankle. Int Orthop. 2013;37(9):1697–706. https://doi.org/10.1007/s00264-013-2076-1.
92. Pagenstert GI, Hintermann B, Barg A, Leumann A, Valderrabano V. Realignment surgery as alternative treatment of varus and valgus ankle osteoarthritis. Clin Orthop Relat Res. 2007;462:156–68. https://doi.org/10.1097/BLO.0b013e318124a462.
93. Tol JL, Verheyen CP, van Dijk CN. Arthroscopic treatment of anterior impingement in the ankle. J Bone Joint Surg Br. 2001;83(1):9–13.
94. Tol JL, Slim E, van Soest AJ, van Dijk CN. The relationship of the kicking action in soccer and anterior ankle impingement syndrome. A biomechanical analysis. Am J Sports Med. 2002;30(1):45–50. https://doi.org/10.1177/03635465020300012101.
95. van Dijk CN, Wessel RN, Tol JL, Maas M. Oblique radiograph for the detection of bone spurs in anterior ankle impingement. Skelet Radiol. 2002;31(4):214–21. https://doi.org/10.1007/s00256-002-0477-0.
96. Miyamoto W, Miki S, Kawano H, Takao M. Surgical outcome of posterior ankle impingement syndrome with concomitant ankle disorders treated simultaneously in patient engaged in athletic activity. J Orthop Sci. 2017;22(3):463–7. https://doi.org/10.1016/j.jos.2016.12.017.
97. Kose O, Okan AN, Durakbasa MO, Emrem K, Islam NC. Fracture of the os trigonum: a case report. J Orthop Surg (Hong Kong). 2006;14(3):354–6. https://doi.org/10.1177/230949900601400326.
98. Lees A, Asai T, Andersen TB, Nunome H, Sterzing T. The biomechanics of kicking in soccer: a review. J Sports Sci. 2010;28(8):805–17. https://doi.org/10.1080/02640414.2010.481305.
99. Walls RJ, Ross KA, Fraser EJ, Hodgkins CW, Smyth NA, Egan CJ, Calder J, Kennedy JG. Football injuries of the ankle: a review of injury mechanisms, diagnosis and management. World J Orthop. 2016;7(1):8–19. https://doi.org/10.5312/wjo.v7.i1.8.
100. Niek van Dijk C. Anterior and posterior ankle impingement. Foot Ankle Clin. 2006;11(3):663–83. https://doi.org/10.1016/j.fcl.2006.06.003.
101. de Leeuw PA, Golano P, Clavero JA, van Dijk CN. Anterior ankle arthroscopy, distraction or dorsiflexion? Knee Surg Sports Traumatol Arthrosc. 2010;18(5):594–600. https://doi.org/10.1007/s00167-010-1089-1.
102. de Leeuw PA, Golano P, Sierevelt IN, van Dijk CN. The course of the superficial peroneal nerve in relation to the ankle position: anatomical study with ankle arthroscopic implications. Knee Surg Sports Traumatol Arthrosc. 2010;18(5):612–7. https://doi.org/10.1007/s00167-010-1099-z.
103. van Dijk CN, Scholten PE, Krips R. A 2-portal endoscopic approach for diagnosis and treatment of posterior ankle pathology. Arthroscopy. 2000;16(8):871–6. https://doi.org/10.1053/jars.2000.19430.
104. Haverkamp D, Bech N, de Leeuw P, d'Hooghe P, Kynsburg A, Calder J, Ogut T, Batista J, Pereira H. Posterior compartment of the ankle joint: a focus on arthroscopic treatment (ICL 17). In: Becker R, Kerkhoffs GMMJ, Gelber PE, Denti M, Seil R, editors. ESSKA instructional course

lecture book. Berlin: Springer; 2016. https://doi.org/10.1007/978-3-662-49114-0_15.

105. Schafer D, Hintermann B. Arthroscopic assessment of the chronic unstable ankle joint. Knee Surg Sports Traumatol Arthrosc. 1996;4(1):48–52.

106. Vega J, Allmendinger J, Malagelada F, Guelfi M, Dalmau-Pastor M. Combined arthroscopic all-inside repair of lateral and medial ankle ligaments is an effective treatment for rotational ankle instability. Knee Surg Sports Traumatol Arthrosc. 2017;28:132. https://doi.org/10.1007/s00167-017-4736-y.

107. Pereira H, Ripoll P, Oliveira JM, Reis RL, Espregueira-Mendes J, van Dijk C. Peroneal and posterior tibial tendon pathology. The Ankle in Football. Heidelberg: Springer; 2014.

108. Chauhan B, Panchal P, Szabo E, Wilkins T. Split peroneus brevis tendon: an unusual cause of ankle pain and instability. J Am Board Fam Med. 2014;27(2):297–302. https://doi.org/10.3122/jabfm.2014.02.130009.

109. van Zoest WJ, Janssen RP, Tseng CM. An uncommon ankle sprain. Br J Sports Med. 2007;41(11):849–50. https://doi.org/10.1136/bjsm.2007.035295.

110. Ahmad M, John Gray A. Ruptured tibialis posterior tendon, presenting as a lateral ligament sprain. Eur J Emerg Med. 2003;10(1):42–3. https://doi.org/10.1097/01.mej.0000058249.71227.88.

111. Evans JM, Schucany WG. Radiological evaluation of a high ankle sprain. Proc (Bayl Univ Med Cent). 2006;19(4):402–5.

Nonbiological Adjuncts for Ankle Stabilization

39

Hélder Pereira, Manuel Resende Sousa, Daniel Mendes, Matt Solan, J. Acevedo, Ibrahim Fatih Cengiz, Rui L. Reis, and Joaquim M. Oliveira

39.1 Introduction

Ankle sprain is an extremely common injury which might lead to functional limitations and absence to work or sports participation. It has been stated among the most frequent injuries during sports activity (either in professional or recreational athletes or even in general population) [1].

Usually after an inversion ankle sprain, there is a significant risk of development of chronic anterolateral ankle instability (CLAI).

H. Pereira (✉)
Orthopedic Department of Póvoa de Varzim, Vila do Conde Hospital Centre, Vila do Conde, Portugal

Ripoll y De Prado Sports Clinic: Murcia-Madrid FIFA Medical Centre of Excellence, Murcia-Madrid, Spain

International Centre of Sports Traumatology of the Ave, Vila do Conde, Portugal

3B's Research Group, I3Bs – Research Institute on Biomaterials, Biodegradables and Biomimetics, University of Minho, Headquarters of the European Institute of Excellence on Tissue Engineering and Regenerative Medicine, Barco GMR, Portugal

ICVS/3B's - PT Government Associate Laboratory, University of Minho, Braga-Guimarães, Portugal

M. R. Sousa
Foot and Ankle Unit, Hospital Beatriz Ângelo, Lisbon, Portugal

Foot and Ankle Unit, Hospital da Luz, Lisbon, Portugal

D. Mendes
Foot and Ankle Unit, Hospital Beatriz Ângelo, Lisbon, Portugal

Foot and Ankle Unit, Hospital da Luz Setúbal, Setubal, Portugal

M. Solan
London Foot and Ankle Centre, London, UK

J. Acevedo
Department of Orthopedics, Southeast Orthopedic Specialists, Jacksonville, FL, USA

I. F. Cengiz
3B's Research Group, I3Bs – Research Institute on Biomaterials, Biodegradables and Biomimetics, University of Minho, Headquarters of the European Institute of Excellence on Tissue Engineering and Regenerative Medicine, Barco GMR, Portugal

ICVS/3B's - PT Government Associate Laboratory, University of Minho, Braga-Guimarães, Portugal
e-mail: fatih.cengiz@i3bs.uminho.pt

R. L. Reis · J. M. Oliveira
3B's Research Group, I3Bs – Research Institute on Biomaterials, Biodegradables and Biomimetics, University of Minho, Headquarters of the European Institute of Excellence on Tissue Engineering and Regenerative Medicine, Barco GMR, Portugal

ICVS/3B's - PT Government Associate Laboratory, University of Minho, Braga-Guimarães, Portugal

The Discoveries Centre for Regenerative and Precision Medicine, Headquarters at University of Minho, Barco, Guimarães, Portugal
e-mail: rgreis@i3bs.uminho.pt; miguel.oliveira@i3bs.uminho.pt

H. Pereira et al. (eds.), *Lateral Ankle Instability*, https://doi.org/10.1007/978-3-662-62763-1_39

Concerning CLAI, 50% of these patients will have concomitant or subsequent injuries in the affected ankle (medial ligaments injuries, impingements, syndesmotic injuries, loose bodies, osteochondral defects (OCD), synovitis, ankle arthritis) [2–6].

Furthermore, patients with CAI have changed joint kinematics which leads to higher risk for further recurrence of ankle sprains [7].

Traditionally, conservative treatment is the first option; however a relevant percentage with persistent symptoms will require surgical treatment [8, 9].

Multiple studies demonstrated describe high rate of favorable outcome (over 90%) after Broström procedure in any of its several modifications [10]. Although Broström repair procedure is largely considered a successful surgical treatment, the recovery might require a prolonged period of immobilization and rehabilitation, with functional impairment and socioeconomical implications [9, 11–13].

Aiming to diminish the possible risk of acute reinjury and chronic damage of the repaired anterior talofibular ligament (ATFL) which could lead to recurrence of joint instability and further damage, as well as pursue a more aggressive rehabilitation [8, 14], enabling a faster return to activity, augmentation techniques have been proposed.

Herein it will be described a technique of augmentation suitable either for open, mini-open, or endoscopic-assisted CLAI repair by means of use of a high-molecular-weight polyethylene "suture-tape augmentation," also known as "internal brace" (plus anchor/small inference screw's), to augment ligament repair [9–11, 13, 15–19].

The most frequently used device has been stated to permit a greater resistance of the final construct (250 N) than the native ATFL (154 N), which is around the triple of the resistance of the average achieved by the Broström repair procedure (68 N) [12, 13, 17]. Still, it is not a biological approach at this time (acellular); thus, it has no favorable effect in proprioception or vascularization. Biocompatibility of the so-called "biomaterials" is of paramount importance [20].

However, recent works have been reporting favorable results without major complications in the setting of CLAI but also in other pathologies around the ankle [19, 21]. The principles of the surgical technique are described herein.

39.2 Surgical Technique

As before mentioned, this augmentation can be used for most modification of the Broström repair procedure (open, mini-open, or endoscopic-assisted) (Fig. 39.1).

For clarification purposes, the open technique will be herein described [18].

Several authors use two small anchors in the distal fibula, slightly proximal than the tunnel used for the suture tape for reinforcement of the ATFL repair.

For the open Broström, a linear incision is done starting around 1 cm proximal to the tip of the fibula, in line with the orientation of the anterior talofibular ligament (ATFL), in order to enable access to the fibular and talar attachment of the ATFL and inspection of the peroneal tendons.

Sharp dissection is performed from the skin and subcutaneous tissue until the inferior extensor retinaculum and lateral ligament complex are identified. The anterolateral fat pad is removed/reduced according to the needs for proper visualization. The ATFL is identified and removed along with its surrounding periosteum and surrounding joint capsule from its attachment on the distal fibula with the inferior extensor retinaculum, as described elsewhere [10]. This will be used for later reinsertion. The distal fibula bone is prepared to bleeding bone with a rongeur or similar. The ATFL and evolving tissue is retracted distally to expose its talar insertion.

The nonarticular side of the talar lateral ridge will be the site for tunnel drilling and placement of the 3.5-mm biocomposite suture anchor with the suture tape (Fig. 39.2).

A 2.7-mm drill bit with a suitable guide is used. This guide is of paramount relevance for surrounding tissue protection and particularly in mini-open or endoscopic techniques.

The tunnel has usually a 45° medial and cephalad orientation for placement of the 3.5-mm

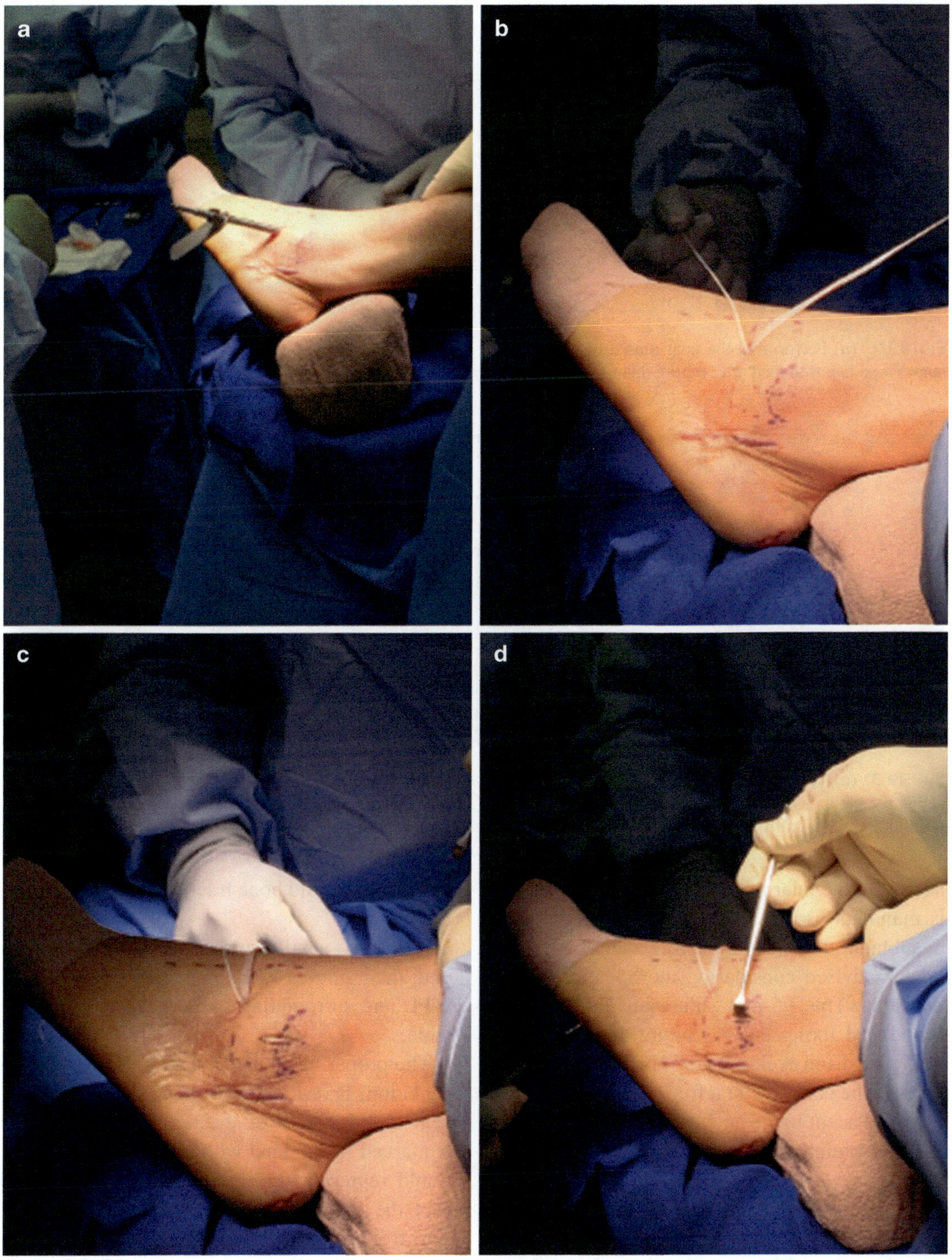

Fig. 39.1 Mini-open (percutaneous) technique. (**a**) Performing the talar tunnel using adequate guide. Fluoroscopy can be useful. (**b**) The suture tape is held in the talus. (**c** and **d**) Mini-incision to permit the fibular tunnel while the tape will slide extra-articularly

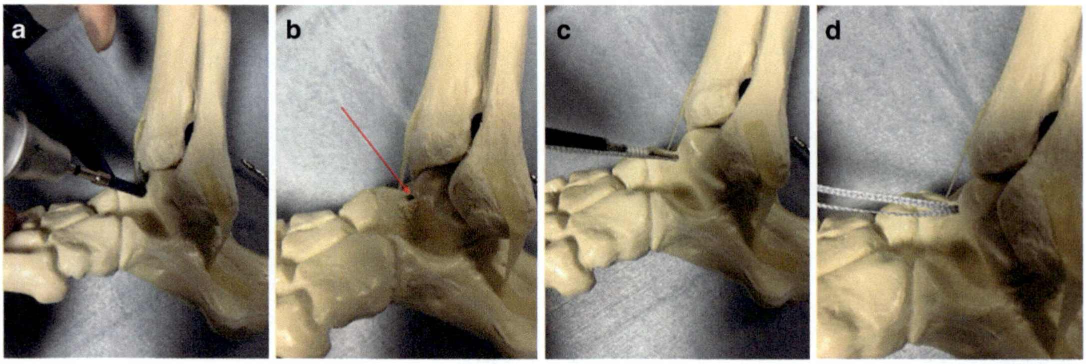

Fig. 39.2 (**a**) Performing the talar tunnel using adequate guide. (**b**) Talar tunnel (red arrow). (**c** and **d**) Anchor with suture tape is introduced after taping due to bone density in the talus

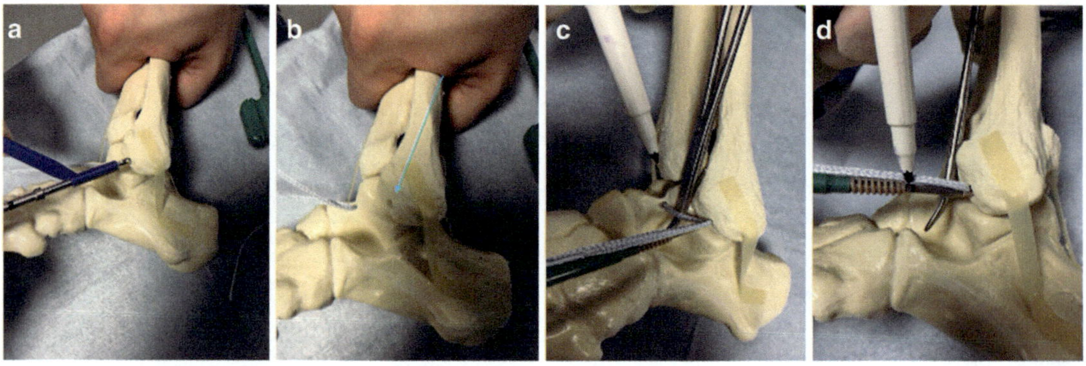

Fig. 39.3 (**a**) Tunnel in the distal tip of the fibula (replicating the native ATFL insertion) is oriented from distal to proximal at 45° and from medial to lateral 30–45° (avoid bone fracture or joint damage); (**b**) fibular tunnel (light blue arrow); (**c**) the mosquito clamp is used to avoid overtension; and (**d**) preparation for final fixation

anchor in the talar body (Figs. 39.1 and 39.2). It is mandatory to avoid damage on the tibiotalar or subtalar joints. Taping before anchor introduction is advised considering the bone density of the talus. The 3.5-mm suture anchor is finally introduced fixing the #2 Suture Tape (attached through a distal eyelet). In the open technique, the tape can be passed with a free needle through the tissue adjacent to the anchor including the extensor retinaculum. This will ensure that the augmentation will lie extra-articularly, as intended; however this is not mandatory and can be ensured by palpation or direct visualization. The fibular tunnel for the 4.75 mm anchor is performed centrally in the distal tip of the fibula (replicating the native ATFL insertion), oriented from distal to proximal around 45° and from medial to lateral 30–45° (avoid bone fracture or joint damage) (Fig. 39.3).

If the two small proximal anchors have been used, their sutures will now be used to bring the ATFL and surrounding tissue back to the distal fibula.

The proper tension of the #2 suture-tape augmentation is critical. This includes measurement of the length of the tunnel which should be marked in the tape with a marker. One mark should represent the place where the tape will meet the end of the tunnel and a second one, apart from the first the exact length of the tunnel will be used by the surgeon to control if the augmentation tape is properly adapted to the tunnel length. A mosquito clamp can be used to ensure that there will be no overtension of the polyethyl-

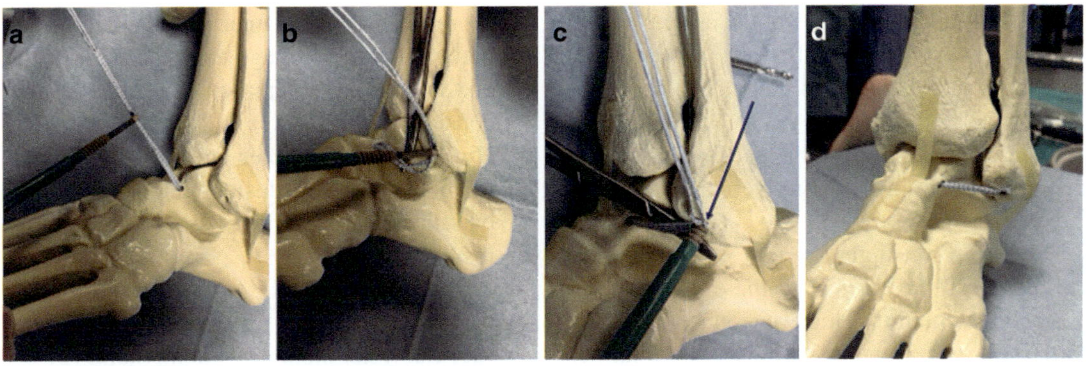

Fig. 39.4 (**a**) A mark is made in the tape representing the length of the ATFL; (**b**) The tunnel length is measured and a second mark is made in the tape (distally to the first mark the equivalent of the tunnel length); (**c**) The second mark will be visible once the anchor is fully introduced (dark blue arrow). (**d**) Final aspect of the suture-tape augmentation

ene tape once it has no inherent elasticity. Putting the tip of the mosquito clamp beneath, the augmentation tape will ensure that some desired slight laxity is maintained (Fig. 39.4). The excess tape is removed and adequate wound closure performed. A posterior splint is applied and used in the first week.

Postoperative care: patients are advised to use a Walker boot with immediate full weight-bearing from day 1. Dressings are changed after 1 week, and dorsiflexion/plantarflexion exercises start at that point. The boot is removed at 4 weeks and a soft brace (Fig. 39.5) is used in regular shoe wear. Rehabilitation starts focused on strengthening and proprioception. Sports-specific exercises might be reintroduced from 6 weeks. And full return to activity might be achieved from 8 to 12 weeks.

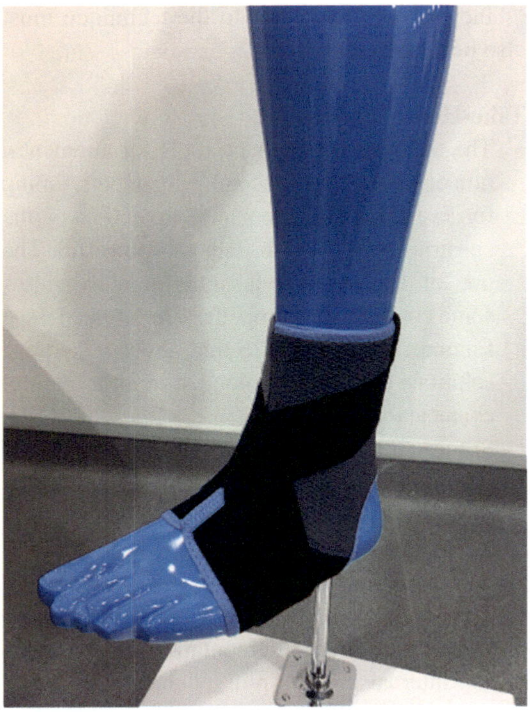

Fig. 39.5 Example of an ankle soft brace

39.3 Clinical Outcome

Besides the fact that this approach does not bring biological enhancement to the surgical repair, several authors have reported compliance with accelerated rehabilitation and return to activities of daily living.

An example is the return to cycling at 2 weeks and running at 8 weeks, which have been reported [18]. A small case series enrolling 15 running athletes stated that all returned to running within 12 weeks.

It has been stated that results are at least as good as any of the modifications of the Broström repair technique [9–11, 15–19].

A faster rehabilitation and return to activity are important goals to pursuit.

Similarly, lowering the "low" failure rate, particularly through long follow-up after surgery in high-level athletes, is also worth all efforts.

For the moment, most studies report to small case series and short follow-up, and most are related to authors involved in the development of the implants or technique.

Larger series with longer follow-ups are required before more definitive conclusions can be made.

However, we might say that it is as effective as "classical" treatment and there is a trend for faster rehabilitation. However, one must recognize that several studies with classical treatment without suture-tape augmentation report very similar timings for return to activity [10].

We will need to wait to know more about the biological reaction to the material itself, as it has been reported in other orthopedic examples [20].

Increased costs related to the technique must also be considered.

Take-Home Messages

- The trend for finding new tools for augmentation of surgical repair of ankle ligaments aiming for faster rehabilitation and protection of the construct is very up to date and powerful. The use of synthetic devices traditionally raises some concerns in orthopedics. In future, Tissue Engineering promises to find new regenerative solutions by joining biological input to biomechanical reinforcement.
- Suture-tape augmentation of surgical repair of chronic anterolateral ankle instability (CLAI) promises to achieve "stronger" repairs, with inferior risk of failure and allowing a faster rehabilitation.
- This includes high-molecular-weight polyethylene "suture-tape augmentation," also known as "internal brace" (plus anchor/small inference screws), to augment ligament repair in modified Broström repair.
- Technically, once this technique does not improve biology, nor proprioception and the synthetic material has very low compliance it is mandatory to avoid overtension—the "mosquito clamp" is quite effective (see Sect. 39.2).
- Moreover, careful tunnel positioning is mandatory to avoid damage to distal fibula, talus, and ankle joint. Increased cost must also be considered.
- Higher quality studies are required before more definitive conclusions can be established but this technique has shown promising results.

Fact Box 1: Nonbiological Augmentation of ATFL Repair—Tips and Tricks

- There is a recent trend for augmentation of surgical repair of ankle ligaments aiming for faster rehabilitation.
- Synthetic high-molecular-weight polyethylene "suture-tape augmentation," also known as "internal brace," has become popular.
- Use of adequate material including proper guide is advised.
- The tunnel has usually a 45° medial and cephalad orientation for placement of the 3.5-mm anchor in the talar body (avoid damage on the tibiotalar or subtalar joints).
- Taping before anchor introduction is advised considering the bone density of the talus.
- Tunnel in the distal tip of the fibula (replicating the native ATFL insertion) is oriented from distal to proximal at 45° and from medial to lateral 30–45° (avoid bone fracture or joint damage).
- The proper tension of the #2 suture-tape augmentation is critical. A mosquito clamp can be used (see Sect. 39.2).
- Synthetic materials for ligament repair traditionally raises some concerns in orthopedics. Tissue Engineering promises to find new solutions by joining biological input to biomechanical reinforcement.

References

1. Hunt KJ, Fuld RS, Sutphin BS, Pereira H, D'Hooghe P. Return to sport following lateral ankle ligament repair is under-reported: a systematic review. J ISAKOS Joint Disord Orthopaed Sports Med. 2017; https://doi.org/10.1136/jisakos-2016-000064.
2. van Dijk CN, Bossuyt PM, Marti RK. Medial ankle pain after lateral ligament rupture. J Bone Joint Surg Br. 1996;78(4):562–7.
3. Ferkel RD, Chams RN. Chronic lateral instability: arthroscopic findings and long-term results. Foot Ankle Int. 2007;28(1):24–31. https://doi.org/10.3113/fai.2007.0005.
4. Lee J, Hamilton G, Ford L. Associated intra-articular ankle pathologies in patients with chronic lateral ankle instability: arthroscopic findings at the time of lateral ankle reconstruction. Foot Ankle Spec. 2011;4(5):284–9.
5. Liszka H, Depukat P, Gadek A. Intra-articular pathologies associated with chronic ankle instability. Folia Med Cracov. 2016;56(2):95–100.
6. Harrington KD. Degenerative arthritis of the ankle secondary to long-standing lateral ligament instability. J Bone Joint Surg Am. 1979;61(3):354–61.
7. Kobayashi T, Gamada K. Lateral ankle sprain and chronic ankle instability: a critical review. Foot Ankle Spec. 2014;7(4):298–326. https://doi.org/10.1177/1938640014539813.
8. Karlsson J, Rudholm O, Bergsten T, Faxen E, Styf J. Early range of motion training after ligament reconstruction of the ankle joint. Knee Surg Sports Traumatol Arthrosc. 1995;3(3):173–7. https://doi.org/10.1007/BF01565478.
9. Ramirez-Gomez VJ, Gomez-Carlin LA, Ortega-Orozco R, Zazueta-Arnaud CA, Patino-Fernandez JP. Clinical and functional results of Brostrom-Gould procedure with suture tape augmentation: an evaluation using three scales. J Foot Ankle Surg. 2020; https://doi.org/10.1053/j.jfas.2020.01.005.
10. Schuh R, Benca E, Willegger M, Hirtler L, Zandieh S, Holinka J, Windhager R. Comparison of Brostrom technique, suture anchor repair, and tape augmentation for reconstruction of the anterior talofibular ligament. Knee Surg Sports Traumatol Arthrosc. 2016;24(4):1101–7. https://doi.org/10.1007/s00167-015-3631-7.
11. Petrera M, Dwyer T, Theodoropoulos JS, Ogilvie-Harris DJ. Short- to medium-term outcomes after a modified Brostrom repair for lateral ankle instability with immediate postoperative weightbearing. Am J Sports Med. 2014;42(7):1542–8. https://doi.org/10.1177/0363546514530668.
12. Viens NA, Wijdicks CA, Campbell KJ, Laprade RF, Clanton TO. Anterior talofibular ligament ruptures, Part 1: Biomechanical comparison of augmented Brostrom repair techniques with the intact anterior talofibular ligament. Am J Sports Med. 2014;42(2):405–11. https://doi.org/10.1177/0363546513510141.
13. Willegger M, Benca E, Hirtler L, Hradecky K, Holinka J, Windhager R, Schuh R. Biomechanical stability of tape augmentation for anterior talofibular ligament (ATFL) repair compared to the native ATFL. Knee Surg Sports Traumatol Arthrosc. 2016;24(4):1015–21. https://doi.org/10.1007/s00167-016-4048-7.
14. Maffulli N, Del Buono A, Maffulli GD, Oliva F, Testa V, Capasso G, Denaro V. Isolated anterior talofibular ligament Brostrom repair for chronic lateral ankle instability: 9-year follow-up. Am J Sports Med. 2013;41(4):858–64. https://doi.org/10.1177/0363546512474967.
15. Cho BK, Kim YM, Choi SM, Park HW, SooHoo NF. Revision anatomical reconstruction of the lateral ligaments of the ankle augmented with suture tape for patients with a failed Brostrom procedure. Bone Joint J. 2017;99-B(9):1183–9. https://doi.org/10.1302/0301-620X.99B9.BJJ-2017-0144.R1.
16. Cho BK, Park KJ, Kim SW, Lee HJ, Choi SM. Minimal invasive suture-tape augmentation for chronic ankle instability. Foot Ankle Int. 2015;36(11):1330–8. https://doi.org/10.1177/1071100715592217.
17. Mackay GM, Blyth MJ, Anthony I, Hopper GP, Ribbans WJ. A review of ligament augmentation with the InternalBrace: the surgical principle is described for the lateral ankle ligament and ACL repair in particular, and a comprehensive review of other surgical applications and techniques is presented. Surg Technol Int. 2015;26:239–55.
18. Mackay GM, Ribbans WJ. The addition of an "internal brace" to augment the Brostrom technique for lateral ankle ligament instability. Tech Foot Ankle Surg. 2016;15(1):47–56.
19. Ulku TK, Kocaoglu B, Tok O, Irgit K, Nalbantoglu U. Arthroscopic suture-tape internal bracing is safe as arthroscopic modified Brostrom repair in the treatment of chronic ankle instability. Knee Surg Sports Traumatol Arthrosc. 2020;28(1):227–32. https://doi.org/10.1007/s00167-019-05552-w.
20. Pereira H, Correlo VM, Silva-Correia J, Oliveira JM, Reis RL, Espregueira-Mendes J. Migration of "bioabsorbable" screws in ACL repair. How much do we know? A systematic review. Knee Surg Sports Traumatol Arthrosc. 2013;21(4):986–94. https://doi.org/10.1007/s00167-013-2414-2.
21. Acevedo J, Vora A. Anatomical reconstruction of the spring ligament complex "internal brace" augmentation. Foot Ankle Spec. 2013;6(6):441–5. https://doi.org/10.1177/1938640013499404.

Unique Perspective of Care of the Elite Athlete

40

C de V. Marais, J. D. F. Calder, and G. A. McCollum

40.1 Introduction

It is estimated that 25% of all musculoskeletal injuries involve inversion injuries of the ankle and constitute 7–10% of emergency departments visits [1]. Up to 50% of these are sport-related injuries in individuals under 35 years of age [2–7]. In the systemic review by Fong et al. the ankle was the most commonly injured part of the body in 24 of the 70 sports included [8]. The incidence varies for different sports but ankle injuries are commonly seen in athletes participating in basketball, soccer, running and ballet or dancing [9–11]. Up to 53% of injuries sustained during basketball and 29% of soccer injuries can be attributed to ankle injuries [12]. Though multiple structures around the ankle are at risk of injury, three-quarters of ankle injuries involve the lateral ligamentous complex [3, 6].

Therefore, athletes are a high-risk population for ankle injuries, specifically lateral ligamentous complex injuries. For high-level athletes, the absence from key sporting events or matches can have great economic impact and negatively affect ranking and future selections. Athletes have significantly greater load and demand on their ankle joint than the average population, and sports performed at the highest level may be an unfavourable prognostic factor for the development of residual complaints [13].

Treating an elite athlete with a lateral ankle injury provides an extra challenge. The goal of treatment would be the accurate diagnosis and effective treatment to facilitate a safe return to sport in the shortest time frame possible without an increase in risk of future re-injury, chronic instability and osteoarthritis.

40.2 Mechanism of Injury

In the neutral position, the bony architecture greatly contributes to the stability of the ankle joint, especially when coupled with the compressive load of weight bearing. As the foot goes into plantar flexion, this inherent stability decreases and the ligamentous structures assume a greater role in providing stability to the ankle. It is therefore during plantar flexion that the ligamentous structures around the ankle are more vulnerable to injury [14].

C de V. Marais (✉) · G. A. McCollum
Groote Schuur Hospital, University of Cape Town, Cape Town, Western Cape, South Africa
e-mail: christoff@drchristoffmarais.com; Ga.mccollum@uct.ac.za; grahammac@discoverymail.co.za

J. D. F. Calder
Department of Bioengineering, Imperial College London, London, UK

Fortius Clinic London, London, UK
e-mail: jamescalder@fortius.com

H. Pereira et al. (eds.), *Lateral Ankle Instability*, https://doi.org/10.1007/978-3-662-62763-1_40

The most common mechanism of injury is internal rotation or inversion of the plantarflexed foot. Due to the biomechanics of the lateral ligamentous complex, the anterior talofibular ligament (ATFL) is under maximum tension during plantar flexion and is therefore the first ligament injured, followed by the calcaneofibular ligament (CFL). The posterior talofibular ligament (PTFL) is usually not injured in inversion injuries as the maximal load to failure is three times that of the ATFL and is lax during plantarflexion [1].

Isolated ATFL injuries occur in about 65% of all ankle sprains, and combined rupture of ATFL and CFL occurred in 20% of cases [5].

The majority of ankle sprains during soccer are sustained during player contact [15]. Video analysis of ankle supination injuries demonstrated two main mechanisms of injury: impact on the medial aspect of the leg before or at foot strike, resulting in a lateral directed force causing the player to land with the ankle in an inverted position; forced plantar flexion when the injured player hits the opponent's foot when attempting to shoot or clear the ball [16].

40.3 Evaluation

Delayed examination after 3–5 days of treatment with rest, immobilization, elevation and compression following an injury have been shown to surpass stress radiography and ultrasound in identifying athletes with a significant lateral ligament injury [17, 18], with a sensitivity of 96% and a specificity of 84%.

However, the initial evaluation is still very important and in the case of most elite athletes will in all likelihood be performed immediately after the injury by an attending medical professional. The goal of the initial evaluation is to rule out associated injuries that may need to be addressed more urgently and to prevent further injury [14].

A thorough history is important following an inversion injury, specifically regarding the mechanism of injury, a history of previous injuries and treatment and what treatment modalities have already been initiated. It is common for athletes to report that they heard a "snap" at the time of the injury. However, feeling a tearing sensation or hearing a snap does not correlate with the severity of the injury [7].

Several hours after the injury, generalized pain and swelling can make examination more difficult and less reliable [14]. However, in the initial period following the injury, key features such as swelling, bruising and localized pain on palpation can provide important information regarding underlying pathology. Pain and swelling over the area of the ATFL may be indicative of an ATFL injury, but of more importance, if there is no pain over the ATFL, it is highly unlikely that there is an ATFL injury [16–18].

It is important to examine the entire leg to ensure that no other injuries are missed. Applying the Ottawa Ankle/Foot Rule helps to guide if further imaging is needed to rule out fractures in the acute setting and has been proven to have a sensitivity of 99.6% if applied within the first 48 h [19]. In reality, when treating professional athletes there is a trend to over-investigate. This is understandable as the consequences of missing a diagnosis or delaying diagnosis have economic and team performance consequences [19].

As mentioned previously, clinical tests to establish the integrity of the lateral ligamentous complex and assess the stability of the ankle are best performed 3–5 days after the injury when the pain and swelling have decreased [20].

The anterior draw test is more specific for assessing the integrity of the ATFL and the talar tilt test more specific to detect CFL injury.

The anterior draw test evaluates the integrity of the ATFL by the amount of anterior translation that can be produced in the sagittal plane. An increase in the anterior translation of the talus in relation to the tibia, compared to the uninjured side, is considered a positive sign and indicate an ATFL injury. The amount of translation that would be considered as physiological normal is a subject of debate and a range from 2 to 9 mm has been reported [14, 21].

The talar tilt test is defined as the angle produced by the tibial plafond and the dome of the talus when an inversion force is applied to the hindfoot. Once again, a wide range has been reported as normal but it is generally accepted that a 10° difference from the normal side is considered as a positive sign of a CFL injury [14].

Localized pain on palpation and haematoma discolouration gives 90% chance that there is an acute lateral ligament injury, while a positive anterior draw test in combination with pain on palpation at the ATFL and haematoma discolouration has a sensitivity of 98% and specificity of 84% for having an ATFL injury [1].

Pain on palpation at the level of the medial malleolus is present in about 60% of patients with a lateral ligament injury and 40% have pain over the anterior syndesmosis without rupture of the ligament, probably due to an anterior capsular tear [1].

40.4 Imaging

Plain X-rays will obviously not show the extent of ligament injury, but they can be a dynamic investigation if performed weight bearing. Tibia fibula diastasis or gross instability may be demonstrated.

Stress radiography has no role in the diagnosis of acute lateral ligament injuries [1]. These techniques are more often used to distinguish between mechanical instability and functional instability in patients with chronic instability and has no bearing on the treatment protocols for acute injuries [14].

Magnetic resonance imaging (MRI) has limited indications in the general population due to the high cost and high incidence of ankle sprains, despite having a sensitivity of 75–100% to diagnose lateral ligament ruptures and should be reserved patients that have persistent symptoms and complaint following an ankle injury that does not resolve with conservative treatment [19].

However, MRI should be part of the routine investigation for athletes to rule out associated injuries such as osteochondral lesions and occult fractures that may have a detrimental impact on their recovery and time to return to play [1].

40.5 Classification

The term ankle sprain is used to describe a broad spectrum of pathology ranging from a stretch injury of a ligament to a complete rupture leading to instability of the joint. The classification system proposed by Hamilton and Keikkonen in 1982 grades injuries from I to III. A grade I injury constitute a sprain with intact ATFL and CFL and no clinical findings suggestive of instability. With a grade II injury the ATFL ruptures but the CFL remains intact. An anterior draw test is positive but talar tilt negative. Grade III injuries have both the ATFL and CFL ruptures and anterior draw test as well as talar tilt test are positive.

In clinical practice, it is only relevant to distinguish between a sprain (grade I) and real instability (grade II or III) as this will have an impact on the treatment protocols. Injuries can only be accurately classified during a delayed physical examination as previously discussed [17, 18, 20].

40.6 Management

The treatment for acute lateral ligament injuries are dictated by the severity of the injury. Non-operative treatment has been found to be effective in treating grade I and II injuries in the general population as well as high-demand athletes. However, controversy exist regarding the treatment of grade III injuries especially in athletes [22].

All connective tissue injuries, including the lateral ligament of the ankle, undergo the same phased healing process. These phases consist of (1) haemorrhage and inflammation, (2) fibroblastic proliferation, (3) collagen protein formation and (4) collagen maturation.

Non-operative treatment is based on individualized measures based on these stages of healing with the aim to minimize effusion and haemorrhage, early protected motion, early protected weight bearing and protected return to activity while preventing re-injury.

The greater the severity of the injury, the greater the time will be to progress through each of the phases [1, 22].

40.6.1 Acute Phase

Immediately after the injury the goal of treatment is to limit the inflammatory phase. Minimizing swelling and haematoma formation will reduce the amount of extracellular fluid that would need to be reabsorbed during the healing process.

Treatment methods during this phase can be described by the mnemonic RICE (Rest, Ice, Compression and Elevation). Although some authors recommend early mobilization, others recommend a short period of immobilization for 5–7 days in a below-knee cast or removable boot [23, 24]. When immobilized, the ankle should be placed in maximal dorsiflexion as tolerated. This would place the joint in the position of greatest congruency to minimize capsular distention, approximate torn ligament ends and reduce the tension in sprained ligaments [22]. Prolonged immobilization is however not recommended as it will result in a prolonged rehabilitation period and an inferior outcome [25].

The method of immobilization would be guided by the severity of the injury. In the case of grade I, an elastic bandage or neoprene brace may provide adequate support, while a grade II injury may require a stirrup brace or an air cast boot. Grade III injuries require more protection and support and a functional walking orthosis should be considered.

Weight bearing is encouraged as long as it is pain free and well tolerated with the use of appropriate assistive devises as needed.

40.6.2 Subacute Phase

During the proliferation phase following the 5–7 days of immobilization, protected range of motion is added to the treatment regime. This is to reduce muscle atrophy, maintain full range of motion and prevent arthrofibrosis.

Early motion also facilitates the correct collagen bundle orientation in line with the forces applied. Active and passive range of motion activities are performed within the athletes pain-free range. Initial range of motion in the sagittal plane is introduced first to improve plantar and dorsiflexion without subjecting the injured ligaments to unnecessary stress. Later, as healing progresses, gentle inversion and eversion may be added. During ambulation, the joint should still be protected by means of a brace or functional walking orthosis, and crutches are used till the athlete has a pain-free uncompensated gait pattern [22].

40.6.3 Rehabilitation Phase

A more aggressive rehabilitation programme can be pursued to regain lost strength and range of motion once the healing ligament starts to mature around 4–6 weeks. This should be sport specific and coordinated by the team medical staff. The goal is to re-integrate the player to his/her pre-injury role in the team or the individual sport. Activities should be weight bearing and multi-directional in nature and should progressively simulate the athlete's activities required during training and competing. All activities should be pain and symptom free [22].

40.6.4 Preventative Measures

Whether some form of protective tape or brace should be used once an athlete returns to sporting activities should be considered on a case to case bases for each individual athlete. Athletes should be counselled that they should allow 6–12 months for full maturation and remodelling of the injured ligaments, and a semi-rigid or lace-up brace during high-risk activities has been shown to reduce recurrent injuries [26, 27].

Treatment of grade III ligament injuries in high-level athletes requires discussion. It has been reported that lateral ankle ligament injuries of all grades that are treated conservatively have good to excellent results in 80–90% of patients [28]. Surgical repair should be reserved for patients with persistent symptoms after completion of a functional rehabilitation programme [29]. Particular since delayed surgical reconstruction of ruptured ligaments is possible even years after the initial injury with equal results to a primary repair [19].

A Cochran systemic review of the literature regarding the comparison of surgical and conservative treatment of lateral ligament injuries failed to demonstrate a superiority of one treatment over the other. Due to the higher incidence of stiffness, impaired ankle mobility and higher complication rate associated with surgery, it is concluded that the best option would be conservative treatment with functional rehabilitation and close follow-up to identify athletes with complaints of chronic ligament laxity [30].

However the same Cochran review did report that surgical repair resulted in greater objective ankle stability and a quicker return to activity [30]. Residual ankle instability, as defined by a positive tilt test on stress radiography or a positive anterior draw test, has been reported as a predictor of repeat injury [31].

The goal for high-level athletes following an injury is to return to the same level of activity as before the injury in the shortest time possible without residual symptoms. The risk of recurrent injury should be at a minimum, as repeated absence from training and events will have a detrimental effect on their sporting career. Therefore, the treatment of every high-level athlete should be considered on an individual basis, but a lower threshold for surgical repair should be considered than for the general population. A counter argument for surgery is that the professional athlete has the most loose from a complication such as a deep infection, nerve injury, CRPS or others. Although rare, one of these could end a career.

Excellent long-term results have been reported at a mean follow-up of 10.6 years after a Brostrom repair of the lateral ligament complex, with 28 of the 30 patients returning to pre-injury level of activities, 24 of the 30 being high-level athletes [32].

40.7 Conclusion

The clinical diagnosis and classification of lateral ligament injuries should be made by delayed evaluation 3–5 days after the initial injury. Radiological investigations should be utilized if at any stage there is a suspicion of an associated injury and perhaps more liberally in the professional. An MRI scan is recommended for all high-level athletes with lateral ligament injuries to exclude concomitant soft tissue, cartilage and bony injuries.

The majority of lateral ligament complex injuries sustained by high-level athletes can be treated by non-surgical means with excellent results, especially grade I and II injuries. High-level athletes with grade III injuries may be considered for surgical repair, particularly if there is an acute on chronic picture, features of generalized ligament laxity, critical time frames to return to play as it may have a get them back to play a few weeks sooner, and have less long-term objective instability.

References

1. van den Bekerom MPJ, Kerkhoffs GMMJ, McCollum GA, Calder JDF, van Dijk CN. Management of acute lateral ankle ligament injury in the athlete. Knee Surg Sport Traumatol Arthrosc. 2013;21(6):1390–5.
2. Glick JM, Gordon RB. The prevention and treatment of ankle injuries. Am J Sports Med. 1976;4(4):136–41.
3. Garrick JG. The frequency of injury, mechanism of injury, and epidemiology of ankle sprains. Am J Sports Med. 1977;5(6):241–2.
4. Bosien WR, Staples OS, Russell SW. Residual disability following acute ankle sprains. J Bone Joint Surg Am. 1955;37(6):1237–43.
5. Broström L. Sprained ankles. V. Treatment and prognosis in recent ligament ruptures. Acta Chir Scand. 1966;132(5):537–50.
6. Hosea TM, Carey CC, Harrer MF. The gender issue: epidemiology of ankle injuries in athletes who participate in basketball. Clin Orthop Relat Res. 2000;372:45–9.
7. Nilsson S. Sprains of the lateral ankle ligaments II. Epidemiology and clinical study with special reference to different forms of conservative treatment. J Oslo City Hosp. 1983;33:13–36.
8. Fong D, Hong Y, Chan L-K, Yung P, Chan K-M. A systematic review on ankle injury and ankle sprain in sports. Sport Med. 2007;37:73–94.

9. Balduini FC. Management and rehabilitation of ligamentous injuries to the ankle. Sport Med. 1987;4:364–80.
10. Ekstrand J, Gillquist J, Möller M, Oberg B, Liljedahl S-O. Incidence of soccer injuries and their relation to training and team success. Am J Sports Med. 1983;11(2):63–7.
11. Lindenfeld TN, Schmitt DJ, Hendy MP, Mangine RE, Noyes FR. Incidence of injury in indoor soccer. Am J Sports Med. 1994;22(3):364–71.
12. Garrick JG, Requa RK. Role of external support in the prevention of ankle sprains. Med Sci Sports. 1973;5(3):200.
13. Linde F, Hvass I, Jürgensen U, Madsen F. Early mobilizing treatment in lateral ankle sprains. Course and risk factors for chronic painful or function-limiting ankle. Scand J Rehabil Med. 1985;18(1):17–21.
14. Lynch SA. Assessment of the injured ankle in the athlete. J Athl Train. 2002;37(4):406–12.
15. Wood C, Hawkins R, Hulse M, Hodson A. The Football Association Medical Research Programme: an audit of injuries in professional football: an analysis of ankle sprains. Br J Sports Med. 2003;37:233–7.
16. Andersen TE, Floerenes TW, Arnason A. Video analysis of the mechanisms for ankle injuries in football. Am J Sports Med. 2000;32:69–79.
17. van Dijk CN, Lim LSL, Bossuyt PMM, Marti RK. Physical examination is sufficient for the diagnosis of sprained ankles. J Bone Joint Surg. 1996;78:958–62.
18. Van Dijk CN, Mol BWJ, Lim LSL, Marti RK, Patrick M. Diagnosis of ligament rupture of the ankle joint: physical examination, arthrography, stress radiography and sonography compared in 160 patients after inversion trauma. Acta Orthop Scand. 1996;67(6):566–70.
19. Polzer H, et al. Diagnosis and treatment of acute ankle injuries: development of an evidence-based algorithm. Orthop Rev (Pavia). 2012;4(1):e5.
20. van Dijk CN. On diagnostic strategies in patients with severe ankle sprain. Amsterdam: Rodopi; 1994.
21. Johannsen A. Radiological diagnosis of lateral ligament lesion of the ankle: a comparison between talar tilt and anterior drawer sign. Acta Orthop Scand. 1978;49:295–301.
22. Safran MR, Zachazewski JE, Benedetti RS, Bartolozzi R, Mandelbaum R. Lateral ankle sprains: a comprehensive review Part 2: Treatment and rehabilitation with an emphasis on the athlete. Med Sci Sports Exerc. 1999;31(7):S438–47.
23. Bleakley CM, et al. Effect of accelerated rehabilitation on function after ankle sprain: randomised controlled trial. Br Med J. 2010;340:c1964.
24. Lamb SE, Marsh JL, Hutton JL, Nakash R, Cooke MW, CAST Group. Mechanical supports for acute, severe ankle sprain: a pragmatic, multicentre, randomised controlled trial. Lancet. 2009;373(9663):575–81.
25. Chan KW, Ding BC, Mroczek KJ. Acute and chronic lateral ankle instability in the athlete. Bull NYU Hosp Jt Dis. 2011;69(1):17–26.
26. Sitler M, et al. The efficacy of a semirigid ankle stabilizer to reduce acute ankle injuries in basketball: a randomized clinical study at West Point. Am J Sports Med. 1994;22(4):454–61.
27. Surve I, Schwellnus MP, Noakes T, Lombard C. A fivefold reduction in the incidence of recurrent ankle sprains in soccer players using the sport-stirrup orthosis. Am J Sport Med. 1994;22(5):601–6.
28. Kannus P, Renström P. Treatment for acute tears of the lateral ligaments of the ankle. Operation, cast, or early controlled mobilization. JBJS. 1991;73(2):305–12.
29. Baumhauer J, O'Brien T. Surgical considerations in the treatment of ankle instability. J Athl Train. 2002;37(4):458–62.
30. Kerkhoffs GMMJ, et al. Surgical versus conservative treatment for acute injuries of the lateral ligament complex of the ankle in adults (Review). Science. 2010;2:2–4.
31. Verhagen EALM, Van der Beek AJ, Bouter LM, Bahr RM, Van Mechelen W. A one season prospective cohort study of volleyball injuries. Br J Sports Med. 2004;38(4):477–81.
32. Lee KT, Park YU, Kim JS, Kim JB, Kim KC, Kang SK. Long-term results after modified Brostrom procedure without calcaneofibular ligament reconstruction. Foot Ankle Int. 2011;32(2):153–7.

Assessing Outcomes for Treatment of Chronic Ankle Instability

41

Gwendolyn Vuurberg, A. Perera, G. M. M. J. Kerkhoffs, and Jón Karlsson

41.1 Outcomes in Chronic Ankle Instability

41.1.1 Measurement Challenges

Chronic ankle instability (CAI) may be considered complex due to the many issues associated with this common injury. In addition to persisting instability [1] consisting of mechanical instability [2, 3], functional instability [2] or both, CAI can be associated with musculoskeletal, neuromuscular and psychological deficiencies such as pain, fear of giving way or recurrent sprains [4, 5].

Proper assessment of injury severity and recovery is important for three reasons; firstly, in the day-to-day management of patients; secondly, for auditing the quality of treatment and third, in analysing and comparing new treatments. This requires valid and reliable instruments that can be used both at baseline, for follow-up of symptoms or exacerbation factors associated with CAI. These three different scenarios require high levels of sensitivity and specificity. For instance patients are generally clear about whether they require intervention or not and also whether they have improved after treatment or not, simply by asking them how they feel.

However, for research purposes the ability to compare different patient populations sounds more respectful requires much more accuracy with greater sensitivity and specificity than the description of the ankle being weak or the source of (functional) disability or not. The difficulty here is that the basic building block of instability is the concept of 'giving way'. This is a very subjective feeling and is therefore difficult to quantify. Most patients will not actually get to the point of falling over, rather they will avoid activities that put them at risk and will carefully watch the floor as they move [6].

Assessing CAI is further complicated by the fact that different patients have different levels of stability that they can cope with, and that this

G. Vuurberg (✉) · G. M. M. J. Kerkhoffs
Department of Orthopedic Surgery, Amsterdam UMC, Location AMC, Amsterdam Movement Sciences, University of Amsterdam, Amsterdam, The Netherlands

Academic Center for Evidence Based Sports Medicine (ACES), Amsterdam, The Netherlands

Amsterdam Collaboration for Health and Safety in Sports (ACHSS), Amsterdam UMC, Amsterdam, The Netherlands
e-mail: g.vuurberg@amsterdamumc.nl; g.m.kerkhoffs@amsterdamumc.nl

A. Perera
Foot and Ankle Clinic, Spire Cardiff Hospital, Cardiff, UK

J. Karlsson
Department of Orthopaedics, Sahlgrenska University Hospital, Sahlgrenska Academy, Gothenburg University, Gothenburg, Sweden
e-mail: jon.karlsson@vgregion.se

H. Pereira et al. (eds.), *Lateral Ankle Instability*, https://doi.org/10.1007/978-3-662-62763-1_41

is not per se based on the degree of instability demonstrable on an anterior drawer test [7, 8]. The degree of (in)stability a patient can cope with may, for example, vary with the demands placed on the ankle (such as sports and work), the degree of overall function and their ability to compensate through other mechanisms [9]. The concept of instability is much more than simply the presence or absence of ligament laxity and is a composition of many factors and not always of a binary nature [10].

41.2 Quantifying Ankle Instability

41.2.1 Measurable Features of Chronic Ankle Instability

The challenge is to have a quantifiable overall impression of a patient's complaints that is as objective as possible despite the number of subjective parameters involved. In order to structure this process we have identified six different methods to assess ankle function (Box 41.1).

Box 41.1 Assessment Methods

1. History
2. Physical Examination (including assessment of risk factors)
3. Physical Tests (instrumented and non-instrumented)
4. Supplementary Diagnostics (such as radiographs, CT and MRI investigations)
5. Self-Administered Functional Outcome Scores (generic and instability specific)
6. Activity Level Scores

The ideal assessment can identify and quantify the key features rapidly in a clinical setting, using validated parameters at low costs and ideally in the form of a self-administered instrument [11]. Historically, we have relied upon the first three steps for day-to-day decision-making with perhaps some reference to the use of physical tests in the more specialized environment of sports medicine [9]. Outcome scores are increasingly used in general orthopaedics, but foot and ankle surgery has been less well served. Their use is mainly restricted to quality audits and the research context. The use of instrumented physical tests, which may be used to enhance the diagnostic process or evaluate treatment effects, is also typically restricted to use in a research context.

Identification of risk factors is essential to the day-to-day treatment decision-making per individual. Also in a research context it is vital that we have an understanding of the type of patient that will be operated on. Through risk factor identification additionally expectations can be managed. Realistic expectations are of great importance in a good rehabilitation process. It should be kept in mind expectations and needs vary between individuals; they are different in the young athlete compared with the older sedentary patient. For this reason it is important to understand the nature of disability and the activities that patients wish to return to using the assessment methods mentioned in Box 41.1.

41.2.1.1 History

At the present time Patient Reported Outcome Measures (PROMs) do not always cover all aspects or dimensions in which patients experience complaints sufficiently. For this reason patient history is of vital importance in assessing the patient's functional level. It is, however, a challenge to take this largely qualitative information and have this in a format that is both objective and quantifiable.

Of course the number of episodes of falling over is readily measurable, but for most patients this is a rare occurrence. As a result they will avoid challenging scenarios or stop themselves from falling, so instead they will have episodes of giving way or feelings of insecurity which are less well measurable. For these reasons the Ankle Instability Group set some definitions and highlighted the importance to document the presence and frequency of these symptoms (Table 41.1) [12].

Other features to document are the activity avoidance (uneven surfaces, slopes, sport, walk-

Table 41.1 Definitions according to the Ankle Instability Group [12]

Acute Ankle Sprain	Traumatic injury to the lateral ligament complex following a twisting injury that results in pain, swelling and bruising for more than 1 day
Ankle Instability	Ankle joint feels vulnerable during activity
Giving way	Regular occurrence of uncontrolled ankle joint inversion episodes that do not necessarily result in ankle joint sprain
Recurrent Ankle Sprain	More than 2 episodes of Acute Ankle Sprain on the same side within 6 months
Mechanical Instability	Excessive inversion or anterior laxity on manual strain testing
Functional Ankle Instability	Giving way in the absence of mechanical deficit
Chronic Ankle Instability	Giving way or ankle instability for more than 1 year after the original ankle sprain

ing in the dark), ability to wear heels, sporting/work function, brace/support/walking aid usage, and whether the ankle gives way despite these.

41.2.1.2 Physical Examination

The role of physical examination may be in multiple dimensions. It may be used to assess recovery after treatment, but also to assess risk factors for (recurrent) injury. Physical examination is difficult to quantify in an objective way. Whereas there is little discussion on age or sex, height, weight and BMI must and can be measured according to standardized protocols to subsequently assess these as they are potential prognostic factors for recurrent ankle sprains [13–15]. Other potentially prognostic variables also related to treatment evaluation include strength and range of motion (ROM) as strength diminishes over time if patients are going to avoid certain types of loading such as sports in order to avoid an ankle sprain, or surgery which may result in joint stiffness. In order to get a reliable impression of these variables, they should be measured using a dynamometer and goniometer rather than getting an impression without adequate recording, making future comparison impossible [16].

Apart from these demographic variables, the site of pain should be assessed for pain on palpation to estimate the degree of recovery. Additionally, sites of occult injury, such as the peroneal muscles and tendons, anterior process of the calcaneus and fifth metatarsal should not be forgotten [12, 17].

As there is a low correlation between functional instability and the degree of mechanical laxity, first discrimination should be made between functional ankle instability, which is mainly based on the feeling of giving way [2], and mechanical laxity. To define whether a patient suffers from mechanical laxity or functional instability, the anterior drawer test may be performed. By fixation of the tibia, the calcaneus is pulled in a forward position (Fig. 41.1). A greater laxity of the anterior talofibular ligament (ATFL) will allow greater subluxation of the talus together with the calcaneus. To define the range of laxity, different grades may be reported: Grade 0 (0–2 mm); 1 (3–5 mm); 2 (6–10 mm) and 3 (11–15 mm). Using the Dynamic Anterior Ankle Tester (DAAT) showed lower sensitivity to change and low reliability in assessment of the ATFL in a clinical setting and therefore the ADT is preferred. A sensitivity rate of 0.8 and specificity rate of 0.75 has been reported for the anterior drawer test [7].

41.2.1.3 Special Physical Tests

Special physical tests are assessment methods with the aim to provide the most accurate information in patients with CAI as they directly test the balance. These balance deficits in a patient are often the reason of disability. Balance deficits may be the result of multiple deficiencies, such as (or combinations of) mechanical laxity, functional instability, proprioceptive deficits and hypermobility [18]. The more complex combinations are often closer to the real-life situations. Hence very precise assessment of balance deficiencies and a patient's ability to cope with these challenges in sport as well as day-to-day life is of great importance.

The need of specialist equipment often complicates the use of physical tests in an outpatient setting in addition to the fact that they

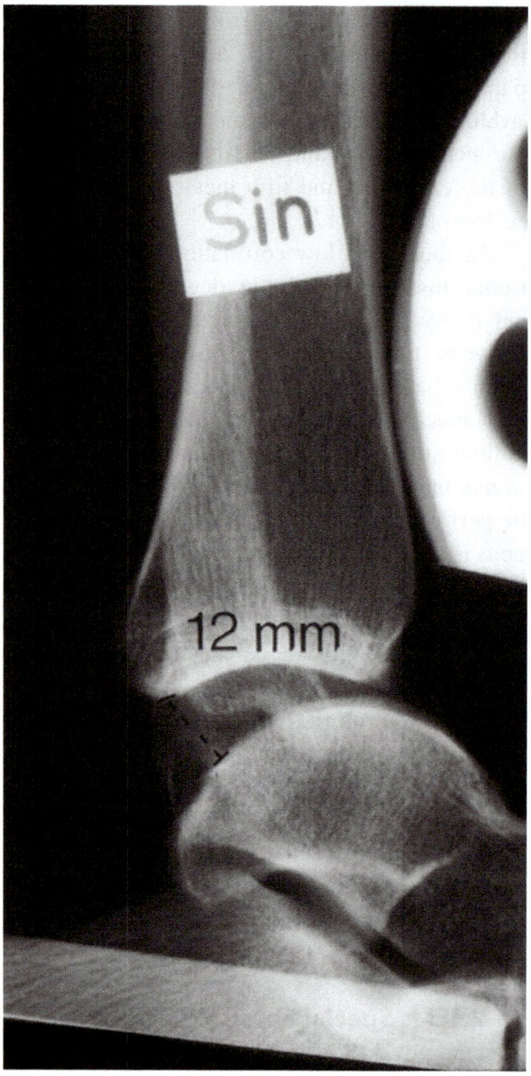

Fig. 41.1 Anterior translation of the talus in relation to the tibia on a lateral radiograph while performing the anterior drawer test

Table 41.2 Physical tests

	Instrumented	Non-instrumented
Static	Centre of Pressure (COP) [22, 23] – Area – Velocity	Balance error scoring system (BESS) [22] – Double legged – Single legged – Tandem
	Single-legged stance Measured balance surface by EMG [20]	Foot lift test [22]
	Star Excursion Balance Test (SEBT) [19, 22]	Time in balance test [22]
	Sway [21] – COP anteroposterior and mediolateral displacements and 95% CI for sway area (ellipse)	Single/double leg balance test [26] – Eyes Open – Eyes Closed
	Time to Boundary (TTB) [22]	Single-legged stance [22] – Eyes Open – Eyes Closed
Dynamic	Time to Stabilization (TTS) [24]	Single leg hop test [27] – Time – Distance
		Hop (for distance) [22, 27] – Crossover – Figure-of-eight – Side – Single – Triple
		Single leg vertical jump [28]

Note: Instrumented tests are measured using, for example, force platforms or other hardware and software assessing deviations. Non-instrumented tests are assessed manually for time, distance, etc., leaving more room for measurement bias

are time consuming when performed appropriately [19–24]. For this reason currently use is mainly restricted to research and sports medicine. Particularly at professional level they are used as criteria for determining Return To Play (RTP), i.e. when a player is sufficiently stable or recovered and functional to be able to play safely and effectively [25]. Most regularly these physical tests are performed by physical therapists as they have both the required equipment and room in their practise. Despite that these are mostly performed by a sports or rehabilitation physician or physical therapist, knowledge on these tests and interpretation is important.

The physical tests can be divided into *static* and *dynamic*, and further into *instrumented* and *non-instrumented* (Table 41.2). Of these perhaps the Y balance has the best combination of accuracy, reproducibility, ease of performance and duration to be most practical.

Apart from assessment of balance, which is one of the main issues in patients with CAI, they may also report on giving way during walking or running on a flat or uneven surface [29].

In case the ankle instability affects the patient during daily living and sporting activities it may also be beneficial to assess the patient's walking pattern according to the 'Walking Cycle' [30]. This cycle is used to analyse the full walking pattern from heel-strike to heel-strike assessing one leg at the time, providing information not only about weight-bearing but also joint kinematics and dynamics (e.g. active Range of Motion, joint momentum) of the full lower extremity (Table 41.3 and Fig. 41.2) [30]. To improve reliability on reporting, aberrations should be reported per phase.

41.2.1.4 Supplementary Diagnostics

Supplementary diagnostics may include imaging such as a radiograph, CT- or MRI scan. In terms of outcome assessment these investigations only have a little role to play. However, in case of an osteochondral defect (OCD), bone marrow oedema or another type of injury a CT-scan or MRI may be relevant to assess the defect size and to define a prognosis on recovery (time) [31]. In case of an OCD a CT-scan may be preferred to avoid overestimation of the defect due to oedema [31, 32]. Ultrasonography (USG) and MRI may also be used to quantify involvement of soft tissues and the ankle joint, but due to a lower specificity of USG and lower availability in combination with high costs these are often not used, unless only these tools can be used to visualize specific structures or, for example, joint effusion [33, 34].

Initially a radiograph will have no extra function, unless a weight-bearing alignment view is chosen, which may identify malalignment as a reason for a shift of the mechanical leg axis in turn potentially predisposing a patient at recurrent ankle sprains and therefore CAI [35]. Also a radiograph with inversion stress may be used to objectively quantify persisting mechanical instability. By stressing the ankle in an inversion position while fixating the tibia the talar tilt may be measured: the angle between the distal tibial joint line and proximal talar joint line [36]. This test is, however, not specific for the tibiotalar joint. A stress view may also help assess the calcaneocuboid laxity, which also plays a role in instability complaints (Fig. 41.3) [37].

Table 41.3 Phases Walking Cycle

Phase	Sub-phase	Action
Stance phase	Shock absorption phase	Heel-strike (HS)
		Foot-flat (FF)
	Mid-stance phase	Mid-stance (MS)
		Heel-off (HO)
		Toe-off (TO)
	Push-off phase	
Swing phase		Mid-swing (MSW)
Double support		Heel-strike (HS)

41.2.1.5 Functional Outcome Scores

The most common and popular approach for measuring subjective outcome measures as systematic and valid as possible is by means of questionnaires. Patient reported outcome measures (PROMs) are gaining popularity due to their efficient assessment of complaints as experiences by patients accompanied by low costs [11]. PROMs usually cover multiple areas of interest such as

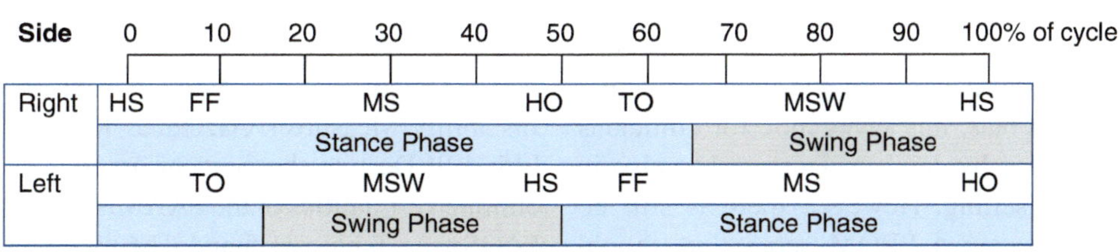

Fig. 41.2 Schematic distribution phases walking cycle. The stance phase includes 60% of the walking cycle. The bipedal phase (the phase during which two feet touch the ground) is seen during the HS, FF, HO and TO phases

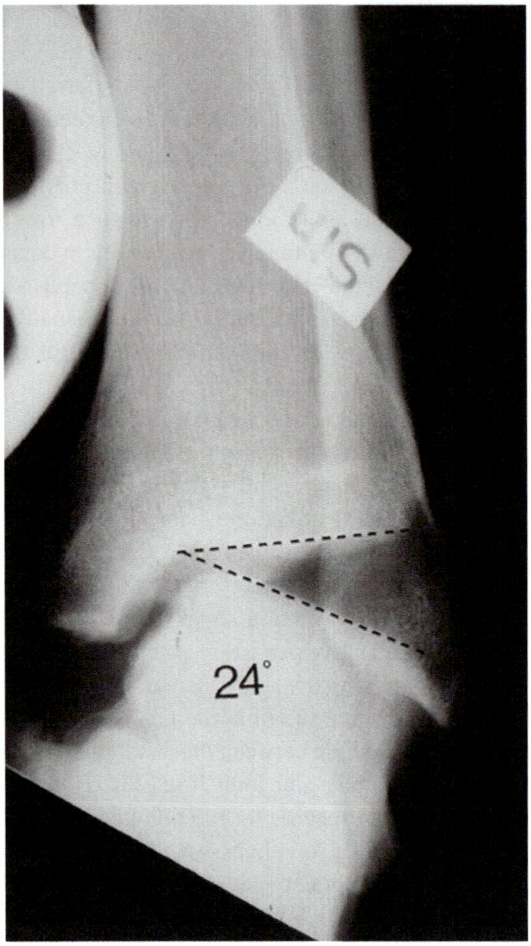

Fig. 41.3 Assessment of mechanical instability by performing inversion stress on the tibiotalar joint while fixating the tibia: the talar tilt test. The angle between the distal tibial and proximal talar joint line objectifies the degree of tibiotalar instability

pain, functional impairment, quality of life globally or in detail inquiring on specific complaints such as the feeling of instability or recovery time after an ankle sprain [29, 38].

The ideal instrument is one that the patient can complete rather than relying on a clinician's determination of balance. In addition to avoiding interpretation bias, this saves time for clinicians not only in day-by-day management but also in the research setting. However, there is still no universally accepted PROM score that should always be used in case of chronic ankle instability. The large amount of PROMs available and

Table 41.4 Questionnaires in ankle assessment

Domain	Questionnaire
General Health Scores	Short-Form 36 (SF-36) [39]
	EuroQualy of Life—5 Dimensions (EQ-5D) [40]
General Foot and Ankle Scores	American Orthopedic Foot and Ankle Society Score (AOFAS) [41]
	Foot and Ankle Ability Measure (FAAM) [42]
	Foot and Ankle Disability Index (FADI) [43]
	Foot and Ankle Outcome Score (FAOS) [38]
	Foot Function Index (FFI) [44]
	Karlsson score [45]
	Self-reported Foot and Ankle Score (SEFAS) [41]
Ankle Instability-Specific Scores	Ankle Instability Instrument (AII) [46]
	Chronic Ankle Instability Scale (CAIS) [47]
	Cumberland Ankle Instability Tool (CAIT) [29]
	Identification of Functional Ankle Instability (IdFAI) [48]

Note: These are only a few examples of the many foot and ankle questionnaires that may be used in the evaluation of complaints and treatment covering multiple sub-domains on complaints and patients' perception

the lack of a score that can differentiate between stable and unstable or between functional instability and mechanical laxity limits usability and comparability (Table 41.4).

To ensure PROMs are fit to assess severity of ankle instability, they need to be validated for the specific target population and need to have a high inter-observer reliability to minimize interpretation and measurement errors. Some of the PROM scores that have proven to fulfil these requirements for CAI are the Ankle Joint Functional Assessment Tool (AJFAT), Foot and Ankle Ability Measure (FAAM), Foot and Ankle Outcome Score (FAOS), Foot and Ankle Instability Measure (FADI) and Karlsson Score [45, 49]. Despite the need of assessment of the clinimetric qualities of the FAAM, the FAAM and FAOS (see Tables 41.5 and 41.6) are considered most appropriate to assess functional disability in patients with ankle instability [49]. Later stud-

Table 41.5 Questions Foot and Ankle Ability Measure [42]

FAAM[a] Questionnaire	
Activities of daily living subscale	Standing
	Walking on even ground
	Walking on even ground without shoes
	Walking up hills
	Walking down hills
	Going upstairs
	Going downstairs
	Walking on uneven ground
	Stepping up and down curbs
	Squatting
	Coming up on your toes
	Walking initially
	Walking 5 min or less
	Walking approximately 10 min
	Walking 15 min or greater
	Home responsibilities
	Activities of daily living
	Personal care
	Light to moderate work (standing, walking)
	Heavy work (push/pulling, climbing, carrying)
	Recreational activities
	How would you rate your current level of functioning during your usual activities of daily living from 0 to 100 with 100 being your level of function prior to your foot or ankle problem and 0 being the inability to perform any of your usual daily activities?
Sports subscale	Running
	Jumping
	Landing
	Starting and stopping quickly
	Cutting/lateral movements
	Ability to perform activity with your normal technique
	Ability to participate in your desired sport as long as you like
	How would you rate your current level of functioning during your sports related activities from 0 to 100 with 100 being your level of function prior to your foot or ankle problem and 0 being the inability to perform any of your sports related activities?

[a]Every question needs to be responded to by checking *one* box on a 5-point Likert scale that most closely fits the patient's condition during the past week ranging from 'no difficulty' to 'unable to do' or 'N/A'. Score calculation: 'no difficulty' is scored as 4 points; 'slight difficulty' = 3; 'moderate difficulty' = 2; 'extreme difficulty' = 1; 'unable to do' = 0. The total score is calculated by adding up all the numbers and divide these by the highest score possible (116 in case none of the questions are answered by N/A) (total score = sum of scores/max. score)

Table 41.6 Foot and Ankle Outcome Score [38]

FAOS[a] Questionnaire	
Subscale Symptoms To what degree have you suffered from the following foot/ankle symptoms during the last week?	Do you have swelling in your foot/ankle?
	Do you feel grinding; hear clicking or any other type of noise when your foot/ankle moves?
	Does your foot/ankle catch or hang up when moving?
	Can you straighten your foot/ankle fully?
	Can you bend your foot/ankle fully?
	How severe is your foot/ankle stiffness after first wakening in the morning?
	How severe is your foot/ankle stiffness after sitting, lying or resting later in the day?
Subscale Pain What amount of foot/ankle pain have you experienced in the last week during the following activities?	How often do you experience foot/ankle pain?
	Twisting/pivoting on your foot/ankle
	Straightening foot/ankle fully
	Bending foot/ankle fully
	Walking on flat surface
	Going up or down stairs
	At night while in bed
	Sitting or lying
	Standing upright
Subscale Function, Daily Living (ADL) Please indicate the degree of difficulty you have experienced in the last week due to your foot/ankle	Descending stairs
	Ascending stairs
	Rising from sitting
	Standing
	Bending to floor/pick up an object
	Walking on flat surface
	Getting in/out of car
	Going shopping
	Putting on socks/stockings
	Rising from bed
	Taking off socks/stockings
	Lying in bed (turning over, maintaining foot/ankle position)
	Getting in/out of bath
	Sitting
	Getting on/off toiler
	Heavy domestic duties (moving heavy boxes, scrubbing floors, etc.)
	Light domestic duties (cooking, dusting, etc.)

(continued)

Table 41.6 (continued)

FAOS[a] Questionnaire	
Subscale Function, Sports and Recreational Activities What degree of difficulty have you experienced during the last week due to your foot/ankle	Squatting
	Running
	Jumping
	Twisting/pivoting on your injured foot/ankle
	Kneeling
Subscale Quality of Life (QoL)	How often are you aware of your foot/ankle problem?
	Have you modified your life style to avoid potentially damaging activities to your foot/ankle?
	How much are you troubled with lack of confidence in your foot/ankle?
	In general, how much difficulty do you have with your foot/ankle?

[a]Questions address complaints they experienced during the past week which patients rate on a five-item scale (0–4 points) ranging from 'never/none/not at all' to 'always/extreme/constantly/totally'. Score calculation per subscale. Pain: 100 − (current score × 100)/36; Symptoms: 100 − (current score × 100)/28; ADL: 100 − (current score × 100)/68; Sport: 100 − (current score × 100)/20; QoL: 100 − (current score × 100)/16

ies show the Cumberland Ankle Instability Tool (CAIT) is also a valid and reliable tool to assess the severity of ankle instability and a cut-off point was determined to assess whether patients suffer from CAI or not. The cut-off values range between 11.5 [50], 25 [51] and 27.5 [29]. Despite correct calculation of all three cut-off points, the difference lies in the basic outcome on which it was determined, feeling of instability (i.e. FAI), or an ankle sprain, respectively, and which study population was used (outpatient clinic vs. healthy volunteers). For this reason, even if outcome measures have been validated, a physician needs to be critical to whether this validation applies to their healthcare setting and patients.

More recently instability-specific instrument have gained an increasing interest. Despite the great body of work from experts in this field there is still no widely accepted score. The IdFAI may provide outcome in identifying cases with functional instability, but is not used widely in the literature yet. Potentially combining three questionnaires (one from each domain, see Table 41.4) may provide the most complete evaluation for a patient. However, this additionally increases patient burden when asking them to fill out the questionnaires completely.

The degree of objectivity may be up for discussion as the variables of interest are measured based on the feeling of the patient on disability-related issues. Therefore PROM scores should always be used in combination with objective (physical) assessment tools.

41.2.1.6 Ankle Activity Scores

In case of ankle instability patients are often tempted to avoid activities that cause risk of spraining the ankle or falling and subsequently (sometimes unnoticeably) lower their activity level both for sports. Also work related they may search for alternatives. This may lead to a decrease if work functionality and with that increase the socio-economic burden [9]. After the activity and participation level of the patient prior to the ankle disability is recorded, wishes on return to activity and participation should be asked and expectations managed. In this step ankle activity scores such as the Ankle Activity Score (AAS) [52] as a validated tool for ankle disability may be helpful. The Tegner score [53], despite initial development for knee problems, has also proven to be of great value to assess activity levels in patients with ankle complaints. If complaints mainly concern sport, an 11-point Likert scale may be used to ask on effort and complaints during practising sports/work and for specific tasks. Specifically for sports also a 4-point scale can be used to define the level of sports practised: no sports; amateur; competitive or professional; with additional questions related to the number of hours practised per week.

41.3 Complications and Recurrence

In case of surgical treatment, complications and recurrence of instability are important outcome measures to assess procedure safety and effectiveness and should always be included in the treatment evaluation. The range and variation of complications should always be assessed in relation to patient-specific characteristics to ensure patients with a greater risk at complications receive a fair risk-benefit analysis prior to undergoing a certain stabilization procedure. Additionally some patients may be prone to recurrence, failed treatment or the assigned treatment may not be sufficient to resolve the degree of instability complaints experienced by a patient. Registration of recurrent sprains is required to indicate the duration of the treatment effect and may help indicate whether reoperation is necessary. Especially recurrence is underreported and in combination with a lack of long-term follow-up of surgical ankle stabilization, long-term effectiveness is unknown [54].

41.4 Psychometric Properties

Depending on what needs to be measured an instrument can be used or developed. When selecting an instrument for physical examination, to measure an outcome, evaluate treatment or for another objective, the properties of the chosen instrument need to measure the intended outcome. Whether an instrument is fit for its intended purpose may be concluded from its psychometric properties. Some of these properties include validity, reliability, reproducibility, responsiveness over time and internal consistency.

41.4.1 Interpretability

If an instrument proves to be valid and reliable, interpretability may still be an issue. Especially in questionnaires interpretability must be known. This is often defined by assessing floor and ceiling effects. A clinician wants to be sure that when patient scores maximally, he or she actually does not experience any complaints, instead of having a problem with the questionnaire's construct. This can be easily assessed. In a heterogeneous population (including the patients' of choice) no more than 15% can have a score equal to the highest or lowest score possible [55].

41.4.2 Reliability

For reliability, differentiation should be made between two types of reliability, namely inter- and intra-observer reliability. Inter-observer reliability includes the reliability comparing measurements between different observers. This is of great importance as a tool/test or device should be able to be used by different professionals individually of each other all measuring the same outcome. Intra-observer reliability includes the reliability within an observer as an observer should be able to measure the same outcome twice without finding any difference, if nothing has changed. To assess reliability the Intraclass Correlation Coefficient (ICC) can be used in case of normally distributed data with the cut-off values of poor reliability if the ICC was ≤40; moderate if 0.40–0.75, substantial from 0.75 to 0.90 and excellent if >0.90 [55]. In case of skewed data the Cronbach's alpha should be used, where 0.70–0.95 indicates good reliability and >0.95 represents excellent reliability [55].

A third type of reliability is test-retest reliability, commonly used in questionnaire validation. This includes retesting a questionnaire in the same population at two different time intervals and finding the same outcome in case patients indicated they experienced no change in complaints [56].

Internal consistency may also be regarded as a measure of reliability as it concerns the consistency within a tool. This measure also mainly concerns questionnaires measuring whether the topics addressed by the questionnaire do not variate too much leading to potential discongruency in patient's response. Internal consistency is measured using the Cronbach's alpha which is a derivative of the comparison of all the questions within a questionnaire. Again the Cronbach's alpha is considered moderate when it ranged from 0.70 to 0.95 and good if it exceeded the 0.95 [55, 56]. In case of a low alpha value, an additional analysis may be performed on whether removal of questions may improve the internal consistency.

Finally a large measurement error may reduce reliability and should therefore also be assessed. This may be easily done by calculating the Standard Error of Measurement (SEM = SD × $\sqrt{(1 - ICC)}$). Here the standard deviation (SD) is derived from the same calculation from which the ICC is derived (e.g. the inter- or intra-observer reliability or test-retest reliability). Additionally the Minimal Detectable Change (MDC = 1.96 × $\sqrt{2}$ – SEM) can provide an indication on what change can be measured and identified by an observer as a 'real' change (based on the used SEM) [57].

41.4.3 Repeatability and Reproducibility

Repeatability refers to measuring the same outcome when there is no variation in observer, location, measurement procedure, exact same measuring instrument (for example, questionnaire format), overall conditions and repetition over a short period of time.

Reproducibility can be assessed when the assessment is performed by different individuals, at different locations with different instruments assessing the ability to replicate findings.

For these two concepts the degree of agreement can be assessed using measures such as the ICC or another method to assess correlation [55].

41.4.4 Responsiveness Over Time

Responsivity is nothing more than the ability of an instrument to detect changes over time if change actually occurred [58]. This is easiest measured by letting patients fill out the questionnaire after some form of treatment and additionally including the question whether they experienced change.

41.4.5 Sensitivity and Specificity

Sensitivity, or true positive rate, is the measure of the proportion of positive outcomes, for example, number of patients suffering from mechanical instability as defined by the questionnaire, that are also defined as such using the golden standard (for example, the anterior drawer test) [59].

Specificity, or true negative rate, measures the ability of a tool (expressed as a percentage) to measure the true negatives, i.e. the proportion of patients that score negatively for mechanical ankle instability that do not suffer from mechanical ankle instability [59].

41.4.6 Validity

To ensure a tool is valid, only translation to the language in which the tool will be used is insufficient. In case needed to ensure comprehensibility of the questionnaire, questions may need to be changed (cross-cultural adaptation). If a tool or questionnaire is translated and tested, this should be done in the target population in which the tool or questionnaire will be used in future practise [52]. A tool should always be tested against a reference tool that has already been (translated) validated to assess construct validity. For example, the FAOS and FAAM could be compared when validating one of the two, while the other has already been validated. Construct validity is assessed using the Spearman's correlation coefficient (CC). A CC of ≤0.30 is considered poor, whereas 0.30–0.60 is moderate and >0.60 strong [55, 60].

41.5 Conclusion

Outcomes after treatment of CAI can be defined and measured in many ways. Objective tools such as physical examination and imaging should be used, especially in case of suspicion of concomitant bone or joint injuries. Additionally to assess the patients' perspective of complaints PROMs provide an efficient and cost-effective tool to assess both complaints and recovery according to the patient. All these tools require local translation, validation and reliability assessment prior to use in local clinics. In case of surgical stabilization, precise reports on complications and recurrence should be implemented in the main outcome measures, ensuring procedure safety and effectiveness.

Take-Home Message

- Depending on the intended outcome, many different measures can be chosen. The choice of outcomes should be patient based. Despite difficulty in orthopaedic practise of performance and adequate measurement of (special) physical tests, these may be of great value in the rehabilitation process and may help decide on whether a patient is fit to return to play.

References

1. Gribble PA, Bleakley CM, Caulfield BM, Docherty CL, Fourchet F, Fong DT, et al. 2016 consensus statement of the International Ankle Consortium: prevalence, impact and long-term consequences of lateral ankle sprains. Br J Sports Med. 2016; https://doi.org/10.1136/bjsports-2016-096188.
2. Ferran NA, Oliva F, Maffulli N. Ankle instability. Sports Med Arthrosc. 2009;17:139–45.
3. Kobayashi T, Gamada K. Lateral ankle sprain and chronic ankle instability: a critical review. Foot Ankle Spec. 2014;7:298–326.
4. Kobayashi T, Suzuki E, Yamazaki N, Suzukawa M, Akaike A, Shimizu K, et al. Fibular malalignment in individuals with chronic ankle instability. J Orthop Sports Phys Ther. 2014;44:872–8.
5. Kobayashi T, Tanaka M, Shida M. Intrinsic risk factors of lateral ankle sprain: a systematic review and meta-analysis. Sports Health. 2016;8:190–3.
6. Baumhauer JF, O'Brien T. Surgical considerations in the treatment of ankle instability. J Athl Train. 2002;37:458–62.
7. de Vries JS, Kerkhoffs GM, Blankevoort L, van Dijk CN. Clinical evaluation of a dynamic test for lateral ankle ligament laxity. Knee Surg Sports Traumatol Arthrosc. 2010;18:628–33.
8. de Vries JS, Krips R, Blankevoort L, Fievez AW, van Dijk CN. Arthroscopic capsular shrinkage for chronic ankle instability with thermal radiofrequency: prospective multicenter trial. Orthopedics. 2008;31:655.
9. Kerkhoffs GM, van den Bekerom M, Elders LA, van Beek PA, Hullegie WA, Bloemers GM, et al. Diagnosis, treatment and prevention of ankle sprains: an evidence-based clinical guideline. Br J Sports Med. 2012;46:854–60.
10. Gribble PA, Bleakley CM, Caulfield BM, Docherty CL, Fourchet F, Fong DT, et al. Evidence review for the 2016 International Ankle Consortium consensus statement on the prevalence, impact and long-term consequences of lateral ankle sprains. Br J Sports Med. 2016; https://doi.org/10.1136/bjsports-2016-096189.
11. De Noronha M, Refshauge KM, Kilbreath SL, Figueiredo VG. Cross-cultural adaptation of the Brazilian-Portuguese version of the Cumberland Ankle Instability Tool (CAIT). Disabil Rehabil. 2008;30:1959–65.
12. Guillo S, Bauer T, Lee J, Takao M, Kong S, Stone J, et al. Consensus in chronic ankle instability: aetiology, assessment, surgical indications and place for arthroscopy. Orthop Traumatol Surg Res. 2013;99:S411–9.
13. Fousekis K, Tsepis E, Vagenas G. Intrinsic risk factors of noncontact ankle sprains in soccer: a prospective study on 100 professional players. Am J Sports Med. 2012;40:1842–50.
14. Milgrom C, Shlamkovitch N, Finestone A, Eldad A, Laor A, Danon YL, et al. Risk factors for lateral ankle sprain: a prospective study among military recruits. Foot Ankle. 1991;12:26–30.
15. Rice H, Nunns M, House C, Fallowfield J, Allsopp A, Dixon S. High medial plantar pressures during barefoot running are associated with increased risk of ankle inversion injury in Royal Marine recruits. Gait Posture. 2013;38:614–8.
16. Toumi A, Leteneur S, Gillet C, Debril JF, Decoufour N, Barbier F, et al. Enhanced precision of ankle torque measure with an open-unit dynamometer mounted with a 3D force-torque sensor. Eur J Appl Physiol. 2015;115:2303–10.
17. van Dijk CN, Lim LS, Bossuyt PM, Marti RK. Physical examination is sufficient for the diagnosis of sprained ankles. J Bone Joint Surg Br. 1996;78:958–62.
18. Zwiers R, Vuurberg G, Blankevoort L, Kerkhoffs GMMJ. Taping and bracing in the prevention of ankle sprains: current concepts. J ISAKOS Joint Disord Orthopaed Sport Med. 2016; https://doi.org/10.1136/jisakos-2016-000104.
19. Collins CK, Masaracchio M, Cleland JA. The effectiveness of strain counterstrain in the treatment of patients with chronic ankle instability: a randomized clinical trial. J Man Manip Ther. 2014;22:119–28.
20. De Ridder R, Willems T, Vanrenterghem J, Roosen P. Influence of balance surface on ankle stabilizing muscle activity in subjects with chronic ankle instability. J Rehabil Med. 2015;47:632–8.
21. dos Santos MJ, Gorges AL, Rios JL. Individuals with chronic ankle instability exhibit decreased postural sway while kicking in a single-leg stance. Gait Posture. 2014;40:231–6.
22. Linens SW, Ross SE, Arnold BL, Gayle R, Pidcoe P. Postural-stability tests that identify individuals with chronic ankle instability. J Athl Train. 2014;49:15–23.
23. Mettler A, Chinn L, Saliba SA, McKeon PO, Hertel J. Balance training and center-of-pressure location in participants with chronic ankle instability. J Athl Train. 2015;50:343–9.
24. Nunes GS, de Noronha M. Postural stabilization after single-leg vertical jump in individuals with chronic ankle instability. Phys Ther Sport. 2016;22:88–93.
25. Clanton TO, Matheny LM, Jarvis HC, Jeronimus AB. Return to play in athletes following ankle injuries. Sports Health. 2012;4:471–4.

26. Trojian TH, McKeag DB. Single leg balance test to identify risk of ankle sprains. Br J Sports Med. 2006;40:610–613; discussion 613.
27. Ross MD, Langford B, Whelan PJ. Test-retest reliability of 4 single-leg horizontal hop tests. J Strength Cond Res. 2002;16:617–22.
28. Stephens TM II, Lawson BR, Reiser RF II. Bilateral asymmetries in max effort single-leg vertical jumps. Biomed Sci Instrum. 2005;41:317–22.
29. Hiller CE, Refshauge KM, Bundy AC, Herbert RD, Kilbreath SL. The Cumberland ankle instability tool: a report of validity and reliability testing. Arch Phys Med Rehabil. 2006;87:1235–41.
30. Deckers JHMB, D.M.L. Ganganalyse en looptraining voor de paramedicus. Houten: Bohn Stafleu Van Loghum; 1996.
31. van Dijk CN, Vuurberg G, Amendola A, Lee JW. Anterior ankle arthroscopy: state of the art. J ISAKOS Joint Disord Orthopaed Sport Med. 2016; https://doi.org/10.1136/jisakos-2015-000009.
32. Verhagen RA, Maas M, Dijkgraaf MG, Tol JL, Krips R, van Dijk CN. Prospective study on diagnostic strategies in osteochondral lesions of the talus. Is MRI superior to helical CT? J Bone Joint Surg Br. 2005;87:41–6.
33. Polzer H, Kanz KG, Prall WC, Haasters F, Ockert B, Mutschler W, et al. Diagnosis and treatment of acute ankle injuries: development of an evidence-based algorithm. Orthop Rev (Pavia). 2012;4:e5.
34. van Dijk CN, Mol BW, Lim LS, Marti RK, Bossuyt PM. Diagnosis of ligament rupture of the ankle joint. Physical examination, arthrography, stress radiography and sonography compared in 160 patients after inversion trauma. Acta Orthop Scand. 1996;67:566–70.
35. Bosman HA, Robinson AH. Treatment of ankle instability with an associated cavus deformity. Foot Ankle Clin. 2013;18:643–57.
36. Cox JS, Hewes TF. "Normal" talar tilt angle. Clin Orthop Relat Res. 1979;(140):37–41.
37. Lohrer H, Nauck T, Arentz S, Scholl J. Observer reliability in ankle and calcaneocuboid stress radiography. Am J Sports Med. 2008;36:1143–9.
38. Roos EM, Brandsson S, Karlsson J. Validation of the foot and ankle outcome score for ankle ligament reconstruction. Foot Ankle Int. 2001;22:788–94.
39. Ware JE Jr, Gandek B, Kosinski M, Aaronson NK, Apolone G, Brazier J, et al. The equivalence of SF-36 summary health scores estimated using standard and country-specific algorithms in 10 countries: results from the IQOLA Project. J Clin Epidemiol. 1998;51:1167–70.
40. Balestroni G, Bertolotti G. [EuroQol-5D (EQ-5D): an instrument for measuring quality of life]. Monaldi Arch Chest Dis. 2012;78:155–9.
41. Coster MC, Rosengren BE, Bremander A, Brudin L, Karlsson MK. Comparison of the Self-reported Foot and Ankle Score (SEFAS) and the American Orthopedic Foot and Ankle Society Score (AOFAS). Foot Ankle Int. 2014;35:1031–6.
42. Martin RL, Irrgang JJ, Burdett RG, Conti SF, Van Swearingen JM. Evidence of validity for the Foot and Ankle Ability Measure (FAAM). Foot Ankle Int. 2005;26:968–83.
43. Hale SA, Hertel J. Reliability and sensitivity of the Foot and Ankle Disability Index in subjects with chronic ankle instability. J Athl Train. 2005;40:35–40.
44. Budiman-Mak E, Conrad KJ, Roach KE. The Foot Function Index: a measure of foot pain and disability. J Clin Epidemiol. 1991;44:561–70.
45. Karlsson J, Peterson L. Evaluation of ankle joint function: the use of a scoring scale. Foot. 1991;1:15–9.
46. Docherty CL, Gansneder BM, Arnold BL, Hurwitz SR. Development and reliability of the ankle instability instrument. J Athl Train. 2006;41:154–8.
47. Eechaute C, Vaes P, Duquet W. The chronic ankle instability scale: clinimetric properties of a multidimensional, patient-assessed instrument. Phys Ther Sport. 2008;9:57–66.
48. Simon J, Donahue M, Docherty C. Development of the Identification of Functional Ankle Instability (IdFAI). Foot Ankle Int. 2012;33:755–63.
49. Eechaute C, Vaes P, Van Aerschot L, Asman S, Duquet W. The clinimetric qualities of patient-assessed instruments for measuring chronic ankle instability: a systematic review. BMC Musculoskelet Disord. 2007;8:6.
50. Vuurberg G, Kluit L, van Dijk CN. The Cumberland Ankle Instability Tool (CAIT) in the Dutch population with and without complaints of ankle instability. Knee Surg Sports Traumatol Arthrosc. 2016; https://doi.org/10.1007/s00167-016-4350-4.
51. Wright CJ, Arnold BL, Ross SE, Linens SW. Recalibration and validation of the Cumberland Ankle Instability Tool cutoff score for individuals with chronic ankle instability. Arch Phys Med Rehabil. 2014;95:1853–9.
52. Halasi T, Kynsburg A, Tallay A, Berkes I. Development of a new activity score for the evaluation of ankle instability. Am J Sports Med. 2004;32:899–908.
53. Tegner Y, Lysholm J. Rating systems in the evaluation of knee ligament injuries. Clin Orthop Relat Res. 1985;(198):43–9.
54. Vuurberg G, Veen OC, Pereira H, Blankevoort L, van Dijk CN. Tenodesis reconstruction in patients with chronic lateral ankle instability is associated with a high risk at complications compared to anatomic repair and reconstruction: a systematic review and meta-analysis. J ISAKOS Joint Disord Orthopaed Sport Med. 2017; https://doi.org/10.1136/jisakos-2016-000121.
55. Terwee CB, Bot SD, de Boer MR, van der Windt DA, Knol DL, Dekker J, et al. Quality criteria were proposed for measurement properties of health status questionnaires. J Clin Epidemiol. 2007;60:34–42.
56. Sierevelt IN, Beimers L, van Bergen CJ, Haverkamp D, Terwee CB, Kerkhoffs GM. Validation of the Dutch language version of the Foot and Ankle Outcome Score. Knee Surg Sports Traumatol Arthrosc. 2015;23:2413–9.

57. de Boer MR, de Vet HC, Terwee CB, Moll AC, Volker-Dieben HJ, van Rens GH. Changes to the subscales of two vision-related quality of life questionnaires are proposed. J Clin Epidemiol. 2005;58:1260–8.
58. Mokkink LB, Terwee CB, Patrick DL, Alonso J, Stratford PW, Knol DL, et al. The COSMIN study reached international consensus on taxonomy, terminology, and definitions of measurement properties for health-related patient-reported outcomes. J Clin Epidemiol. 2010;63:737–45.
59. Lalkhen AG, McCluskey A. Clinical tests: sensitivity and specificity. Contin Educ Anaesth Crit Care Pain. 2008;8:221–3.
60. Hinkle DE, Wiersma W, Jurs SG. Applied statistics for the behavioral sciences, vol. 663. 5th ed. Boston: Houghton MiZin; 2003.

42 Consensus and Algorithm in the Approach to Patients with Chronic Lateral Ankle Instability

Frederick Michels, Hélder Pereira, and Giovanni Matricali

42.1 Introduction

In recent years, minimally invasive and endoscopic techniques to treat chronic lateral ankle instability (CLAI) have emerged [1–11]. Those new techniques offer new opportunities, but several questions remain unanswered. Interesting questions are: Which patients should be operated on? How long proceeding with non-surgical treatment before considering surgery? Can we consider surgical treatment in patients with functional ankle instability? Which preoperative tests are useful? In which cases do we perform a ligament repair and in which cases a reconstruction? Which techniques are used to evaluate subtalar instability? When do we reconstruct both ATFL and CFL?

Some questions are difficult to answer with the currently available evidence-based studies. Awaiting these evidence-based studies, it is of great interest to see if there are points of agreement between surgeons specialized in this pathology. These can be used as guidelines to less experienced surgeons.

Points of disagreement are also interesting because they highlight the hot discussion points.

The purpose of this chapter is to provide guidelines related to these questions, based on the current literature and a questionnaire (Table 42.1) sent to 32 orthopaedic surgeons. All participating surgeons have been trained in foot and ankle surgery or sports surgery. They have an extensive clinical experience with surgical treatment of patients with CLAI and have published about the subject.

An overall response rate of 94% was obtained (30/32). Most of them are member of the ESSKA-AFAS Ankle Instability Group and participants were involved in a total of 123 peer-reviewed publications related to ankle instability.

This chapter is based on a study recently published in KSSTA [12]. A distinction was made between ligament repair and ligament reconstruction. We used the following definitions. A

F. Michels (✉)
Orthopaedic Department AZ Groeninge, Kortrijk, Belgium

MIFAS by GRECMIP (Minimally Invasive Foot and Ankle Society), Merignac, France

H. Pereira
International Sports Traumatology Centre of Ave, Taipas Termal, Vila do Conde, Portugal

G. Matricali
Department of Development and Regeneration, KU Leuven, Leuven, Belgium

Department of Orthopaedics, Foot and Ankle Unit, University Hospitals Leuven, KU Leuven, Leuven, Belgium

Institute of Orthopaedic Research and Training, KU Leuven, Leuven, Belgium

H. Pereira et al. (eds.), *Lateral Ankle Instability*, https://doi.org/10.1007/978-3-662-62763-1_42

Table 42.1 Questionnaire

Imaging
• When considering surgery in a patient with chronic ankle instability, do you request preoperative stress radiographs? YES/NO
• When considering surgery in a patient with chronic ankle instability, do you request a preoperative MRI? YES/NO
Functional ankle instability
We present a patient with only functional instability (the subjective feeling of ankle instability, recurrent, symptomatic ankle sprains; or both) but without mechanical instability (no instability at physical examination, negative stress radiographs), no other abnormalities.
• Is there a place for surgical treatment? YES/NO
• How long should non-surgical treatment be attempted before considering surgical treatment?
• What surgical treatment should be considered as first choice? Open, arthroscopic? debridement, repair, reconstruction, other?
Mechanical ankle instability
We present a patient with symptomatic mechanical instability (clear instability on physical examination, positive stress X-rays), no other abnormalities.
• How long should non-surgical treatment be attempted before considering surgical treatment?
• What surgical treatment should be considered as first choice? Open, arthroscopic? debridement, repair, reconstruction, other?
Patient related issues
In which patients do you prefer to perform a reconstruction above a repair?
• Obesity: Repair/Reconstruction
• Ossicle >1 cm diameter: Repair/Reconstruction
• High-level sports: Repair/Reconstruction
• Generalized hyperlaxity: Repair/Reconstruction
• Positive stress radiographs: Repair/Reconstruction
• MRI finding of CFL injury: Repair/Reconstruction
• Poor ligament quality during surgery: Repair/Reconstruction
• Suspicion of subtalar instability: Repair/Reconstruction
Subtalar instability
• How do you assess subtalar instability? Physical examination? What kind of imaging do you perform?
Reconstruction of ATF and CFL?
If you consider a reconstruction of the ATFL, do you perform a reconstruction of the CFL? Almost always, almost never, it depends on…?

ligament repair is a suturing of the torn lateral ligaments, e.g. Broström-repair [13, 14]. A reconstruction is defined as a replacement of the chronically deficient lateral ligaments with local tissues or with autograft or allograft tissue. A reconstruction may be anatomical or non-anatomical.

42.2 Preoperative Planning

Standard plain radiographs should include standing anteroposterior, lateral and mortise views and a comparative Saltzmann view [14].

The use of preoperative stress radiographs is not standard. Sixty percent of the participating surgeons did not use preoperative *stress radiographs* because they were more confident with their physical examination skills (Fig. 42.1). Stress radiographs have a high specificity but low sensitivity [15–17].

MRI also has a positive predictive value because of a high specificity [18, 19]. However the sensitivity is low and ligament lesions can be underestimated [20]. MRI is valuable to assess associated pathology. Almost all (86.7%) participants used MRI routinely (Fig. 42.2).

42.3 Functional Ankle Instability

Functional ankle instability has been defined as a subjective feeling of giving way that may occur despite an absence of deviation beyond the normal physiological range of motion of the talus [21]. The exact cause of functional ankle instability is still under debate. Multiple possibilities are described: proprioceptive and neuromuscular deficits, scar tissue, damaged ligaments, unrecognized subtalar instability, and micro-instability [20, 22–24]. The last two (or even three) can also be considered as unnoticed mechanical instability.

Most participating surgeons (86.7%) agreed that surgery can be considered in patients with functional ankle instability. A period of at least 3–6 months of non-surgical treatment (physiotherapist-supervised rehabilitation, consisting of strengthening exercises of the active stabilizers of the ankle and proprioceptive training) is recommended (Fig. 42.3). Before consid-

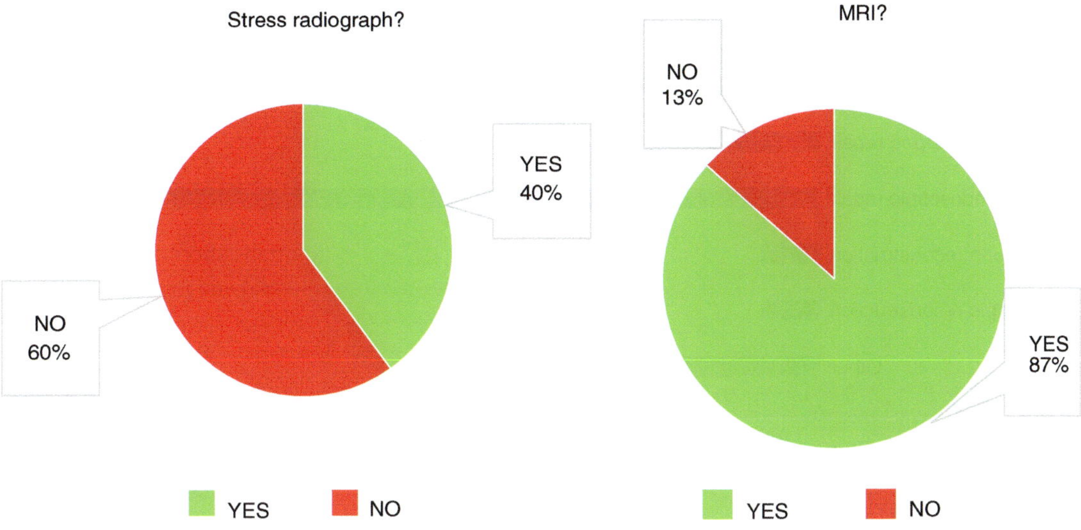

Fig. 42.1 and 42.2 Preoperative stress radiograph and MRI

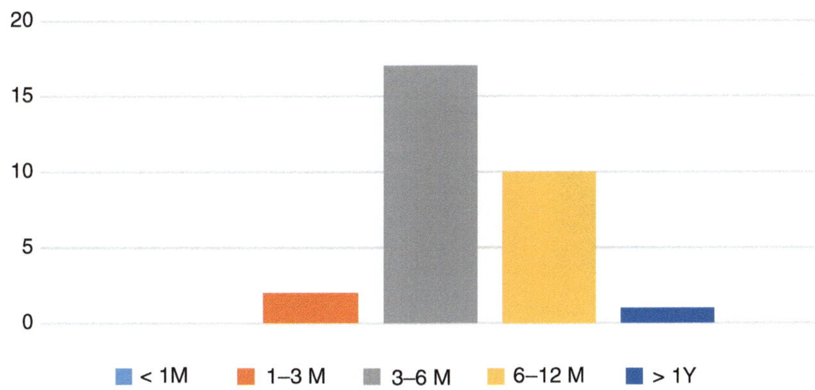

Fig. 42.3 Recommended duration of non-surgical treatment in patients with functional ankle instability

ering surgery, a reassessment of aetiology is recommend to ensure that all possible causes of the ankle problems had been ruled out, e.g. tight gastrocnemius, soft tissue impingement, lesions of the peroneal tendons, missed osteochondral lesions, and tarsal coalition.

There was no consensus about the surgical technique to be used (Fig. 42.4). An arthroscopic approach seemed valuable to assess the ligaments and concomitant pathologic lesions.

42.4 Mechanical Ankle Instability

Mechanical instability is defined as a pathologic laxity of the tibiotalar joint (with reproducible increased motion) in association with complaints of giving way [14]. In contrast to patients with functional ankle instability, most surgeons consider earlier surgery in patients with clinical signs of instability. 36.7% of the participants consider surgery within the first 3 months, 40.0% between

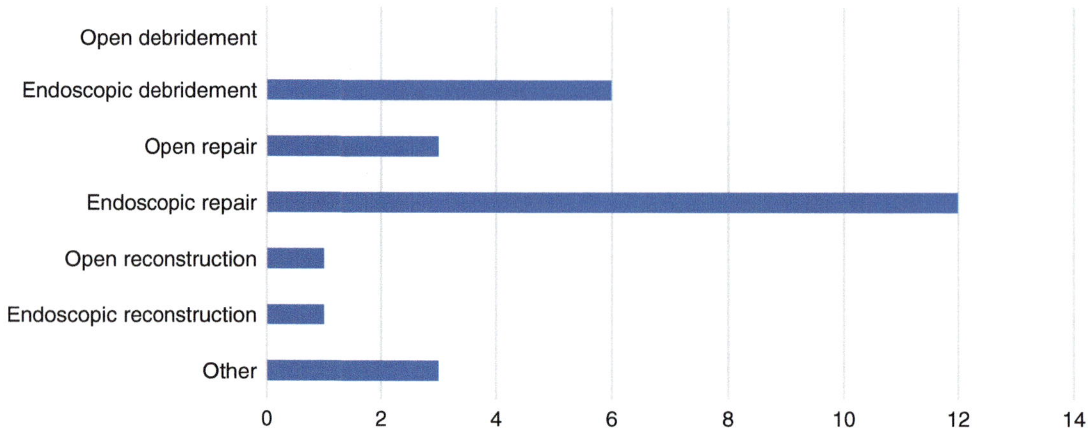

Fig. 42.4 Possible surgical techniques to treat patients with functional ankle instability

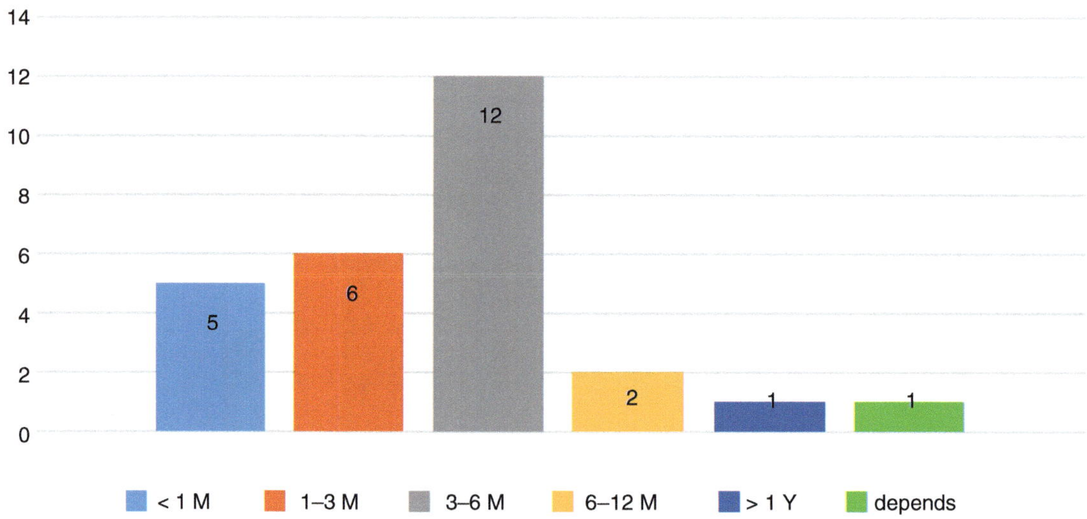

Fig. 42.5 Recommended duration of non-surgical treatment in patients with mechanical ankle instability

3 and 6 months (Fig. 42.5). Although the timing of transition from acute to chronic lateral ankle instability is not clearly defined in literature, this study gives recommendations about the timing of the treatment [12].

Considering the techniques that can be used to treat patients with chronic lateral ankle instability after failure of non-surgical treatment, a distinction was made between ligament repair and ligament reconstruction. As non-anatomical reconstructions may alter the joint biomechanics, resulting in joint loading alterations that may lead to joint degeneration over time [14], we did only consider anatomical reconstructions.

In our study based on the survey, a ligament repair is still considered the gold-standard first-line treatment (agreement of 76.7%) (Fig. 42.6). The fact that most participating surgeons are doing research on less invasive techniques explains the relative high answer focusing endoscopic techniques.

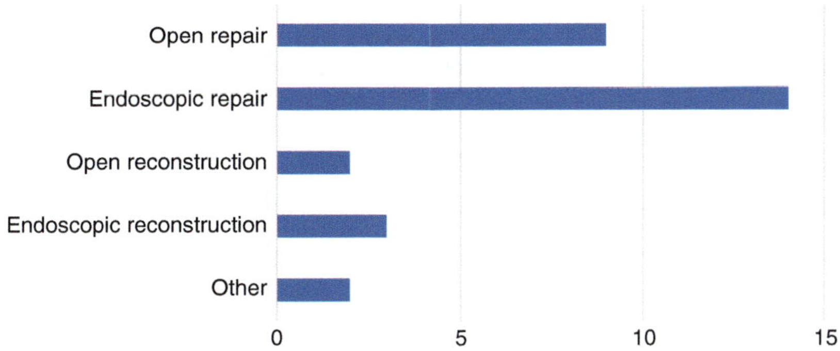

Fig. 42.6 Possible surgical techniques to treat patients with mechanical ankle instability

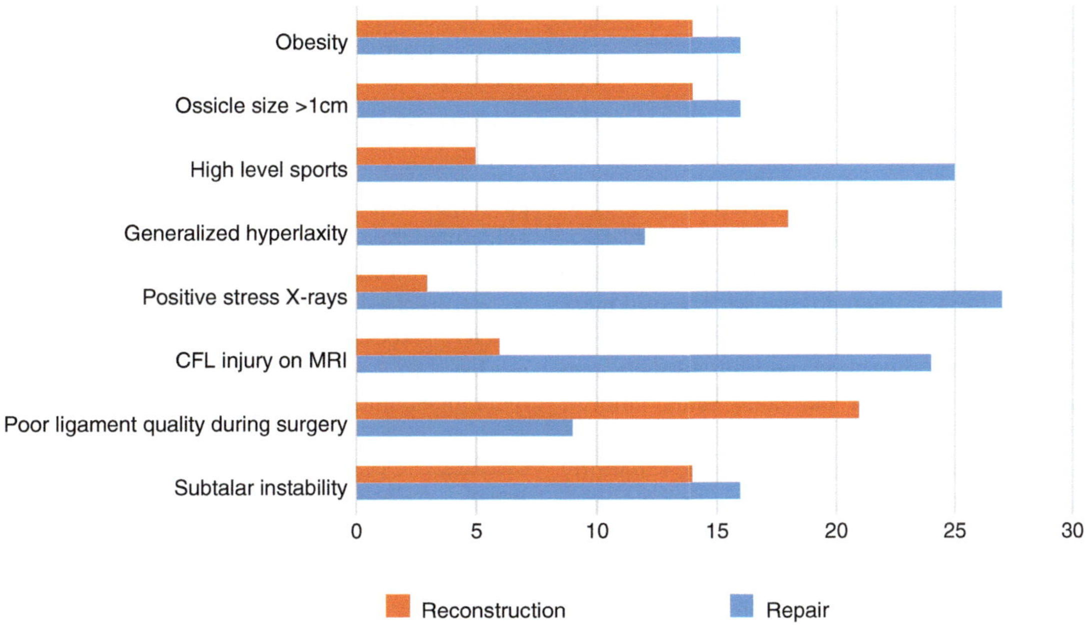

Fig. 42.7 Surgical technique depending on patient-related factors

42.5 Patient-Related Factors Influencing the Choice of Treatment

In literature several important patient-related factors have been described as a good indication to consider a ligament reconstruction instead of a ligament repair as a first-choice procedure [14]. Those factors are: obesity, ossicle size >1 cm, high-level sports, generalized laxity, positive stress radiographs, MRI finding of injury, poor ligament quality during surgery, and suspicion of subtalar instability. However, according to the questionnaire only in patients with generalized laxity and poor ligament quality during surgery, a reconstruction by grafting was the preferred technique (Fig. 42.7). When performing a reconstruction, most surgeons recommended reconstructing both ATFL and CFL.

42.6 Subtalar Ankle Instability

Subtalar instability, often associated with talocrural instability, is still difficult to assess and often overlooked [25, 26]. Among the participants there was no consensus on which diagnostic test is recommended to assess this problem.

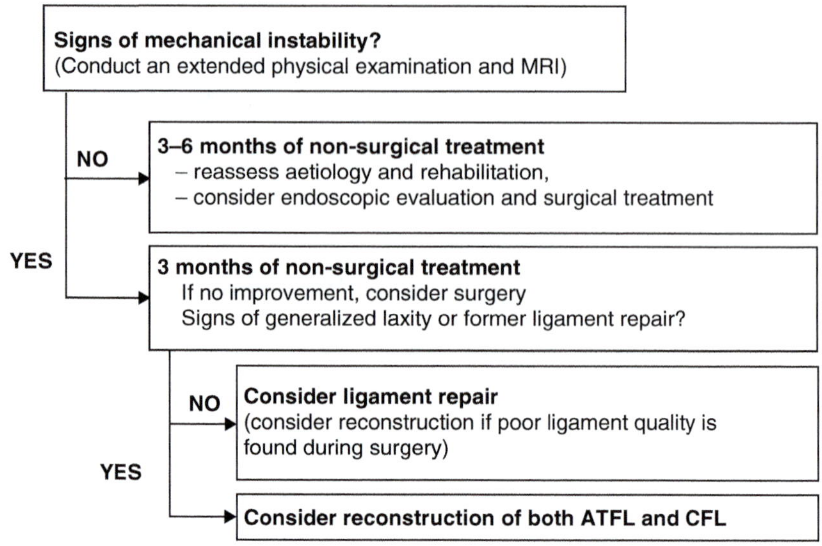

Fig. 42.8 Algorithm

With physical examination it is difficult to distinct talocrural instability from combined talocrural and subtalar instability. Historically, Brodén stress radiographs are widely used measuring medial displacement and subtalar tilt [27–30]. Kato measured anterior displacement of the calcaneus on the talus using anterior stress radiographs [31]. Other studies did not find any subtalar tilt and question the reliability of stress radiographs [27, 32, 33]. Arthrography was used for diagnosis of CFL injury [34]. MRI and MRI arthrography are useful to visualize the course of the subtalar ligaments [35, 36]. More recently MRI stress examination has been described as a valuable diagnostic tool [37]. Further studies are needed to reveal the value of the different tests. Recently, five diagnostic criteria were proposed to diagnose subtalar instability: recurrent ankle sprain, sinus tarsi pain and tenderness, hindfoot looseness or giving way, hindfoot instability on clinical examination, and abnormal anterior drawer-supination radiographs or abnormalities on MRI [38].

42.7 Algorithm

Based on the points of agreement determined by the survey and the currently available literature, a treatment algorithm is proposed (Fig. 42.8). This algorithm has been agreed by the surgeons who participated in this study and may be useful as a guideline in clinical practice when treating patients with chronic lateral ankle instability.

We emphasize that this algorithm is largely based on expert opinions. Future studies are still needed to provide more evidence-based recommendations.

42.8 Conclusion

Concerning the treatment of patients with chronic lateral ankle instability, a survey was conducted among 32 expert surgeons. The reactions showed a clear agreement between experts concerning several scientifically unanswered questions. This allows to present a treatment algorithm that can be used as a guideline. Ligament repair is still considered the gold-standard treatment. However, a ligament reconstruction is recommended in patients with former ligament repair, generalized hyperlaxity or poor ligament quality found at surgery.

Acknowledgement We thank the following surgeons who collaborated in this questionnaire: Jorge Acevedo, Jorge Batista, Thomas Bauer, James Calder, Dominic Carreira, Woojin Choi, Nuno Corte-Real, Mark Glazebrook, Ali Ghorbani, Eric Giza, Stéphane Guillo, Kenneth Hunt, Jón Karlsson, SW Kong, Jin Woo Lee, Frederick Michels, Andy Molloy, Peter Mangone, Kentaro Matsui, Caio Nery, Saturo Ozeki, Chris Pearce, Hélder Pereira, Anthony Perera, Bas Pijnenburg, Fernando Raduan, James Stone, Masato Takao, Yves Tourné, and Jordi Vega.

References

1. Acevedo JI, Mangone PG. Arthroscopic lateral ligament reconstruction. Tech Foot Ankle. 2011;10:111–6.
2. Corte-Real NM, Moreira RM. Arthroscopic repair of chronic lateral ankle instability. Foot Ankle Int. 2009;30:213–7.
3. Giza E, Shin EC, Wong SE, et al. Arthroscopic suture anchor repair of the lateral ligament ankle complex: a cadaveric study. Am J Sports Med. 2013;41:2567–72.
4. Glazebrook M, Stone J, Matsui K, et al. Percutaneous ankle reconstruction of lateral ligaments (Perc-Anti RoLL). Foot Ankle Int. 2016;37:659–64.
5. Kim ES, Lee KT, Park JS, et al. Arthroscopic anterior talofibular ligament repair for chronic ankle instability with a suture anchor technique. Orthopedics. 2011;34(4):273.
6. Matsui K, Burgesson B, Takao M, et al. Minimally invasive surgical treatment of chronic ankle instability: a systematic review. Knee Surg Traumatol Arthrosc. 2016;24:1040–8.
7. Michels F, Cordier G, Burssens A, et al. Endoscopic reconstruction of CFL and the ATFL with a gracilis graft: a cadaveric study. Knee Surg Sports Traumatol Arthrosc. 2016;24:1007–14.
8. Michels F, Cordier G, Guillo S, et al. Endoscopic ankle lateral ligament graft anatomic reconstruction. Foot Ankle Clin. 2016;21:665–80.
9. Nery C, Raduan F, Del Buono A, et al. Arthroscopic-assisted Broström-Gould for chronic ankle instability: a long-term follow-up. Am J Sports Med. 2011;39:2381–8.
10. Takao M, Glazebrook M, Stone J, et al. Ankle arthroscopic reconstruction of lateral ligaments (Ankle Anti-ROLL). Arthrosc Tech. 2015;4:5696–00.
11. Takao M, Matsui K, Stone JW, et al. Arthroscopic anterior talofibular ligament repair for lateral instability of the ankle. Knee Surg Sports Traumatol Arthrosc. 2016;24:1003–6.
12. Michels F, Pereira H, Calder J, et al. Searching for consensus in the approach to patients with chronic lateral ankle instability: ask the expert. Knee Surg Sports Traumatol Arthrosc. 2017; https://doi.org/10.1007/s00167-017-4556-0.
13. Broström L. Sprained ankles. V. Treatment and prognosis in recent ligament ruptures. Acta Chir Scand. 1966;132:537–50.
14. Guillo S, Bauer T, Lee JW, et al. Consensus in chronic ankle instability: aetiology, assessment, surgical indications and place for arthroscopy. Orthop Traumatol Surg Res. 2013;99:S411–9.
15. Frost SC, Amendola A. Is stress radiography necessary in the diagnosis of acute or chronic ankle instability? Clin J Sport Med. 1999;9:40–5.
16. Fujii T, Luo ZP, Kitaoka HB, et al. The manual stress test may not be sufficient to differentiate ankle ligament injuries. Clin Biomech. 2000;15:619–23.
17. Tourné Y, Besse JL, Mabit C. Chronic ankle instability. Which tests to assess the lesions? Which therapeutic options? Orthop Traumatol Surg Res. 2010;96:433–46.
18. Joshy S, Abdulkadir U, Chaganti S, et al. Accuracy of MRI scan in the diagnosis of ligamentous and chondral pathology in the ankle. J Foot Ankle Surg. 2010;16:78–80.
19. Park HJ, Cha SD, Kim SS, et al. Accuracy of MRI findings in chronic lateral ankle ligament injury: comparison with surgical findings. Clin Radiol. 2012;67:313–8.
20. Takao M, Innami K, Matsushita T, et al. Arthroscopic and magnetic resonance image appearance and reconstruction of the anterior talofibular ligament in cases of apparent functional ankle instability. Am J Sports Med. 2008;36:1542–7.
21. Freeman DA, Dean MR, Hanham IW. The etiology and prevention of functional instability of the foot. J Bone Joint Surg. 1965;47-B:678–85.
22. Hertel J. Functional anatomy, pathomechanics, and pathophysiology of lateral ankle instability. J Athl Train. 2002;37:364–75.
23. Kerr H, Bayley E, Jackson R, et al. The role of arthroscopy in the treatment of functional instability of the ankle. Foot Ankle Surg. 2013;19:273–5.
24. Vega J, Pena F, Golano P. Minor or occult ankle instability as a cause of anterolateral pain after ankle sprain. Knee Surg Sports Traumatol Arthrosc. 2016;24:1116–23.
25. Aynardi M, Pedowitz D, Raikin SM. Subtalar instability. Foot Ankle Clin N Am. 2015;20:243–52.
26. Barg A, Tochigi Y, Amendola A, et al. Subtalar instability: diagnosis and treatment. Foot Ankle Int. 2012;33:151–60.
27. Harper MC. Stress radiographs in the diagnosis of lateral instability of the ankle and hindfoot. Foot Ankle Int. 1993;13:435–8.
28. Lee BH, Choi KH, Seo DY, et al. Diagnostic validity of alternative manual stress radiographic technique detecting subtalar instability with concomitant ankle instability. Knee Surg Sports Traumatol Arthrosc. 2016;24:1029–39.
29. Yamamoto H, Yagishita K, Ogiuchi T, et al. Subtalar instability following lateral ligament injuries of the ankle. Injury. 1982;29:265–8.
30. Zwipp H, Tscherne H. Radiological diagnosis of instability of the subtalar joint. Unfallheilkunde. 1982;85:494–8.
31. Kato T. The diagnosis and treatment of instability of the subtalar joint. J Bone Joint Surg Br. 1995;77:400–6.
32. Louwerens JW, Ginai AZ, van Linge B, et al. Stress radiography of the talocrural and subtalar joints. Foot Ankle Int. 1995;16:148–55.
33. Sijbrandy ES, van Gils APG, van Hellemondt FJ, et al. Assessing the subtalar joint: the Brodén view revisited. Foot Ankle Int. 2001;22:329–34.
34. Sugimoto K, Takakura Y, Samoto N, et al. Subtalar arthrography in recurrent instability of the ankle. Clin Orthop Relat Res. 2002;394:169–76.

35. Lee KB, Bai LB, Park JG, et al. Efficacy of MRI versus arthroscopy for evaluation of sinus tarsi syndrome. Foot Ankle Int. 2008;29:1111–6.
36. Lektrakul N, Chung CB, Lai YM, et al. Tarsal sinus: arthrographic, MR imaging, MR arthrographic, and pathologic findings in cadavers and retrospective study data in patients with sinus tarsi syndrome. Radiology. 2001;219:802–10.
37. Seebauer JC, Bail HJ, Rump JC, Hamm B, et al. Ankle laxity: stress investigation under MRI control. Am J Roentgenol. 2013;201:496–504.
38. Michels F, Clockaerts S, Van Der Bauwhede J, Stockmans F, Matricali G. Does subtalar instability really exist? A systematic review. J Foot Ankle Surg. 2019;26:119. https://doi.org/10.1016/j.fas.2019.02.001.

GPSR Compliance

The European Union's (EU) General Product Safety Regulation (GPSR) is a set of rules that requires consumer products to be safe and our obligations to ensure this.

If you have any concerns about our products, you can contact us on ProductSafety@springernature.com

In case Publisher is established outside the EU, the EU authorized representative is:

Springer Nature Customer Service Center GmbH
Europaplatz 3
69115 Heidelberg, Germany

Batch number: 10732799

Printed by Printforce, the Netherlands